PATHOPHYSIOLOGY OF HEART DISEASE

Dr. Karthik Natarajan

ALLIED
HEALTH
PRESS

Pathophysiology of Heart Disease

Author: **Dr. Karthik Natarajan**

Allied Health Press
4164 Lakeshore Road
Burlington ON L7L 1A4
Canada
www.alliedhealthpress.com
Email: orders@arclereducation.com

ISBN: 978-1-77956-807-6

General Disclaimer:

This book is a summation of information from different sources and encompasses a wide range of medical conditions, the latest therapy methods, principals and techniques that are used in current practice, at the time of publication. This book offers general information with educational purposes, it is not to be applied or relied on for any diagnostic or treatment purposes. Please do not use the data/matter as a substitute for professional diagnosis and treatment. Please consult your healthcare provider or a licensed physician before making any healthcare queries or treatment choices. The medical information and research findings presented in this book are for educational purposes only and should not be used for the treatment of specific individual patients, as individual cases may vary. The author(s), editors(s) and publisher cannot be held accountable and make no guarantees that the information provided in this book will apply to each and individual patient. This book is meant to serve as a basic guideline and other relevant literature sources should be used for more specific information. This text can be a vital resource for students, trainees, and practitioners, covering essential topics. This book encompasses a wide range of medical conditions and the latest therapy options used in current practice. Through the utilization of many different medical studies this book provides the basics of different medical conditions, which can be used as a basic guide from where medical students, trainees and practitioners can extract necessary information. Further, some of the books have graphic images to explain anatomy for medical/educational purposes only. Hence, the book is intended for students or teachers/staff or individuals with a mature outlook looking to learn or enhance their knowledge.

ABOUT THE AUTHOR

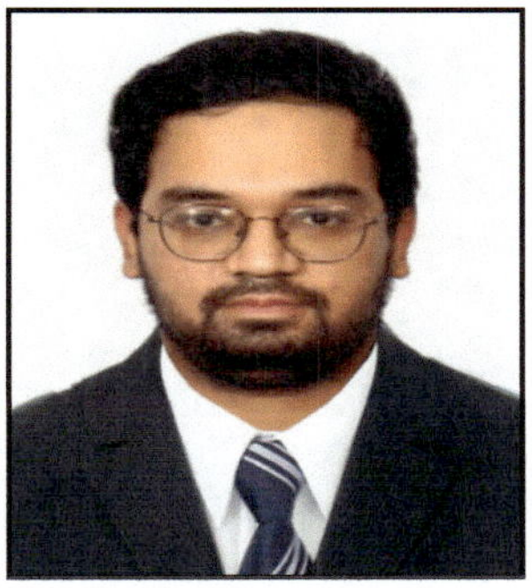

Dr Karthik Natarajan is presently serving as Professor of Cardiology at U N Mehta Institute of Cardiology and Research Centre. He obtained his MBBS and MD(Medicine) from Smt NHL Municipal Medical College, Gujarat University. He obtained his DM(Cardiology) degree from U N Mehta Institute of Cardiology and Research Centre. He has been serving at the institute for the past 7 years. He has vast experience in performing complex coronary interventions. His particular interest lies in LMCA Bifurcations, CHIP interventions, CTO PCI, TAVI, ASD device closure, PDA device closure and Pacemakers. He has also assisted and performed multiple peripheral and carotid interventions. He has performed more than 1000 PCIs and more than 5000 coronary angiographies. He has multiple research publications in national and international journals. He has been involved as a course coordinator and been invited as guest faculty at several national Interventional conferences. He has a keen interest in Cardiovascular Imaging and is an integral part of the transplant program at UN Mehta Institute. He also won the best case presenter award at IJCTO 2023.

Brief Table of Contents

Detailed Table of Contents

CHAPTER 3

Mechanisms of Cardiac Arrhythmias 65

CHAPTER 4

Ischemic Heart Disease 101

CHAPTER 8

Valvular Heart Diseases 233

CHAPTER 9

Congenital Heart Diseases 263

CHAPTER 10

Inflammatory Heart Diseases 289

LIST OF FIGURES

PREFACE

Preface

Understanding how the heart and its associated vessels operate under both healthy and diseased states is fundamental to all fields of medicine. The cardiovascular system sustains life by delivering oxygen and nutrients to tissues, removing waste products, and supporting homeostasis. Alterations in blood flow, cellular function, or structural integrity can precipitate a cascade of events that culminate in clinical syndromes ranging from mild discomfort to sudden cardiac death. A thorough grasp of these physiological changes equips clinicians and researchers to recognize early signs of dysfunction, tailor interventions, and advance therapeutic strategies that improve patient outcomes.

Over the last several decades, research has uncovered the molecular and cellular underpinnings of many cardiac conditions. Inflammation, genetic mutations, hemodynamic stress, and metabolic imbalances each contribute uniquely to disease progression. Such knowledge has transformed how practitioners approach diagnosis and management, providing precision medicine approaches that consider individual risk profiles. Furthermore, advances in imaging, biomarkers, and minimally invasive techniques continue to refine our ability to detect and treat pathology before irreversible damage occurs.

This text, *Pathophysiology of Heart Disease*, provides a systematic examination of the processes that underlie cardiovascular disorders. Drawing on contributions from leading experts, it integrates foundational concepts with current research findings. Readers will find clear explanations of mechanisms as well as discussions of clinical implications and emerging therapies. The title underscores the commitment to linking bench discoveries with bedside applications, ensuring that theoretical knowledge is translated into improved patient care.

- Chapter 1 presents an overview of the standard cardiovascular system, detailing anatomical structures, cardiac cycle dynamics, and regulatory mechanisms that maintain circulatory balance.
- Chapter 2 focuses based on disease processes, exploring how cellular injury, oxidative stress, and neurohormonal activation contribute to vascular and myocardial dysfunction.
- Chapter 3 examines the origins of cardiac arrhythmias, including alterations in ion channel function, conduction pathways, and autonomic influences that lead to rhythm disturbances.

- Chapter 4 addresses ischemic heart disease, tracing the path from coronary artery obstruction to myocardial injury, repair, and scar formation.
- Chapter 5 analyzes the development of atherosclerosis, highlighting lipid deposition, endothelial activation, and plaque vulnerability.
- Chapter 6 discusses heart failure, contrasting systolic and diastolic dysfunction and evaluating compensatory responses that both sustain and ultimately overwhelm cardiac performance.
- Chapter 7 explores hypertension and hypertensive heart disease, covering mechanisms of blood pressure regulation, vascular remodeling, and end-organ effects.
- Chapter 8 reviews valvular pathologies, describing stenotic and regurgitant lesions, their hemodynamic consequences, and options for repair and replacement.
- Chapter 9 surveys congenital heart diseases, from simple septal defects to complex malformations, with attention to developmental biology and clinical management.
- Chapter 10 considers inflammatory heart conditions, including myocarditis and rheumatic carditis, with a focus on immune responses and long-term sequelae.
- Chapter 11 focuses on cardiomyopathies, differentiating hypertrophic, dilated, and restrictive forms, and discussing genetic and acquired etiologies.
- Chapter 12 examines vascular disorders beyond the coronary circulation, addressing aneurysms, vasculitis, and peripheral arterial disease.
- Chapter 13 highlights pulmonary heart disease, or cor pulmonale, analyzing how lung pathology leads to right ventricular strain and failure.
- Chapter 14 covers diseases of the pericardium, such as pericarditis and tamponade, and the impact of fluid accumulation and fibrotic changes on cardiac function.
- Finally, Chapter 15 addresses critical heart disease in infants and children, integrating congenital and acquired disorders unique to the pediatric population, and emphasizing tailored diagnostic and therapeutic approaches.

This text is written for medical students, who will find its clear explanations an ideal supplement to courses in physiology and pathology. Residents and practicing clinicians can use it as a quick reference to refresh their understanding of disease mechanisms and to inform evidence-based decision making. Researchers will appreciate the synthesis of basic science and clinical insights, which may inspire new avenues of investigation. Additionally, allied health professionals—such as nurses, physician assistants, and pharmacists—will benefit from a more profound comprehension of cardiovascular pathophysiology, enabling more effective collaboration in patient care.

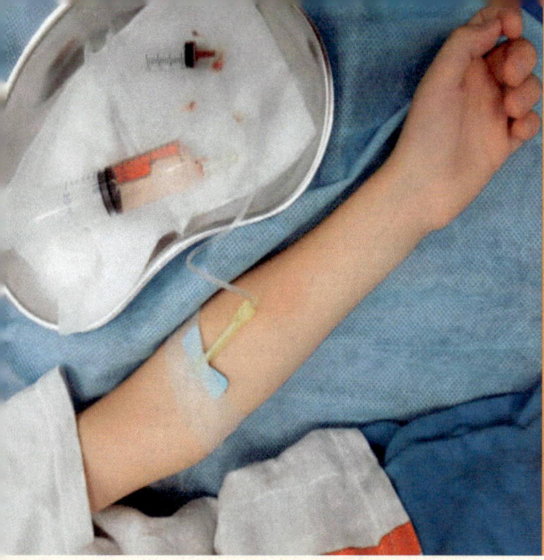

Chapter 1

INTRODUCTION TO CARDIOVASCULAR SYSTEM

Contents

Introduction

The cardiovascular system is one of the supports of human physiology, regulating a complex system that keeps life alive through the circulation of blood. The system includes the heart, blood vessels, and blood and is charged with the distribution of nutrients, oxygen, and hormones to other tissues. At the same time, it picks up waste products generated by metabolism. The heart is a muscular organ that serves as a forceful pump for blood, which travels in two significant circuits: the pulmonary circuit, a circulating blood circuit and CO_2 exchanged for O_2 in the lungs, and the systemic circuit, which works to deliver blood to the remainder of the body. Knowledge of the cardiovascular system is not only vital to understanding how it works healthily but also the implications of cardiovascular disease, which is a significant global problem for health, as detailed in studies outlining its prevalence and impact on human health (Spoială et al., 2022). Additional research has also considered more advanced interrelations of cardiovascular wellness with external agents such as viral infection. The recent COVID-19 pandemic has put into focus the degree to which respiratory illness can impair cardiovascular functioning, questioning the protection and care of individuals with pre-existing cardiovascular disease. Facts indicate that cardiovascular disease sufferers have increased chances of further serious complications if they catch the coronavirus, as it illustrates the interconnectedness of body systems and the requirements of more integrated healthcare approaches. For instance, insightful comments regarding the COVID-19 implications for cardiovascular disease have spurred research on novel methods for rejuvenating virus-infected heart tissue, employing biopolymers like alginate for developing new biomaterials to be used therapeutically (Spoială et al., 2022). The cardiovascular function is also accentuated in specific health situations, e.g., Ramadan fasting, wherein physiological adaptation occurs that can impact blood pressure and general cardiovascular health. Studies have proven that lifestyle interventions, such as fasting, impact cardiovascular risk factors, making it crucial to study how such activities interact with personal health profiles. Epidemiological studies of cardiovascular dynamics during periods like Ramadan have discovered variations in fluid balance, electrolyte levels, and vascular responsiveness, highlighting the need for an integrative concept of health that accounts for cultural practices and their physiological implications. This broad scope of cardiovascular health studies requires an interdisciplinary approach that incorporates basic sciences, clinical uses, and public health perspectives to build a deeper understanding of how various factors interact to shape cardiovascular outcomes (Figure 1.1).

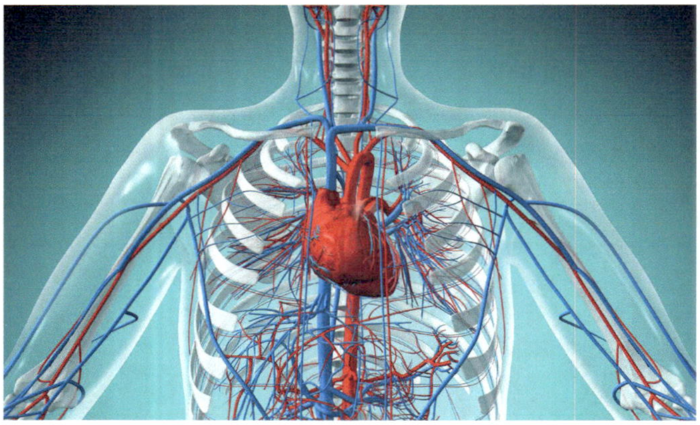

Figure 1.1. Cardiovascular system.

Source: https://www.thoughtco.com/thmb/OEO7Xy_TJ1_E5z1ZJp926gYMdFI=/1500x0/filters:no_upscale():max_bytes(150000):strip_icc()/GettyImages-97537745-59efa47d6f53ba0011c0070b.jpg.

Definition and Function

The cardiovascular system is important because it moves blood to all parts of the body, delivering nutrients, oxygen, and hormones, and also helps remove waste products. The main parts of the system are the heart, the blood vessels, and the blood, which all work together to support life. Blood is pumped throughout the body by the heart, which consists of four chambers—two atria and two ventricles—that cooperate to do the job. Because of this well-organized process, oxygen-rich blood is distributed to the body's organs and tissues through arteries and veins, bringing the used blood back to the heart to be reoxygenated in the lungs. Therefore, the cardiovascular system is important for cellular function and maintaining balance in the body, underlining its central role in human physiology. The cardiovascular system must work properly to support good health and to avoid chronic diseases. If the cardiovascular system is weakened, it can cause hypertension, heart failure, and cardiovascular disease, which can significantly reduce quality of life. For instance, individuals with diabetes face increased risks of progressive chronic kidney disease and cardiovascular complications, primarily due to hypertension, which serves as a reversible risk factor (Banerjee et al., 2022). Maintaining a healthy blood pressure is crucial, as it can help prevent kidney disease and reduce the risk of heart problems. It underlines the need to know both the meaning and role of the cardiovascular system for good health and for designing effective treatments against diseases. New studies suggest that interventions such as specially designed exercise programs can strengthen the heart and improve the lives of people affected by heart disease. Notably, studies examining the effects of an Individualized Activity Program (IAP) on patients with chronic fatigue syndrome revealed significant improvements in fatigue levels and autonomic function, indicating the potential of exercise to stimulate cardiovascular health (Sławomir Kujawski et al., 2021). It points out that the cardiovascular system plays many roles, including those in health management and rehabilitation, not only in circulation. Besides, new drugs, including RAAS blockers and SGLT-2 inhibitors, are showing how cardiovascular care for people with diabetes is being improved. Hence, the understanding of the cardiovascular system's definition and functions can inform comprehensive approaches to health promotion and disease prevention (Figure 1.2).

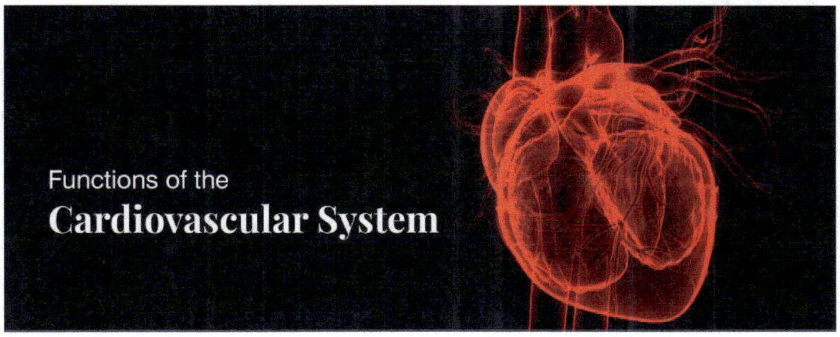

Figure 1.2. Function of the cardiovascular system.

Source: https://www.relainstitute.com/wp-content/uploads/2023/09/cardio-vascular.jpg.

Components of the Cardiovascular System

The cardiovascular system, which is sometimes called the circulatory system, is made up of several essential parts that cooperate to keep the body functioning normally. The heart is mainly a muscular pump that moves blood all over the body. The heart has two chambers: the atria and the ventricles, and these chambers contract together to make sure blood is pumped through the body effectively. Deoxygenated blood from the body enters the right side of the heart, which pumps it to the lungs via the pulmonary arteries, and oxygenated blood from the lungs enters the left side of the heart, which pumps it to the rest of the body through the aorta. It facilitates gas exchange and ensures that blood consistently reaches the organs, enabling them to function correctly. The blood vessels, which are part of the cardiovascular system, work with the heart to move blood around the body. The three types of blood vessels are arteries, veins, and capillaries, and each one has its role. Blood leaves the heart through muscular arteries, carrying oxygen to the tissues, and returns through veins, which bring deoxygenated blood back to the heart. The smallest blood vessels, called capillaries, allow nutrients, gases, and waste to be exchanged between blood and tissues. Because of this , vast network of blood vessels, the body can maintain its balance by controlling blood pressure, the flow of blood, and body temperature. They demonstrate how the cardiovascular system can change to meet the body's requirements, whether someone is resting or exercising. Blood is an essential component in the cardiovascular system because it carries important materials to all parts of the body.

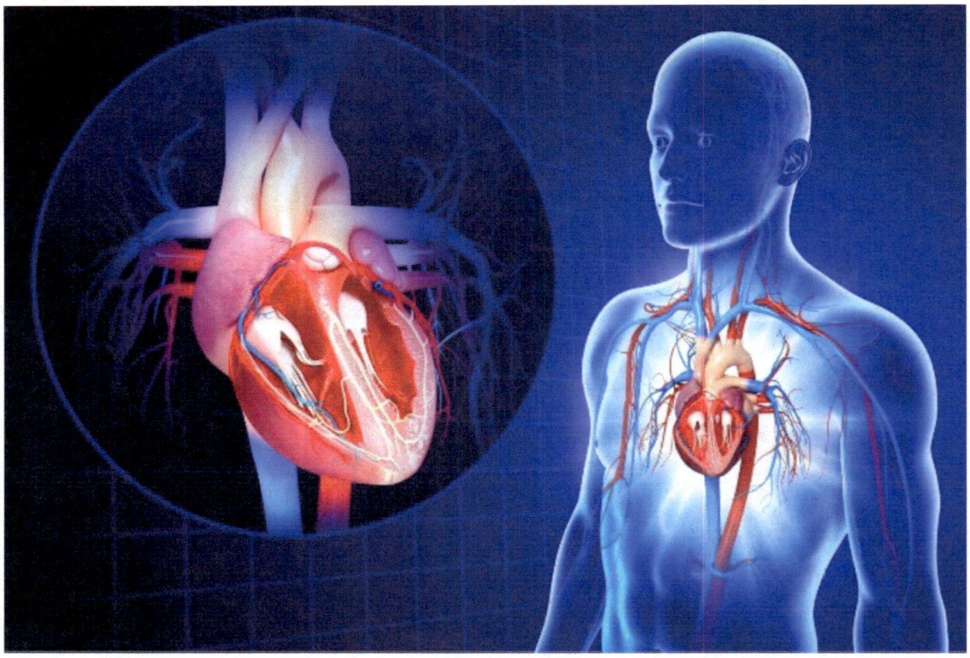

Figure 1.3. Understanding Cardiovascular System.

Source: https://www.thoughtco.com/thmb/trPfovZS2IZLtR7QBwo2rxoARfw=/1500x0/filters:no_upscale():max_bytes(150000):strip_icc()/cardiovascular_system-57f6d56a3df78c690f77c7c7.jpg.

Because blood contains plasma, red blood cells, white blood cells, and platelets, it plays a part in giving oxygen and nutrients while carrying off waste for excretion. The liquid part of plasma contains water, electrolytes and proteins which help keep blood thick and steady. Red blood cells take oxygen from the lungs and attach it to hemoglobin, and white blood cells help protect the body from infections. Platelets play a crucial role in hemostasis, stopping bleeding when someone gets hurt. Collectively, these elements of blood ensure the effective functioning of the cardiovascular system, as they interact continuously with the heart and blood vessels to sustain life at the cellular level and maintain overall homeostasis within the organism (Oki et al., 2018; Azzalini et al., 2019) (Figure 1.3)

Importance in Human Health

In human health, trace elements play a crucial role, particularly in cardiovascular health. Selenium, for instance, is a determinant in maintaining the numerous functions of the body through being incorporated into selenoproteins. Selenoproteins such as glutathione peroxidases play a critical role in neutralizing oxidative stress, which is a known risk factor for cardiovascular disease.

Selenium's antioxidant action has been linked to the inhibition of free radical-induced cell injury and thus to a protective action on the cardiovascular system. Selenium also plays an important role in modulating immune responses, which may influence cardiovascular events. Because deficiency and toxicity of selenium both pose harmful health consequences, maintaining the ideal intake of this valuable element is essential to promote cardiovascular wellness and health (Bai et al., 2024). As significant as cardiovascular wellness is, the awareness of the gut microbiome's role in maintaining physiological homeostasis. The gut microbiota exists in a complicated interplay with all body systems, including the nervous and immune systems, to create an interconnected network that influences cardiovascular function. Dysbiosis or intestinal microbiome abnormalities have been implicated in the etiology of cardiovascular disease, proving that a perfect microbiota plays a critical role in preventing the occurrence of such diseases. This exchange highlights the need for more research into how nutritional choices and the environment affect the makeup of gut microbiota and, subsequently, cardiovascular disease. Gut bacterium metabolites can modulate systemic inflammation and metabolism, and thus the gut-cardiovascular axis is highly relevant. Sustaining a healthy gut microbiome through proper nutrition may therefore support cardiovascular health and decrease disease risk (Riehl et al., 2024). Moreover, the gut health interaction with trace elements is a good example of the complexities in human health, including in the case of the cardiovascular system. Selenium and gut microbiota interact to sustain homeostasis since the two variables control oxidative stress as well as inflammation in the body. For instance, the gut microbiota can control the bioavailability of nutrients and trace elements like selenium and consequently impact their respective roles in cardiovascular protection. Dysbiosis of gut microbiota can compromise the absorption of such nutrients, which exacerbates cardiovascular disease risk. It is therefore crucial to adopt an all-around philosophy of health through assessing nutritional intake and maintaining a healthy gut microbiome to enhance cardiovascular health outcomes. Further understanding of the interactions involved can pave the way for novel therapeutic and dietary interventions designed to promote cardiovascular health and cure allied disorders (Bai et al., 2024; Riehl et al., 2024).

1.1. Anatomy of the Heart

The heart, the cardiovascular system's central organ, is comprised primarily of specialized muscular tissue known as the myocardium, with the help of which effective pumping of blood to various parts of the body is brought about. The heart operates under the law of rhythmical contraction, initiation of which by electrical stimuli occurs from the sinoatrial (SA) node, also referred to as the heart's natural pacemaker. The cardiac anatomy consists of four chambers: the left and right atrium and ventricle. The right and left atria accept blood, while the right and left ventricles eject blood. The four chambers all play an essential role in maintaining an efficient circulatory system by supplying oxygen-rich blood to the tissues and concurrently sending deoxygenated blood to the lungs to be oxygenated. This intricate structure plays a central role to sustain life, and therefore it is important that health professionals as well as students understand this structural and functional aspect of the heart. In addition to chambers, the heart also has several valves, which regulate the movement of blood by preventing backflow upon contraction. Atrioventricular valves, or tricuspid and mitral (or bicuspid) valves, lie between atria and ventricles, whereas semilunar valves such as pulmonary and aortic valves control blood flow exiting the heart. Such architectural configuration is that of one-way flow-permitting blood, thereby facilitating proper circulation without unwanted features like regurgitation. In addition, understanding the relationship between heart structure and function is essential in reacting to cardiovascular disease. According to recent research, cardiovascular health is inextricably linked with lifestyles, including diet, that can influence blood pressure. Evidence indicates that moderate consumption of coffee may be associated with lower systolic blood pressure, and therefore, the learning of heart anatomy and physiology is further pertinent to public health interventions concerned with disease prevention and health promotion (Cicero et al., 2023). Beyond just structure, cardiac anatomy has a significant impact on the issues facing modern healthcare, especially concerning cardiovascular diseases (CVD). Given an unprecedented population of individuals with CVD globally, accurate heart anatomy knowledge can inform prevention as well as treatment measures. For instance, in China alone, where nearly 330 million individuals reside with a cardiovascular disease, there exists an urgent need for professional medical equipment and care provision (The Writing Committee of the Report on Cardiovascular in China and Sheng-shou Hu, 2023). As the population increases with each passing year, and risk factors like diabetes and hypertension, understanding the anatomy of the heart is essential. An educated healthcare provider establishes appropriate guidelines for early intervention and screening, thus promoting patient outcomes among high-risk individuals for heart disorders. Consequently, the study of the heart's anatomy is essential not just for purposes of knowledge in academia but also for practical uses in clinics (Figure 1.4).

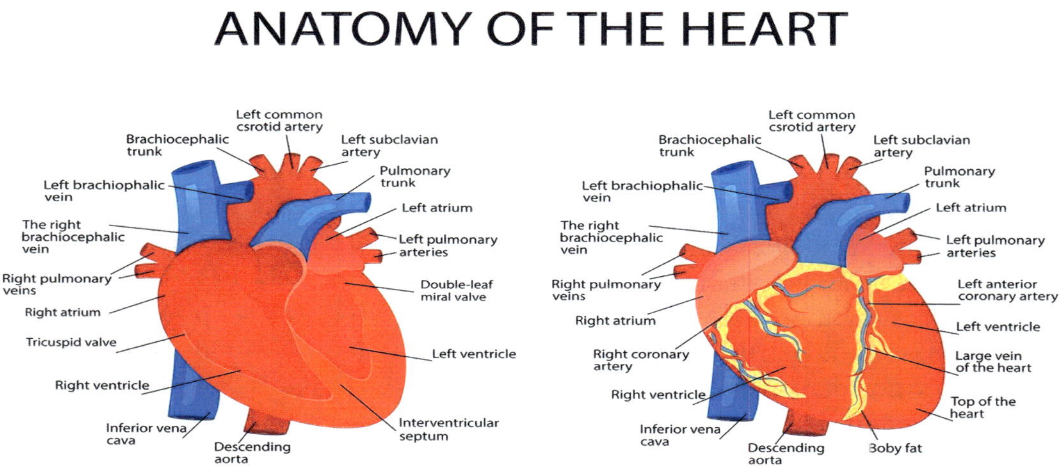

Figure 1.4. Anatomy of the heart.

Source: https://static.vecteezy.com/system/resources/previews/034/605/575/non_2x/anatomy-of-the-heart-of-the-human-heart-on-a-white-background-illustration-for-poster-vector.jpg.

1.1.1. Structure of the Heart

The heart, a fascinating organ that is found in the center of the cardiovascular system, has a complex composition that is designed to facilitate it to carry out its basic functions. Comprising four central chambers—the right atrium and left atrium, and the right ventricle and left ventricle—the heart functions to distribute oxygenated and deoxygenated blood throughout the body. This chamber separation allows for efficient separation of oxygen-rich blood from oxygen-poor blood to provide overall physiological equilibrium. In addition, the muscular walls of the heart, most significantly the myocardium, are responsible for the contractions that propel blood. This intricate anatomical structure highlights the prominence of the heart as a vital organ. It demonstrates its necessity in sustaining life through the upkeep of all tissues in a well-oxygenated state to enable metabolic activity. The structure of the heart is complemented by a set of valves that regulate blood flow, ensuring unidirectional movement and preventing backflow. The atrioventricular valves (mitral and tricuspid) control the blood flow from the atria into the ventricles, while the semilunar valves (pulmonary and aortic) control the ejection of blood from the ventricles into the pulmonary artery and aorta, respectively. Such an arrangement maximizes the cardiac cycle and increases the efficiency of the heart. During heart pumping, coordinated opening and closing of these valves generate a rhythmic sound which can be heard using auscultation and provides valuable information about cardiac health. Understanding the structural role of these valves is vital, since failure in their function can cause significant cardiovascular illnesses, and thus, an organized cardiac architecture plays an important role in overall cardiovascular integrity. A more detailed study of the structure of the heart reveals the significance of the electrical conduction system, which controls the rhythmic contractions of the heart. The SA node, or natural pacemaker as it is otherwise called, is responsible for initiating the electrical impulses that pass through the atria, causing them to contract. The electric impulse extends through to the atrioventricular (AV) node, and then finally passes through the His-Purkinje network, contracting the ventricles in a synchronized fashion. Consequently, this tightly regulated electrical system allows the heart's capability to maintain an adequate heart rate and rhythm, which are crucial for effective blood circulation. Electrical impulse interactions with structural components highlight the complex functional character of the heart, with implications toward the understanding of various cardiovascular diseases. Notably, features such as fractal geometry in the electrical pathways of the heart (Almog et al., 2025) show deeper correlations between structure and function, which again enhance our conception of cardiac physiology (Figure 1.5)

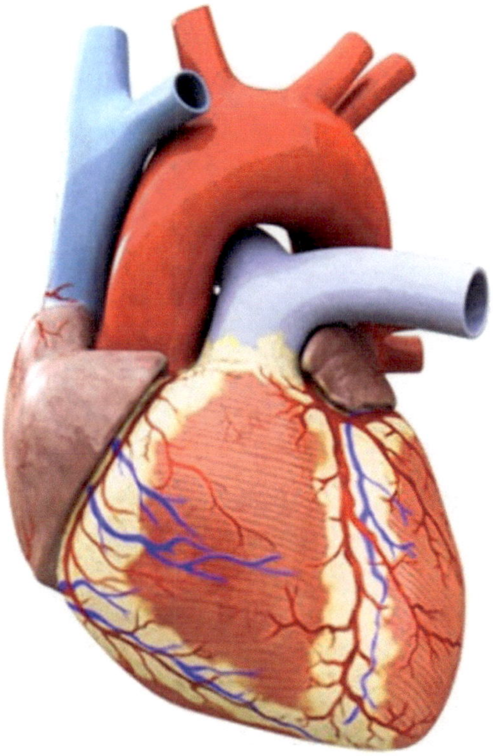

Figure 1.5. Heart structure.

Source: https://onlinesciencenotes.com/wp-content/uploads/2017/09/heart-human.jpg.

1.1.2. Chambers and Valves

The human heart is a remarkable organ composed of four chambers—two atria and two ventricles—each playing a vital role in the circulation of blood throughout the body. The right atrium receives deoxygenated blood from the systemic circulation via the superior and inferior venae cavae, directing it into the right ventricle. After that, the pulmonary arteries allow the right ventricle to pump this blood into the lungs for oxygenation. The left atrium, on the other hand, collects oxygen-rich blood from the lungs via the pulmonary veins, which it forwards to the left ventricle. This coordinated movement between the chambers ensures efficient blood flow, crucial for maintaining adequate oxygen delivery to tissues and organs. Understanding the anatomy and function of these chambers is essential for comprehending various cardiac pathologies and their implications on overall cardiovascular health. Integral to the heart's function are its valves, which regulate blood flow between the chambers and prevent backflow.

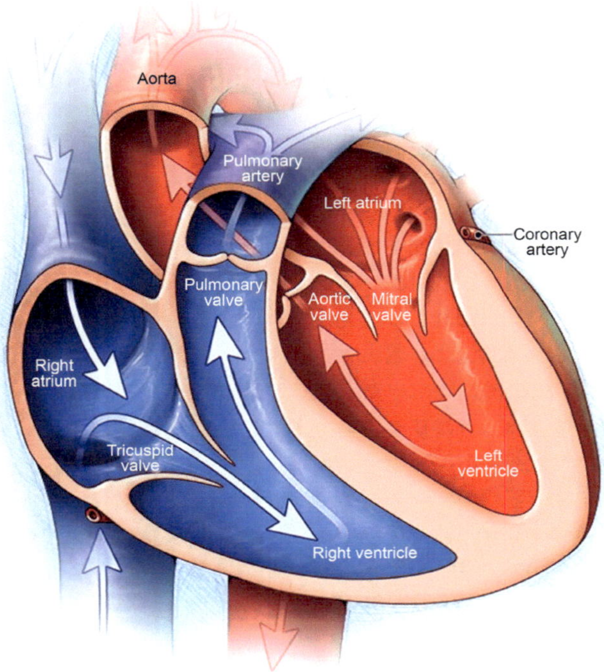

Figure 1.6. Chambers and valves of the heart.

Source: https://www.mayoclinic.org/-/media/kcms/gbs/patient-consumer/images/2014/09/22/12/43/mcdc7_theheart.jpg.

The heart contains four primary valves: the tricuspid valve, the pulmonary valve, the mitral valve, and the aortic valve. The tricuspid valve, located between the right atrium and right ventricle, is particularly vulnerable to dysfunction, often due to conditions such as tricuspid regurgitation (TR). TR can manifest as primary, resulting from structural abnormalities, or secondary, linked to right ventricular enlargement due to pulmonary hypertension or left-sided heart disease (Praz et al., 2021). TR presence leads to volume overload and increased wall stress, subsequently resulting in detrimental cardiac remodeling. The condition is critical to treat because it may jeopardize survival and exacerbate the symptoms of heart failure. Proper examination and intervention strategies are thus central to valve-related disorder management. Advances in medical technology over the past few decades have significantly contributed to the diagnosis and treatment of cardiac diseases, particularly those related to chambers and valves. New technologies such as transcatheter interventions represent a significant development in valve disease treatment without the surgical hazards of standard open-heart surgery. Transcatheter interventions are minimally invasive with the potential to target therapy in disease conditions such as TR, which has hitherto been treated suboptimally due to surgical risk and delayed presentations (Chen et al., 2020). In addition, with growing artificial intelligence and deep learning enhancing cardiac imaging segmentation, cardiologists are now better equipped to evaluate anatomical structures, facilitating accurate diagnosis and treatment planning. The multimodal strategy, including expert heart teams, is central to maximizing the potential of these technical advancements and best patient selection for emerging therapeutic strategies. Better patient outcomes for a range of cardiovascular conditions, especially those involving the chambers and valves, can result from the intelligent integration of these innovations. (Figure 1.6).

1.1.3. Blood Flow Pathway

The direction of blood circulation is a sophisticated network that is required to sustain life through the delivery of oxygen, nutrients, and waste products throughout the body. It begins with the heart, from which the oxygenated blood is pumped into the aorta, the body's largest artery, marking the start of systemic circulation. Blood then passes through progressively narrower arteries, arterioles, and finally arrives in the capillary beds, where nutrients and gases are transferred at the cellular level. The design of this circuit is not only helpful but dynamic as well, in that it adjusts to accommodate the body's needs during varying degrees of activity, rest, or stress. Understanding these intricate pathways enables possible innovations in clinical interventions and therapy procedures, especially with the advent of the complicated hemodynamics that can be replicated using sophisticated mock circulation models, as shown by current studies (Lu et al., 2025).

Once there has been an exchange of nutrients and gases at the capillary level, deoxygenated blood is captured by venules and veins and then returned to the heart. The venous system operates at a lower pressure than the arterial system and requires it. It requires the assistance of skeletal muscle contractions and the presence of one-way valves to enable blood to return towards the heart. This section of the pathway of blood flow plays a crucial role in ensuring that venous pooling is avoided and circulation is adequate. The anatomical and physiological properties of veins, e.g., their elasticity and lumen diameter, are significant in the return of the blood under various physiological conditions. It is this need to return deoxygenated blood to the heart that renders it pertinent to investigate hemodynamic alterations throughout the circulatory system, especially in cases of pathological diseases like heart failure, where these adaptations are typically lost (Lu et al., 2025). In addition, recent research has highlighted the function fulfilled by specialized pathways of blood circulation, such as the vascular portal systems, in regulating the transmission of hormones and other messengers throughout the body. For instance, the recognition of a portal system between the brain's suprachiasmatic nucleus (SCN) and the organum vasculosum of the lamina terminalis (OVLT) finds a complex route for neuroendocrine signaling, which can operate unidirectionally and vary in blood flow with a time-of-day dependency. These findings not only increase our information on the interrelatedness of various processes at the physiological level but also predict potential applications for clinical trials in the cure of endocrine disorders. These results highlight the intricacies of blood circulation, extending beyond current understanding to facilitate an integrated approach to cardiovascular processes and their impact on health (Figure 1.7).

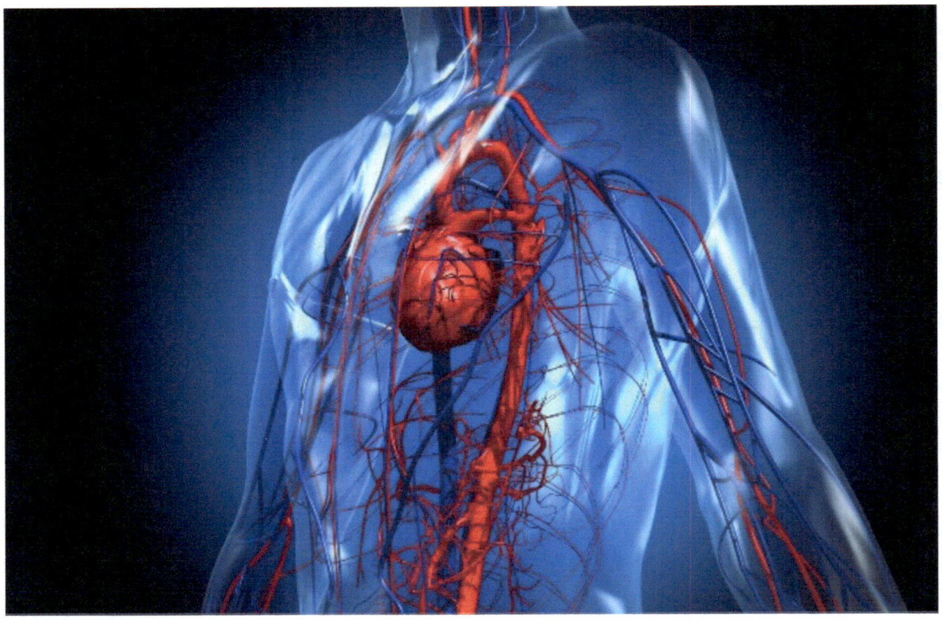

Figure 1.7. Blood flow through the heart.

Source: https://www.verywellhealth.com/thmb/q-DE1yH8q4m1eG34Yy4YKntzt2Q=/1500x0/filters:no_upscale():max_bytes(150000):strip_icc()/GettyImages-626974567-defc9220866c4e679c8d244dfbb997bb.jpg.

1.2. Blood Vessels and Circulation

The cardiovascular system is a complete system through which blood is transported throughout the body, and blood vessels are the conduits via which this bodily system of transport is achieved. Arteries, veins, and capillaries are the three main categories of blood vessels. Each vessel is present to serve a distinct but synchronized purpose in achieving adequate circulation and delivery of nutrients. Arteries, with their thick muscular walls, carry oxygenated blood from the heart to other parts of the body under pressure. Veins, on the other hand, return deoxygenated blood to the heart with thin walls and backflow-preventing valves. Capillaries are the micro-exchange sites where blood and tissues exchange gases and nutrients to support general cellular function and homeostasis. An appreciation of the hemodynamics of blood vessels is necessary to understand circulation complexities. Elasticity of vessels, vessel diameter, and viscosity of blood all contribute to hemodynamics and can have a significant influence on flow patterns and blood pressure. The Starling principle, initially proposed by Ernest Starling, has been modified to consider improved fluid balance within the environment of microvessels under varied physiological states. It has now been established in the current times that vascular health goes hand in hand with organ function, particularly in organs such as the kidneys, where blood pressure drives filtration and also overall renal function. When the blood pressure drops as a result of vascular blockage or inadequate venous return, the kidneys are particularly susceptible to damage, further compounding the body's fluid balance mechanisms (Ding et al., 2017). Furthermore, controlling blood flow and pressure requires complex hormonal and neurological regulation in addition to mechanical modification, which alters the vascular response to physical demands. For example, when the body is under more physical strain, the muscles dilate to increase blood flow, and the non-essential parts vasoconstrict to maximize the use of available resources. Understanding these regulatory systems not only has broad implications for the physiology of sports but also in the clinical setting, where regulation of blood flow can be decisive for the care of patients. Harmonizing these concepts about the cardiovascular system emphasizes how important healthy blood vessels are to sustain functions necessary to the body and emphasizes how mandatory ongoing research and guidelines in cardiovascular health are (Mach et al., 2019) (Figure 1.8).

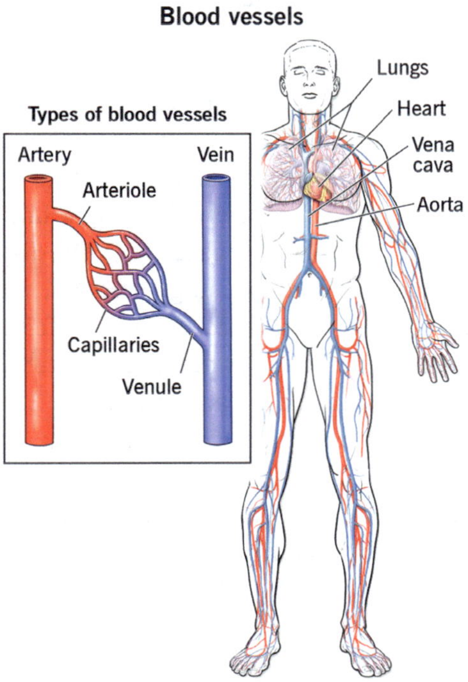

Figure 1.8. Blood vessels of various sizes and types transport blood through your body. They bring your cells what they need.

Source: https://my.clevelandclinic.org/-/scassets/images/org/health/articles/blood-vessels.

1.2.1. Types of Blood Vessels

The cardiovascular system is strictly organized and relies on three broad types of blood vessels: arteries, veins, and capillaries. All three are necessary in the process of circulating blood, ensuring nutrients, oxygen, and waste products are transported efficiently throughout the body. Arteries carry oxygenated blood from the heart to other tissues and possess thick, elastic walls to withstand the high pressure put on them during heart contractions. The aorta, the largest artery, branches into numerous small arteries, which in turn branch into arterioles, with the ultimate effect being the extensive network of capillaries that facilitate the exchange of nutrients and gases at the cellular level. Such supply is required for tissue viability and general physiological balance. Veins, however, have the function of returning deoxygenated blood to the heart, with a particular anatomic structure with thinner walls and larger lumens compared to arteries. The lower venous pressure is sustained by the presence of specific structures known as valves, which prevent backward blood flow, thereby allowing effective venous return despite the effect of gravity. Venous blood is constantly aided by the contraction of adjacent skeletal muscles, which compress veins and push blood toward the heart. Prominent veins such as the superior and inferior vena cavae collect blood from various regions of the body, reflecting the coordinated effort of the venous system within the broader framework of cardiovascular health and function. Capillaries are the largest in number and smallest blood vessels, being a vital interface between venous and arterial systems. Because of their single layer of endothelium, their thin walls facilitate rapid transfer of gases, nutrients, and waste products from tissues to blood and vice versa. This diffusion-dependent and osmosis-based process is vital for cellular metabolism and homeostasis. Capillary beds vary in density with the metabolic activity of the tissue, and higher densities are found in highly active organs such as muscles and the brain.

Also, capillary bed regulation by precapillary sphincters allows dynamic control of blood flow based on body physiological demand, underlining their vital role in the overall functioning of the cardiovascular system (Azzalini et al., 2019; Liu et al., 2020) (Figure 1.9).

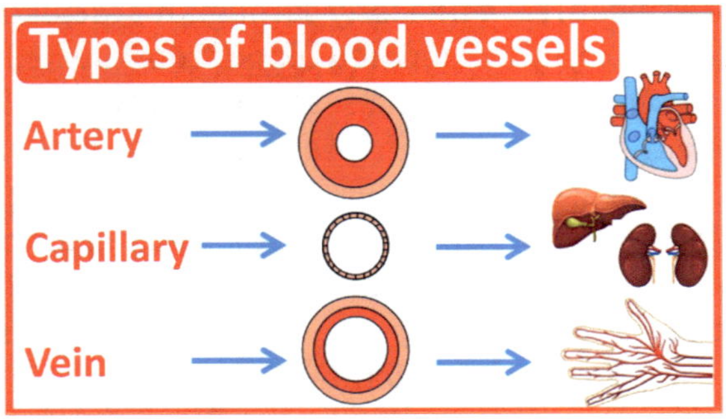

Figure 1.9. Types of blood vessels.

Source: https://i.ytimg.com/vi/0q3SbxO8RB0/maxresdefault.jpg.

1.2.2. Systemic Versus Pulmonary Circulation

The most basic element of the cardiovascular system is the closely interdependent relationship between systemic and pulmonary circulation, the two essential circuits whereby the delivery and exchange of blood throughout the entire body happens. Systemic circulation is responsible for distributing oxygenated blood from the left ventricle of the heart to organs and tissues scattered throughout the body and distributing deoxygenated blood to the right atrium. This complex process is made up of an enormous network of veins and arteries, with the arteries tasked with carrying oxygenated blood away from the heart and, through branching route paths, end up at the capillary beds. In this process, oxygen and nutrients are exchanged for waste and carbon dioxide, respectively, which are then expelled through the venous system to the heart, creating a dynamic cycle required to support cellular metabolism and general physiological integrity. Pulmonary circulation, in contrast, is a unique system in which the gas exchange takes place in the lungs. This process is triggered when deoxygenated blood from the body returns to the heart's right atrium and then is pumped into the right ventricle. The blood then continues to be forced out through pulmonary arteries into the lungs, where it undergoes a crucial process; carbon dioxide is expelled from the blood cells, and oxygen is absorbed into the bloodstream. The oxygenated blood, now returned to the left atrium through pulmonary veins, signifies the end of this critical cycle.

Pulmonary circulation efficiency not only guarantees that tissues are adequately supplied with oxygen but also contributes to acid-base balance by governing carbon dioxide content in the blood. Grasping the distinctiveness of these two circulatory systems is essential to better appreciate their specialized functions and interdependence as part of the cardiovascular system. For example, whereas systemic circulation requires increased pressure to deliver blood over longer distances efficiently, pulmonary circulation uses less pressure, meeting the requirement for gas exchange without putting the sensitive lung tissues through inordinate stress. Abnormalities within each system have important implications for general health, with disease states like pulmonary embolism having the potential to cause severe hemodynamic compromise as reflected in cases where right ventricular strain is implicated through imaging studies (Qureshi et al., 2020). Furthermore, new methods like artificial placenta therapy also emphasize the perseverance in research towards the enhancement of systemic circulation in high-risk groups like extremely preterm infants, thereby highlighting the primacy of these circulatory systems to the regulation of health and disease (Usuda et al., 2023) (Figure 1.10).

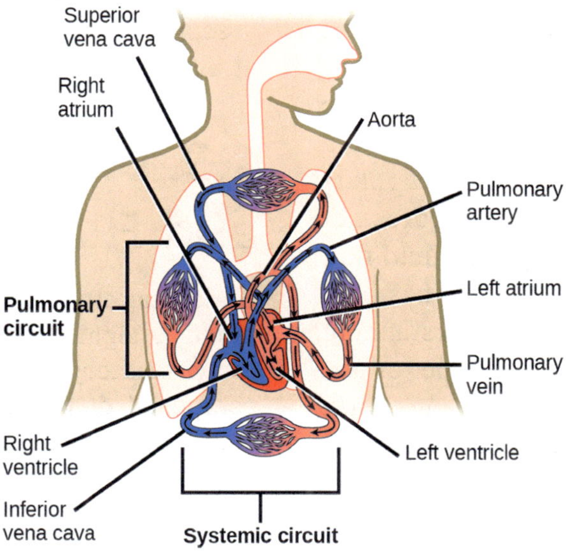

Figure 1.10. Pulmonary and systemic circulation.

Source: https://i2.wp.com/s3-us-west-2.amazonaws.com/courses-images/wp-content/uploads/sites/1842/2017/05/26234511/figure-40-03-01ab.png?w=1025&ssl=1.

1.2.3. Role of Capillaries

Capillaries, the cardiovascular system's finest vessels, are crucial for the exchange of gases and nutrients between blood and tissues. The single structure made of a single endothelial cell layer is ideal for the diffusion of carbon dioxide, oxygen, and other metabolites. This fine boundary not only serves to maximize the exchange rate but also demarcates the physiological environment to perform cellular functions. Capillary beds, whose density varies among tissues, are variable to a great extent to accommodate changes in perfusion as a function of metabolic demand.

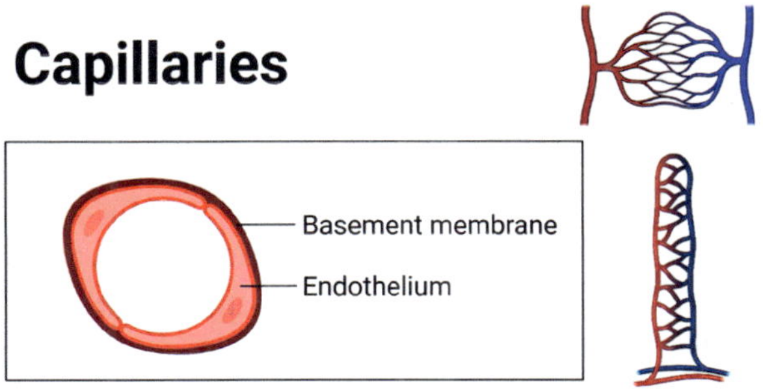

Figure 1.11. Capillaries.

Source: https://microbenotes.com/wp-content/uploads/2023/06/Capillaries.jpg.

For instance, in contracting tissues that require an increased supply of oxygen, the capillary density is elevated, emphasizing the dynamic role played by capillaries for maintaining homeostasis. The Starling principle, a central concept associated with capillary physiology, illustrates the balance of hydrostatic and osmotic pressures that regulate fluid flow between capillary walls. The concept has been developed into a higher level of understanding, including consideration of the role of the endothelial surface layer in water and solute movement. Permeability of capillaries has also been shown to be modified by a myriad of factors like inflammation and integrity of endothelial cells, which can regulate fluid homeostasis. Any dysfunction in this finely regulated process can lead to disease conditions such as edema or impaired perfusion.

Hence, understanding capillary dynamics will enable a better feeling for cardiovascular health and its influence on systemic fluid balance, particularly in tissues such as the kidney that are extremely highly responsive to alterations in blood flow (Ding et al., 2017). Moreover, capillaries are not mere passive tubes but also play an active role in blood flow regulation and tissue perfusion. They also communicate with surrounding cells, influencing signals controlling local blood flow.

Capillaries also play a significant role in hematopoiesis, notably in the bone marrow, where they create microenvironments required for hematopoietic stem cell (HSC) cultivation. Hypoxia and capillary-related factors have been proven to play vital roles in preserving HSC quiescence, pivotal for optimal cellular performance under stress. This is the representation of cellular dynamics and capillary function's interdependence and multifaceted contribution to the cardiovascular system. Sanitizing these protocols not only adds to our knowledge of normal physiology but also sets the stage for therapeutic strategies against vascular dysfunction-related diseases (Locatelli et al., 2017) (Figure 1.11).

1.3. Blood Composition and Function

Understanding the chemical composition of blood is significant in appreciating its role in the circulatory system. Blood is predominantly composed of plasma, red blood cells (RBCs), white blood cells (WBCs), and platelets. Plasma, which makes up about 55% of the volume of blood, is comprised of water, electrolytes, proteins, nutrients, and waste products. As a vehicle for the transportation of essential substances such as hormones and nutrients and the excretion of metabolic waste, plasma serves various purposes. The cellular elements of blood are the RBCs, the oxygen carriers, in that they have hemoglobin, the WBCs, the airlines of the immune system, and platelets, the carriers of clotting.

The interaction of these elements is required to ensure homeostasis, immunity, and repair functions, all of which the body needs to be well and the cardiovascular system properly functioning. Furthermore, the cross-talk between blood composition and cardiovascular disease has also been the focus of ongoing research. Specifically, body composition, as characterized by lean body mass, has been found to influence cardiovascular events, especially in specific patient groups. For instance, evidence has established that variations in lean body mass have a strong association with left ventricular mass index and renal resistive index in normotensive renal transplant recipients. This suggests that the composition of an individual's body can be an indicator of graft function as well as overall cardiovascular risk. By examining indicators like blood composition and left ventricular function, doctors can develop interventions to support improved cardiovascular health and determine the effectiveness of patient-tailored treatment protocols based on each patient's physiological condition (Demirci et al., 2024). Additionally, technology has introduced new windows to investigate blood's involvement in cardiovascular wellness. Photoplethysmogram signal-based equipment provides rich information above and beyond traditional heart rate and oxygen saturation. This equipment can quantify cardiovascular parameters such as systolic augmentation and waveform variability and report on an individual's cardiovascular status through their blood composition and function. These technologies also hold promise for personalizing health interventions in the context of monitoring cardiovascular behavior in real-time across various settings, including daily physical activity. Though studies continue to advance these approaches, these may potentially inform anticipatory healthcare decisions, further closing the gap in the connection between blood composition, function, and cardiovascular disease care (Mathieu et al., 2024) (Figure 1.12).

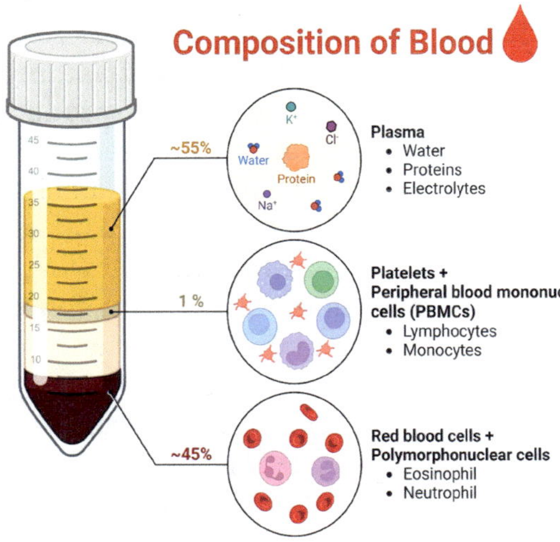

Figure 1.12. Composition of blood.

Source: https://microbenotes.com/wp-content/uploads/2023/04/Composition-of-Blood.jpg.

1.3.1. Components of Blood

The blood components are critical to the general functions of the cardiovascular system. Blood consists primarily of plasma, RBCs, WBCs, and platelets. Plasma, the liquid portion, comprises about 55% of the total blood volume and serves as a vehicle for the transport of nutrients, hormones, and waste products. RBCs, or erythrocytes, are designed to carry oxygen, oxygenating in lungs and deoxygenating in tissues, thereby sustaining cellular respiration. WBCs, or leukocytes, are responsible for immune defense, combating infection and foreign substances, and platelets, or thrombocytes, bring about blood clotting. This subtle interaction among these components not only sustains homeostasis but also considers the cardiovascular system's ability to respond to physiological and pathological stressors and identifies the need to consider each component's independent role. The function of blood components extends beyond transport and delivery of nutrients; they are also involved in regulatory mechanisms essential for cardiovascular health. Plasma proteins and hormones play a crucial role in regulating blood pressure and fluid balance, thereby enhancing the efficiency of the heart and blood vessels in creating the most efficient blood circulation and tissue perfusion. The operation and number of RBCs, stimulated by erythropoiesis in the bone marrow, show another complexity level as their numbers must adapt to variations in altitude and exercise. Platelets, which are products of the megakaryocytes, not only cause clotting but also release growth factors that are essential for the repair and healing of tissues after vascular trauma. Consequently, malfunction in any of them can trigger severe cardiovascular conditions, underlining the need for further research and clinical focus on the upkeep of blood component health, most notably in light of increasing cardiovascular disease (Li et al., 2024). Current advances in clinical science have consistently revealed how the intricate behavior of blood constituents contributes to the management and prevention of cardiovascular disease. The potential of many substances as therapeutic agents in regulating blood component behavior has been explored by research. For instance, angiotensin II receptor blockers (ARBs) and angiotensin-converting enzyme inhibitors (ACEIs) have been challenged concerning their opposing effect on cardiovascular outcomes, which has further clarified how blood components react to pharmacotherapy (King et al., 2023). Such observations reflect the need for customized treatment approaches based on an individual's blood component profiles and suspected deficiencies. With advancing knowledge of blood components and their significance in cardiovascular health, there is potential for more individualized regimens aimed at correcting underlying physiological dysfunctions, ultimately leading to better patient outcomes and a lessened overall burden of cardiovascular disease (Figure 1.13).

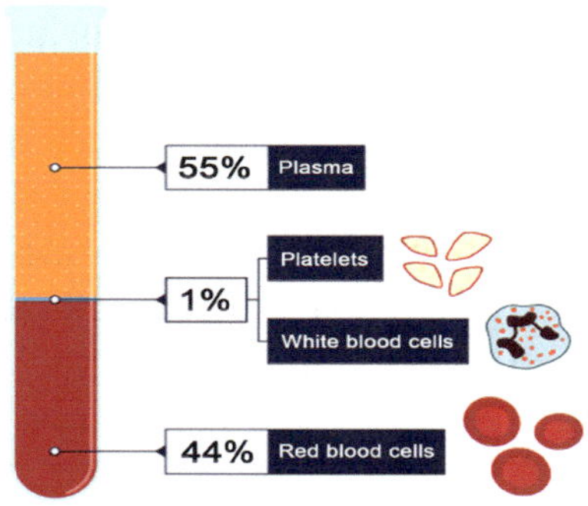

Figure 1.13. The components of the blood shown as percentages.

Source: https://bam.files.bbci.co.uk/bam/live/content/znsntrd/large.

1.3.2. Functions of Blood Cells

The body of humans is mainly reliant on blood cells, which carry out many essential activities in the circulatory system. Among such cells, erythrocytes or red blood cells play a vital role in the delivery of oxygen from the lungs to the tissues and the carriage of carbon dioxide back to be exhaled. Such gas exchange is essential in cellular metabolism and ensuring maximum tissue function. In addition, erythrocytes also regulate blood pH through the bicarbonate buffer system. The red blood cells' biconcave shape allows them to have increased surface area for efficient gas exchange, as well as flexibility to move through the most minute capillaries. Such a function emphasizes the fundamental nature of erythrocytes in sustaining life, and the fact that any alteration in their quantity or quality can lead to severe health issues, highlighting the vulnerability of the cardiovascular system to blood composition alterations. In addition to erythrocytes, leukocytes, or white blood cells, are significant in the immune response as well as in the general health of the cardiovascular system. These cells are of various types, including neutrophils, lymphocytes, monocytes, eosinophils, and basophils, each playing unique immune defense roles. Neutrophils, for instance, are the ones that initially respond to infection by migrating quickly into inflammatory sites to engulf and destroy microbes by phagocytosis. Lymphocytes, however, play a critical role in adaptive immunity, with T cells participating in cell-mediated immunity and B cells producing antibodies. Furthermore, the presence of immune cells in the vascular network and blood strengthens the body's ability to respond to injuries and infections efficiently, showing the way that the mechanics of leukocyte function engage with the circulatory dynamics. Thus, understanding the varied roles of leukocytes strengthens our insight into cardiovascular health and disease. Platelets, or thrombocytes, serve another crucial function by inducing hemostasis, the mechanism that stops bleeding once injuries occur. Platelets are disk-shaped cell fragments that are generated from megakaryocytes in the bone marrow. Platelets are activated when the blood vessels are damaged, aggregating rapidly to form a transient plug at the injury site. This clumping is also augmented by the release of chemically active molecules that activate additional platelets, giving an aggressive response to vascular insult. Platelets further aid tissue repair and wound healing by the release of growth factors and cytokines that promote healing and regulate inflammation.

As platelets are of vital importance in hemostasis and inflammation, dysregulation can lead to catastrophic cardiovascular complications such as thrombosis or hemorrhage. It is therefore critical to understand the roles of the blood cells to unravel the complexities of cardiovascular well-being and the mechanisms that control heterogeneous diseases, providing insights valuable for effective therapeutic intervention.

1.3.3. Importance of Plasma

Plasma is the core component of the cardiovascular system, facilitating many of the physiological activities required to maintain homeostasis. Constituting approximately 55% of blood volume, plasma is a straw-colored liquid that facilitates the transport of nutrients, hormones, and waste products throughout the body.

The high plasma content in the form of water, proteins, electrolytes, and gases facilitates efficient delivery and elimination of various substances crucial to cellular processes. Particularly, the contribution of plasma proteins such as albumin and globulins to maintaining osmotic pressure and immune activity is essential. This functional heterogeneity is a reflection of plasma's significance not just in circulation, but also in the pathophysiology of many cardiovascular disorders, where plasma composition alterations can influence disease causation and therapeutic responses. Further contributing to the significance of plasma in cardiovascular wellness is the connection it bears with genetic differences that impact cardiovascular characteristics. For instance, the apolipoprotein A5 gene plays a significant role in modulating plasma lipid concentrations and, consequently, cardiovascular disease risk. One of the gene polymorphisms, rs662799, has been associated with increased body mass index and blood pressure, both of which are risk factors for cardiovascular disease. Individuals that carry the minor allele G have an outstandingly higher risk of developing these diseases, demonstrating the way in which genetic susceptibility can instantaneously impact plasma traits and, by extension, cardiovascular health. These genetic interactions offer essential clues to the ways in which personalized medicine approaches minimizing cardiovascular risks linked to plasma biochemistry (Fatma et al., 2023). In addition, the role of plasma extends to the pathogenesis of atherosclerosis, one of the leading reasons for cardiovascular disease. Atherosclerosis is characterized by the accumulation of plaque within arterial walls, a process regulated by molecular interactions present in plasma membranes across all cells. These mechanisms relate plasma composition to the progression of disease and include lipid transport, immunological response, and blood flow dynamics modulation. In this way, a more sophisticated comprehension of these relationships improves the precision of atherosclerosis diagnosis and treatment plans for atherosclerosis risk individuals. Through research into the role of plasma in merging various biological processes, scientists can devise new therapeutic modalities that counteract cardiovascular disease endpoints (Kotlyarov et al., 2022). This nuanced role of plasma recognizes its irreplaceable position in the cardiovascular system, worthy of more investigation and understanding (Figure 1.14).

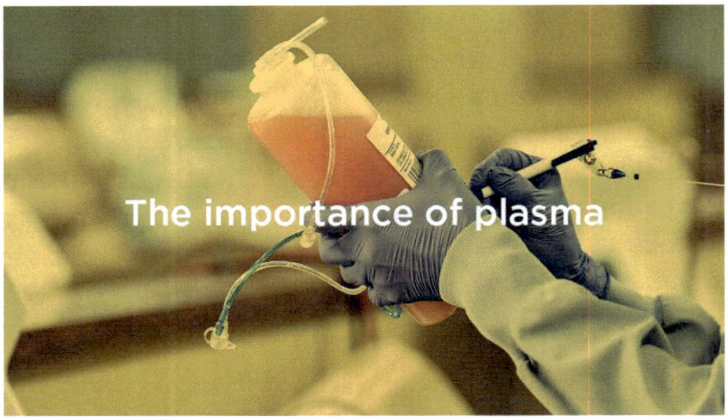

Figure 1.14. Importance of plasma.

Source: https://i.ytimg.com/vi/2wNRK87ucPs/maxresdefault.jpg.

1.4. Electrical System of the Heart

The electrical system of the heart is vital in the control of synchronized cardiac contractions and adequate blood perfusion of the body. Unlike skeletal muscle, which relies on nerve innervation for contraction, the heart possesses an intrinsic electrical system that is controlled by specialized pacemaker cells. They are located predominantly in the SA node, which is typically defined as the heart's natural pacemaker. The SA node generates electrical impulses that travel through the atria, causing them to contract and push blood into the ventricles. The impulses then move to the AV node, a vital holding point, pausing the electrical signal before it continues to the ventricles. This intricate timing enhances coordinated heartbeating that makes for efficient blood flow, which is required for cardiovascular fitness as a whole. As the electrical impulses pass through the heart, they induce mechanical contractions, which are measured quantitatively by electrocardiographic (ECG) parameters. ECG is a valuable diagnostic test, tracing intervals like RR, PR, and QTc, which are the electrical propagation and cardiac contraction timing. Abnormalities in these parameters can indicate concomitant arrhythmias or other cardiac illnesses. Recent focus has been on the genetic influences on these ECG parameters. Impressive studies employing HXB/BXH recombinant rat inbred strains have identified quantitative trait loci (QTL) for significant ECG parameters and linked provided gene expressions to cardiac conduction variability (Adriaens et al., 2018). Identification of these loci not only provides insights into the heart's electrical system but also expresses the capability of personalized treatment schemes in the management of cardiac ailments as genetic predispositions can influence the way individuals react to interventions (Adriaens et al., 2018). Understanding of the electric heart system exceeds functional knowledge; it also directs therapeutic interventions and tactics. Pathological conditions, such as myocardial infarction (MI), may lead to abnormal electrical conduction, arrhythmias, and unfavorable outcomes. Studies have started to elucidate pathways including sympathetic hyperactivity and neuroimmune responses targeted at heart remodeling after MI. In particular, decreased sympathetic activity and enhanced cardiac function following MI have been linked to microglial depletion in the central nervous system. This seminal work implies that interventions targeting the heart's electrical system and its regulatory controls might be able to notably limit harmful cardiac remodeling and enable recovery from ischemic injury.

Through an understanding of both systemic and genetic factors influencing electrical activity, the potential for treating cardiovascular disease more efficiently is increased (Wang et al., 2023) (Figure 1.15).

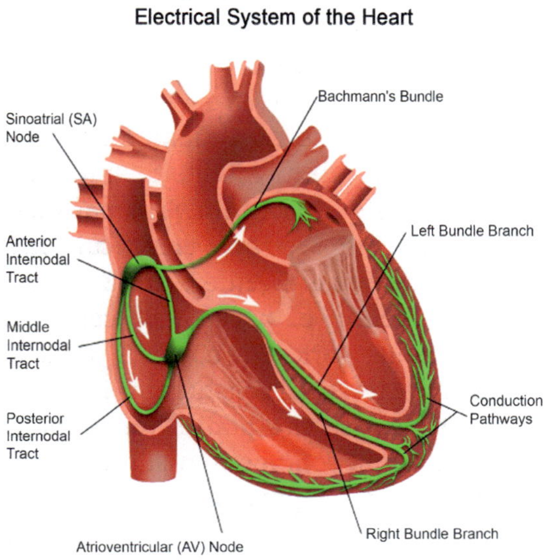

Figure 1.15. Electrical system of the heart.

Source: https://www.stanfordchildrens.org/content-public/topic/images/77/125477.gif.

1.4.1. Cardiac Conduction System

The cardiac conduction system is a critical mechanism that regulates the rhythm of the heart and allows coordinated contractions for adequate blood circulation. The system of specialized cells that includes cardiac pacemaker cells pervades the heart and regulates the sequence of electrical impulses, resulting in the activation of cardiac contraction. The system is primarily made up of the SA node, AV node, Bundle of His, and Purkinje fibers. All of these structures are inserted with precision to transmit electrical impulses, starting from the SA node, often referred to as the heart's natural pacemaker. This generates impulses that travel all over the atria, leading to their contraction and then channelling the electrical impulse to the ventricles, where there is synchronized contraction. This intricate timing is of tremendous significance in facilitating maximum cardiac output and in making the heart function at an optimal rate under various physiological demands. Dysfunction in any part of the cardiac conduction system can lead to an array of arrhythmias that can have significant clinical presentations in terms of patient health. These dysfunctions can manifest as bradycardia, tachycardia, or even blockage, and can lead to symptoms ranging from palpitations to syncope. Realizing the interconnectivity of the conduction system, particularly in patients with possible complications from concomitant disease such as rheumatic diseases, is vital. According to emerging evidence, inflammatory rheumatic diseases have a substantial impact on cardiovascular health, extending beyond the myocardial function to the integrity of conduction pathways. Furthermore, the relationship between systemic inflammation and electrical disturbances emphasizes the need for thorough cardiovascular assessment in such populations since early detection can enable timely interventions (Buleu et al., 2019). Furthermore, therapeutic management of conduction disorders is of utmost importance, and the development of therapeutic interventions for managing conduction disorders underlines the importance of multidisciplinary practice within the healthcare setting. Therapeutic management may be attained using pharmacologic therapy in the guise of antiarrhythmic drugs or procedural management in the guise of pacemaker implantation aimed at normalizing rhythm. Additionally, research on cardiovascular comorbidities in inflammatory rheumatic diseases informs clinical practice, emphasizing repeated electrocardiographic and echocardiographic checks. These measurements are essential to detect potential electrical changes early so that healthcare workers can customize management schemes appropriately. The more that we learn concerning the cardiac conduction system and its vulnerabilities, the better we are equipped to observe improved patient outcomes, particularly in those at higher risk for cardiovascular morbidity due to chronic inflammatory conditions (Zeppenfeld et al., 2022) (Figure 1.16).

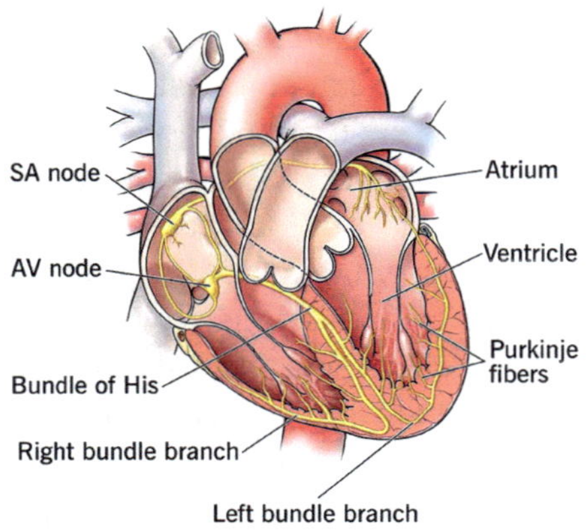

Figure 1.16. Cardiac conduction system.

Source: https://my.clevelandclinic.org/-/scassets/images/org/health/articles/heart-conduction-system.

1.4.2. Role of the Sinoatrial Node (SAN)

The SAN is the primary pacemaker of the heart, and it is the master organ that creates a normal cardiac rhythm. The SAN lies within the right atrium and emits electrical impulses that initiate each heartbeat. It is through the intrinsic electrical activity that cardiac muscle contraction is synchronized, ensuring rhythmic and efficient blood circulation within the body. The electrical signals from the SANs cascade through the atria, stimulating these chambers to contract and push the blood into the ventricles. Irregularities in the functioning of the SAN can lead to arrhythmias, such as atrial fibrillation, a condition of unsynchronized electrical activity that impairs the heart's ability to pump effectively. This shows the pivotal role of the SAN in ensuring not only rhythm, but overall cardiovascular health and function, as emphasized by studies that identify its roles in both healthy and pathological states of cardiac activity (Elsayed, 2024). More recent research has also explained the complex mechanisms of the pacemaking ability of the SAN and emphasized its intricate cellular structure. The coupled-clock theory provides a framework for describing how SAN cells coordinate to generate rhythmic impulses via intracellular calcium dynamics and transmembrane voltage changes in concert. It highlights the function of local calcium releases within SAN pacemaker cells, synchronizing to propel electrical activity throughout the node. Besides, the SAN is not merely a collection of pacemaker cells but a sophisticated network that consists of various cell types and interstitial constituents interacting and contributing to the node's function. This multi-dimensional composition allows the SAN to adapt to varying physiological conditions so that heart rate can increase or decrease according to the body's demands (Donald et al., 2023). Understanding the role of the sinoatrial node involves more than the pacemaker role; it consists of an appreciation of its role in broader cardiovascular dynamics. As an example, with diseases like atrial fibrillation, the SAN's regular electrical activity can be overcome by chaotic electrical activity from another source, e.g., pulmonary veins. This disturbance underlines the importance of therapeutic methods of reclaiming normal sinus rhythm, which is essential for maximum cardiac output. The determination of the SAN's capacity to sustain its functions, even under disturbances, signals the way forward for research on devising interventions to improve its resilience. Through understanding the intricate dynamics of the SANs structure and function, a more profound comprehension of its role in the cardiovascular system is brought about, substantiating the role of this node in ensuring heart well-being and effective circulation (Elsayed, 2024) (Figure 1.17).

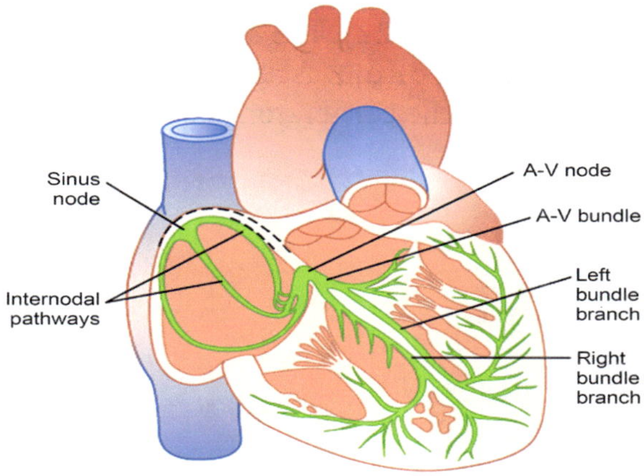

Figure 1.17. Sinoatrial node (SAN).

Source: https://img.brainkart.com/imagebk20/Xsqopzi.png.

1.4.3. Electrocardiogram (ECG) Basics

The ECG is a vital piece of equipment utilized in the assessment of cardiovascular health, reporting on the electrical activity of the heart. By recording rhythm patterns of electrical impulses that are generated during each heartbeat, an ECG allows physicians to identify many cardiac abnormalities. The graphic output, based on electrodes placed on the body surface, makes it possible to measure heart rate, rhythm, and the size and location of cardiac chambers. Understanding of the main structures of an ECG, namely the P wave, QRS complex, and T wave, is required to interpret the findings effectively. An understanding of this basic fact not only assists in developing an appreciation of a normally beating heart but also aids in the detection of abnormalities such as arrhythmias, ischemia, and remote myocardial infarctions, thereby making ECGs a cornerstone of cardiovascular diagnosis and assessment. The technological innovations are substantially influencing ECG practices and readings in the cardiovascular field. The technological advancements in devices, such as portable and digital ECG devices, have enhanced cardiac monitoring to be more convenient and accessible. The portable devices can send data wirelessly to healthcare professionals, enabling real-time monitoring and immediate interventions. Furthermore, the use of artificial intelligence and deep learning algorithms has revolutionized ECG analysis. Current studies highlight how deep learning algorithms enhance diagnostic accuracy, identifying patterns that elude even experienced clinicians (Egger et al., 2022). These developments not only shorten the time to analyze but also make sophisticated diagnostic equipment accessible to more people, especially in remote or underprivileged areas. This shift illustrates the new face of cardiovascular health care, ensuring ECGs are still the central hub of patient care. Aside from this, the incorporation of ECG technology into telemedicine has also transformed the monitoring and maintenance of cardiovascular health. With the growing popularity of telemedicine in clinics, especially post-COVID-19, it has facilitated virtual consultations as well as the remote monitoring of patients. With ECG technology used under this system, perpetual heart health monitoring is possible without the requirement of on-site visits, thereby supporting complete patient convenience and follow-up care compliance. Moreover, as medical practitioners increasingly rely on digital platforms, the future for platforms like the

CardioVerse is feasible, bringing together augmented and virtual reality in cardiovascular education and patient empowerment (Skalidis et al., 2022). The integration of these latest technologies with traditional ECG practice marks a new era in cardiovascular medicine in which efficiency, accessibility, and patient-centered care continue to be the cornerstones of promoting heart health (Figure 1.18).

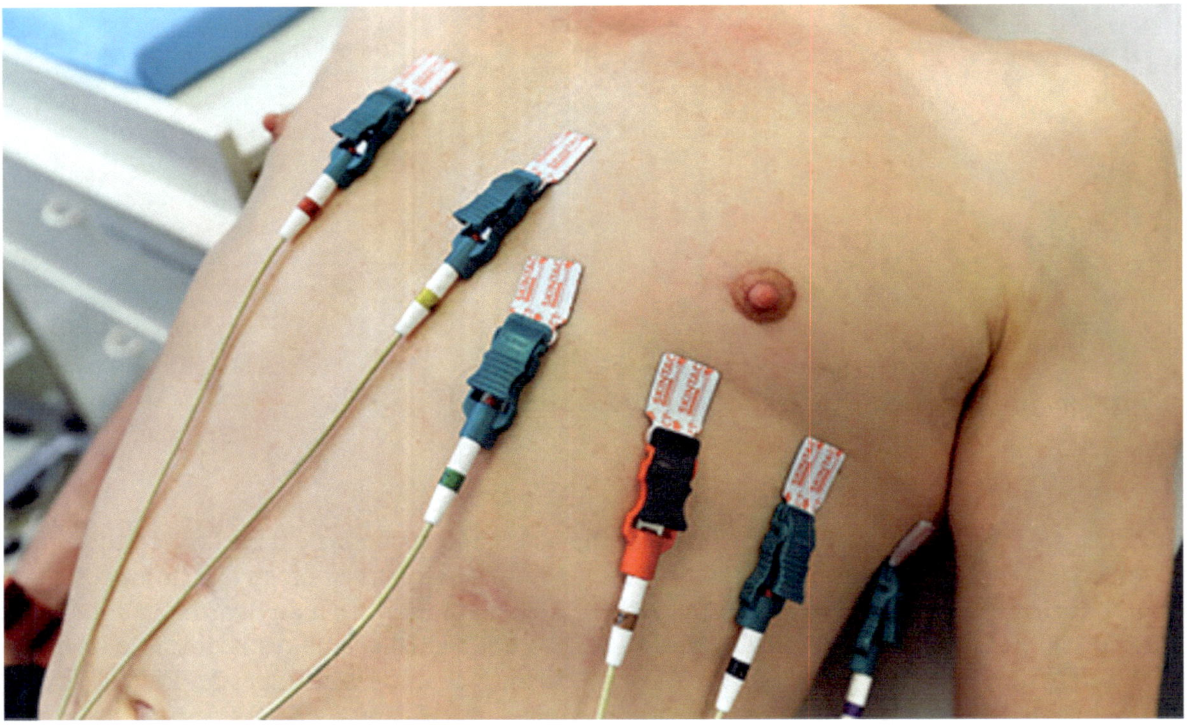

Figure 1.18. Electrocardiogram (ECG).

Source: https://media.healthdirect.org.au/images/inline/original/ecg-electrodes-attached-chest-dc55ff.jpg.

SUMMARY

The strategy of this chapter illustrates the utmost importance of studying the cardiovascular system, its structure, and function to maintain the whole body in a healthy condition. The network complexity of veins and arteries, the pump function of the heart, and the regulation mechanisms in place are indicative of the network complexity present within this system. The data on how lifestyle behaviors, including diet and exercise, impact the cardiovascular system highlight the need for health-conscious choices. As emphasized further recently by breakthroughs in health guidelines, including the WHO 2020 recommendation, exercise is the foundation for reducing cardiovascular disease risk. Compliance with the above advice can deliver improved cardiovascular health outcomes, ultimately to a healthier population overall (Bull et al., 2020). Furthermore, research continues to identify the complexities and harms of other products, e.g., electronic nicotine delivery systems. Smokers show varying degrees of exposure to harmful volatile organic compounds, and therefore, although some alternatives are seemingly less dangerous, they are still of concern to the cardiovascular system. These. Dangers must be addressed, particularly by young adults, as they are most likely to experiment with such substances. products. This awareness leads toward the direction of future research on the long-term effects of other nicotine devices and on how they affect cardiovascular well-being (Keith et al., 2019). Overall, a comprehensive understanding of the heart and circulatory system and knowledge of external factors that influence its well-being opens doors to prevention and treatment avenues. The interaction between physical activity, smoking, and cardiovascular health is essential, and public policy needs to be attuned to the forces at work. Effective health education can facilitate individuals in making lifestyle choices favorable to their cardiovascular health, and ongoing research can guide policymaking. Thus, it becomes of utmost priority in the quest for a healthy society to turn towards cardiovascular health as far as well-educated decision-making is concerned, and also listen to the potential danger of newer drugs. The findings of the investigation of the prevailing traditional practices and ongoing trends in health behavior verify the necessity for an active strategy towards cardiovascular health.

The cardiovascular system is a highly interconnected entity required for the accomplishment of homeostasis and the maintenance of physiological processes. Based on recent research, neurodevelopmental disabilities (NDD) have been found to be highly related to poorer cardiovascular health (CVH) status among children and adolescents. A comparative study based on the National Survey of Children's Health indicates that children with NDD exhibit high percentages of unfavorable cardiovascular outcomes, such as obesity and diabetes mellitus, when compared with their non-NDD counterparts. This inconsistency emphasizes the need to target interventions for improving CVH among this high-risk population. Changing modifiable lifestyle determinants of cardiovascular risk is a way through which it may be possible to achieve better health and quality of life among adolescents with NDD. Strategic public health initiatives are imperative for generating awareness and establishing effective preventive measures. Moreover, understanding physiological responses to environmental stressors such as the application of lower body negative pressure (LBNP) comes into play with regard to cardiovascular health. Research has shown that LBNP is a potential countermeasure to utilize in combating cardiovascular deconditioning due to exposure to microgravity. Through the systematic determination of the cardiovascular impacts of various doses of LBNP, scientists have established a system quantitatively analyzing responses of numerous cardiovascular variables. Notably, the study found that LBNP is effective in an advantageous influence on jugular venous circulation to counteract stagnation danger, particularly for use with individuals who experience phenomena like spaceflight. Such findings are of considerable use in developing methods of maintaining cardiovascular integrity in atypical physical environments. Integration of the cardiovascular system with other physiological processes is illustrated to call attention to the importance of a holistic perception of cardiovascular health. The study of determinants of CVH in neurodevelopmental environments and conditions like microgravity proposes a multi-modal strategy for cardiovascular risk control. Interventions for improved lifestyle behaviors combined with new countermeasures through means like LBNP present opportunities for enhanced cardiovascular outcomes on multiple fronts. The collective knowledge acquired through research on youth with NDD and the physiological reactions to LBNP creates avenues for future research and public health initiatives towards optimizing cardiovascular wellness among heterogeneous populations. Implementation of such information into community and clinical practice is essential for creating a healthier society.

A CLOSER LOOK

CARDIOVASCULAR DISEASES

Valve diseases and malformations are the cause of a tremendous number of deaths each year. Stenosis, which is the obstructed outflow of blood and regurgitation or backflow of blood due to defective closure of valves, is a presentation of valve disease.

Heart sounds result from vibrations that are produced on valve closure. Abnormal heart sounds, or heart murmurs, indicate valve malfunction.

The most common valve malformations are mitral valve prolapse and bicuspid aortic valve. The degeneration of elastin, proteoglycan, and collagen layers of the extracellular matrix of valves can also cause valve disease.

Coronary heart diseases (CHD) or ischemic heart disease also progress over some time. Atherosclerosis, or the accumulation of fat, cholesterol, or calcium on coronary artery walls that supply blood to the heart, is responsible for coronary heart disease. This results in a diminishing flow of oxygenated blood to the heart. Pieces of these fat deposits may also break away, forming a blood clot that may block the coronary artery, denying blood supply to the heart, and resulting in a heart attack.

The signs of CHD are chest pain, nausea, traveling limb pain, and shortness of breath. The risk factors include high blood pressure, smoking, high cholesterol, diabetes, and obesity (Figure 1.19).

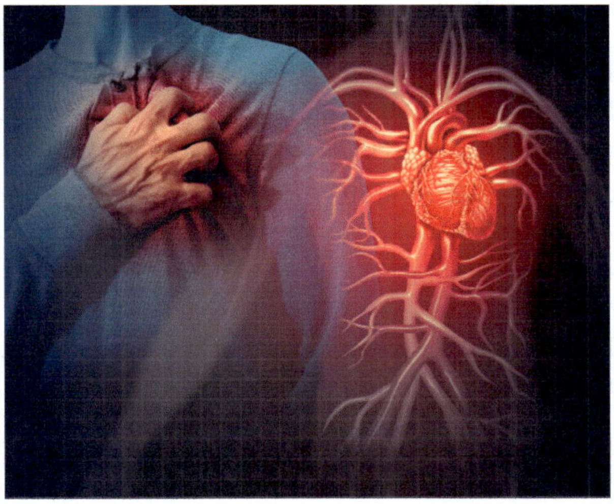

Figure 1.19. Cardiovascular Diseases.

Source: https://images.ctfassets.net/eexbcii1ci83/3AGUUtHuXuzHKu1O5PFKhh/b76f6b4e18105209f858886462de28f0/Cardiovascular_disease_3.png.

References

1. Adriaens, M. E., Lodder, E. M., Moreno-Moral, A., Šilhavý, J., Heinig, M., Glinge, C., Belterman, C., Wolswinkel, R., Petretto, E., Pravenec, M., Remme, C. A., & Bezzina, C. R. (2018). Systems genetics approaches in RAT identify novel genes and gene networks associated with cardiac conduction. *Journal of the American Heart Association, 7*(21). https://doi.org/10.1161/jaha.118.009243Almog, Y., Aon, M. A., Aon, M. A., Barabasi, A. L., Bhalla, U. S., Bigger, J. T. Jr., Boxenbaum, H., et al. (2025). Deterministic chaos and fractal complexity in the dynamics of cardiovascular behavior: Perspectives on a new frontier. *Open Cardiovasc. Med. J.* https://core.ac.uk/download/pdf/8336146.pdf (accessed on 29th May 2025).

2. Andreassi, M. G., & Vassalle, C. (2009). Genetic polymorphisms of the natriuretic peptide system in the pathogenesis of cardiovascular disease: What lies on the horizon? *Clinical Chemistry.* https://core.ac.uk/download/pdf/37831226.pdf (accessed on 29th May 2025).

3. Azzalini, D., Rebollo, I., & Tallon-Baudry, C. (2019). Visceral signals shape brain dynamics and cognition. *Trends in Cognitive Sciences, 23*, 488–509. https://doi.org/10.1016/j.tics.2019.03.007 (accessed on 29th May 2025).

4. Bai, S., Zhang, M., Tang, S., Li, M., Wu, R., Wan, S., Chen, L., et al. (2024). Effects and impact of selenium on human health: A review. *Molecules, 30.* https://www.semanticscholar.org/paper/08676b4f8045bc3282bd1d2bfeb7bc0db0c81d4a (accessed on 29th May 2025).

5. Baker-Smith, C., Zhang, Z., Robson, S. M., Patterson, F., Brewer, B., Tsai, J. M., & Bhat, A. (2024). Abstract 4144597: Cardiovascular health among youth with neurodevelopmental disability: Analysis of National Survey of Children's Health (NSCH) – 2021. *Circulation.* https://www.semanticscholar.org/paper/e10aa11cda2b78a97e9527b17e73dcffd967fe4a (accessed on 29th May 2025).

6. Banerjee, D., Winocour, P., Chowdhury, T., De, P., Wahba, M., Montero, R., Fogarty, D., et al. (2022). Management of hypertension and renin-angiotensin-aldosterone system blockade in adults with diabetic kidney disease: Association of British Clinical Diabetologists and the Renal Association UK guideline update 2021. *BMC Nephrology, 23.* https://www.semanticscholar.org/paper/6ae17910eef88141a71a3e6aaea42687dd418cc9 (accessed on 29th May 2025).

7. Berezin, A., & Berezin, A. (2022). Point-of-care heart failure platform: Where are we now and where are we going to? *Expert Review of Cardiovascular Therapy, 20*, 419–429. https://www.semanticscholar.org/paper/924f4dd4982dc51d1b8ad31c2209c64db0ae4b9f (accessed on 29th May 2025).

8. Bikbov, B., Purcell, C., Levey, A. S., Smith, M., Abdoli, A., Abebe, M., Adebayo, O., et al. (2020). Global, regional, and national burden of chronic kidney disease, 1990–2017: A systematic analysis for the Global Burden of Disease Study 2017. *The Lancet, 395*, 709–733. https://doi.org/10.1016/s0140-6736(20)30045-3 (accessed on 29th May 2025).

9. Bokou, N. M., Dimitriadis, N., Arnaoutis, G., & Panagiotakos, D. (2025). The effect of aerobic and resistance exercise on markers of atherosclerosis: A narrative review of meta-analyses and systematic reviews. *Health & Research Journal.* https://www.semanticscholar.org/paper/4dc2b12706b6aa1381bc8ca5d38a7a15f294b11b (accessed on 29th May 2025).

10. Borghi, C., Grassi, G., Rosei, E. A., Savoia, C., et al. (2017). *Personalized Medicine—A Modern Approach for the Diagnosis and Management of Hypertension.* https://core.ac.uk/download/96884785.pdf (accessed on 29th May 2025).

11. Buleu, F., Sîrbu, E., Caraba, A., & Drăgan, S. (2019). Heart involvement in inflammatory rheumatic diseases: A systematic literature review. *Medicina, 55*, 249–249. https://doi.org/10.3390/medicina55060249 (accessed on 29th May 2025).

12. Bull, F., Al-Ansari, S. S., Biddle, S., Borodulin, K., Buman, M. P., Cardon, G., Carty, C., et al. (2020). World Health Organization 2020 guidelines on physical activity and sedentary behavior. *British Journal of Sports Medicine, 54*, 1451–1462. https://doi.org/10.1136/bjsports-2020-102955 (accessed on 29th May 2025).

13. Chen, C., Qin, C., Qiu, H., Tarroni, G., Duan, J., Bai, W., & Rueckert, D. (2020). Deep learning for cardiac image segmentation: A review. *Frontiers in Cardiovascular Medicine, 7*. https://doi.org/10.3389/fcvm.2020.00025 (accessed on 29th May 2025).

14. Cicero, A., Fogacci, F., D'Addato, S., Grandi, E., Rizzoli, E., Borghi, C., & On Behalf of the Brisighella Heart Study. (2023). Self-reported coffee consumption and central and peripheral blood pressure in the cohort of the Brisighella Heart Study. *Nutrients, 15*. https://www.semanticscholar.org/paper/6afc6c1c344e3edbe78fbae3a44e665e2a17bbee (accessed on 29th May 2025).

15. Coste, B., & Delmas, P. (2024). PIEZO ion channels in cardiovascular functions and diseases. *Circulation Research, 134*, 572–591. https://www.semanticscholar.org/paper/1e8ca252fdf45d4a67bf1ddca77acbaa7d2a76be (accessed on 29th May 2025).

16. Cześnikiewicz-Guzik, M., Dróżdż, M., Filip, M., Guzik, T. J., et al. (2014). *Denture-Related Stomatitis is Associated with Endothelial Dysfunction.* https://core.ac.uk/download/42353840.pdf (accessed on 29th May 2025).

17. Demirci, B. G., & Karakan, M. S. (2024). Effect of body composition on graft function and cardiovascular outcomes in normotensive renal transplant recipients. *Experimental and Clinical Transplantation: Official Journal of the Middle East Society for Organ Transplantation, 22*(2), 108–113. https://www.semanticscholar.org/paper/ea8e99b5d882f5ebca5d4c1b7ffd1310119287e7 (accessed on 29th May 2025).

18. Ding, X., Cheng, Z., & Qian, Q. (2017). Intravenous fluids and acute kidney injury. *Blood Purification, 43*, 163–172. https://doi.org/10.1159/000452702 (accessed on 29th May 2025).

19. Donald, L., & Lakatta, E. (2023). What makes the sinoatrial node tick? A question not for the faint of heart. *Philosophical Transactions of the Royal Society B: Biological Sciences, 378*. https://www.semanticscholar.org/paper/d0ebd7ee14aedcf529659b18bb831847f99c2d1a (accessed on 29th May 2025).

20. Egger, J., Gsaxner, C., Pepe, A., Pomykala, K. L., Jonske, F., Kurz, M., Li, J., et al. (2022). Medical deep learning—A systematic meta-review. *Computer Methods and Programs in Biomedicine, 221*, 106874. https://doi.org/10.1016/j.cmpb.2022.106874 (accessed on 29th May 2025).

21. Elsayed, Y. M. H. (2024). Sinusoidal atrial fibrillation (Yasser's fibrillation) and partial SAN function in COVID-19 pneumonia; a new cardiovascular discovery change in atrial fibrillation directory. *International Journal of Cardiovascular Medicine*. https://www.semanticscholar.org/paper/9d61cc3ff1ec844d2943fa0ccbf2ebbdfe1027f9 (accessed on 29th May 2025).

22. Fatma, R., Chauhan, W., Riyaz, S., Rasheed, K., & Afzal, M. (2023). Genetic association analysis of rs662799 (−1131A > G) polymorphism of *APOA5* gene with morphometric and physiometric traits using multiplex PCR. *Egyptian Journal of Medical Human Genetics, 24*. https://

www.semanticscholar.org/paper/7e3532761406444c73d4eb93376c217f459da029 (accessed on 29th May 2025).

23. Hassan-Beck, R., Hafidh, K., Badi, A., Dougman, K., Karmo, M., Mir, R., & Beshyah, S. (2022). Ramadan fasting in health and disease in 2021: A narrative review. *Ibnosina Journal of Medicine and Biomedical Sciences, 14*, 050–067. https://www.semanticscholar.org/paper/55020fc679fb2ddc00581e7da055ffa768f66641 (accessed on 29th May 2025).

24. Karim, Z., Reese, R. A., Smith, A. N., Blackadar, M. E., Arora, V., Moore, N. M., & Johnson, E. A. (2024). Positive impact of nutrition in the prevention of peripheral vascular disease and severe acute respiratory syndrome coronavirus 2: Review. *Frontiers in Nutrition, 11*. https://www.semanticscholar.org/paper/52d2fdf6d1f8d7f127fde9c389b8e26fba80659f (accessed on 29th May 2025).

25. Keith, R. J., Fetterman, J. L., Orimoloye, O. A., Dardari, Z., Lorkiewicz, P., Hamburg, N. M., DeFilippis, A. P., et al. (2019). Characterization of volatile organic compound metabolites in cigarette smokers, electronic nicotine device users, dual users, and nonusers of tobacco. *Nicotine & Tobacco Research, 22*, 264–272. https://doi.org/10.1093/ntr/ntz021 (accessed on 29th May 2025).

26. King, J. B., Berchie, R. O., Derington, C., Marcum, Z., Scharfstein, D., Greene, T. H., Herrick, J. S., et al. (2023). New users of angiotensin II receptor blocker–versus angiotensin-converting enzyme inhibitor–based antihypertensive medication regimens and cardiovascular disease events: A secondary analysis of ACCORD-BP and SPRINT. *Journal of the American Heart Association: Cardiovascular and Cerebrovascular Disease, 12*. https://www.semanticscholar.org/paper/e67546c8e14f21402867372a9154e5a0107e5986 (accessed on 29th May 2025).

27. Kotlyarov, S., & Kotlyarova, A. (2022). The importance of the plasma membrane in atherogenesis. *Membranes, 12*. https://www.semanticscholar.org/paper/04c01796de90073e9ff1feda8d8e4ab48caba5b7 (accessed on 29th May 2025).

28. Krishnan, G., Tamkhade, J., Arul, K. V. P., Kandhari, H., Rathika, S., & Swarup, L. (2024). Hyperparameter optimization and its impact on machine learning performance for heart disease prediction. *2024 IEEE 4th International Conference on ICT in Business Industry & Government (ICTBIG)*. https://www.semanticscholar.org/paper/af6e9972806d3805f2f3bad68d1d55ce326fccca (accessed on 29th May 2025).

29. Kujawski, S., Cossington, J., Słomko, J., Zawadka-Kunikowska, M., Tafil-Klawe, M., Klawe, J., Buszko, K., et al. (2021). Relationship between cardiopulmonary, mitochondrial and autonomic nervous system function improvement after an individualized activity program upon chronic fatigue syndrome patients. *Journal of Clinical Medicine, 10*. https://www.semanticscholar.org/paper/7b997dd6ebf6eba32d33729c4d52e029f8a19d59 (accessed on 29th May 2025).

30. Li, J., Lin, M., Xie, Z., Chen, L., Qi, J., & Yu, B. (2024). Target cell extraction and spectrum–effect relationship coupled with BP neural network classification for screening potential bioactive components in ginseng extract with a protective effect against myocardial damage. *Molecules, 29*. https://www.semanticscholar.org/paper/97f5a5fb50146d59b34e9db0d02677b3ccf21b8c (accessed on 29th May 2025).

31. Liu, W., Zhang, G., Wu, J., Zhang, Y., Liu, J., Luo, H., & Shao, L. (2020). Insights into the angiogenic effects of nanomaterials: Mechanisms involved and potential applications. *Journal of Nanobiotechnology, 18*. https://doi.org/10.1186/s12951-019-0570-3 (accessed on 29th May 2025).

32. Locatelli, F., Fishbane, S., Block, G. A., & Macdougall, I. C. (2017). Targeting hypoxia-inducible factors for the treatment of anemia in chronic kidney disease patients. *American Journal of Nephrology, 45*, 187–199. https://doi.org/10.1159/000455166 (accessed on 29th May 2025).

33. Lu, P., Chan, M., Tsui, S., Shen, T. T., & Chang, J. C. (2025). Development of an anatomy-mimicking, wave transport-preserving mock circulation loop for evaluating pulsatile hemodynamics as supported by cardiovascular assist devices. *Cardiovascular Engineering and Technology*. https://www.semanticscholar.org/paper/828dfc4478d497f045198a1b0d0db681651ce8ec (accessed on 29th May 2025).

34. Mach, F., Baigent, C., Catapano, A. L., Koskinas, K. C., Casula, M., Badimón, L., Chapman, M. J., et al. (2019). 2019 ESC/EAS guidelines for the management of dyslipidemias: Lipid modification to reduce cardiovascular risk. *European Heart Journal, 41*, 111–188. https://doi.org/10.1093/eurheartj/ehz455 (accessed on 29th May 2025).

35. Mathieu, A. J. W., Pascual, M. S., Charlton, P. H., Volovaya, M., Venton, J., Aston, P., Nandi, M., et al. (2024). Advanced waveform analysis of the photoplethysmogram signal using complementary signal processing techniques for the extraction of biomarkers of cardiovascular function. *JRSM Cardiovascular Disease, 13*. https://www.semanticscholar.org/paper/7d3912d4912353c5297b1f4935ed8746aec7e78e (accessed on 29th May 2025).

36. Mirzahosseini, H. K., Esmaeili, M., & Mirakhorli, A. (2025). Factors affecting gut microbiota and its relationship with cardiovascular diseases: A narrative review. *Journal of Microbiota*. https://www.semanticscholar.org/paper/e962bf54b733d8dd2ed8ef7c92b64b848b99b1be (accessed on 29th May 2025).

37. Nordanstig, J., Behrendt, C. A., Baumgärtner, I., Belch, J. J. F., Bäck, M., Fitridge, R., Hinchliffe, R. J., et al. (2023). Editor's Choice — European Society for Vascular Surgery (ESVS) 2024 clinical practice guidelines on the management of asymptomatic lower limb peripheral arterial disease and intermittent claudication. *European Journal of Vascular and Endovascular Surgery, 67*, 9–96. https://doi.org/10.1016/j.ejvs.2023.08.067 (accessed on 29th May 2025).

38. Oki, S., Ohta, T., Shioi, G., Hatanaka, H., Ogasawara, O., Okuda, Y., Kawaji, H., et al. (2018). ChIP-Atlas: A data-mining suite powered by full integration of public ChIP-seq data. *EMBO Reports, 19*. https://doi.org/10.15252/embr.201846255 (accessed on 29th May 2025).

39. Praz, F., Muraru, D., Kreidel, F., Lurz, P., Hahn, R. T., Delgado, V., Senni, M., et al. (2021). Transcatheter treatment for tricuspid valve disease. *EuroIntervention, 17*, 791–808. https://doi.org/10.4244/eij-d-21-00695 (accessed on 29th May 2025).

40. Qureshi, M., & Alsarraj, M. B. (2020). Massive pulmonary embolism presents as a seizure – Role of PERT team & catheter directed thrombectomy. *Trauma and Emergency Care*. https://www.semanticscholar.org/paper/16dbbf7dbf616f8b3e1ff0dbe2acbed3567412f7 (accessed on 29th May 2025).

41. Rahaman, M. M., Hossain, R., Herrera-Bravo, J., Islam, M. T., Atolanı, O., Adeyemı, O. S., Owolodun, O. A., et al. (2023). Natural antioxidants from some fruits, seeds, foods, natural products, and associated health benefits: An update. *Food Science & Nutrition, 11*, 1657–1670. https://doi.org/10.1002/fsn3.3217 (accessed on 29th May 2025).

42. Riehl, L., Fürst, J., Kress, M., & Rykalo, N. (2024). The importance of the gut microbiome and its signals for a healthy nervous system and the multifaceted mechanisms of neuropsychiatric disorders. *Frontiers in Neuroscience, 17*. https://www.semanticscholar.org/paper/1fbed278467f04a103172a07840207b9049446d0 (accessed on 29th May 2025).

43. Roy, R. K., Yao, Y., Silver, R., & Stern, J. (2023). In vivo determination of direction of blood flow in the newly discovered SCN-OVLT vascular portal system in rat. *Physiology*. https://www.semanticscholar.org/paper/76577b7237c509d07013fb317b5e545d1de73bfd (accessed on 29th May 2025).

44. Skalidis, I., Müller, O., & Fournier, S. (2022). CardioVerse: The cardiovascular medicine in the era of Metaverse. *Trends in Cardiovascular Medicine, 33*, 471–476. https://doi.org/10.1016/j.tcm.2022.05.004 (accessed on 29th May 2025).

45. Sobhy, M., Eletriby, A., Ragy, H., Kandil, H., Saleh, M., Farag, N., Guindy, R., et al. (2024). ACE inhibitors and angiotensin receptor blockers for the primary and secondary prevention of cardiovascular outcomes: Recommendations from the 2024 Egyptian Cardiology Expert Consensus in collaboration with the CVREP Foundation. *Cardiology and Therapy, 13*, 707–736. https://www.semanticscholar.org/paper/30b3dbbdb4da5b6fd4fcdecb4c00ed4d186d0ffc (accessed on 29th May 2025).

46. Spoială, A., Ilie, C., Ficai, D., Ficai, A., & Andronescu, E. (2022). From biomedical applications of alginate towards CVD implications linked to COVID-19. *Pharmaceuticals, 15*. https://www.semanticscholar.org/paper/6e3b4826f635c9aeaf7c8a92d0434ae6357cffdf (accessed on 29th May 2025).

47. Sun, Y., Peng, Z., & Liang, H. (2025). Role of physical activity in cardiovascular disease prevention: Impact of epigenetic modifications. *Frontiers in Cardiovascular Medicine, 12*. https://www.semanticscholar.org/paper/d3019f25e622def13256c4e2ba1a9a0b6340477c (accessed on 29th May 2025).

48. Tan, B. Y.-Q., Chew, N., Lee, G. K. H., Jing, M., Goh, Y., Yeo, L. L. L., Zhang, K., et al. (2020). Psychological impact of the COVID-19 pandemic on health care workers in Singapore. *Annals of Internal Medicine, 173*, 317–320. https://doi.org/10.7326/m20-1083 (accessed on 29th May 2025).

49. The Writing Committee of the Report on Cardiovascular in China Sheng-Shou Hu. (2023). Report on cardiovascular health and diseases in China 2021: An updated summary. *Journal of Geriatric Cardiology: JGC, 20*(6), 399–430. https://www.semanticscholar.org/paper/b3da8bacf180f6e35d727cc389a5a67cf39fb90d (accessed on 29th May 2025).

50. Totoń-Żurańska, J., Mikolajczyk, T. P., Saju, B., & Guzik, T. J. (2024). Vascular remodeling in cardiovascular diseases: Hypertension, oxidation, and inflammation. *Clinical Science, 138*(13), 817–850. https://www.semanticscholar.org/paper/5d9381ccc05a2bc3d3eb01d2940964a6efb2d00e (accessed on 29th May 2025).

51. Usuda, H., Ikeda, H., Watanabe, S., Sato, S., Fee, E. L., Carter, S., Kumagai, Y., et al. (2023). Artificial placenta support of extremely preterm ovine fetuses at the border of viability for up to 336 hours with maintenance of systemic circulation but reduced somatic and organ growth. *Frontiers in Physiology, 14*. https://www.semanticscholar.org/paper/65765bed68af4cb03e29e06292803ad10ba0d9d4 (accessed on 29th May 2025).

52. Wang, M., Zhang, J., Yin, Z., Ding, W., Zhao, M., Liu, J., Xu, Y., et al. (2023). Microglia-mediated neuroimmune response regulates cardiac remodeling after myocardial infarction. *Journal of the American Heart Association: Cardiovascular and Cerebrovascular Disease, 12*. https://www.semanticscholar.org/paper/a51e64c4b63321ae953a196ba1df6702a21cc10e (accessed on 29th May 2025).

53. Whittle, R., Keller, N., Hall, E. A., Patanam, S., Dunbar, B. J., & Diaz-Artiles, A. (2024). Integrative cardiovascular dose-response to graded lower body negative pressure. *bioRxiv*. https://www.semanticscholar.org/paper/a9abdea3fba467474540198fae9439cb745615cf (accessed on 29th May 2025).

54. Wickramasinghe, S. C., Wickramasinghe, S. W. A. D. A., & Senaratne, P. A. S. (2024). Cardiovascular disease risk assessment by medical officers according to the guidelines at healthy lifestyle centers in Western and North Western Provinces and the factors affecting implementation of guidelines. *Sri Lankan Journal of Medical Administration*. https://www.semanticscholar.org/paper/7e771ff927b2c72d85c11057e4e8d51d6301d5c0 (accessed on 29th May 2025).

55. Zeppenfeld, K., Tfelt-Hansen, J., Riva, M., Winkel, B. G., Behr, E. R., Blom, N. A., Charron, P., et al. (2022). 2022 ESC guidelines for the management of patients with ventricular arrhythmias and the prevention of sudden cardiac death. *European Heart Journal, 43*, 3997–4126. https://doi.org/10.1093/eurheartj/ehac262 (accessed on 29th May 2025).

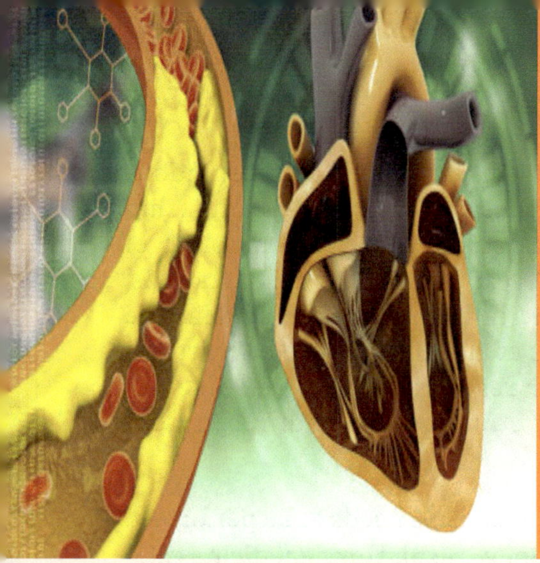

Chapter 2

MECHANISMS OF CARDIOVASCULAR PATHOPHYSIOLOGY

Contents

Introduction

It is essential to understand the pathophysiological mechanism of the cardiovascular system in an attempt to combat the growing incidence of cardiovascular disease (CVD) globally. CVD remains the leading cause of morbidity and mortality globally, with chronic inflammation as one of the most important modifiable risk factors. Recent research increasingly suggests that the innate immune system, particularly through components such as Toll-like receptors (TLRs), plays a pivotal part in mediating the inflammatory response that accompanies cardiovascular events. TLRs, being present in most immune and non-immune cells, recognize pathogens and self-derived molecules, triggering an inflammatory cytokine cascade that contributes to systemic inflammation and atherosclerosis (Simons et al., 2024). This multi-dimensional interaction means that cardiovascular health cannot fully be explained without considering the inflammatory processes that disrupt homeostasis and cause disease in vulnerable individuals. In addition, the sophistication of this association is additionally demarcated within specific patient populations, i.e., chronic obstructive pulmonary disease (COPD). Exacerbations of COPD dramatically augment cardiovascular event risk, bearing witness to a close relationship between respiratory and cardiovascular pathophysiology. Recent studies elucidate a series of interrelated processes by which acute exacerbations can initiate cardiovascular complications, including ventilation/perfusion mismatch and sustained systemic inflammation far beyond the respiratory manifestations of the acute event have resolved (Simons et al., 2024). These interactions not only emphasize the polyfactorial nature of the cardiovascular responses to lung disease but also serve to highlight the necessity of coordinated management strategies for both respiratory and cardiovascular health for improvement in patient outcomes.

Consequently, studying the cardiovascular pathophysiological mechanisms needs to be performed through a multidisciplinary approach, with input from immunology, respiratory medicine, and cardiovascular science. The interaction between TLR-induced inflammation and the progression of conditions like COPD needs to incorporate an improved understanding of these processes in sustaining enhanced cardiovascular risk. Evidence also suggests that preventive interventions targeting these inflammatory pathways could have significant therapeutic significance to the reduction of cardiovascular morbidity and mortality (Tabatabaei et al., 2024).

Further studies in outlining the temporal dynamics of pathophysiological states involved in exacerbations and their contribution to long-term cardiovascular health are still critical, paving the way for new treatment and management highlighting holistic patient care across various clinical settings (Figure 2.1).

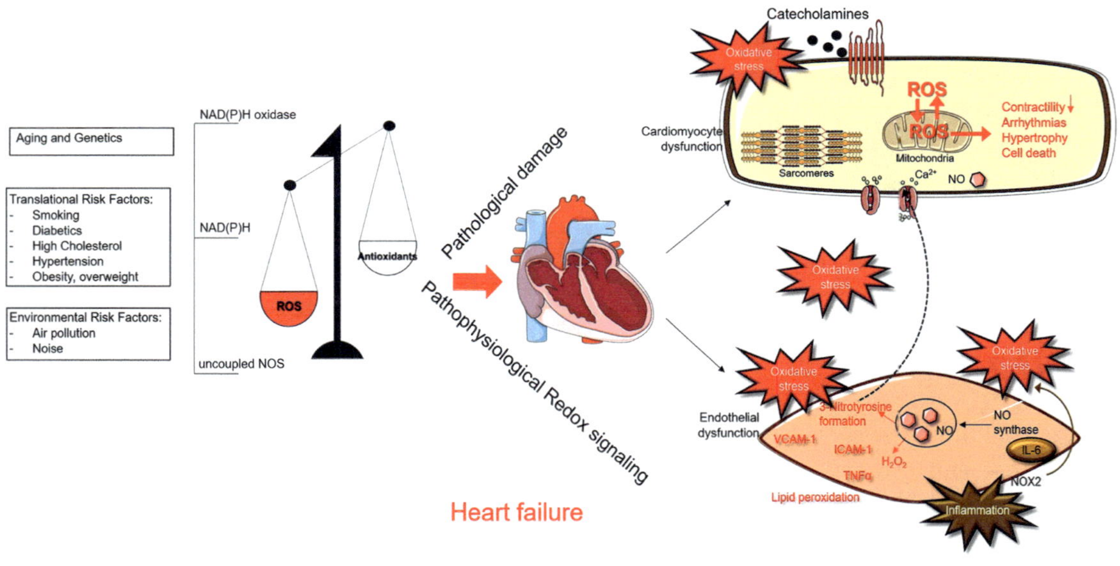

Figure 2.1. Mechanisms, sources, and implications of oxidative stress in cardiovascular disease and heart failure.

Source: https://media.springernature.com/full/springer-static/image/art%3A10.1007%2Fs12551-020-00742-0/MediaObjects/12551_2020_742_Fig1_HTML.png?as=webp.

Definition of Cardiovascular Pathophysiology

Cardiovascular pathophysiology is the complex biological and physiological mechanisms behind cardiovascular disease. It is inherently changes in cardiac and vascular function that evolve into disorders such as hypertension, heart failure, and atherosclerosis. These changes are typically founded on a multifaceted amalgamation of genetic predispositions, environmental exposures, and behaviors, leading to an individualized interaction that potentiates cardiovascular dysfunction. As an example, inflammatory processes and endothelial dysfunction usually play a crucial role in atherosclerosis. This arterial wall plaque leads to reduced blood flow and oxygen delivery to essential organs. With a cardiovascular pathophysiology framework, the scientists and clinicians comprehend the mechanisms and determine therapeutic targets that can arrest cardiovascular disease progression. In cardiovascular pathophysiology, statin effectiveness points to the multifactorial interaction that will define the outcome of therapy. While statins are powerful lipid- and cardiovascular event-rate reducers, they also come with adverse effects such as statin-associated muscle symptoms (SAMS). The development of SAMS underscores the multifactorial nature of responses to cardiovascular pharmacology, where precise pathophysiologic mechanisms are not well delineated. Understanding SAMS is significant not merely for effective management of those patients requiring cholesterol-lowering treatment but also for designating treatments taking into account side effects. Such a complication advocates the role of tailored interventions in cardiovascular treatment, following the assumption that cardiovascular pathophysiology is not a collection of azygous processes but an interactive play of elements that shape outcomes (Shah et al., 2024). The cardiogenic shock phenomenon is also a good example of critical aspects of cardiovascular pathophysiology and what it entails in terms of its effects on patient management and prognosis. Featuring as a profound reduction in cardiac output occasioned by some underlying factor or factors, cardiogenic shock poses serious challenges that significantly affect mortality rates regardless of advances in therapies offered by medicine. Inflammation and microvascular abnormalities are key issues in this condition, presenting the need for better diagnostic and therapeutic approaches. Increased understanding of these pathophysiological mechanisms may drive the creation of new interventions for improving survival following cardiogenic shock. This explains why an understanding of cardiovascular pathophysiology is worth knowing in developing successful interventions, since it is where clinical practice and improved patient care in cardiovascular medicine are derived (Krychtiuk et al., 2022).

2.1. Common Cardiovascular Diseases (CVDs)

The prevalence of common CVDs reflects a health crisis in populations across the globe. Coronary artery disease, hypertension, heart failure, and stroke comprise the leading causes of morbidity and mortality rates across the world. CAD, primarily due to atherosclerosis, is an example of arteries that deliver blood to the heart constricting and limiting blood circulation. This condition can lead to myocardial infarction, commonly known as a heart attack, thus the importance of early diagnosis and treatment. Hypertension, as characterized by chronically elevated arterial blood pressure, also significantly increases the risk of developing a variety of cardiovascular complications, including stroke and heart failure. It is thus essential to learn about the pathophysiology of these diseases since it plays a pivotal role in characterizing effective prevention and intervention measures. The intricate relationship between cardiovascular disease and oral health has been of more interest in recent years. The evidence has shown that oral infection, particularly periodontitis, is associated with endothelial dysfunction, a key feature in the pathogenesis of vascular and atherosclerosis disease. For instance, patients with denture stomatitis (DRS) have dramatic variability in endothelial function compared to healthy subjects who do not have this condition. This relationship illustrates ways in which systemic inflammatory processes can exacerbate cardiovascular threats and the way that oral health is a significant component of overall cardiovascular health. Risk factors such as diabetes and smoking increase not only the risk for developing DRS but also significantly magnify the risks of cardiovascular disease. Thus, the correlation of oral health with cardiovascular disease must be emphasized in preventive health care for better outcomes among patients and to reduce the impact of such diseases (Cześnikiewicz-Guzik et al., 2014). The ultimate control of hypertension is at the heart of decreasing the occurrence of cardiovascular disorders. Despite the improvement in antihypertensive treatment, optimal blood pressure control is still missing in the majority of patients. The traditional approach to the treatment of hypertension is a general, trial-and-error therapeutic strategy that ignores patient heterogeneity. Consequently, more emphasis on individualized medicine is revolutionizing how the condition is managed. By considering genetic predisposition, lifestyle factors, and patient-specific response to pharmacotherapy, healthcare providers can craft treatment strategies that are more effective and best tailored to patient needs. Discoveries in systems biology and integration of high-throughput technologies make this shift to personalized treatment possible, ultimately aiming to reduce the burden of cardiovascular disease from uncontrolled hypertension (Borghi et al., 2017). With these customized strategies, there are possibilities for significant reduction in cardiovascular morbidity and mortality, fostering public health initiatives (Figure 2.2).

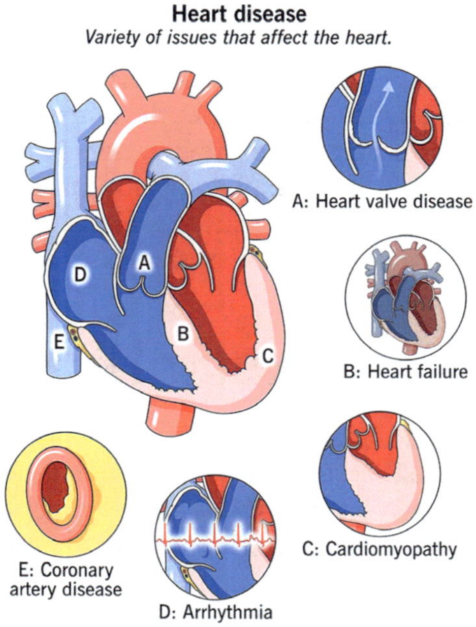

Figure 2.2. Heart disease has many types and can affect various parts of your heart.

Source: https://my.clevelandclinic.org/-/scassets/images/org/health/articles/24129-heart-disease-illustration.

2.1.1. Hypertension

Hypertension, or high blood pressure, is a significant public health issue that impacts millions of individuals worldwide. Hypertension relates to elevated arterial pressure and, if left untreated, can lead to serious health conditions like heart disease, stroke, and kidney disease. Hypertension is frequently not diagnosed because it does not come with noticeable symptoms and is therefore also referred to as the silent killer. Routine screening for blood pressure is essential for the detection of those who are at risk. Knowing the risk factors for hypertension, including obesity, physical inactivity, smoking, and heavy alcohol use, is essential in prevention. Furthermore, these risk factors may lead to conditions such as chronic kidney disease that further augment the cardiovascular burden, underlining the importance of comprehensive health surveys and treatments for controlling and restricting hypertension on a wide population basis. Hypertension must be controlled by a multi-faceted approach, including lifestyle modifications and, as an alternative, drug treatment.

The World Health Organizations (2020) also highlight the role of physical activity as one of the critical components in blood pressure control. The habitual engagement in moderate-intensity activity for at least 150 minutes weekly has been demonstrated to reduce blood pressure and promote cardiovascular well-being, valuing individualized health interventions. Apart from physical activity, lifestyle modifications such as reduction of sodium and consumption of a potassium-rich diet can contribute to successful hypertension management. Besides, nutrition for weight management is also crucial in the prevention and control of high blood pressure. Through embracing lifestyle adjustments and clinical intervention, patients have a better ability to control hypertension, thereby reducing the risk of ensuing cardiovascular complications, including occurrences that compromise renal functioning alongside overall wellbeing (Bull et al., 2020). The relationship between hypertension and chronic kidney disease is particularly significant, prompting concern from clinicians as well as policymakers. Evidence has confirmed that increased blood pressure produces kidney damage and a vicious cycle of ill health.

In 2017, a shocking percentage of cardiovascular disease and mortality could be related to impaired kidney function, with a significant percentage of these being due to hypertension (Bikbov et al., 2020). This association calls for holistic healthcare models addressing both the dual burden of hypertension and kidney disease. Increasing awareness of such comorbidities will facilitate preventive measures, which in turn will encourage individuals to practice proactive health habits. Proper communication of risk conditions and their health implications will help propel better health habits among populations, ultimately decreasing the incidence of hypertension as well as its corresponding complications through evidence-based and effective healthcare policies (Figure 2.3).

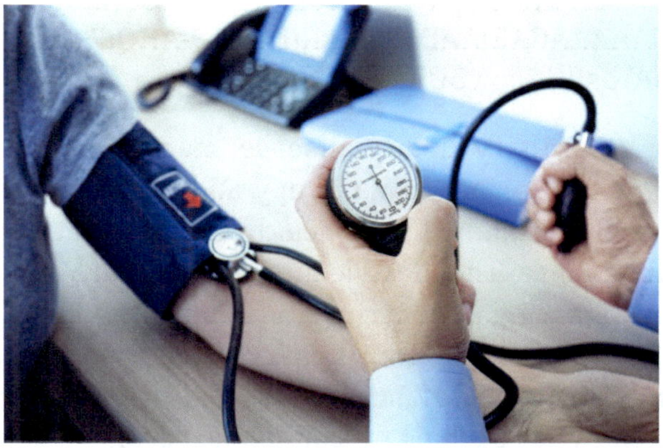

Figure 2.3. High blood pressure.

Source: https://www.bda.uk.com/static/fe771c94-80de-45bc-86457396ed810af3/BloodPressure.jpg.

2.1.2. Coronary Artery Disease (CAD)

CAD is a leading cause of significant health issues among cardiovascular diseases and accounts for a major proportion of morbidity and mortality worldwide. CAD is primarily characterized by constricting or obstruction of coronary arteries, most commonly by atherosclerosis, where fat material builds up in the artery walls. The illness decreases blood flow to the heart muscle, leading to ischemia, which is felt as chest pain or angina. Additionally, its most severe form can culminate in myocardial infarction (heart attack) due to complete occlusion of one of the coronary arteries. CAD prevalence is also influenced by an enormous pool of risk factors like age, hypertension, smoking, diabetes, and hyperlipidemia, highlighting the intricate interaction between susceptibility genes and lifestyle variables in the etiology of the disease (Nordanstig et al., 2023).

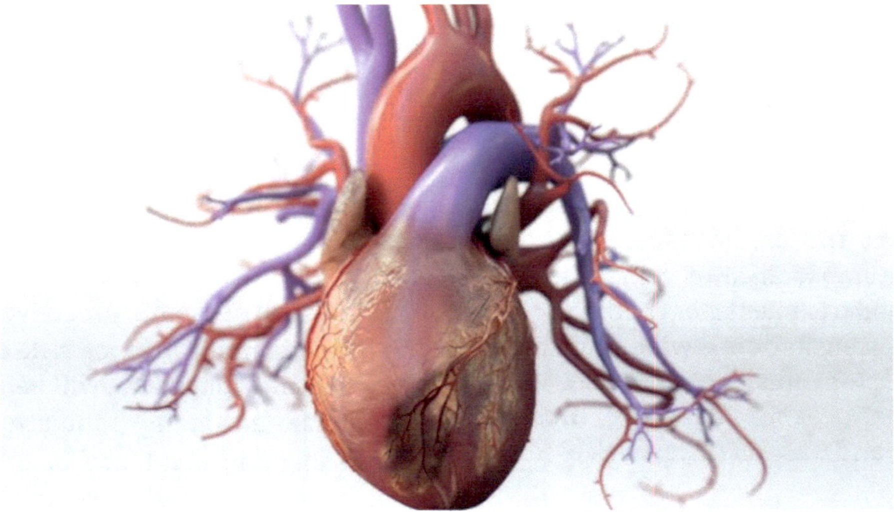

Figure 2.4. Coronary artery disease (CAD).

Source: https://i.ytimg.com/vi/flJsXOMhuK0/hq720.jpg?sqp=-oaymwE7CK4FEIIDSFryq4qpAy0IARUAAAAAGAElAADIQj0AgKJD8AEB-AHQCYAC0AWKAgwIABABGHIgPyhBMA8=&rs=AOn4CLD2ug58XpAYdsRGGfayy5UKkx7vUg.

Coronary artery disease management involves a multi-disciplinary strategy of lifestyle modification, medical therapy, and, in selected instances, surgical intervention. Primary prevention is simply attaining a heart-healthy lifestyle that encompasses exercise, dietary modification, and smoking abstinence. The lifestyle modifications are crucial not only in preventing CAD development but also in enhancing patients' overall health, particularly for those with existing conditions. Pharmacological therapies usually encompass the use of antiplatelet medications, statins, and antihypertensive drugs to manage symptoms and prevent disease progression. Advanced cases are handled with invasive techniques such as percutaneous coronary interventions (angioplasty) or CABG for re-establishing normal blood flow to the cardiac muscle (François Mach et al., 2019). Besides, the recent advances in the pathophysiology of coronary artery disease have further emphasized the role of targeted treatment modalities according to the individual needs of the patient. Recent studies have created a platform for the introduction of innovative therapeutic agents and interventions that enhance cardiovascular results. For instance, studies have elucidated the role of dual antiplatelet therapy in those with high risk after coronary intervention and thereby reduced the likelihood of further detrimental cardiovascular events. These are matched pairs with developments in imaging technologies, such as computed tomography angiography, providing enhanced diagnostic alternatives for early detection and intervention. Accompanying this are current clinical trials and updated clinical guidelines, such as the latter by the European Society of Cardiology, that increasingly fine-tune management approaches for CAD following the latest evidence-based practices (François Mach et al., 2019) (Figure 2.4).

2.1.3. Heart Failure (HF)

HF is a clinical syndrome with multiple facets in which the heart's inability to supply sufficient blood to meet the body's metabolic requirements leads to incapacitating illness. This incapacitating illness is most often produced by numerous underlying cardiovascular diseases, such as coronary artery disease and hypertension, and leads to structural and functional heart abnormalities. It may be classified into several phenotypes, most commonly based on left ventricular ejection fraction (LVEF), which is a measure of the percentage of blood that is pumped by each pump. Patients with heart failure with reduced ejection fraction (HFrEF) usually have a poorer prognosis than patients with heart failure with preserved ejection fraction (HFpEF), and hence the necessity for successful measures of control. It is essential to recognize the multifactorial origin of heart failures to plan targeted therapeutic interventions and improve patient outcomes. Pharmacological intervention in heart failure is essential, and various studies have highlighted the role of the renin–angiotensin–aldosterone system (RAAS) in this regard. Dysregulation of RAAS can go a long way in propelling hypertension, myocardial infarction, and ultimately heart failure, which highlights the need for adequate blood pressure control. Of all the different types of therapies, angiotensin-converting enzyme inhibitors (ACEis) and angiotensin receptor blockers (ARBs) have emerged as pillars in managing patients with heart failure. Evidences indicate that ACEis are particularly worthwhile, with superior protective effects compared to ARBs in reducing mortality and morbidity associated with heart failure and cardiovascular events. The choice of RAAS inhibitors is not only predicated upon their efficacy but also based on the general clinical presentation of patients, thereby personalizing therapies to individual requirements (Sobhy et al., 2024). The use of point-of-care (POC) heart failure platforms further complements heart failure management by enabling early diagnosis and personalized treatment strategies.

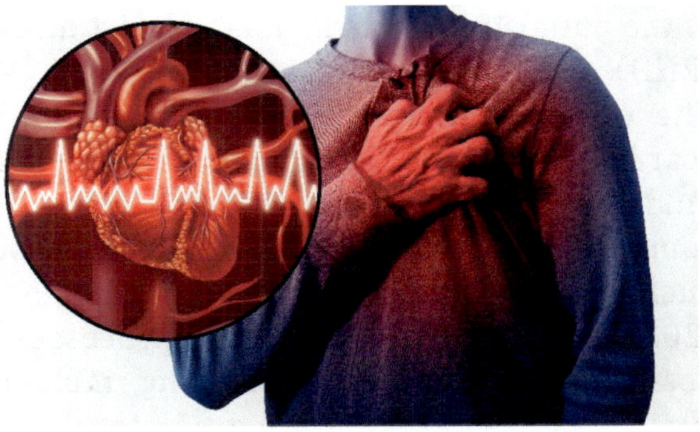

Figure 2.5. Heart Failure.

Source: https://hinduja-prod-assets.s3.ap-south-1.amazonaws.com/s3fs-public/2024-03/Heart%20Failure%20and%20Symptoms.jpg.

By using diagnostic algorithms and biomarker testing, these advanced technologies enable medical professionals to precisely assess risk, control comorbidities, and give prompt intervention. Furthermore, the use of POC designs to improve clinical outcomes is becoming more and more recommended by current standards, especially in the complex field of managing heart failure. Notwithstanding the difficulties in achieving widespread implementation of POC systems, including disparities in health care access and provider education, their possible value in maximizing clinical decision optimization must not be underestimated. Continuous investigation and strict scrutiny will be vital to confirm the effectiveness of POC heart failure platforms as a change agent in contemporary cardiovascular care (Berezin et al., 2022) (Figure 2.5).

2.2. Pathophysiological Mechanisms

Pathophysiological mechanisms underlying CVDs are often multifactorial, with a dynamic interaction between several biological pathways. Inflammatory responses and structural modification of heart valve tissues are central to the pathogenesis of rheumatic heart disease (RHD) and degenerative aortic stenosis (AS). The chronic inflammation of RHD leads to scarring and cardiac valve derangement, hindering regular blood flow and leading to compensatory hypertrophy of cardiac tissue. Such work, as delineated in Mutithu et al. (2024), aims to describe these processes in detail via comprehensive profiling, including clinical assessments, imaging, and molecular biomarkers. This multifactorial approach not only enhances our understanding of the disease but also enables us to formulate specific therapeutic interventions directed against specific pathophysiological changes seen in disease patients. Obstructive sleep apnea (OSA) offers another pathway through which cardiovascular pathophysiology is manifested, further blurring the cardiovascular disease (CVD) landscape. OSA is defined by recurrent upper airway collapses, leading to intermittent hypoxia and increased sympathetic drive. This resulting elevation in oxidative stress, chronic inflammation, and endothelial dysfunction creates a permissive environment for the development of hypertension, coronary artery disease, and other cardiovascular complications, as seen in Pisklak et al. (2024). The interplay between these factors results in the chronicity and advancement of cardiovascular diseases among the affected population. Explanation of these intersecting mechanisms not only sheds light on the secondary complications of OSA but also points to major areas for intervention, validating the necessity of management guidelines grounded in a holistic approach. Additionally, discovery and validation of new biomarkers are essential in progressing our understanding of cardiovascular pathophysiology. Biomarkers can potentially provide information about disease mechanisms, facilitate early detection, and guide therapy. The cited work in Mutithu et al. (2024) describes the use of multiparametric cardiovascular magnetic resonance (CMR) imaging and tissue analysis in the discovery of putative circulatory and tissue-specific biomarkers in individuals with RHD and AS. Its combination with high-throughput proteomic and metabolomic profiling has the potential to unravel specific pathophysiological pathways, enable phenotyping of CVDs, and guide personalized treatment paradigms. Ultimately, such advancements underscore the need to integrate new technologies into cardiovascular science, as they hold much potential for improving outcomes for patients and controlling disease progression effectively.

2.2.1. Inflammation and Its Role in Cardiovascular Disease (CVD)

Inflammation's key role in CVD needs to be understood to appreciate cardiovascular disease's pathophysiological mechanisms. Inflammation contributes predominantly to all forms of CVD by mechanisms involving endothelial dysfunction, atherosclerosis, and myocardial injury. The activation of the immune response in the vascular setting leads to leukocyte recruitment and the secretion of pro-inflammatory cytokines, such as IL-1β and IL-18, which lie at the core of the inflammatory cascade. This response creates a pathological setting conducive to plaque development and expansion in atherosclerosis and underscores the necessity of comprehending the mechanisms through which chronic inflammation exacerbates cardiovascular disease. As research continues to advance, greater emphasis has been placed on targeting the inflammation pathway to enhance CVD outcomes, highlighting that inflammation is a hallmark and therapeutic target for treatment of such diseases (Saadh et al., 2025). The NLRP3 inflammasome has emerged at the forefront of the inflammation-cardiovascular disease interaction. This poly-protein inflammasome complex responds to several stressors, such as ion fluxes and mitochondrial injury, triggering the activation of inflammatory pathways leading to elevated cardiovascular risk.

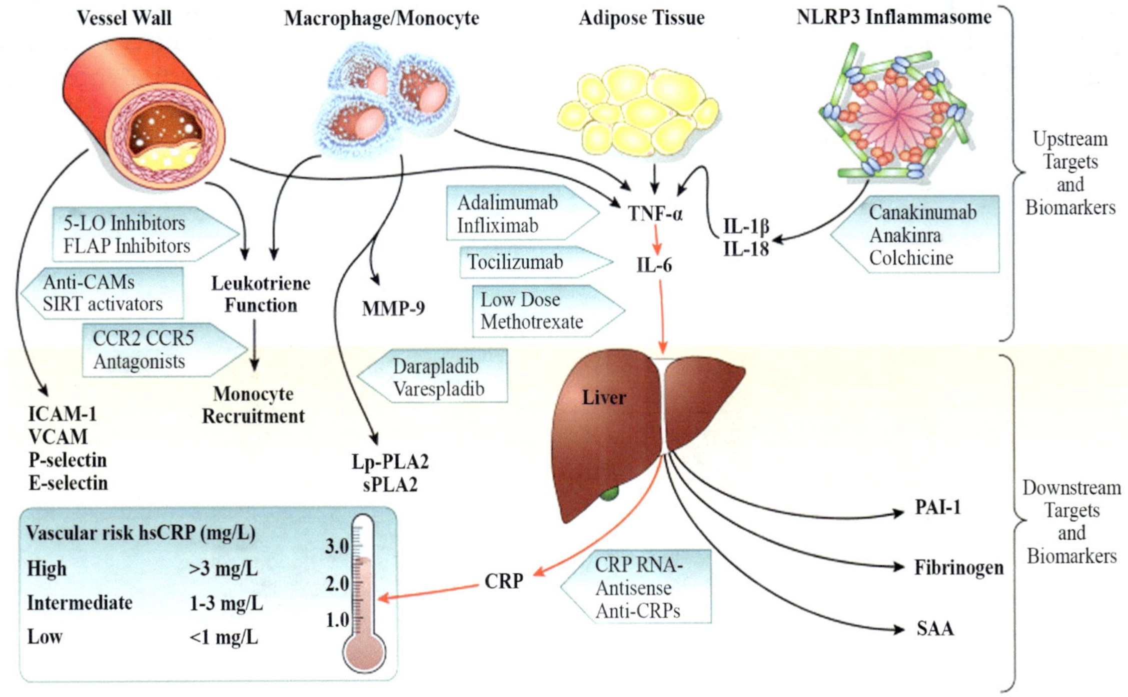

Figure 2.6. Inflammatory pathways as potential targets for atherosclerosis therapies.

Source: https://ijcscardiol.org/wp-content/uploads/2020/09/Visual-abstract_20200048.x61798.png.

By facilitating the production of IL-1β and other cytokines, NLRP3 is responsible for the inflammatory setting observed in hypertension and heart failure. The inflammation not only maintains endothelial dysfunction but also enhances vascular permeability, facilitating atherosclerotic plaque growth. With the therapeutic potential of NLRP3 as a drug target, research is now focused on small-molecule and biologic inhibitors that may demonstrate evidence against inflammation-induced damage in CVD. Thus, elucidating the mechanisms of NLRP3 may open up new possibilities for cardiovascular disease prevention (Saadh et al., 2025). The effects of inflammation also extend beyond atherosclerosis to reach across a wide spectrum of cardiovascular pathologies. A unifying understanding of the interface between inflammation and cardiovascular health guides preventive as well as therapeutic intervention. Importantly, long-term inflammation plays a role in acute cardiovascular disease, making novel research studies crucial to unravel the very molecular mechanisms involved. More contemporary data highlight the role of macrophages and other immune cells in augmenting plaque inflammation and atherosclerosis development, and provide new therapeutic options that potentially may stop these deleterious processes. Progress in the field also comes with the potential to develop anti-inflammatory strategies that target the mechanisms of cardiovascular disease, ultimately yielding benefits to the patient. Lastly, the research being conducted on inflammatory processes today has the potential to advance knowledge of CVD and facilitate the identification of beneficial therapeutic interventions in the future (Figure 2.6).

2.2.2. Endothelial Dysfunction

Endothelial dysfunction is a key mechanism in the pathophysiology of most cardiovascular diseases and a prelude to numerous disorders, including atherosclerosis and heart failure. Endothelium, a monolayer of cells that covers blood vessels, plays an essential role in vascular homeostasis. Its key function is the regulation of vascular tone through the release of nitric oxide (NO), which causes vasodilation. But whenever the endothelium ceases to function, this homeostatic control is lost, leading to a decrease in NO bioavailability.

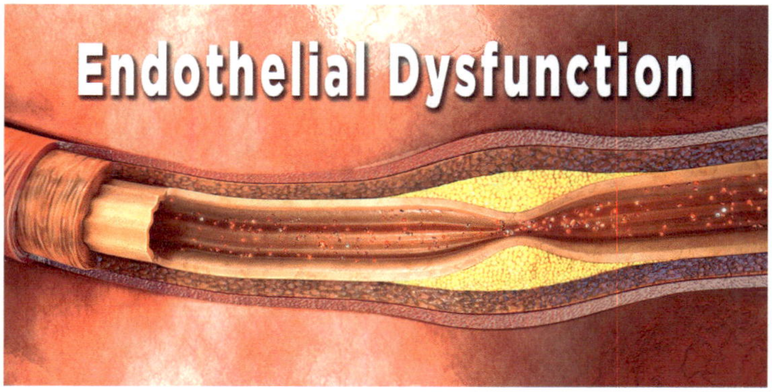

Figure 2.7. Endothelial dysfunction.

Source: https://www.optimaldx.com/hubfs/endothelial_dysfunction_1000x500.jpg.

Thus, this imbalance starts a cascade of events that increase oxidative stress and inflammation within the vessel wall. These reactions not only exacerbate endothelial dysfunction but also create a self-reinforcing process that facilitates the progression of cardiovascular diseases, thereby complicating patient outcomes (Higashi, 2022). The interconnectedness between endothelial dysfunction and diabetes has been the subject of considerable interest in recent research, particularly in terms of diabetic cardiomyopathy (DCM) pathogenesis. Diabetes mellitus induces barrier dysfunction in the endothelium by hyperglycemia and insulin resistance, resulting in enhanced generation of reactive oxygen species (ROS). The dysfunction creates a pro-inflammatory environment responsible for myocardial injury in an ischemia injury-independent fashion. Notably, the structural and functional cardiomyopathy of the heart in DCM can manifest as stiffness and fibrosis, which will eventually become diastolic and systolic dysfunction. Hence, endothelial dysfunction is not just an aftereffect but also an essential player in the pathologic process of cardiac complications of diabetes, a fact that highlights drug treatment aimed at endothelial recovery as a proper practice (Wang et al., 2022). Furthermore, clinical treatments aiming to reverse the effects of endothelial dysfunction remain inadequate despite their pivotal role in cardiovascular pathophysiology. Traditional management is more in favor of controlling risk factors such as hypertension and hyperlipidemia without direct interference with endothelial status. More recent drugs for endothelial function facilitation, such as the reversal of oxidative stress with antioxidants, are encouraging but require in-depth studies to determine their effectiveness. Besides, understanding the interlinked interaction between endothelial dysfunction, inflammation, and cardiovascular events will mean novel therapeutic regimens that not just recover endothelial function but also arrest the progression of cardiovascular disease. Clarification of the mechanisms causing endothelial dysfunction can help in the improvement of interventions capable of revolutionizing the management of patients with cardiovascular risk (Higashi, 2022; Wang et al., 2022) (Figure 2.7).

2.2.3. Neurohormonal Activation

The neurohormonal activation hypothesis is at the core of cardiovascular pathophysiology mechanisms. The phenomenon has been termed a dynamic interaction of neural and hormonal mechanisms that respond to physiological stressors such as hypertension and heart failure. Neurohormonal pathways, including the sympathetic nervous system and the RAAS, are activated by hemodynamic instability or tissue injury to produce augmentation of norepinephrine and angiotensin II. These neurohormonal substances act to oppose threatened cardiac function with vasoconstriction, renal sodium retention, and increased cardiac contractility. However, while initially compensatory, prolonged activation of the neurohormonal systems can result in maladaptive sequelae, including cardiac fibrosis and remodeling, which may exacerbate heart failure and establish a cascade of additional cardiovascular deterioration. Activation of the neurohormonal pathways is most striking in conditions such as hypertension and obesity, both of which are leading major etiologies of cardiovascular disease. In hypertension, chronic stress associated with increased vascular resistance triggers neurohormonal remodeling leading to cardiac hypertrophy and renal damage. Two types of fibrosis associated with neurohormonal activation have been newly defined: replacement and reactive fibrosis. Replacement fibrosis is a response to tissue damage, but reactive fibrosis occurs due to chronic mechanical and neurohormonal stress.

This identification is necessary because it demonstrates that, although these adaptive responses work to benefit healing, they are detrimental when stressors are chronic. Myofibroblasts, a type of activated fibroblasts, gain contractile functions that further complicate tissue restructuring in hypertensive states, which necessitates targeted intervention in attenuating this maladaptive response (Torimoto et al., 2024). Obesity also raises another dimension along which neurohormonal activation encroaches into cardiovascular health, particularly in the case of HFpEF.

Obese patients exhibit unique phenotypes with abnormal diastolic dysfunction and elevated left ventricular filling pressures. This is partially due to mechanisms at the level of the neurohormones that lead to fluid retention and enhancement of pre-load, contributing to the cardiac load. Further, interaction between neurohormonal stimulation and obesity results in increased sympathetic nervous activity and an increase in circulating hormones, leading to increased cardiac remodeling and dysfunction. As more than 80% of HFpEF patients are either overweight or obese, there is a need to unravel such neurohormonal interactions for the design of effective treatment strategies directed towards this group of patients. Further investigation is needed elucidate the precise mechanisms involved in the interaction between obesity, activation of neurohormones, and the pathophysiology of cardiovascular disease (Lee, 2022) (Figure 2.8).

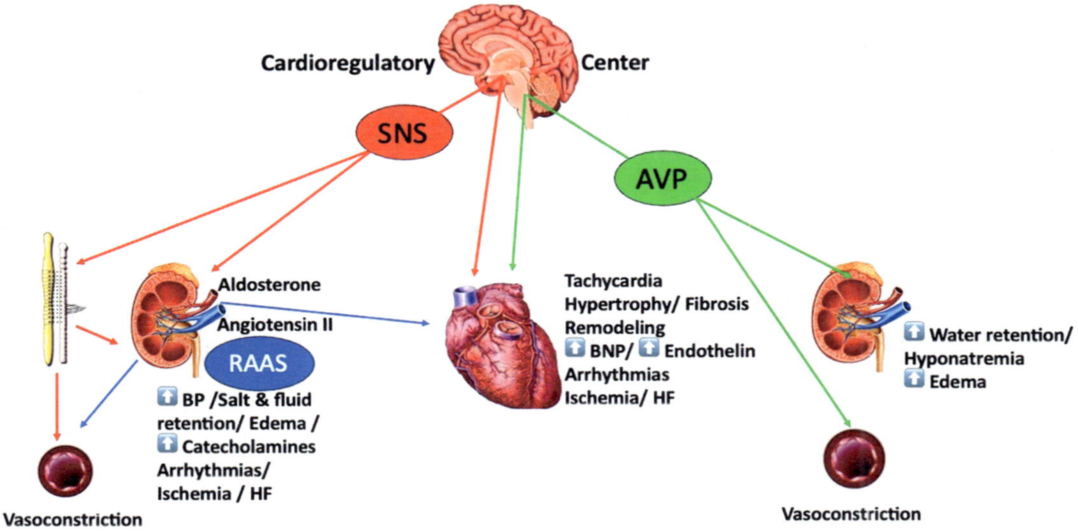

Figure 2.8. Neurohumoral activation in heart failure (HF).

Source: https://pub.mdpi-res.com/ijms/ijms-24-15472/article_deploy/html/images/ijms-24-15472-ag.png?1699350055.

2.3. Risk Factors for Cardiovascular Disease (CVD)

CVD constitutes a broad category of disorders, the majority of which are multifactorial in origin and may either be modifiable or non-modifiable. Amongst the most crucial modifiable factors is hypertension. The term "hypertensive disorders of pregnancy" (HDP) specifically highlights a salient complication occurring in many pregnant women. HDP-exposed females have increased long-term hazards of cardiovascular disease irrespective of traditional criteria such as age and family history. Despite the risks having been identified, the United States has seen minimal change in its protocols for treating HDP over the years. The absence of revolution in the way HDP treatment is done raises questions regarding the advantages of having standardized treatment for the women diagnosed with HDP, especially considering that the long-term effects of this condition have on the health of the mother and the fetus (Garovic et al., 2021). Elevated lipoprotein(a), which is known to play a separate role in the pathophysiology of cardiovascular disease, is another very significant risk factor to take into account. Lp(a) is an atherogenic lipoprotein whose architecture and genetic variability determine its role in cardiovascular processes. Elevated levels of Lp(a) are associated with increased atherogenesis, inflammation, and thrombosis and represent an independent and causal risk factor for atherosclerotic cardiovascular disease. Notably, Lp(a) is also under substantial genetic control, and thus the disparity seen between populations is not unexpected. Besides efficient control of other lipid conditions like low-density lipoprotein cholesterol, elevated

Lp(a) has been a challenging condition to treat due to the lack of uniform diagnostic criteria and treatment protocols (Reyes-Soffer et al., 2021). This necessitates further studies to comprehend better the genetic and biological determinants involved in contributing to cardiovascular disease risk with Lp(a). The interplay of genetic and lifestyle factors adds to the complexity of risk factors in cardiovascular disease. For instance, individuals with genetic predispositions can be augmented by inappropriate lifestyle practices, e.g., bad diet, physical inactivity, and smoking, that can increase underlying risk factors, e.g., hypertension and dyslipidemia. The additive effect of these modifiable risk factors can significantly enhance the risk of developing cardiovascular diseases. Moreover, attention must be directed towards addressing socioeconomic and racial disparities that could impact access to healthcare and the management of these risks. Understanding the implications of these factors is vital in designing effective public health interventions that will respond to the burden of cardiovascular disease among population groups. Recognition of these layers does not simply contribute to our knowledge of cardiovascular pathophysiology but also facilitates the design of targeted interventions for high-risk individuals (Figure 2.9).

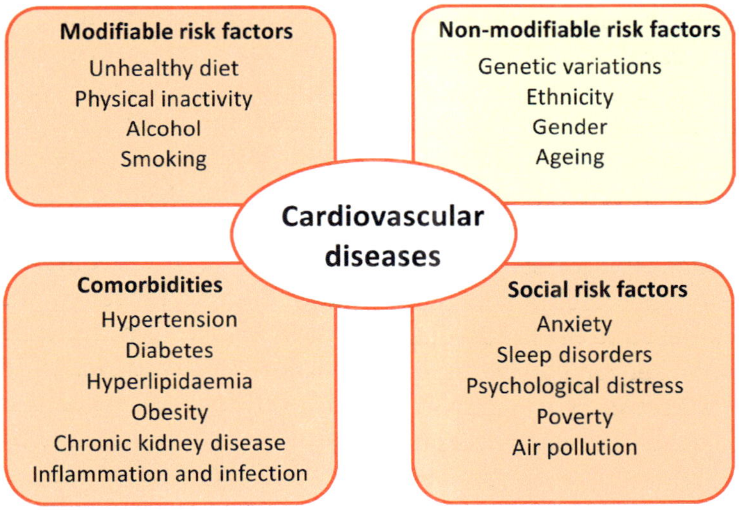

Figure 2.9. Main risk factors for cardiovascular diseases (CVDs).

Source: https://www.mdpi.com/biomolecules/biomolecules-14-01032/article_deploy/html/images/biomolecules-14-01032-g001.png.

2.3.1. Modifiable Risk Factors

Understanding cardiovascular pathophysiology mechanisms is highly reliant on the investigation of modifiable risk factors. The latter includes hypertension, diabetes, smoking, and dyslipidemia, and they have profound cardiovascular impacts. Of all the factors mentioned, hypertension is the most modifiable risk factor with the highest rate of cardiovascular mortality in the world. Interestingly, men and women are affected by hypertension differently. Women, by the way, may be at higher cardiovascular risk at lower blood pressure levels than men, and therefore must adopt personalized management. Mechanistic treatment protocols have been found to overlook such differences, highlighting the shortcomings in current clinical practice that overlook sex differences in hypertension pathophysiology (Lazaridis et al., 2025). Erasure of these differences is at the core of designing successful interventions and optimizing therapeutic response between the genders, and therefore in reducing the incidence of cardiovascular disease and also in augmenting population health. In light of interactions among modifiable risk factors, they can be viewed to play a crucial role in precipitating and promoting atherosclerotic cardiovascular diseases. It has been established through studies that traditional modifiable cardiovascular risk factors (SMuRFs) are inversely related to acute myocardial infarction (MI) in the sense that their presence aggravates the severity of the disease. But when patients have acute MI but no risk factor, some interesting findings have been noted, which point towards the fact that the effect of modifiable factors on cardiovascular events is not linear but complex (Saito et al., 2024). These events stimulate additional investigation into underlying mechanisms, and hypotheses are formed regarding potential genetic, environmental, or psychosocial determinants that potentially counteract typical risk profiles. In-depth examination of these cases is essential in optimizing risk assessment and cardiovascular occurrence prevention. Moreover, correction of reversible risk factors is necessary not only for the prevention of first cardiovascular events but also for secondary prevention in compromised status. Therapeutic interventions against SMuRFs can potentially decrease recurrent myocardial infarction risk significantly and offer health systems an essential potential to enhance patient outcomes. However, the literature has validated that the efficacy of such interventions will also be subject to certain aspects like sex, age, and comorbidities. Women, for example, typically struggle with blood pressure control and experience differential drug-related side effects compared to men, hence finding it hard to follow and manage treatment (Lazaridis et al., 2025). This necessitates the application of personalized medicine in cardiovascular therapy, where practitioners are forced to consider each patient's profile in order to maximize the effectiveness of treatment. In managing modifiable risk factors using a targeted strategy, healthcare providers can significantly influence the long-term health trajectories of patients with an increased risk of developing cardiovascular diseases.

2.3.2. Non-Modifiable Risk Factors

The pathophysiology of cardiovascular disease indicates that non-modifiable risk factors play a critical role in defining an individual's risk of developing cardiovascular diseases. Age is a topmost non-modifiable risk factor; the higher the age, the greater the risk of developing various heart conditions, including heart attacks and strokes. This augmented risk is a consequence of the additive effect of environmental and lifestyle exposures over many years, as well as to age-related intrinsic changes. Vascular elasticity declines and augmented arterial stiffness with aging account for the development of hypertension, which is an established precursor of cardiovascular events. Genetic predispositions may also enhance an individual's risk, with some inherited conditions causing early-onset cardiovascular diseases. An understanding of the influences of age and genetic factors on cardiovascular health is relevant since it forms the basis of disease mechanisms and highlights the need for specific prevention strategies in those groups at risk. Race and ethnicity are another crucial non-modifiable risk factor, wherein they can lead to both prevalence and types of cardiovascular diseases observed within groups. Certain racial groups have been discovered to have higher levels of hypertension and its related cardiovascular conditions. An example is that African Americans are more likely to suffer from hypertension as well as its secondary cardiovascular conditions, including heart disease and stroke. Lifestyle factors alone cannot explain this discrepancy; rather, a mix of environmental, socioeconomic, and genetic factors must be considered. Furthermore, the current study also reveals that such racial differences in cardiovascular health may be due to different responses in the cardiovascular system to stressors and varying inflammatory biomarkers. The understanding of the racial and ethnic variations in cardiovascular health is crucial to formulate efficient public health interventions that consider these unique vulnerabilities and the related mechanistic pathways. Finally, although lifestyle changes can profoundly influence the risk of cardiovascular diseases, the existence of some genetic or congenital factors cannot be altered and are therefore still essential areas of consideration. Diseases like familial hypercholesterolemia reflect the influence of non-modifiable risk factors on cardiovascular health.

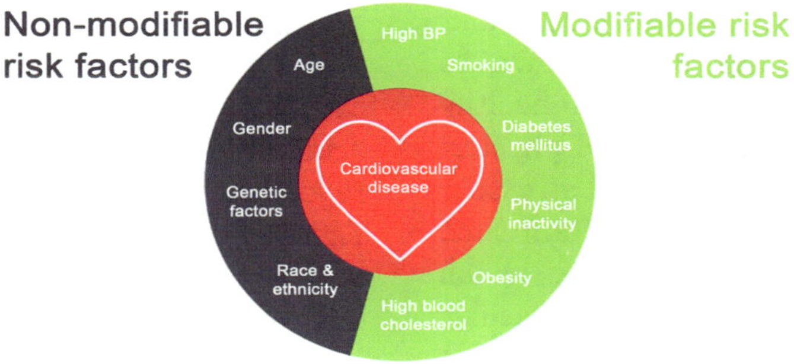

Figure 2.10. Modifiable and non-modifiable risk factors of cardiovascular disease.

Source: https://www.researchgate.net/profile/Arun-Kumar-495/publication/330099579/figure/fig1/AS:710797210681345@1546478669785/Risk-factors-of-cardiovascular-disease.png.

People who are born with a genetic disorder of this condition are at increased risk of high cholesterol levels, and this makes them susceptible to premature cardiovascular events regardless of any lifestyle modifications. Moreover, non-modifiable risk factors are also responsible for developing other complications such as coronary artery disease. Understanding the mechanisms by which such genetic predispositions operate accounts for the pathophysiological mechanisms in cardiovascular diseases. Heightening awareness of these immutables as risk factors can enable medical practitioners to implement more effective intervention and screening tactics, focusing, ultimately, on cardiovascular risk management in population groups that are significantly impacted by such immutables, as highlighted by recent findings of molecular underpinnings of the risks as mentioned earlier (Breijyeh et al., 2020; Alkahtani, 2022) (Figure 2.10).

2.3.3. Socioeconomic Influences on Cardiovascular Health

Socioeconomic status (SES) profoundly influences cardiovascular well-being through various mechanisms that are interrelated with access to health care, education, and lifestyle. Individuals of lower SES face constraints, including restricted access to preventive care and inadequate financial means to sustain a healthy lifestyle. This inequality generates a situation where the prevalence rate of hypertension and related cardiovascular diseases is disproportionately increased. For instance, as implied by existing evidence, the connection between socioeconomic deprivation and hypertension is articulated through compromised health habits and low risk factor awareness. Furthermore, SES not only defines the quantity of care consumed but also the quality, with those in lower economic statuses potentially being offered healthcare systems that are ineffective in delivering aid for chronic care like hypertension (Connelly et al., 2022). These disparities must be addressed to regulate cardiovascular disease in different population groups. Psychosocial determinants, including stress and social support further complicate the linkage between socioeconomic status and cardiovascular health. These patients can experience high levels of stress related to financial insecurity, job loss, and social isolation, all of which can be detrimental to cardiovascular health. Chronic stress has been shown to heighten blood pressure and induce unhealthy lifestyle habits such as poor diet and physical inactivity. Moreover, the psychosocial stressors associated with lower SES will maintain such chronic diseases as obesity and diabetes, which are notorious risk predictors of cardiovascular disease. It is evidenced that socioeconomic adversity might exacerbate these illnesses, prevalence, and severity (Rivera-Mancilla et al., 2021). Therefore, an integrated synthesis of the psychosocial determinants of SES is critical to developing effective interventions for the determinants of cardiovascular risk. Addressing the socioeconomic determinants of cardiovascular health necessitates a multi-level approach that goes beyond treatment in the medical setting to include community and public health. Improving health education and ensuring equitable access to resources can help enable individuals in lower SES groups to make informed health choices. Public health interventions encouraging nutrition and physical exercise are essential in bridging the gap in cardiovascular disease incidence. In addition, policymakers must prioritize structural change in order to reduce barriers to healthcare accessibility such that everyone can manage risk factors. By adopting a comprehensive approach that integrates socioeconomic factors into cardiovascular health strategies, it is possible to mitigate the disparities in cardiovascular disease outcomes, thereby improving public well-being (Rivera-Mancilla et al., 2021; Connelly et al., 2022;).

2.4. Diagnostic Approaches

The diagnostic methods for cardiovascular pathophysiology have undergone significant transformations, utilizing the finest of technological advances for better identification and characterization of cardiac ailments. The groundbreaking advances in non-invasive imaging modalities like echocardiography and cardiac MRI have been an immense gift in bringing valuable information to the clinician regarding cardiac structure and function. These imaging modalities allow visualization of cardiac chamber, valve, and adjacent arterial bed pathology, allowing early diagnosis of cardiovascular disease. In addition, the presence of biomarker analysis maximally enhances diagnostics as it provides analysis of specific cardiac injury or stress. For example, biomarkers such as troponins and natriuretic peptides are crucial in diagnosing myocardial infarction and heart failure. Ongoing evolution of these diagnostic instruments allows for the ability to acquire more cardiovascular health knowledge and thus enhances patient management techniques. Beyond traditional imaging and biomarker approaches, there is a growing recognition of the significance of microvascular dysfunction in cardiovascular disease. Existing research underscores the significance of assessing microvascular function within the larger context of cardiovascular disease pathology. Diagnostic procedures to identify microvascular dysfunction, such as skin perfusion testing and advanced echocardiographic methods, are being developed and standardized to enhance diagnostic sensitivity. As noted in recent reports, microvascular detection imaging appears to uncover early signs of cardiovascular injury commonly not detected using conventional imaging. These advancements raise the significance of adding microvascular tests to standard diagnosis protocols and thereby filling an essential mechanistic gap in cardiovascular pathophysiology knowledge. Such integration can finally enable identification of at-risk populations and inform targeted intervention policy (Masi et al., 2020). Furthermore, use of uniform guideline models in cardiovascular diagnosis enables evidence-based and standardized patient therapy. The ESC and EAS guidelines offer integrated advice for prevention, diagnosis, and treatment approaches in cardiovascular medicine. While these guidelines guide clinical practices, they also acknowledge the ever-changing nature of cardiovascular disease and the obligation that clinicians should use judgment in test interpretation. This tension between conforming to guidelines and adapting tests to specific patient situations is vital to maximizing outcomes in cardiovascular practice. As the scientific world continues to develop new diagnostic devices and refine existing modalities, the use of these guidelines will continue to stand at the forefront of enhancing the diagnostic framework of cardiovascular disease, ultimately leading towards the implementation of timely and effective interventions (Mach et al., 2019) (Figure 2.11).

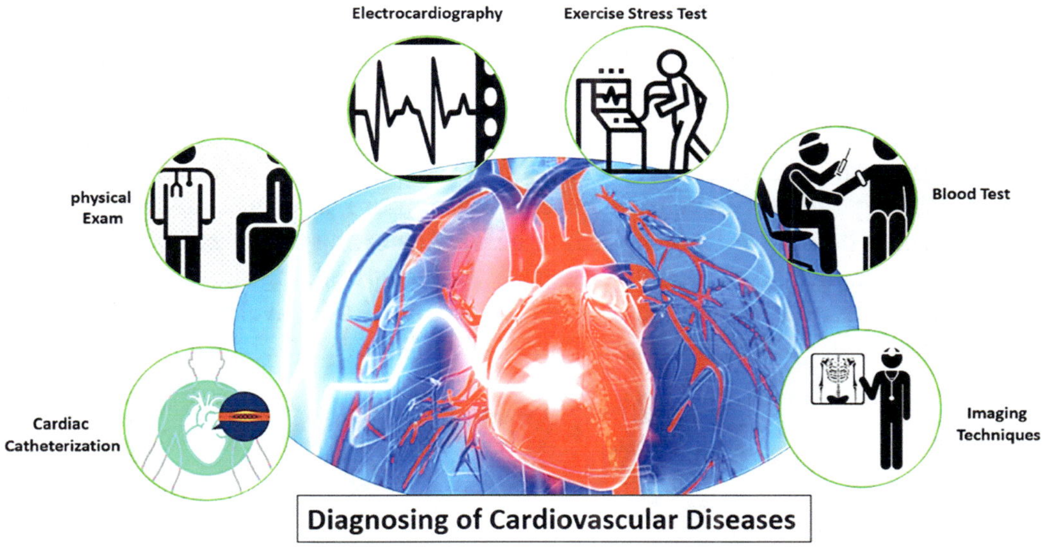

Figure 2.11. Current diagnosis techniques for Cardiovascular diseases (CVDs).

Source: https://www.mdpi.com/chemosensors/chemosensors-09-00067/article_deploy/html/images/chemosensors-09-00067-g002.png.

2.4.1. Imaging Techniques (e.g., Echocardiography (ECG), MRI)

Imaging modalities play a vital role in the understanding of the pathophysiological mechanisms of the cardiovascular system, where cardiac structural and functional derangement is under scrutiny. Of all the numerous modalities available, echocardiography stands out with its non-invasive and multi-modality features. The technique uses ultrasound waves to produce real-time images of the heart and allow assessment of chamber size, wall motion, and valvular mechanism. Such careful evaluations are essential in diagnosing conditions like cardiomyopathy, valvular heart disease, and heart failure. Doppler examination ability further augments echocardiography, enabling clinicians to study patterns of blood flow and detect intracardiac pressure gradients. Overall, echocardiography is a cornerstone in cardiovascular disease diagnostic strategy and is useful in therapeutic decision-making and monitoring disease progression based on the changing pathophysiology of cardiovascular mechanisms. Magnetic resonance imaging (MRI) is an advanced imaging technique that offers panoramic views of the structure and function of the heart and is particularly useful in patients with complex cardiovascular disease. In contrast to echocardiography, MRI employs magnetic fields and radio waves to generate high-quality images, and it is simple to evaluate myocardial infarction, ischemia, and tissue characterization, which are essential in cardiovascular pathophysiology. MRI's capacity to provide information about cardiac function and viability has transformed the way clinicians approach treatment strategies, especially concerning arrhythmias and myocardial diseases. Furthermore, the integration of functional imaging, including late gadolinium enhancement, allows for the detection of areas of scar tissue and fibrosis that are critical in assessing the overall health of the myocardium. Such advanced imaging information provides valuable information, enhancing clinical information and improving patient treatment plans for cardiovascular disease. The advent of advanced imaging technology continues to drive our knowledge of the pathophysiology of the cardiovascular system, validating the usefulness of various approaches in practice. The evolving imaging environment complements traditional techniques, combining data from echocardiography and MRI into established methods such as cardiac computed tomography (CT) and nuclear imaging. This multi-dimensional approach encourages an entire-person image of cardiovascular disease to enable early diagnosis and customized treatment algorithms. With integration of information from heterogeneous imaging modalities, clinicians can make more informed decisions about patient care, particularly when dealing with complicated cases. According to the 2022 ESC/ERS guidelines, such comprehensive diagnostic strategies are required for optimizing therapeutic management so that clinicians may make evidence-based choices based on the best available current and complete information (Glikson et al., 2021; Humbert et al., 2022) (Figure 2.12).

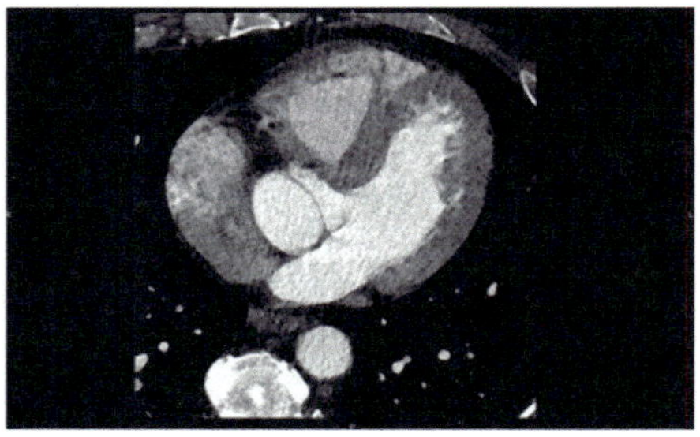

Figure 2.12. Computed tomography (CT) image of the left and right ventricle, left atrium, and ascending aorta.

Source: https://www.mdpi.com/applsci/applsci-11-10549/article_deploy/html/images/applsci-11-10549-g011.png.

2.4.2. Biomarkers In Cardiovascular Disease (CVD)

The study of biomarkers in CVD is at the heart of the unraveling of the mechanisms of pathophysiologic processes of cardiovascular disease. Biomarkers are indicators of physiological functions and can serve as a means to understand the onset and progression of CVDs. Particularly, metabolomic study has become important in the identification of numerous metabolites that represent metabolic perturbations associated with diseases like type 2 diabetes, which is usually co-morbid with

CVD. Current findings in this field are the key to the biological complexity underlying both CVD and type 2 diabetes, revealing various metabolic pathways influencing disease risk and development. By integrating metabolomic data with clinical practice, doctors can enhance the patient's diagnosis and prognosis, paving the way for personalized therapy that considers the individual metabolic signatures of the patients with these related disorders (Silva et al., 2025). Cardiovascular biomarkers can also be categorized based on their specific function in diagnosis or CVD monitoring. For instance, enzyme markers such as cardiac troponins and creatine kinase MB (CK-MB) are critical in myocardial damage detection in acute coronary syndromes. The best marker for identifying myocardial infarction is cardiac troponins, which stand out among the others due to their high specificity and sensitivity. Apart from the conventional enzyme indicators, protein markers such as myeloperoxidase (MPO) and C-reactive protein (CRP) offer crucial information on oxidative stress and inflammation, two factors that are essential in the pathogenesis of atherosclerosis. These biomarkers are not only helpful for short-term clinical decision-making but also for long-term risk stratification and planning of disease management for cardiovascular patients (Netala et al., 2025). The recent research into novel biomarkers is further developing our understanding of CVD, calling for a multidisciplinary approach to the diagnosis of cardiovascular disease. Pioneering biomarkers, such as microRNAs and long non-coding RNAs, are the pathfinders in this respect, offering sensitive markers for early diagnosis and risk stratification of CVD. Such next-generation biomarkers are promising to enhance diagnostic capability and facilitate the design of targeted therapies to alter pathological processes in CVD. In addition, the inclusion of lipid markers and inflammatory markers allows for comprehensive information to be gathered about the interaction between lipid metabolism, chronic inflammation, and cardiovascular health, thus improving our knowledge of the complex process of cardiovascular pathophysiology. The dynamic aspect of biomarker research highlights its significant role in the development of personalized medicine and improved patient outcomes in cardiovascular management (Netala et al., 2025).

2.4.3. Functional Tests (e.g., Stress Testing)

Functional testing, in the form of exercise stress testing, is an important component of evaluating cardiovascular health and making diagnoses for its related conditions. They quantify the physiological responses of the cardiovascular system under exertion, providing valuable information about cardiac function, exercise capacity, and potential ischemic states. By increasing the work of the heart, clinicians can monitor parameters such as heart rate, blood pressure, and electrocardiogram changes that serve as markers to identify non-apparent abnormalities at rest. Stress testing is beneficial in diagnosing CAD in patients who may be presenting with unusual symptoms or those who are asymptomatic. The ability to reproduce actual circumstances in controlled surroundings inspires the reliability of functional testing in everyday clinical settings because not only do they evaluate the cardiovascular response, they also record the systemic effect of effort on overall bodily health. Furthermore, functional testing in the form of stress testing is highly significant in guiding treatment regimens and rehabilitation in patients presenting with intrinsic cardiovascular disorders. Clinicians can create an exercise regimen that is customized for each patient based on their individual risk profile and current level of fitness according to the information obtained from these tests. For instance, after assessing the performance of a patient on stress testing, doctors are in a position to adjust medications, balance surgery, or prescribe lifestyle changes. The findings are of key relevance to disease treatment in conditions such as heart failure or after a myocardial infarction, where exercise prescription has a crucial role to play in functional status and quality of life. The approach aligns with modern patient-centric models of care that focus on tailored treatment approaches based on specific physiological responses induced in functional testing (Cheng et al., 2021).

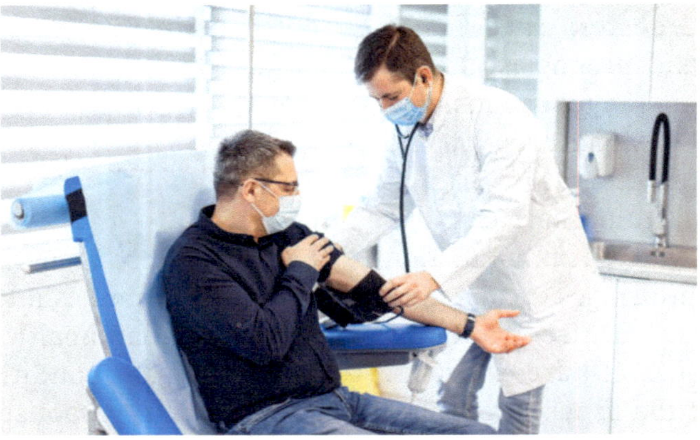

Figure 2.13. Cardiac stress testing for heart failure patients.

Source: https://images-cdn.welcomesoftware.com/Zz03MzE2OGNmMjc0YTIxMWVkYmIzNWNlZWEwODY4ZGZkOA==/image-stress-testing-with-case-and-treadmill-dcar.jpg.

In addition to their prognostic and diagnostic usefulness, functional tests also can elucidate mechanisms of cardiovascular pathophysiology. Under stress testing, the researcher can observe the aerobic function of the heart and its metabolic responses and employ these to establish pathophysiological changes to various conditions such as hypertension or valvular heart disease. For example, changes in the performance of the heart during stress can indicate oxygen delivery and mechanical dysfunction. In addition, understanding how different maneuvers affect cardiac output and vascular integrity helps understand the exercise-myocardial demand relationship. Research combining stress testing with advanced imaging techniques or biomarker assessment can provide more evidence of the molecular underpinnings of cardiovascular disease. In general, all these techniques play crucial roles in furthering cardiovascular medicine and shaping therapeutic interventions (Sabbagh et al., 2017) (Figure 2.13).

2.5. Treatment Strategies

The successful treatment of cardiovascular pathophysiology relies upon a multifunctional design directed toward disease mechanisms. Recent findings have led to endothelial dysfunction being identified as the central process leading to CAD, a widespread condition with serious potential complications. Recent literature indicates that this dysfunction is a result of inflammatory activation and therefore highlights the need to appreciate inflammatory pathways to atherosclerosis. Therapeutic interventions aimed at preserving and restoring endothelial function, thus, form the core of preventing the evolution of CAD and its resulting consequences. Evolution in biomarkers through liquid biopsies and molecular biology techniques presents new avenues for early identification of at-risk patients and, possibly, personalized therapy that would halt disease evolution and improve patient outcomes (Medina-Leyte et al., 2021). Pharmacological treatment still forms the center of the management strategies that seek to reverse cardiovascular disease. The traditional methods include antiplatelet therapy and statins aimed at modifying the lipid profiles and platelet count, countering the risks of acute events such as myocardial infarctions. However, newer therapies are focusing their attention on new anti-inflammatory drugs specifically designed to reverse endothelial dysfunction and, by consequence, atherosclerosis. The determination of specific molecular targets and endothelial health biomarkers opens the door to a precision medicine paradigm shift that can potentially allow clinicians to personalize treatment regimens. Additionally, non-pharmacologic interventions, such as lifestyle modifications through exercise and diet, remain crucial in preventing cardiovascular risk factors and promoting overall vascular well-being, underscoring the need for global treatment strategies to achieve optimal cardiovascular care (Medina-Leyte et al., 2021). As more and more cardiovascular complications of systemic disease, such as COVID-19, are coming into prominence, therapeutic practice has to be suitably altered. Present investigations describe that COVID-19 patients frequently present with cardiovascular complications and should receive cautious anticoagulation therapy for the prevention of thromboembolism. The administration of anticoagulants, particularly during hospitalization, has been recommended for preventing venous thromboembolism in patients with severe disease states, as highlighted by recent assessments in clinical practice. This new clinical scenario mirrors the need for ongoing investigations and refinement of therapeutic strategies to resist acute and chronic forms of cardiovascular strain resulting from external causes, including viral infection. This flexibility not only benefits the patient more effectively but also contributes to the greater goal of reducing cardiovascular pathophysiology-related mortality in diverse clinical settings (Figure 2.14).

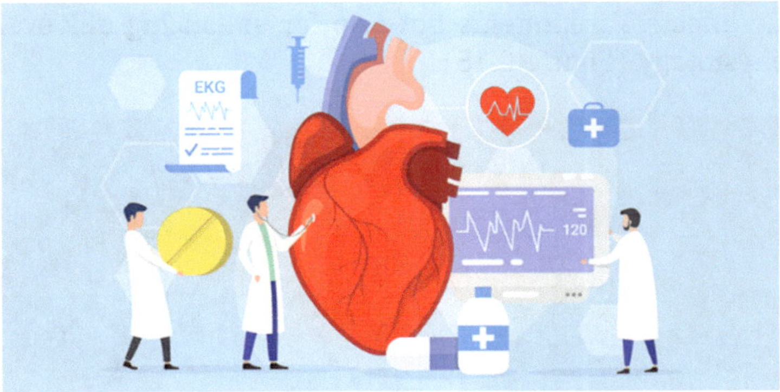

Figure 2.14. Heart Disease Treatment.

Source: https://www.drbennyjose.com/wp-content/uploads/2021/05/heart-disease-treatment-in-baner-800x400.png.

2.5.1. Pharmacological Interventions

Treatments with medications have become very important in managing heart-related diseases as our understanding of them has improved. Medications such as angiotensin-converting enzyme (ACE) inhibitors, beta-blockers, and statins are routinely prescribed to mitigate the effects of hypertension, heart failure, and atherosclerosis. They affect specific routes in the body that control the tightness of blood vessels, the heart's pumping, and the processing of fats. As an example, ACE inhibitors lower the amount of angiotensin II produced, which results in less blood vessel tightening and less fluid buildup. Using these drug strategies is a significant improvement in managing cardiovascular diseases, but it is vital to keep checking the patient's reaction and any side effects. Also, when you combine pharmacological treatments with non-pharmacological approaches such as healthy lifestyle changes, you can have a more complete plan for your heart health. More cases of diabetes mean that traditional drug treatments have to overcome new difficulties. One example is DCM, which can happen in diabetes patients and causes heart muscle changes and worsening heart failure. Because the disease has a complex process, it is hard to use medications effectively since their success varies among patients. Recent research has found that standard treatments may improve symptoms, but they do not always change the course of the disease for everyone. So, it is necessary to discover new drugs that address the specific metabolic problems seen in diabetic patients with DCM. Research suggests that combining pharmacological therapies with lifestyle modifications yields significant cardiovascular benefits, particularly in improving outcomes for individuals at high risk of DCM progression (Zhong et al., 2025). When we see how pharmacotherapy and lifestyle changes affect each other, we can create better personalized treatments. Furthermore, exploring new drugs goes past traditional therapies to target the leading causes of heart problems. One example is the use of targeted biological therapies, for example, monoclonal antibodies and gene therapy, which is a promising area in cardiovascular pharmacology. These therapies aim to modulate pro-inflammatory pathways and improve endothelial function, which are critically involved in the development of conditions like atherosclerosis and intracranial aneurysms (IAs). Genetically modified mice are significant for checking the effectiveness and safety of these new treatments. By observing the effects of pharmacological treatments in a controlled environment, researchers can gain insights into the complex dynamics of cardiovascular diseases, potentially leading to breakthroughs in managing conditions like IAs (Khan et al., 2024). Continued advancement in this area is imperative not only for developing effective treatments but also for enhancing our overall understanding of cardiovascular pathophysiology (Figure 2.15).

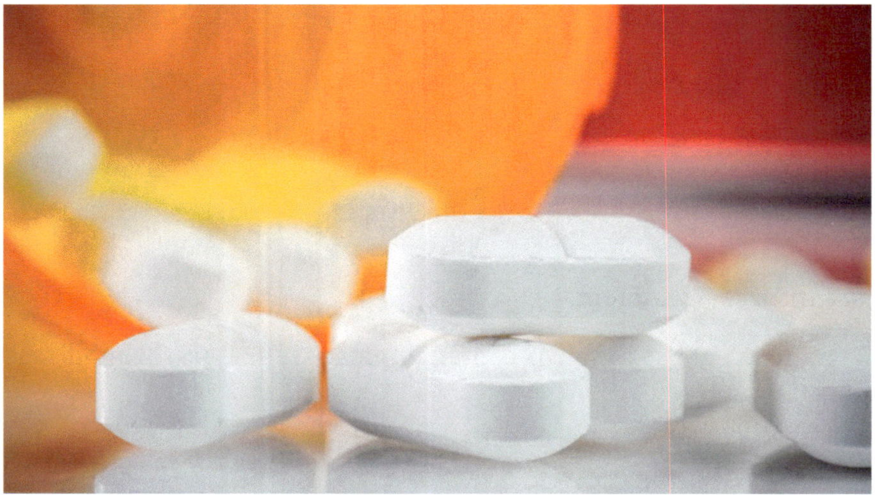

Figure 2.15. Cardiac Rehabilitation Medication.

Source: https://www.heart.org/-/media/Images/Health-Topics/Cardiac-Rehab/medicine-close-up.jpg?h=450&w=800&sc_lang=en&hash=92E38C815278A6F21D6198D019B14EE2.

2.5.2. Lifestyle Modifications

Lifestyle interventions lie at the core of regulating mechanisms of cardiovascular pathophysiology, particularly for individuals at risk of progressing conditions such as Type 2 diabetes mellitus (T2DM). The connection between lifestyle factors and cardiovascular well-being is of considerable note in that behaviors such as dietary modification and an increased level of physical activity may fundamentally restructure oxidative stress, a leading initiator of cardiovascular sequelae related to T2DM. As evident from current studies, hyperglycemia triggers the formation of reactive oxygen species that lead to endothelial dysfunction and vascular inflammation. Accordingly, taking up a healthy diet with antioxidant supplementation and exercise by way of aerobic exercise is capable of reversing the changes and enhancing the body's antioxidant defenses and cardiovascular outcomes. These activities not only improve metabolic control but also provide a healthier environment for vascular function. Concerning lifestyle modifications, these changes carry their implication over into conditions such as DCM in which previous disruptions in metabolism compromise cardiac function. The latest facts show that the combination of exercise with daily activity and a nutritionally balanced diet can effectively improve myocardial contractility and halt the progression of DCM. Pathophysiologic mechanisms governing DCM are a complex interplay between deranged metabolism and impaired cardiovascular function, whose derangement through lifestyle interventions renders them even more critical. By appropriately managing these factors, the risk of heart failure and other cardiovascular events is minimized, maintaining prolonged longevity and better quality of life. These modifications further invite patients to become more engaged in the treatment of their diseases, inducing healthy habits that surpass the adverse effects of their illnesses. The integrative approach of lifestyle modification is now more familiar not only for its protective promise but also as a possible treatment. As research increasingly identifies the molecular pathways influenced by lifestyle, it is clear that exercise and diet are adjuncts to usual medical therapy. The interventional approach mirrors new evidence that these adaptations hold the ability to reduce the burden of oxidative stress and inflammation, villains of the cardiovascular pathophysiologic environment (Caturano et al., 2025; Zhong et al., 2025). Therefore, the development of personalized exercise regimens and diet plans is a top agenda in enhancing therapeutic outcomes. Accordingly, these multidisciplinary life interventions can significantly reduce cardiovascular occurrences among high-risk individuals, underscoring the importance of a holistic strategy in mitigating the impacts of cardiovascular diseases.

2.5.3. Surgical Options and Interventions

Surgical procedures are very imperative in treating cardiovascular disease after simpler options have failed. These surgical procedures are usually indicated for those with severe coronary artery disease, heart defects, or problems that have been acquired as a consequence of conditions such as aneurysms in the coronary arteries. For example, treatment of coronary artery aneurysms with conventional measures may fall short because of the dangers they present, such as risks of rupture and acute coronary syndrome. Various treatments are offered to these conditions, such as surgical procedures and catheter-based procedures consisting of stenting or coil embolization. Through their creative application of such surgery, clinicians aim to restore normal hemodynamics and prevent further cardiovascular complications, thereby reducing the prevalent pathophysiologic processes that cause cardiovascular morbidity and mortality (Khalid et al., 2024). Apart from the treatment of coronary artery disease, metabolic syndrome surgery is essential in managing its effect on the heart. Metabolic syndrome makes an individual prone to having cardiovascular disease and type

2 diabetes mellitus. For those for whom other options are not effective, bariatric surgery is also an option. They help people lose a significant amount of weight, improve insulin utilization, and control cholesterol levels, thereby reducing the heart risk associated with metabolic syndrome. The rise in correlation between improved metabolic status post-surgery and reduction of cardiovascular events is increasingly being recognized, with the central overlap between surgical intervention and cardiovascular pathophysiology management (Dhondge et al., 2024). In addition, new surgical procedures such as minimally invasive and robotic surgeries have dramatically transformed processes of treating cardiovascular disease. With such innovative technologies, treatments become more targeted, less time-consuming to recover from, and result in fewer complications. Examples include procedures like transcatheter aortic valve replacement (TAVR), which is gaining popularity as an alternative to open-heart procedures. It offers a less invasive approach to addressing issues like aortic stenosis. Enhanced cardiovascular pathophysiology understanding allows surgeons to design procedures to suit diverse causes and needs in patients. The implication of this aspect draws attention to ongoing research and clinical trials to optimize surgical strategies, improve patients' outcomes, and, consequently, enhance the quality of cardiovascular care (Khalid et al., 2024) (Figure 2.16).

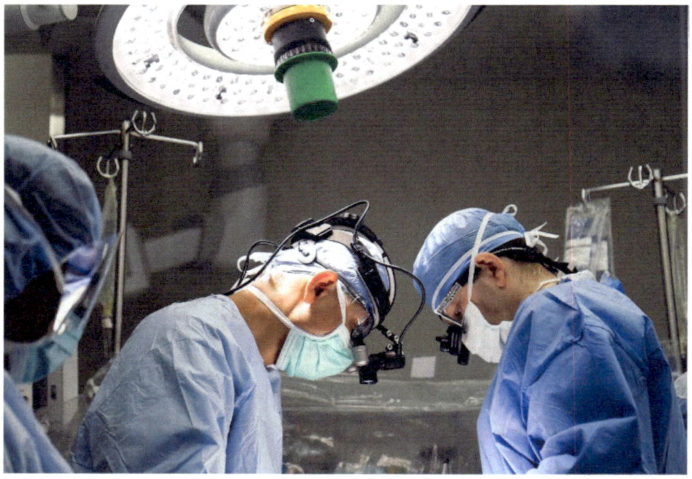

Figure 2.16. Surgical treatment of cardiovascular diseases.

Source: https://dam.northwell.edu/m/1e1fce6349aa6b1f/Drupal-NEWS_lenox-hills-cardiac-program-ranks-among-nys-best-doh-reports.jpg.

SUMMARY

In brief, the mechanisms underlying the pathophysiology of cardiovascular disease involve a multifactorial interaction of various factors, including dyslipidemic metabolism and oxidative stress. The worldwide spread of CVD, as characterized by the coincidence of a diversity of related pathologies, testifies to the necessity of its etiology explanation by a diversity of factors. The reason that CVD is still a major cause of death worldwide is only more reason to emphasize the usefulness of such research towards uncovering these complicated mechanisms. Oxidative stress, which has been postulated as the common ground among the majority of cardiovascular diseases, is observed to be of central importance in the etiology of hypertension and atherosclerosis. Recognition of the role played by such mechanisms is hence essential in terms of improving the treatment policy and implementing effective preventive care management systems in order to prevent the occurrence of cardiovascular disease across the globe. Additionally, inquiry into the impact of lipid profiles and, more importantly, triglyceride levels sheds light on a critical source of information concerning cardiovascular health. Hypertriglyceridemia is becoming more well recognized for its adverse effects on vascular function and metabolism and for inducing such disease states as metabolic syndrome. Emerging literature indicates that hypertriglyceridemia has not only adverse effects in the cardiovascular system but also catastrophic effects in neurovascular health, and this leads to cognitive impairment. Against the background of rising obesity and related hyperlipidemic disorders, public health interventions have to focus on building awareness regarding the role of diet in lipid level regulation. With increasing awareness of such metabolic impairments, it is clear that triglyceride regulation plays a crucial role in modulating cardiovascular risk and preventing the onset of related disorders, as indicated by the results of various studies. In summary, the pathophysiology of cardiovascular disease is multifactorial and necessitates a combined understanding based on multiple contributory processes, including lipid dysregulation and oxidative stress. Further studies are necessary to understand better the mechanism of these interactions and its application in clinical practice. The corpus of literature also emphasizes the importance of using a preventive approach to treating cardiovascular health complications, advocating for lifestyle changes and intervention at an early point that is designed to curtail dangers in high triglycerides and oxidative stress. With a better understanding of the pathophysiological mechanisms of such conditions, health professionals can institute targeted interventions that not only improve patient outcomes but also stem the rising incidence of cardiovascular disease, a public health priority confronting communities and societies today.

An understanding of cardiovascular pathophysiologic mechanisms as multi-dimensional involves an inquiry into the metabolic determinants, particularly the overlap between cardiovascular wellness and diseases such as non-alcoholic fatty liver disease (NAFLD). The etiology of NAFLD, along with other metabolic derangements including insulin resistance, dyslipidemia, and obesity, plays a significant role in exacerbating CVD. The overlap of metabolic syndrome and cardiovascular disease illustrates how pathologies of the liver become equated with cardiovascular pathology. With worsening advanced fibrosis and NASH, predictive hazard risks of CVD mortality increase, and the necessity of early diagnosis and treatment of liver disease to mitigate cardiovascular outcomes becomes an imperative (Rinella et al., 2023). Moreover, there is data that the therapies for improvement in liver function may also act synergistically to enhance cardiovascular wellness, necessitating a combined treatment plan that has both hepatic and cardiovascular targets in mind. Pathophysiology of cardiovascular disease is also controlled by mechanisms of excess oxidative stress, which has been noted to be of core importance in the etiology of various cardiovascular diseases. The ubiquitin-proteasome system (UPS) has been reported to play a significant regulatory function in the amount of oxidative stress and thus plays a vital role in cardiovascular function. As oxidative stress is implicated in endothelial dysfunction, inflammation, and apoptosis of cardiac cells, identification of this pathway is crucial in the development of therapeutic interventions against CVD. It is now apparent that UPS dysfunction can increase oxidative stress, thus linking it to common cardiovascular diseases such as atherosclerosis and heart failure. This link explains the significance of exploring UPS-targeted intervention in minimizing oxidative injury in cardiovascular disease and is an emerging area of future research (Qiu et al., 2022). In addition, cross-talk between metabolic disease, oxidative stress, and cardiovascular pathophysiology reveals an interactive understanding of disease mechanisms. Cardiovascular wellness cannot be envisioned in isolation; metabolic dysregulation can have a cascade of pathophysiological responses that accelerate heart-related issues. Cross-talk between systemic inflammation and dyslipidemia provokes increased oxidative stress, which, combined with other pathways such as hypertension, promotes the risk for CVD events. Therefore, a two-pronged approach to both metabolic control and management of oxidative stress can be of considerable benefit in reducing cardiovascular risks. Through the synthesis of knowledge from various disciplines, including hepatic health and mechanisms of oxidative stress signaling, doctors can better assess patient risk and offer better treatment plans that cure the multicausal complexities of cardiovascular disease (Qiu et al., 2022; Rinella et al., 2023).

A CLOSER LOOK

PREVENTION OF CARDIOVASCULAR DISEASE (CVD)

Prevention of CVD is primarily maintaining a healthy lifestyle and managing risk factors. This includes a heart-healthy diet, physical activity, healthy weight, quitting smoking, and decreasing alcohol consumption. Stress management, good sleep, and regular health check-ups are also highly crucial in the prevention of CVD (Figure 2.17).

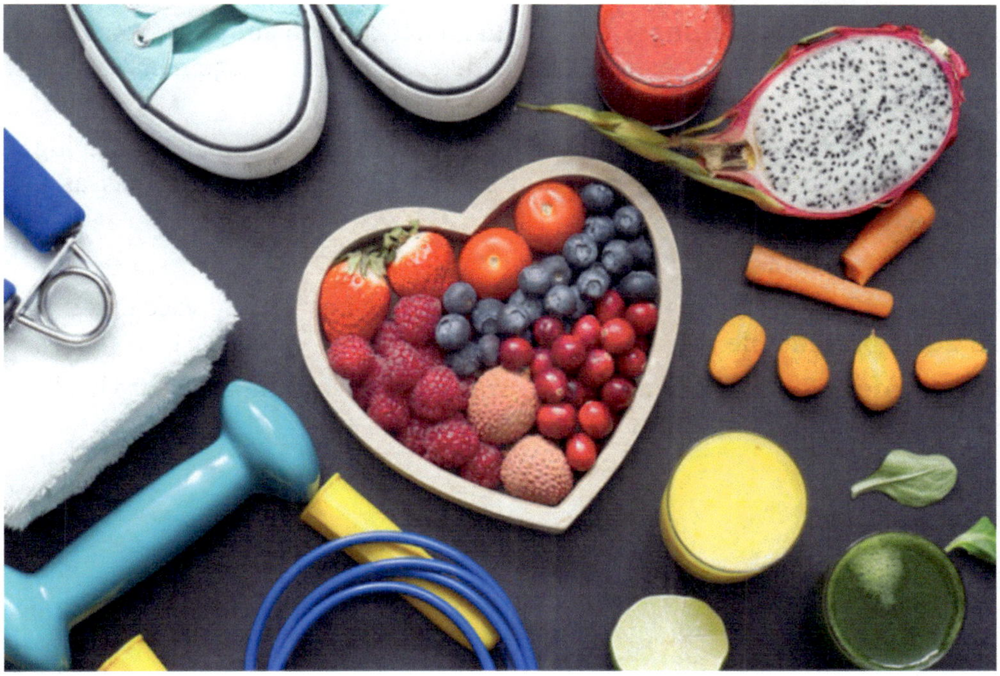

Figure 2.17. Heart healthy diet.

Source: https://domf5oio6qrcr.cloudfront.net/medialibrary/11317/4689519c-af5a-4997-9113-0c13d2b1669f.jpg.

Here's a more detailed breakdown of prevention strategies:

1. **Lifestyle Modifications:**
   a. **Healthy Diet:** Focus on consuming plenty of fruits, vegetables, whole grains, and lean proteins. Limit saturated and trans fats, processed foods, sugary drinks, and excessive salt. The DASH diet is a good example of a heart-healthy eating plan.
   b. **Regular Physical Activity:** Aim for at least 30–60 minutes of moderate-intensity exercise most days of the week. This can include activities like walking, jogging, swimming, or cycling.
   c. **Maintain a Healthy Weight:** Obesity is a significant risk factor for CVD. Weight management can be achieved through a combination of diet and exercise.

d. **Quit Smoking:** Smoking is a significant risk factor for CVD. Quitting can significantly reduce your risk.

e. **Limit Alcohol Consumption:** Excessive alcohol intake can raise blood pressure and increase the risk of heart disease.

f. **Manage Stress:** Stress can contribute to CVD. Practices like meditation, yoga, or spending time in nature can help reduce stress.

g. **Get Quality Sleep:** Lack of sleep can negatively impact heart health. Aim for 7–9 hours of sleep per night.

2. **Early Detection and Management:**

   a. **Regular Health Screenings:** Get regular checkups to monitor your blood pressure, cholesterol, and blood sugar levels. Early detection and management of these risk factors can significantly reduce the risk of CVD.

   b. **Medications as Prescribed:** If you are diagnosed with high blood pressure, high cholesterol, or other conditions that increase your risk of CVD, take medications as prescribed by your doctor.

3. **Specific Considerations:**

   a. **Infections:** Taking steps to prevent infections, such as getting vaccinated against the flu and other preventable diseases, can also help protect your heart.

   b. **Air Pollution:** Exposure to air pollution can negatively impact heart health. If possible, avoid areas with high pollution levels.

References

1. Ajoolabady, A., Pratico, D., Lin, L., Mantzoros, C. S., Bahijri, S., Tuomilehto, J., & Ren, J. (2024). Inflammation in atherosclerosis: pathophysiology and mechanisms. *Cell Death and Disease, 15*(11). https://doi.org/10.1038/s41419-024-07166-8Alkahtani, R. (2022). Molecular mechanisms underlying some major common risk factors of stroke. *Heliyon, 8*, e10218–e10218. https://doi.org/10.1016/j.heliyon.2022.e10218 (accessed on 29th May 2025).

2. Caturano, A., Rocco, M., Tagliaferri, G., Piacevole, A., Nilo, D., Di Lorenzo, G., Iadicicco, I., et al. (2025). Oxidative stress and cardiovascular complications in type 2 diabetes: From pathophysiology to lifestyle modifications. *Antioxidants, 14*. https://www.semanticscholar.org/paper/dd8dc80de2b12e5cfd47e5ecc0011eb3f715360a (accessed on 29th May 2025).

3. Cheng, S., Schumann, M., & Bloch, W. (2021). Translational medicine and exercise prescription (TMEP): Advancing the era of exercise medicine. *Translational Medicine and Exercise Prescription*. https://www.semanticscholar.org/paper/f17111c540081880ef6cc37d4c5d348fd80af874 (accessed on 29th May 2025).

4. Connelly, P., Currie, G., & Delles, C. (2022). Sex differences in the prevalence, outcomes and management of hypertension. *Current Hypertension Reports, 24*, 185–192. https://doi.org/10.1007/s11906-022-01183-8 (accessed on 29th May 2025).

5. Derouiche, S., Guemari, I. Y., & Boulaares, I. (2024). Study of the role of oxidative stress in pathophysiology of cardiovascular diseases. *Collective Journal Cardiovascular Medicine*. https://www.semanticscholar.org/paper/d231a6f7ff8c27df1da7d21f4020ffbbc733471d (accessed on 29th May 2025).

6. Dhondge, R. H., Agrawal, S., Patil, R., Kadu, A., & Kothari, M. (2024). A comprehensive review of metabolic syndrome and its role in cardiovascular disease and type 2 diabetes mellitus: Mechanisms, risk factors, and management. *Cureus, 16*. https://www.semanticscholar.org/paper/3b51ca1ac6ad160004ba7f4ad4fd67ae99f7017b (accessed on 29th May 2025).

7. El Sabbagh, A., & Nishimura, R. (2017). Clinical conundrum of coronary artery disease and aortic valve stenosis. *Journal of the American Heart Association: Cardiovascular and Cerebrovascular Disease, 6*. https://www.semanticscholar.org/paper/6f1ba541b66d74b72e5ec6076f24e4e81f85ebc3 (accessed on 29th May 2025).

8. Garovic, V. D., Dechend, R., Easterling, T. R., Karumanchi, S. A., Baird, S. M., Magee, L. A., Rana, S., et al. (2021). Hypertension in pregnancy: Diagnosis, blood pressure goals, and pharmacotherapy: A scientific statement from the American Heart Association. *Hypertension, 79*. https://doi.org/10.1161/hyp.0000000000000208 (accessed on 29th May 2025).

9. Glikson, M., Nielsen, J. C., Kronborg, M. B., Michowitz, Y., Auricchio, A., Barbash, I. M., Barrabés, J. A., et al. (2021). 2021 ESC guidelines on cardiac pacing and cardiac resynchronization therapy. *European Heart Journal, 42*, 3427–3520. https://doi.org/10.1093/eurheartj/ehab364 (accessed on 29th May 2025).

10. Higashi, Y. (2022). Roles of oxidative stress and inflammation in vascular endothelial dysfunction-related disease. *Antioxidants, 11*, 1958. https://doi.org/10.3390/antiox11101958 (accessed on 29th May 2025).

11. Humbert, M., Kovács, G., Hoeper, M. M., Badagliacca, R., Berger, R. M. F., Brida, M., Carlsen, J., et al. (2022). 2022 ESC/ERS guidelines for the diagnosis and treatment of pulmonary hypertension. *European Respiratory Journal, 61*, 2200879. https://doi.org/10.1183/13993003.00879-2022 (accessed on 29th May 2025).

12. Khalid, N., Kumar, S., Muskula, P., Muhammad, H., & Helmy, T. (2024). Coronary artery aneurysms and acute coronary syndrome: An interventionalist's dilemma. *Methodist DeBakey Cardiovascular Journal, 20*, 33–39. https://www.semanticscholar.org/paper/4a676bd4a298c94dd097b19927ce6de459f9d737 (accessed on 29th May 2025).

13. Khan, D., Li, X., Hashimoto, T., Tanikawa, R., Niemela, M., Lawton, M., & Muhammad, S. (2024). Current mouse models of intracranial aneurysms: Analysis of pharmacological agents used to induce aneurysms and their impact on translational research. *Journal of the American Heart Association*. https://www.semanticscholar.org/paper/38c0e425636123aa533529bde725a0802815f00d (accessed on 29th May 2025).

14. Krychtiuk, K., Vrints, C., Wojta, J., Huber, K., & Speidl, W. (2022). Basic mechanisms in cardiogenic shock: Part 1—Definition and pathophysiology. *European Heart Journal: Acute Cardiovascular Care*. https://www.semanticscholar.org/paper/a2c3be8c34e709b145210c58adddd780fdc1c60c (accessed on 29th May 2025).

15. Lazaridis, A., Malliora, A., & Gkaliagkousi, E. (2025). The particularities of arterial hypertension in female sex: From pathophysiology to therapeutic management. *Journal of Clinical Medicine*. https://www.semanticscholar.org/paper/c993503e1bb9bf0784536f43cc1454f19d64fcd0 (accessed on 29th May 2025).

16. Lee, D. (2022). Obesity and heart failure with preserved ejection fraction: Pathophysiology and clinical significance. *Cardiovascular Prevention and Pharmacotherapy*. https://www.semanticscholar.org/paper/ad63608c24f11b759de41adf8003d40e786216d9 (accessed on 29th May 2025).

17. Mach, F., Baigent, C., Catapano, A. L., Koskinas, K. C., Casula, M., Badimón, L., Chapman, M. J., et al. (2019). 2019 ESC/EAS guidelines for the management of dyslipidemias: Lipid modification to reduce cardiovascular risk. *European Heart Journal, 41*, 111–188. https://doi.org/10.1093/eurheartj/ehz455 (accessed on 29th May 2025).

18. Masi, S., Rizzoni, D., Taddei, S., Widmer, R. J., Montezano, A. C., Lüscher, T. F., Schiffrin, E. L., et al. (2020). Assessment and pathophysiology of microvascular disease: Recent progress and clinical implications. *European Heart Journal, 42*, 2590–2604. https://doi.org/10.1093/eurheartj/ehaa857 (accessed on 29th May 2025).

19. Medina-Leyte, D. J., Zepeda-García, O., Domínguez-Pérez, M., González-Garrido, A., Villarreal-Molina, T., & Jacobo-Albavera, L. (2021). Endothelial dysfunction, inflammation and coronary artery disease: Potential biomarkers and promising therapeutical approaches. *International Journal of Molecular Sciences, 22*, 3850. https://doi.org/10.3390/ijms22083850 (accessed on 29th May 2025).

20. Mutithu, D., Aremu, O. O., Mokaila, D., Bana, T., Familusi, M. A., Taylor, L., Martin, L., et al. (2024). A study protocol to characterize pathophysiological and molecular markers of rheumatic heart disease and degenerative aortic stenosis using multiparametric cardiovascular imaging and multiomics techniques. *PLOS ONE, 19*. https://www.semanticscholar.org/paper/12418e47e15de9db37bebaf9b6d2a5dc5bede84b (accessed on 29th May 2025).

21. Netala, V. R., Hou, T., Wang, Y., Zhang, Z., & Teertam, S. (2025). Cardiovascular biomarkers: Tools for precision diagnosis and prognosis. *International Journal of Molecular Sciences, 26*. https://www.semanticscholar.org/paper/6daf83e324c305abce432b0ea88060aa6e153284 (accessed on 29th May 2025).

22. Pisklak, A., Sykuła, J., Zalewska, N., & Filipek, K. (2024). What is the relationship between obstructive sleep apnea and cardiovascular disease? Pathophysiology and therapeutic strategies: A review of the literature. *Medical Science*. https://www.semanticscholar.org/paper/62fc9bef7818e8a75ea14b98c0d11c6e4110676d (accessed on 29th May 2025).

23. Prabhu, G. S., & Concessao, P. (2024). Triglycerides and metabolic syndrome: From basic to mechanism – A narrative review. *Archives of Physiology and Biochemistry*. https://www.semanticscholar.org/paper/cd324c80589c6642ffe24f0371366f55a5142550 (accessed on 29th May 2025).

24. Qiu, M., Chen, J., Li, X., & Zhuang, J. (2022). Intersection of the ubiquitin–proteasome system with oxidative stress in cardiovascular disease. *International Journal of Molecular Sciences, 23*, 12197. https://doi.org/10.3390/ijms232012197.

25. Reyes-Soffer, G., Ginsberg, H. N., Berglund, L., Duell, P. B., Heffron, S., Kamstrup, P. R., Lloyd-Jones, D. M., et al. (2021). Lipoprotein(a): A genetically determined, causal, and prevalent risk factor for atherosclerotic cardiovascular disease: A scientific statement from the American Heart Association. *Arteriosclerosis, Thrombosis, and Vascular Biology, 42*. https://doi.org/10.1161/atv.0000000000000147.

26. Rinella, M. E., Neuschwander-Tetri, B. A., Siddiqui, M. S., Abdelmalek, M. F., Caldwell, S. H., Barb, D., Kleiner, D. E., et al. (2023). AASLD practice guidance on the clinical assessment and management of nonalcoholic fatty liver disease. *Hepatology, 77*, 1797–1835. https://doi.org/10.1097/hep.0000000000000323.

27. Rivera-Mancilla, E., Al-Hassany, L., Villalón, C. M., & MaassenVanDenBrink, A. (2021). Metabolic aspects of migraine: Association with obesity and diabetes mellitus. *Frontiers in Neurology, 12*. https://doi.org/10.3389/fneur.2021.686398.

28. Saadh, M., Muhammad, F. A., Albadr, R. J., Sanghvi, G., Jyothi, S. R., Kundlas, M., Joshi, K. K., et al. (2025). Inflammasomes and cardiovascular disease: Linking inflammation to cardiovascular pathophysiology. *Scandinavian Journal of Immunology, 101*(4), e70020. https://www.semanticscholar.org/paper/f791c11cab5b5d8eac1a4905a1915678aa3c4643 (accessed on 29th May 2025).

29. Saito, Y., Tsujita, K., & Kobayashi, Y. (2024). No standard modifiable cardiovascular risk factors in acute myocardial infarction: Prevalence, pathophysiology, and prognosis. *Cardiovascular Intervention and Therapeutics, 39*, 403–411. https://www.semanticscholar.org/paper/d71f2c2c8680a4759a1b61201b04452040d809ea (accessed on 29th May 2025).

30. Shah, M., Shrestha, K., Tseng, C. W., Goyal, A., Liewluck, T., & Gupta, L. (2024). Statin-associated muscle symptoms: A comprehensive exploration of epidemiology, pathophysiology, diagnosis, and clinical management strategies. *International Journal of Rheumatic Diseases, 27*(9), e15337. https://www.semanticscholar.org/paper/6eba49da4e74015ca86e0e40daa802bf37461021 (accessed on 29th May 2025).

31. Silva, L. F., & Laakso, M. (2025). Advances in metabolomics: A comprehensive review of type 2 diabetes and cardiovascular disease interactions. *International Journal of Molecular*

Sciences, 26. https://www.semanticscholar.org/paper/1768020c6740abcc3b45c48e5a4049bf87a1aee2 (accessed on 29th May 2025).

32. Simons, S. O., Heptinstall, A. B., Marjenberg, Z., Marshall, J., Mullerova, H., Rogliani, P., Nordon, C., et al. (2024). Temporal dynamics of cardiovascular risk in patients with chronic obstructive pulmonary disease during stable disease and exacerbations: Review of the mechanisms and implications. *International Journal of Chronic Obstructive Pulmonary Disease, 19*, 2259–2271. https://www.semanticscholar.org/paper/594068cd7c7b96c74ab6708624a42fa128e4d19b (accessed on 29th May 2025).
33. Tabatabaei, F. S., Shafeghat, M., Azimi, A., Akrami, A. E., & Rezaei, N. (2024). Endosomal Toll-like receptors intermediate negative impacts of viral diseases, autoimmune diseases, and inflammatory immune responses on the cardiovascular system. *Expert Review of Clinical Immunology*. https://www.semanticscholar.org/paper/d47930c6414216d3ff1c3512dddf7dc3ae028b1e (accessed on 29th May 2025).
34. Torimoto, K., Elliott, K., Nakayama, Y., Yanagisawa, H., & Eguchi, S. (2024). Cardiac and perivascular myofibroblasts, matrifibrocytes, and immune fibrocytes in hypertension; commonalities and differences with myocardial infarction and other cardiovascular diseases. *Cardiovascular Research*. https://www.semanticscholar.org/paper/e07beceb4526d5b9d925676bbe79ae8fac6a0da2 (accessed on 29th May 2025).
35. Wang, M., Li, Y., Li, S., & Lv, J. (2022). Endothelial dysfunction and diabetic cardiomyopathy. *Frontiers in Endocrinology, 13*. https://doi.org/10.3389/fendo.2022.851941.
36. Wichmann, D. (2020). Autopsy findings and venous thromboembolism in patients with COVID-19. *Annals of Internal Medicine, 173*, 1030–1030. https://doi.org/10.7326/l20-1206.
37. Zhong, L., Hou, X., Tian, Y., & Fu, X. (2025). Exercise and dietary interventions in the management of diabetic cardiomyopathy: Mechanisms and implications. *Cardiovascular Diabetology, 24*. https://www.semanticscholar.org/paper/6ce2f4aa2792b7e36e4093a95417b850efff7e46 (accessed on 29th May 2025).

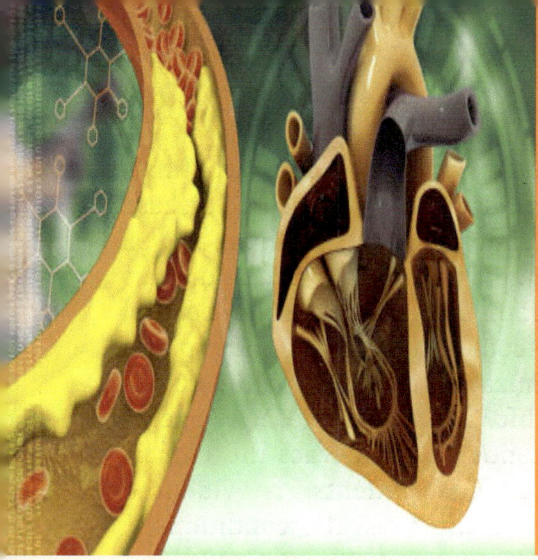

Chapter 3

MECHANISMS OF CARDIAC ARRHYTHMIAS

Contents

Introduction

Cardiac arrhythmias are a significant clinical challenge, particularly in the geriatric population, with a further augmented incidence of comorbid cardiovascular pathology. Understanding the underlying mechanisms causing such abnormal heart rhythms is crucial for successful management and diagnosis. Structural and functional changes in the heart with increasing age, as well as underlying comorbid conditions such as hypertension, diabetes, and heart failure, provide a multifaceted background, making older patients prone to many arrhythmias. In this context , the quest for frequency and type of arrhythmia in elderly patients has highlighted the need for the incorporation of gender-specific health determinants, thereby reflecting priceless insight into treatment and monitoring strategies formulated for the population (Vlasova et al., 2025). Beyond even the sheer number of arrhythmias is the intricacy of the root causes. Pathophysiologic alterations involving cellular electrical remodeling and structural changes to the heart are key to arrhythmogenic potential. One such example is the phenomenon of atrial fibrillation, with much of it occurring in elderly patients, and oftentimes further burdened by the presence of heart enlargement and fibrosis secondary to chronic disease (Houck, 2024). All these underlying pathologies necessitate a good understanding of chronic as well as intermittent arrhythmias, particularly how they relate to well-established cardiovascular disease states. Thus, detailed examination of the heart's electrical conduction system and implications of pacing therapies becomes unavoidable in developing functional outcome-oriented treatment plans. While discussing the treatment of cardiac arrhythmias, with optimization of functional outcomes in the foreground, there is a need to enhance patients' quality of life. The addition of new pacing technologies, along with patient-specific treatment algorithms, tends to counteract the clinical effect of arrhythmias and consider specific clinical profiles of individual patients. As evidenced through more current studies, its capacity to treat a diverse range of cardiovascular conditions in combination with patient-specific pacing goals is very promising in improving patients' outcomes, such as relief of dyspnea and cardiac fatigue symptoms (Houck, 2024). Hence, a concerted approach that involves diligent monitoring and management of reversible risk factors is crucial to address the complexities of arrhythmias in the elderly, offering an inclusive and effective management plan (Figure 3.1).

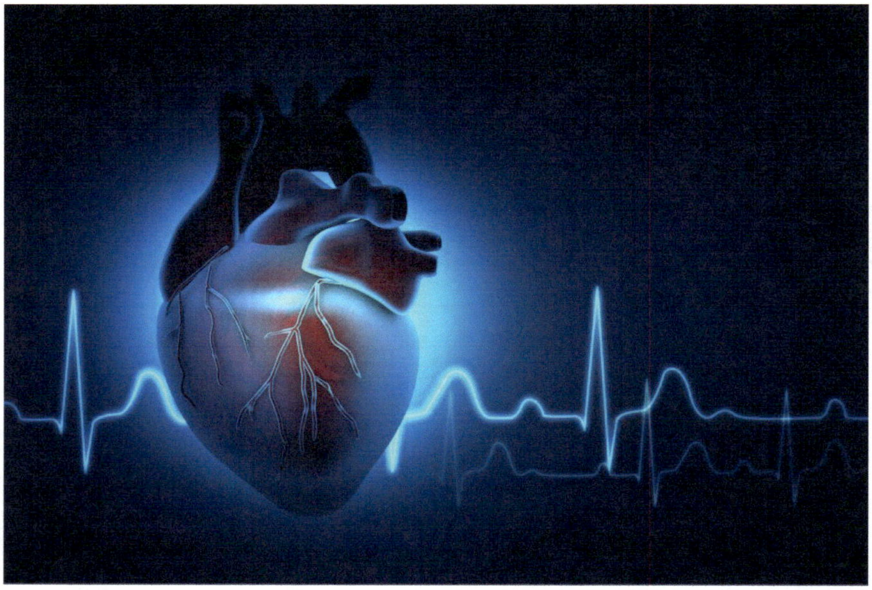

Figure 3.1. Understanding Cardiac Arrhythmias.

Source: https://cvrti.utah.edu/wp-content/uploads/2021/09/Cardiac-Arrhythmia-1024x683.jpeg.

Definition of Cardiac Arrhythmias

Cardiac arrhythmias may be described as a spectrum of disorders characterized by irregularity of the rhythm of the heart, influencing the frequency, regularity, and origin of the heartbeats. Dysrhythmias of the heart can be produced by pathophysiologically diverse mechanisms that range from dysfunction in the conducting apparatus of the heart to structural myocardial defects. They are disparate enough to be roughly classified into supraventricular and ventricular arrhythmias, depending on the location of origin. The clinical effects of arrhythmias are occasionally serious, and some are connected with high morbidity and mortality due to compromised cardiac output and potential development into severe states such as heart failure or stroke. Understanding of these definitions is crucial since they form the basis of understanding mechanisms and clinical management strategies involved in cardiac arrhythmias, which are critical for the patient's treatment and prognosis (Zhang et al., 2025). Cardiac arrhythmia mechanisms could be multifactorial, with electrical, structural, and biochemical changes in the heart. For instance, re-entry mechanisms involve pathological circuit formation in myocardial tissue, facilitating continuous electrical impulses irrespective of the normal pathways of conduction. Automaticity refers to the normal impulse generation by pacemaker cells, excluding sinoatrial node cells, leading to abnormal rhythm. Triggered activity can be induced by afterdepolarizations, which disrupt the normal process of repolarization and can result in ectopic beats. All mechanisms are involved in distinct arrhythmias with distinct clinical presentations. Studies on these mechanisms may lead to new therapies and interventions aiming at restoring normal rhythm and function in patients (Nagpal et al., 2024). The high incidence of cardiac arrhythmias warrants complete understanding and management programs. According to recent reviews, the key to successful management is accurate diagnosis and classification of arrhythmias. Such investigations as electrocardiography (ECG) and electrophysiological studies play a significant role in identifying the precise type and mechanism of arrhythmia in patients. Therapy can also vary significantly, from pharmacological therapy with antiarrhythmic drugs to non-pharmacological treatment with catheter ablation. Familiarity with the definition of cardiac arrhythmias and mechanisms thereof not only directs clinical practice but also sets the stage for further advances in therapeutic approaches. The integration of new technologies, including human cardiac organoids, highlights the necessity for additional research to advance our understanding of these conditions and maximize patient outcomes (Nagpal et al., 2024; Zhang et al., 2025) (Figure 3.2).

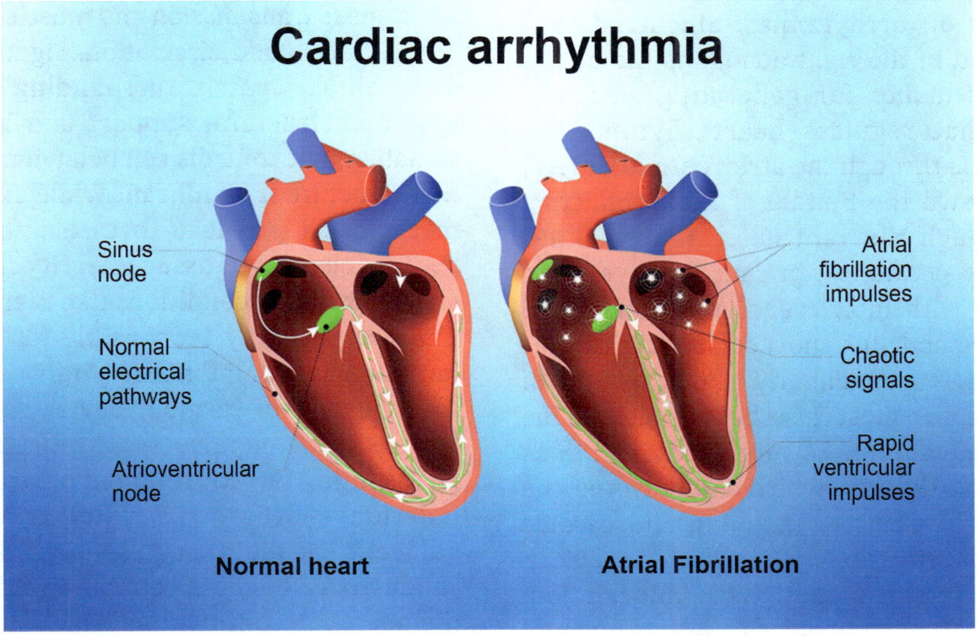

Figure 3.2. Cardiac arrhythmias.

Source: https://gph.ae/contents/uploads/media/cardiac-arrhythmia.png.

3.1. Anatomy of the Heart

Understanding cardiac anatomy comes into play in the context of the mechanism of cardiac arrhythmias. The heart is a muscular organ that has four chambers, namely the right and left atria and the right and left ventricles. There must be a strong interaction between these chambers so that there can be effective hemodynamic performance. Normally, the atria receive blood and pump it to the ventricles, which pump blood to the lungs and the rest of the body. Dysregulation of the intricate system can lead to arrhythmias, particularly in complex congenital heart disease such as tetralogy of Fallot. As indicated, ventricular arrhythmia is the leading cause of death in corrected tetralogy of Fallot Therefore, greater insight into the anatomy of the heart and the functional effects of any abnormal anatomy is required (Krieger et al., 2022). In addition, the contribution made by the conduction pathways in the anatomy of the heart plays a vital role in research on arrhythmias. Sinoatrial (SA) node, located in the right atrium, is the body's natural pacemaker for generating electrical impulses that regulate heart rhythm. The impulses pass through the atrioventricular (AV) node and down the Bundle of His, conducting signals through the ventricles. Abnormalities within these conduits can cause arrhythmias, particularly with interference from structural changes or remodeling, most common in cardiac disease. As noted, the underlying mechanisms of arrhythmia can in most cases be attributed to the anatomical adaptations of surgical interventions or congenital defects, which underscores the importance of accurate mapping and cardiac structure investigation (Krieger et al., 2022). Apart from intrinsic anatomical information, extrinsic factors such as diet can be instrumental in arrhythmia development. Dietary choices are great modifiers of some of the physiological processes, and one of them is cardiovascular function. In aged mouse models that are fed Western diets, changes in expression were observed for specific genes, particularly in cardiac function, inflammatory responses, and oxidative stress pathways. These changes can be viewed of compromised cardiac structure and function, making it more vulnerable to diseases like arrhythmia and hypertension. The identified pathways, coupled with the anatomical tendencies of the heart, highlight the complex interaction between the circumstances of life and the inherent anatomical properties that are accountable for the development of cardiac arrhythmia.

3.1.1. Structure of Cardiac Tissue

The anatomy of the heart is highly intricate, comprising cardiac tissue which is specialized to maintain its rhythmic activity. Cardiac tissue is predominantly composed of cardiac muscle cells or cardiomyocytes, which are interwoven to create a tough, rigid, elastic matrix with an ability to endure contraction and relaxation. The arrangement ensures a convenient route for impulse transmission and muscle contraction to facilitate blood circulation. Significantly, the extracellular matrix surrounding these cells provides structural support and biochemical signaling that controls cell behavior. Identifying this structure is significant while exploring the mechanisms that lead to cardiac arrhythmias because changes in tissue integrity could initiate arrhythmogenic conditions like reentry circuits that are primarily responsible for arrhythmia initiation and maintenance (Aitova et al., 2023). Arrangement of cardiomyocytes also provides for electrical impulse synchronization, which is essential for coordinated heartbeats. Gap junctions—protein assemblies connecting adjacent cardiomyocytes—provide for fast conductivity of the electrical signal, such that the heart can contract uniformly. Malformation or malfunction of these junctions can induce delayed conduction and an increased likelihood of arrhythmias. Also, the composition of the interstitial space, e.g., the content of inflammatory cells or fibrotic tissue, can markedly modulate electrical conduction pathways. It has been shown that cardiac fibrosis, as a tissue architecture modifier, increases the potential for atrial fibrillation, a ubiquitous arrhythmia (Liu et al., 2023). Such structural interactions are paramount in the development of therapeutic interventions against the prevention and treatment of arrhythmias. Furthermore, advances in tissue engineering have created new possibilities for examining the structural intricacy of cardiac tissue and its contribution to arrhythmias.

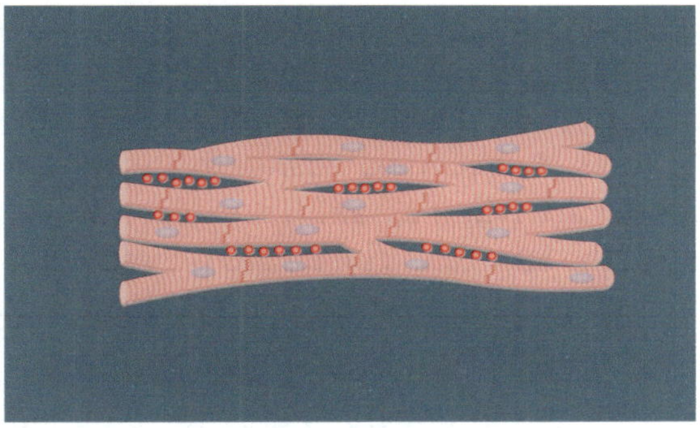

Figure 3.3. The cardiac muscle cell or fiber.

Source: https://www.getbodysmart.com/wp-content/uploads/2017/11/Unlabelled-image-of-the-cardiac-muscle-cells-1-1024x540.png.

Engineered cardiac tissues can reproduce some structural and functional characteristics of native myocardium, thereby enabling the examination of arrhythmogenic mechanisms in a controlled setting. These models allow scientists to more comprehensively study reentry circuits and wave propagation, uncovering the contribution of structural changes to arrhythmia pathways (Aitova et al., 2023). The application of scaffolds that mimic the extracellular matrix of the heart provides further insight into the relationship between cellular structure and electrical activity. With cardiovascular disease still a global concern, ongoing research into the structure of cardiac tissue will be crucial to the design of new treatment strategies for arrhythmias and better patient outcomes (Figure 3.3).

3.1.2. Electrical Conduction System

The heart's electrical system is an essential part for controlling the heart's beats, which aids in proper blood circulation. It consists of specialized heart cells that make and send action potentials, which start the contraction of the heart muscle. The SA node, which is at the heart's apex, is the primary pacemaker and sends electrical signals to the atria. The AV node, bundle of His, and Purkinje fibers help coordinate the subsequent contraction, which makes ventricular contraction more efficient. Any disturbance in this well-organized process may cause cardiac arrhythmias because the regular flow of electrical signals is interrupted. Thus, understanding the conduction pathways is crucial for identifying the origins of such disturbances, which can manifest as various arrhythmias, ranging from atrial fibrillation to more life-threatening ventricular tachycardia (Gönczi et al., 2013). More studies have explained how the electrical conduction system can lead to myocardial ischemia which is often the cause of significant arrhythmias. When blood flow drops, myocardial ischemia happens, and the cells do not get enough oxygen, which causes them to malfunction. Because of this condition, the tissue in the heart can change, leading to gap junctions being separated, which lowers electrical communication between myocytes. Ischemia in the heart can cause the conduction system to malfunction, which may lead to dangerous arrhythmias like reentrant circuits. Different studies have found that opening or closing gap junctions may both protect the heart from ischemic arrhythmias. Given the complex interplay between gap junction function and electrical stability, ongoing research emphasizes the necessity for a nuanced understanding of these dynamics (Gönczi et al., 2013). One must also think about how changes in the way electrical signals move can disturb the heart's regular activity. The generation of action potentials is essential for the coordinated contraction of myocytes; when this process is perturbed, it can result in chaotic wave patterns, such as those seen in atrial fibrillation (AF) and ventricular fibrillation (VF). Both computational models and experiments have pointed out that nonlinear effects in these processes are important, and they can result in reentrant circuits caused by defects in the wavefront. When waves in the heart move erratically, the chance of arrhythmogenesis rises significantly, so learning more about these mechanisms can help find ways to prevent and treat them. Increasing our understanding of the intricacies involved in cardiac electrical dynamics is vital for developing effective therapeutic interventions aimed at addressing complex arrhythmias (Muñoz et al., 2016).

3.1.3. Role of the Autonomic Nervous System (ANS)

The ANS is important, essential for heart rhythm, and has become a key part in understanding cardiac arrhythmias. Two main branches make up the autonomic nervous system: the sympathetic and parasympathetic systems, which manage heart rate and the force of myocardial contractions together. Usually, when the sympathetic nervous system is active, the heart beats faster.

It pumps harder, but when the parasympathetic nervous system is involved, through the vagus nerve, the heart slows down and its strength decreases. If the balance between the autonomic nerves is lost, either by them working more or less than usual, it can cause arrhythmias. An example is that a rise in sympathetic tone often leads to tachycardia, and a sharp decrease in parasympathetic activity can result in abnormal heart rhythms. It is important to know how the ANS influences heart rhythm to develop effective treatments for arrhythmias, which are a major cause of health problems and deaths. In some arrhythmias, the autonomic nervous system plays a crucial role, as activating the sympathetic branch can exacerbate arrhythmias, whereas activating the parasympathetic branch can help control them. Atrial fibrillation often involves both systems working together at the same time, which can set off arrhythmias. If ventricular fibrillation happens due to cardiac ischemia, sympathetic activity usually leads to arrhythmias, whereas parasympathetic stimulation may help to prevent them. Because of these roles, cardiac electrophysiology is complex, and it shows that treating heart problems requires careful strategies. By better understanding these processes, it becomes easier to detect what leads to arrhythmias and to explore ways to control the autonomic system as a treatment for many arrhythmias, which can result in better clinical outcomes.

Advances in understanding the autonomic nervous system's impact on cardiac arrhythmias have led to new treatment options, including neural modulation therapies. By using these approaches, which involve destroying parts of the sympathetic nervous system and stimulating the parasympathetic system, doctors hope to restore balance in the autonomic system and lower the risk of arrhythmias. Some studies have found that using therapies to change the autonomic tone might help reduce the risk of arrhythmias in long QT syndrome. However, the use of neural modulation to address other arrhythmic diseases is still being primarily studied. Although some positive findings have been seen in small studies, more significant clinical studies are needed to confirm them and create guidelines for broader use. This evolving landscape signifies a vital step toward improving arrhythmia management, underscoring the critical role of the autonomic nervous system in maintaining cardiac health and preventing life-threatening arrhythmic events (Shen et al., 2014; Ponikowski et al., 2016) (Figure 3.4).

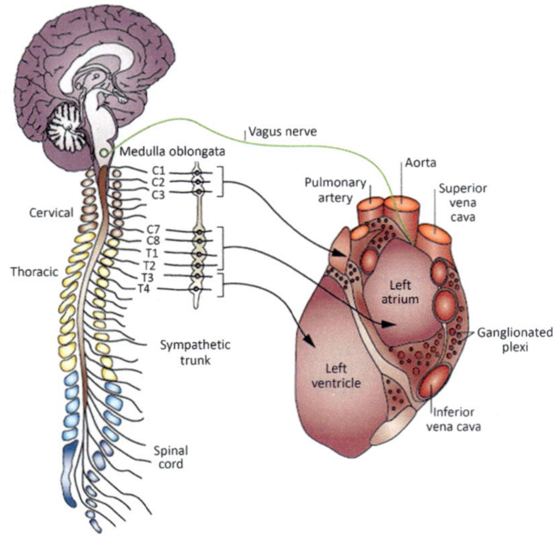

Figure 3.4. Scheme of autonomic innervation of the heart. The cardiac sympathetic ganglia consist of cervical ganglia, stellate (cervicothoracic) ganglia, and thoracic ganglia. Parasympathetic innervation comes from the vagus nerves.

Source: https://www.ahajournals.org/cms/10.1161/CIRCRESAHA.113.302549/asset/7b8d8178-ad8b-496d-8c9c-d195055e14c7/assets/graphic/1004fig01.jpeg.

3.2. Types of Cardiac Arrhythmias

Other types of cardiac arrhythmias can be classified based on their site, rate, and rhythm disturbances. The common ones are supraventricular arrhythmias, such as atrial fibrillation and atrial flutter, and ventricular arrhythmias, such as ventricular tachycardia and ventricular fibrillation. Supraventricular arrhythmias tend to be from above the ventricles and characteristically have palpitations or an irregular heart rhythm. Atrial fibrillation, the most prevalent among them, is characterized by chaotic and fast atrial electrical activity, with a severe risk of stroke and heart failure. Thus, understanding the finer details of these arrhythmias matters while identifying suitable treatment options, which include lifestyle modification and medication therapies (Nagpal et al., 2024). Ventricular arrhythmias, on the other hand, take place in the ventricles and can form imminent threats to life. Ventricular tachycardia is an abnormality in which three or more consecutive heartbeats, arising from the ventricles, are at a fast rate, risking drastic curtailment of cardiac output. Ventricular fibrillation is its acute expression, when the heart's failure to contract leads to immediate cardiac arrest. Early action and diagnosis are imperative, commonly backed by electrocardiogram (ECG) findings and observation in high-risk patients. Treatment may involve antiarrhythmic drugs, implantable cardioverter-defibrillators (ICDs), or catheter ablation for severe cases (Nagpal et al., 2024). These arrhythmias need to be identified early to ensure optimal patient outcomes. Evolving research is elucidating the function of microscopic mediators in cardiac arrhythmia pathophysiology, including the role of microRNAs (miRNAs) in the process of arrhythmogenesis-related gene expression. For example, new research indicates that alterations in the expression of specific miRNAs are essential to the development and progression of arrhythmias like atrial fibrillation. The mechanism by which these miRNAs regulate cell signaling pathways implicated in cardiac function underscores their therapeutic target potential. By developing models meant to drive cardiomyocytes, researchers have identified differential expression of different miRNAs during arrhythmic events, making it clear how gene regulation is connected with electrical dysfunctions. With knowledge of such molecular mechanisms, new doors could be opened up for new therapies aimed explicitly at interfering with pathogenic processes in arrhythmias.

3.2.1. Atrial Arrhythmias

Atrial arrhythmias are multi-causal diseases with abnormal atrial electrical activity and consequent inefficient cardiac function and increased risks of stroke and heart failure. The most prevalent form of atrial arrhythmia, atrial fibrillation, depicts the pathophysiology of these conditions with several mechanisms involving ectopic foci and re-entrant circuits. With advancing research, knowledge of the gene and molecular underpinnings of such arrhythmias has yielded to characterizations of the roles played by dysfunction of ion channels, structural remodeling, and deranged signaling pathways. In particular, transient reactivation of transcription factors such as Notch has been identified to underlie atrial electrophysiological abnormalities, leading to slowed conduction and susceptibility to arrhythmias. Such complex interaction of factors supports the need for continued study of atrial arrhythmias to develop effective therapeutic interventions for the variable etiologies involved. Atrial arrhythmia modeling provides an opportunity and a challenge for the explanation of their mechanisms and treatment. Traditional animal models have been of considerable benefit; however, their flaws, including heterogeneity with human cardiac physiology, necessitate the development of more representative models. New findings show the potential of human cardiac slices, which can support electrical viability and mimic human conditions, to facilitate the investigation of atrial arrhythmias. The slices allow researchers to uncover the intricate changes in gene expression that are associated with atrial fibrillation and other arrhythmias, thus understanding their pathogenesis better. Moreover, enhanced culture conditions provide a solid platform for long-term experimentation, revealing cellular responses to a wide range of pharmacologic agents. This translation of basic science to clinical applications can potentially improve the prognosis of atrial arrhythmia patients. Utilization of novel analytical approaches, i.e., directed network analysis, has emerged as a key tool in the research of atrial arrhythmias. Traditional methods use surface electrocardiography and, at times, obscure the underlying mechanisms of arrhythmias. However, with targeted networks, excitation patterns and interactions among various cardiac electrodes can be precisely characterized, thereby revealing complex information about arrhythmia mechanisms. In simulations and clinical data, scientists have demonstrated that this technique can be more precise and quicker than traditional techniques. Through these procedures becoming integrated into routine clinical practice, they can be expected to lead to earlier diagnosis and more specific treatment strategies for atrial arrhythmia patients. This innovation in diagnostic tools adds richness to the field of cardiac electrophysiology, enabling new methodologies for examining and treating complex arrhythmic disorders (Qiao et al., 2018; Neve et al., 2019) (Figure 3.5.

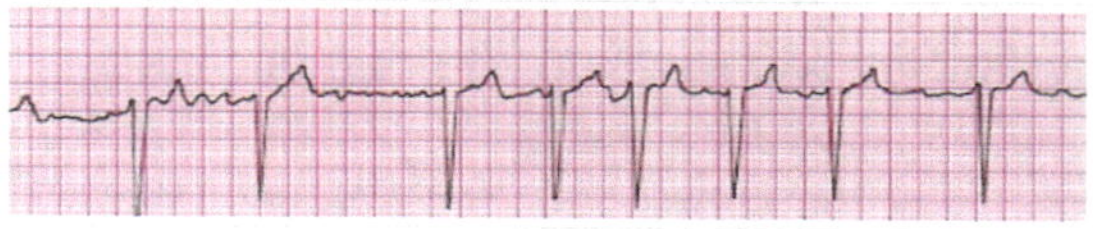

Figure 3.5. Atrial arrhythmias.

Source: https://upload.medbullets.com/topic/108080/images/a-fib..jpg.

3.2.2. Ventricular Arrhythmias

Ventricular arrhythmias are a significant concern in medicine because they are linked to a higher chance of death, mainly for people with heart problems. Arrhythmias cause many cases of sudden cardiac arrest, and these often happen during a myocardial infarction. The process of their development occurs in three phases: during the ischemic event, during healing, and after the scar has matured. Every phase involves different ways the arrhythmias happen, showing the complexity of their causes. Most of the time, ventricular tachycardia is found to be a reentrant arrhythmia that occurs in the scar tissue left after a heart attack. The conduction disturbances, resulting from structural alterations in the cardiac tissue, lead to impaired excitability and abnormal conduction paths that characterize ventricular arrhythmias, highlighting the need for advanced understanding and intervention strategies in at-risk populations (Donahue et al., 2024). Even though structural heart disease is strongly linked to ventricular arrhythmias, these problems can also appear in people whose hearts are structurally normal. Without structural heart disease, ventricular arrhythmias are most often due to a mix of genetic and environmental factors. It has been found through family research that problems with heart ion channels and calcium handling are significant causes of this group of arrhythmias. In addition, using genome-wide association studies, scientists have found certain parts of the genome linked to ventricular tachycardia and ventricular fibrillation, suggesting that these conditions can be inherited. Epigenetics, which involves non-coding RNAs and DNA methylation, is now being studied as a way to influence arrhythmia susceptibility. Understanding these mechanisms provides critical insights into the multifactorial nature of ventricular arrhythmias that extend beyond anatomical anomalies (Wang et al., 2022). Ventricular arrhythmias are very significant in clinical practice since they often lead to serious health problems and death in those who have them. New ways of diagnosing and treating people are necessary to find those who are more likely to develop the disease and take preventive action. The way arrhythmias in the ventricles occur depends on their structure, genes, and epigenetic changes, which all play a role in shaping the clinical picture. Working on research that unites basic and clinical science is necessary to invent new ways to treat and prevent arrhythmias. As the understanding of the pathophysiological mechanisms of ventricular arrhythmias continues to evolve, there is significant potential for improved patient outcomes through personalized medicine approaches that address the underlying causes of these arrhythmias (Wang et al., 2022; Donahue et al., 2024) (Figure 3.6).

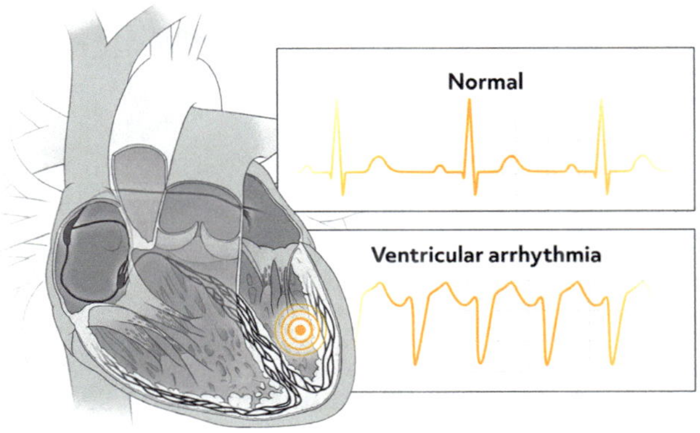

Figure 3.6. Ventricular arrhythmias.

Source: https://cdn-academy.pressidium.com/academy/wp-content/uploads/2025/02/image_365.png.

3.2.3. Conduction Block Arrhythmias

Disruptions in the electrical pathways of the heart cause conduction block arrhythmias, which are essential for many heart problems. Such arrhythmias can happen because of problems in the heart's structure or conduction system, which prevent or delay electrical signals in the heart muscle. Among the most common conduction blocks are first-degree heart block, which shows a prolonged PR interval, second-degree heart block, which is further divided into Mobitz type I and II, and complete heart block, in which atrial and ventricular activities are completely out of sync. Conduction blocks may lead to more severe arrhythmias such as ventricular tachycardia or fibrillation, mainly when someone has ischemia or a scarred heart. It is critical to use electrocardiography and advanced imaging to diagnose and manage these arrhythmias well. Conduction block arrhythmias can be caused by many things, for example, ischemia in the heart muscle, damage to the conduction tissues or inflammation. People with congenital heart defects, for example, Tetralogy of Fallot, can get arrhythmias from structural issues in the heart or due to problems after surgery. Studies suggest that many patients who die suddenly from heart disease have sustained ventricular arrhythmias caused by conduction problems, which stresses the importance of accurate risk assessment. Using signal-averaging ECG and MRI has been very important in identifying high-risk individuals.

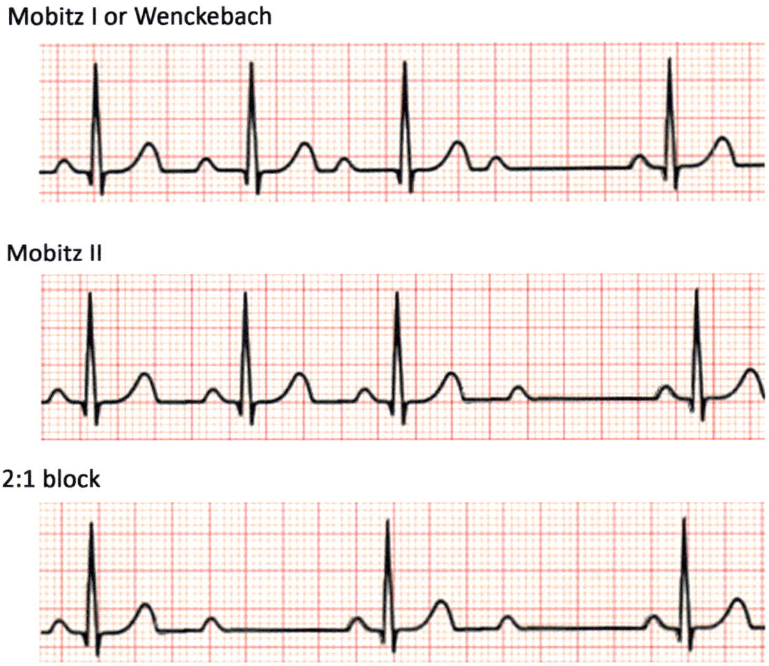

Figure 3.7. Electrocardiograms (ECGs) demonstrating forms of second-degree AV block.

Source: https://upload.wikimedia.org/wikipedia/commons/8/88/Second_degree_heart_block.png.

The results suggest that doctors should use a combination of patient records and advanced tests, such as electroanatomic mapping, to check for the risk of sudden cardiac events due to conduction blocks. The main goal of treatment for conduction block arrhythmias is to restore a normal heartbeat and heart function. A new way of treating arrhythmias is cryothermal ablation, which uses controlled energy to destroy only abnormal pathways and keep nearby conduction structures intact. Observations in the clinic show that cryothermal techniques improve safety during procedures by allowing doctors to see conduction immediately during the procedure. It has proven to be very useful for managing accessory pathways and atrioventricular nodal reentrant tachycardia. Due to the advancements in catheter designs and the flexibility of cryoablation, it is emerging as a viable alternative to radiofrequency ablation. Nevertheless, the complexity inherent to each patient's condition requires a tailored treatment plan, ensuring that the unique anatomical and electrophysiological landscape influences the selection of intervention techniques, contributing to successful outcomes in arrhythmia management (Daliento et al., 2005; Ponti et al., 2005) (Figure 3.7).

3.3. Pathophysiology of Arrhythmias

Pathophysiologically, arrhythmias are caused by the intricate interaction among structural, electrical, and molecular processes that disrupt the normal rhythm of the heart. At the cellular level, ion channel dysfunction, cellular excitability, and conduction velocity are often the root causes of these abnormalities. Changes in the function or expression of sodium, potassium, and calcium channels, for example, can lead to inappropriate automaticity or triggered activity that produces premature excitations or reentrant circuits. In addition, structural changes such as myocardial infarct or ischemia can form fibrotic regions that obstruct the electrical conduction and cause arrhythmogenesis. Scientific studies indicate that these pathophysiological phenomena may be particularly crucial in pulmonary hypertension, and right heart hypertrophy and dysfunction that can significantly alter electrophysiological properties and hence contribute to an enhanced vulnerability to arrhythmias (Abouzaid et al., 2024).

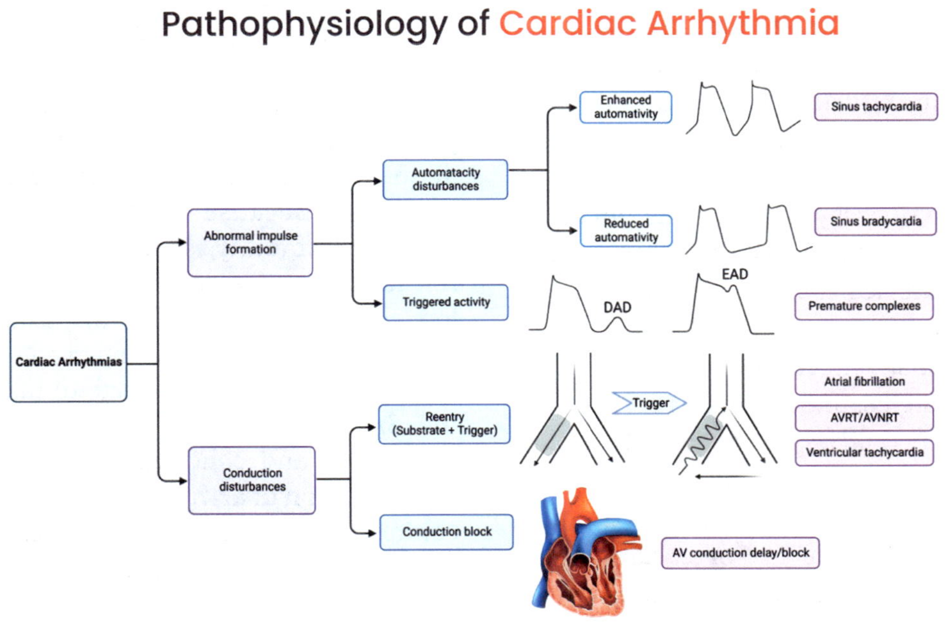

Figure 3.8. Pathophysiology of cardiac arrhythmia.

Source: https://sunfox.in/wp-content/uploads/2024/02/blog-image-3-1-02.jpg.

The clinical implications of these pathophysiological changes are enormous, since arrhythmias by themselves can be responsible for serious morbidity and mortality. For example, atrial fibrillation, the most common arrhythmia, is associated with an increased risk of stroke and heart failure. The deranged electrical impulses in the atria result in blood stasis and thrombus formation, hence highlighting the need for proper risk stratification and treatment interventions. Furthermore, ventricular arrhythmias that result from disturbances in ventricular repolarization or depolarization could lead to fatal occurrences like sudden cardiac arrest. Arrhythmias like these are exacerbated by factors like age and comorbidities, hence being hard to manage and requiring a broad familiarity with their mechanisms of action. This calls for a methodical approach to treating patients that addresses the electrical and structural elements causing cardiac arrhythmias (Nagpal et al., 2024). The occurrence of advanced diagnostic tools and therapeutic options has significantly advanced the treatment of arrhythmias induced by complex pathophysiological mechanisms. Techniques such as ECG monitoring, Holter monitoring, and electrophysiological studies are now an integral part in making an accurate diagnosis of the true nature of arrhythmia and its potential precipitating causes. Moreover, innovative therapeutic strategies, including antiarrhythmic drugs, catheter ablation, and device therapy in the form of ICDs, reflect the advancement of treatment paradigms. Understanding arrhythmia pathophysiology allows physicians to tailor such therapies even better, enhancing patient outcomes. By reconciling clinical expertise and continued research, the art of cardiology is well-positioned to drive treatment approaches for arrhythmias, thus effectively meeting the pressing needs posed by these complex disorders (Abouzaid et al., 2024) (Figure 3.8).

3.3.1. Mechanisms of Electrical Impulse Generation

Electrical impulses generated by the heart are necessary to keep the heartbeat regular. Most of this process happens in specialized groups of cells called pacemakers, which are the SA node, AV node, and Purkinje fibers. The SA node, located in the right atrium, serves as the primary pacemaker because it depolarizes faster than other cells, thereby setting the normal sinus rhythm. This intrinsic pacemaker is controlled by the levels of ions and by the autonomic nervous system. Abnormal electrical impulses outside the SA node or if they travel through the heart's conduction system in the wrong way, can cause different arrhythmias. Understanding these mechanisms of impulse generation is crucial for identifying and managing different types of rhythm disturbances, as they form the basis for the pathology underpinning various cardiac arrhythmias (Sampson, 2016). The movement of ions across the heart cell membranes is made possible by ion channels, which also help produce electrical impulses. When channels open and close, the membrane potential changes, which causes action potentials that are electrical impulses. Sodium, potassium, and calcium channels are essential in the different stages of the cardiac action potential. Because of this interaction, the heart's excitability, speed of conduction, and refractoriness are determined. A problem with ion channels can disrupt the usual electrical signals, which can result in ectopic beats when the ectopic pacemaker starts to take over from the SA node. These disruptions in impulse generation and conduction are pivotal in the manifestation of arrhythmias, creating a clinical context that necessitates further examination of the underlying mechanisms (Sampson, 2016). Advances in genetic and developmental biology point out that changes in gene expression can affect the electrical function of the heart. Changes in how ion channels and gap junction proteins are regulated can cause problems with the structure and function of the heart's electrical system. Genome-wide association studies point out that common genetic variants are linked to arrhythmia, proving that epigenetic changes can influence the health of the heart over time. Such issues may begin in childhood but only become noticeable as arrhythmias later, which shows why we should pay attention to both genetic and environmental factors. Understanding how impulses are generated in the heart is crucial for developing treatments that help patients with cardiac arrhythmias.

3.3.2. Factors Leading Dysfunction

Dysfunction within the cardiac conduction system (CCS) plays a central role in the generation of various arrhythmias, primarily as a result of dysfunction within the signal pathways to ensure expected propagation of the electrical impulse. One central cause of this dysfunction is the presence of blockages within internodal tracts (ITs), which are crucial for effective signal conduction from the sinoatrial node (SAN) to the left atrium and the atrioventricular node (AVN). Research has indicated that dysfunctional IT function can lead to atrial conduction block, a precursor to AF and other arrhythmias.

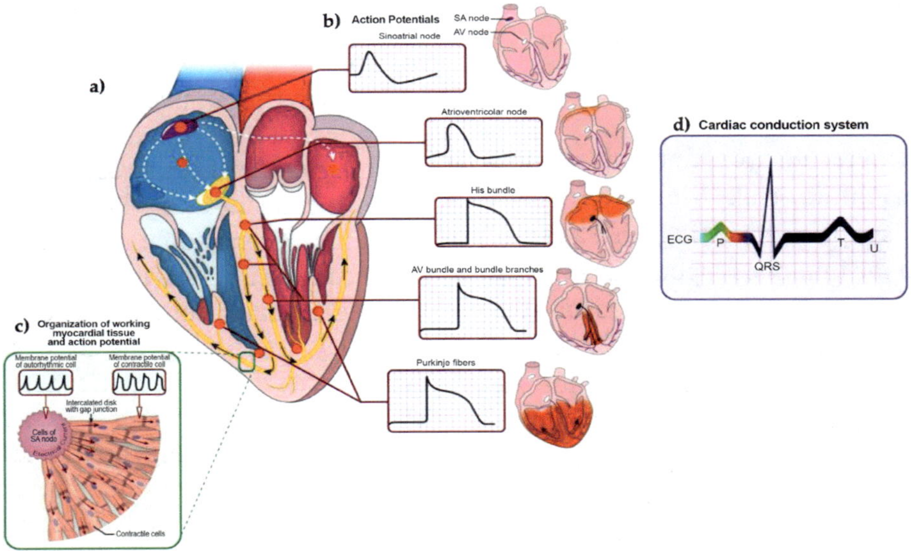

Figure 3.9. The cardiac conduction system (CCS). (a) The stations of the CCS and their typical action potential: sinoatrial node (SAN), atrioventricular node (AVN), His bundle, AV bundle and bundle branches, and, finally, Purkinje fibers; (b) Heart regions activated by the CCS electrophysiological activity during the cardiac cycle; (c) The working myocardium: architecture and action potential; and (d) Electrocardiogram (ECG) of a healthy subject.

Source: https://www.mdpi.com/cells/cells-10-03175/article_deploy/html/images/cells-10-03175-g001.png.

Further, morphogenesis of ITs is regulated by pivotal transcription factors such as NKX2.5 and TBX3, responsible for the formation and differentiation of these structures. An awareness of these mechanisms of development is a prerequisite to understanding the mechanisms behind the prevalence of cardiac rhythm disturbances and the pathogenesis of CCS disorders in general (Zhao et al., 2025). Immune mechanisms have likewise seemed to be critical elements of the mechanisms for altered conduction and resultant arrhythmias. Numbers of circulating leukocytes, such as lymphocytes, have been related to changes in cardiac conduction properties. According to recent studies, a 1-standard deviation increase in lymphocyte count has been associated with a significantly increased risk of atrioventricular block. Such association validates the complex relationship between immune status and cardiac function, suggesting that abnormal immune status has the potential to trigger or exacerbate cardiac conduction defects. Importantly, the association persists even after considering confounding variables by employing methods such as Mendelian randomization.

Thus, leukocyte function not only signals potential arrhythmia risk biomarkers but also provides scope for testing therapeutic interventions to the immune response as a means of limiting conduction disorders and associated risks (Chen et al., 2023). Having structural heart disease is also an essential factor for the altered conduction. These conditions, including myocardial ischemia, hypertrophy, and fibrosis, can disrupt the cardiac tissue architecture to create abnormal electrical conduction channels. Fibrotic tissue, for example, can replace normal myocardium, breaking the electrical continuity needed for a proper contraction sequence. This architectural alteration can allow regions of slow conduction or obstruction, which can result in tachycardias or fibrillation in susceptible subjects. Moreover, lifestyle and aging play a role in cardiac tissue remodeling. With our exploration of the multifactorial causes of altered conduction, the need for explicit prevention and management techniques is apparent, illustrating the need for intervention not only at the electrical and structural heart levels but also to treat arrhythmias properly (Zhao et al., 2025) (Figure 3.9).

3.3.3. Role of Ischemia and Infarction

The role of infarction and ischemia in the pathogenesis of cardiac arrhythmias is of crucial significance since both states comprise an environment conducive to electrical disturbance of the heart. Ischemia, a state of reduced cardiac tissue perfusion, creates a state of oxygen insufficiency. This environment is the substrate of metabolic disturbances and disorders, e.g., the generation of reactive oxygen species (ROS), which may directly affect cardiac myocytes' electrical stability. The injury that occurs during ischemia alters ion channel function and disrupts regular action potential conduction, increasing tachyarrhythmia predisposition. Myocardial infarction, therefore, manifests as a focal process where severe ischemia results in necrosis of the tissue, increasing arrhythmic danger and making the clinical scenario following myocardial injury more complex. Following myocardial infarction, there are many cellular processes that come into play, increasing the arrhythmogenic risk even further. The necrotic tissue is besieged by inflammatory processes, which bring about electrical remodeling in the form of altered conduction pathways and diminution in impulse propagation. Additionally, scarring at the time of healing distorts the heart's structural integrity, transforming erstwhile cohesive myocardial architecture into reentry loop areas. Intriguingly, this remodeling process is accompanied by the entry of calcium and sodium, facilitating aberrant depolarizations that could trigger rapidly fatal arrhythmias. Tracking such events emphasizes the subtle interplay between ischemic injury and arrhythmia generation, emphasizing the pathophysiologic alterations that support acute coronary syndromes for which specific therapeutic interventions are required to modulate arrhythmic risks. Modulation of key signaling pathways engaged in ischemia-reperfusion has been proven, by various studies, to modulate the incidence of arrhythmias effectively. Specifically, L-type blockade of calcium channels, as proven in pharmacologic models by the use of compounds like nifedipine and verapamil, has been demonstrated to be helpful in reducing arrhythmic activity after infarction, highlighting the very significance of calcium entry towards electrical stability in cardiomyocytes (Tallo et al., 2023).

Conversely, attempts to counteract oxidative stress through the utilization of antioxidants like N-acetylcysteine have remained inconclusive, an indication that oxidative events are contributory to reperfusion arrhythmogenesis while systemic intervention might be unable to address the multidimensional nature of arrhythmia formation (Hansen et al., 2023). These findings indicate that comprehension of ischemic processes in more than one dimension is required to advance therapeutic interventions towards addressing the high prevalence of arrhythmias coupled with myocardial infarction.

3.4. Risk Factors for Cardiac Arrhythmias

Obesity, being so common nowadays, is linked to many cardiac problems, including arrhythmias. Having obesity can cause heart diseases such as high blood pressure and heart failure, which are related to arrhythmias. The main reasons are insulin resistance, oxidative stress, and inflammation, which cause the heart to change in harmful ways. For example, these processes cause the left ventricle to change shape and may affect its ability to relax properly, which in turn makes the heart more likely to have arrhythmias. Also, if a person has cardiometabolic risk factors such as dyslipidemia and diabetes, the risk of heart disease increases even more. Thus, addressing obesity through lifestyle modifications and therapeutic interventions is crucial in mitigating the likelihood of arrhythmias and improving overall cardiac health in affected individuals (Gutiérrez-Cuevas et al., 2024). Another significant risk factor for cardiac arrhythmias is the existence of chronic cardiovascular conditions, such as coronary artery disease (CAD) and heart failure. When these conditions are present, the heart's structure and electrical activity may be altered, which increases the risk of arrhythmia.

For example, scar tissue can be caused by ischemic heart disease, and this can disrupt the heart's usual electrical pathways, which increases the risk of tachyarrhythmias and fibrillation. Heart failure also leads to changes in hormones and increases pressure in the atrium, which can directly cause atrial fibrillation, a common type of arrhythmia. Consequently, careful management of chronic cardiovascular conditions, through both pharmacological and non-pharmacological treatments, remains a priority in minimizing arrhythmic risk in this population (Shlobin et al., 2024). Studies are now focusing on how genes contribute to someone's risk of cardiac arrhythmias. Genetic mutations may increase a person's risk of Long QT Syndrome or Brugada Syndrome, and these can cause serious problems without any warning signs. Recent studies have shown that seizures and sudden cardiac death share genetic links which makes it harder to assess the risk of arrhythmias. Genetic testing is now a meaningful way to find out the risk levels of patients, especially those who have a family history of sudden cardiac or arrhythmic events. As the understanding of genetic contributions to arrhythmic phenomena advances, it is essential to incorporate these insights into comprehensive risk stratification and management strategies for better outcomes in at-risk individuals (Gutiérrez-Cuevas et al., 2024; Shlobin et al., 2024) (Figure 3.10).

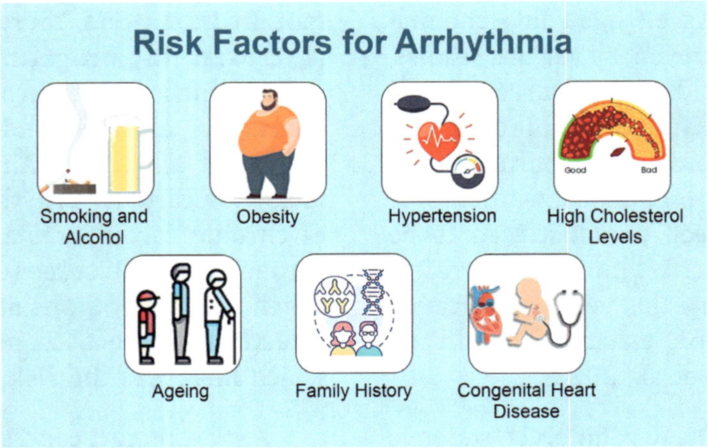

Figure 3.10. Risk factors for cardiac arrhythmia.

Source: https://cdn.hexahealth.com/Image/1726051904027-428208697.webp.

3.4.1. Genetic Predispositions

Genetic predispositions are used directly in the causation of cardiac arrhythmias, which are characterized by irregular rhythms of the heart. The arrhythmias can be caused by many genetic determinants that influence the electrical characteristics of cardiac cells. It has been studied that specific genetic mutations can disrupt the ion channels that aid in maintaining the rhythmic contractions of the heart and thus cause such conditions as Long QT Syndrome and Brugada Syndrome. All of these conditions illustrate the complex interaction among genetic factors and arrhythmogenic processes predisposing patients to a high risk of sudden cardiac events. Furthermore, early detection of high-risk patients and the implementation of preventive measures, which might lower the risk of fatal arrhythmias, depend on knowledge of these genetic predispositions (Reemtsen et al., 2017). The etiology of congenital heart defects (CHDs) being multifactorial once again highlights the intricate relationship between cardiac arrhythmias and genetics. CHDs occur in approximately 1% of live births and make them susceptible to arrhythmic presentations later in life. The etiology of these defects is contributed to by genetic as well as epigenetic factors, which makes our comprehension of the etiologies of CHDs and their associated arrhythmias more complex. Even with the continuing developments in diagnostic methods, most patients are still undiagnosed as to the precise genetic mutations that are causing their diseases. Targeted treatments based on these genetic variants would be a paradigm shift in treatment, improving quality of life and reducing complications associated with both CHDs and their potential arrhythmias. Hence, systematic approaches integrating molecular and phenotypic data are critical in building up knowledge and therapy of such conditions (Duplaga et al., 2024). In examining the broader ramifications of genetic susceptibility to cardiac health, the role of artificial intelligence (AI) becomes increasingly important. Artificial intelligence built into medical diagnostics holds the potential for refining risk stratification techniques, thus enabling early identification of at-risk individuals for cardiovascular diseases, such as arrhythmias. Through analysis of large data sets that include genomic information, AI can tailor treatment regimens to the individual patient profile, ensuring enhanced therapeutic efficacy and safety. Not only does the new approach provide clinicians with live data, but it also enhances our capacity to unravel how genetics are involved in arrhythmia mechanisms. Thus, the application of AI in precision medicine is a pivotal field in the management of cardiac arrhythmias, with the vision to improve overall patient outcomes with individualized care strategies (Duplaga et al., 2024).

3.4.2. Lifestyle Factors (Diet, Exercise, etc.)

When looking at how cardiac arrhythmias happen, what we eat and how much we exercise are very important for our heart health. A healthy diet rich in nutrients can support the heart and lower the chances of arrhythmias. Eating foods rich in omega-3 fatty acids, antioxidants, and fiber has been linked to less inflammation and better stability of the heart muscle's electrical system. Eating a lot of saturated fats and sugar can result in obesity and hypertension, which are both linked to arrhythmias. The intricate interplay between dietary choices and cardiac health underscores the importance of nutritional awareness in formulating preventive strategies against arrhythmogenic conditions, thereby promoting optimal heart rhythm and function (Kitsiou et al., 2013). Exercise is a key part of a lifestyle that can influence cardiac rhythm. Staying physically active regularly improves cardiovascular fitness, which is necessary for a steady heartbeat. Regular exercise helps the autonomic nervous system regulate itself, so there is a good balance between the sympathetic and parasympathetic parts, which is vital for controlling heart rate. In addition, aerobic exercises work well with a proper diet, helping to manage weight and decrease visceral fat, which both help decrease the chances of arrhythmias. Physical activity not only fosters resilience against various cardiovascular diseases but also directly influences the electrophysiological properties of the heart, ultimately supporting the maintenance of a healthy cardiac rhythm (Mattioli et al., 2011). Taking care of diet and physical activity together gives a broader approach to lowering the chances of cardiac arrhythmias. Using both nutritional advice and exercise plans together can explain to people how their decisions affect their heart. If people eat more whole foods and less processed food and are encouraged to exercise often, it can be very helpful. Making these changes in lifestyle reduces the risk of arrhythmias and also improves overall heart health, showing how much lifestyle plays a role in cardiac electrophysiology. As such, prioritizing these factors is imperative in the prevention and management of cardiac arrhythmias within at-risk populations (Kitsiou et al., 2013) (Figure 3.11).

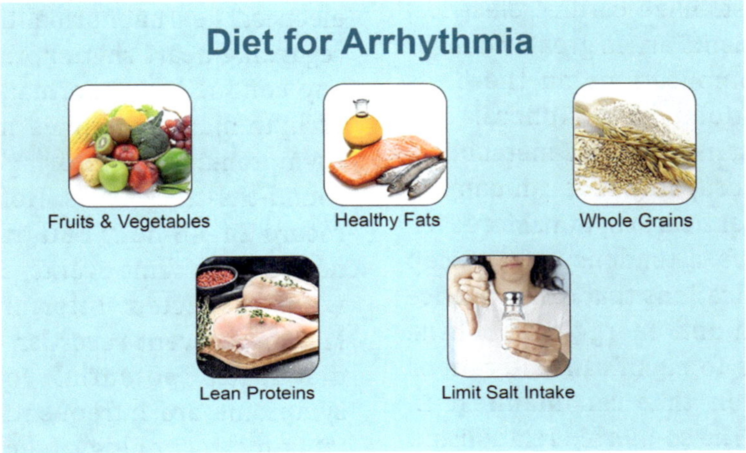

Figure 3.11. Diet of arrhythmia.

Source: https://cdn.hexahealth.com/Image/1726052700434-277738696.webp.

3.4.3. Comorbid Conditions (Hypertension, Diabetes)

The coexistence of comorbidities such as hypertension and diabetes significantly impacts the cardiac arrhythmia mechanisms. Hypertension, as characterized by elevated blood pressure, is capable of inducing structural and electrical remodeling of the heart and thereby triggering arrhythmias. Chronic high blood pressure is associated with left ventricular hypertrophy, which alters the myocardial terrain so that it is vulnerable to arrhythmic events. This remodeling has the potential to disrupt normal electrical conduction patterns and cause situations where arrhythmias, such as atrial fibrillation or ventricular tachycardia, are more likely to occur. Also, hypertensive patients often show different biochemical changes, such as increased sympathetic nervous activity, which will increase arrhythmogenic potential. Therefore, understanding the role of hypertension is essential to take care of patients with a tendency to develop cardiac arrhythmias. Diabetes mellitus is another common comorbidity that complicates the clinical picture of cardiac arrhythmias due to its multifactorial effect on cardiovascular health. Diabetes is associated with a heightened state of inflammation and oxidative stress, which, in turn, can further destabilize cardiac electrical stability. Diabetic patients are in greater danger of cardiovascular complications on the basis primarily of alterations in peripheral and central vascular resistance, glucose metabolism disturbances, and neuropathy that can damage autonomic control over heart rhythm. Moreover, diabetic patients have a tendency to develop microvascular complications that can influence myocardial perfusion and energy metabolism. This ultimately leads to significant alterations in cardiac conduction that can manifest in various arrhythmias. The co-morbid relationship between diabetes and arrhythmias shows the necessity for an integrated policy of management, particularly if such co-morbid conditions occur. The interaction between hypertension and diabetes makes their consolidated effect on cardiac arrhythmias necessitate thorough clinical evaluation. It has been revealed that patients with any two of these conditions are at increased risk of experiencing major arrhythmic events and need a more profound insight into pathophysiological processes. As quoted in literature, comorbidities also enhance unfavorable outcomes for cardiovascular disease, indicating the extreme complexity of treating patients with such sickness (Jakovljević et al., 2009). Even more so, the enhanced vulnerability of arrhythmias with diabetes is augmented by its effect on the autonomic nervous system, tending to manifest differential heart rate regulation (Alyari et al., 2020). This identification is critical to healthcare professionals in the adjustment of effective interventions that encompass diabetes and hypertension, thereby reducing morbidities and mortalities of arrhythmia among patients.

3.5. Diagnostic Techniques

Diagnosis of cardiac arrhythmias is complex and demands a range of advanced diagnostic tests. ECG remains a baseline in identifying electrical heart abnormalities. It offers evidence regarding heart rhythm, rate, and frequency of any conduction abnormalities. However, since arrhythmias sometimes may be transient or asymptomatic, monitoring might be done on a round-the-clock basis. Holter monitors, which record 24–48-hour ECG tracings, enable one to detect these faint events, especially in patients with suspected intermittent arrhythmias. Moreover, event recorder utilization increases diagnostic potential for patients whose symptoms are infrequent. More sophisticated imaging technology, such as transthoracic and transesophageal echocardiography, also helps to evaluate structural heart disease, potentially inducing arrhythmias. These imaging modalities are essential to obtain detailed clinical information that guides further management plans. With the latest advances in cardiac imaging, the detection of arrhythmias and their cause in the early stages has been significantly facilitated. Magnetic resonance imaging (MRI) with T1 and T2 mapping is an emerging diagnostic tool, facilitating accurate visualization of myocardial tissue characteristics. This imaging technique is of particular interest in diseases like Fabry disease, where early detection of cardiac dysfunction is paramount to patient prognosis. Cardiac MRI can detect features such as myocardial inflammation and fibrosis, which are significant in the arrhythmogenic pathophysiology. These imaging modalities can also risk-stratify patients based on arrhythmia, and this will aid focused therapeutic interventions.

As diagnostic methods continue to advance, integration of imaging with more traditional techniques might enhance prognostication and overall care of arrhythmias. Added to these tests is the recognition of electrocardiographic markers of cardiac impending instability. For instance, detection of QT interval prolongation and T-wave alternans (TWA) occurrence are ever-greater determinants of risk stratification for ventricular arrhythmias. The association between chronic kidney disease (CKD) and the prevalence of such markers emphasizes careful assessments among vulnerable populations.

The evidence suggests that CKD patients are prone to electrical instability, leading to arrhythmia and sudden cardiac death (SCD). Therefore, convergence of ECG results with clinical assessments is crucial in enhancing early detection and intervention efforts. With increasing understanding of these correlations, there will be an increasing need for individually specific diagnostic approaches about the risk factors of the patient to allow enhanced prognostic stratification and targeted management to counterbalance the impact of cardiac arrhythmias (Figure 3.12).

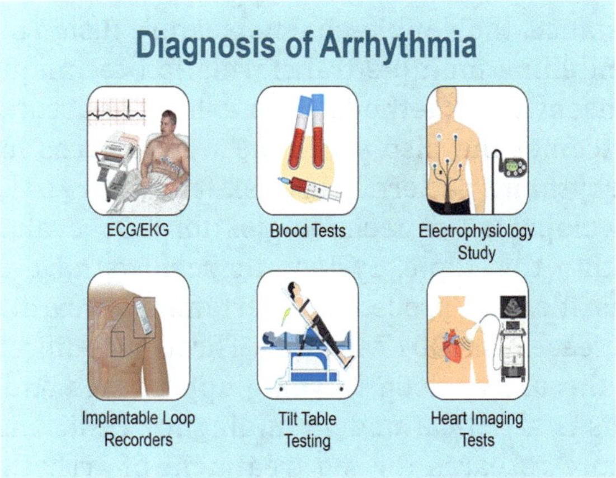

Figure 3.12. Diagnosis of arrhythmia.

Source: https://cdn.hexahealth.com/Image/1726052185895-615262719.webp.

3.5.1. Electrocardiogram (ECG)

ECG is a simple diagnostic and management tool applied in the assessment of cardiac arrhythmias that gives critical information about the electrical activity of the heart. Through tracing the electrical impulses that govern heartbeats, the ECG allows clinicians to identify abnormal heart functions and rhythms. Each component of the ECG waveform — the P wave, QRS complex, and T wave — correlates with specific electrical phases of the cardiac cycle. Thus, irregularities in these stages may be indicative of various types of arrhythmias, such as atrial fibrillation, ventricular tachycardia, or flutter. The contribution of ECG to arrhythmia detection is emphasized through improvements in signal processing and analysis algorithms that enhance the accuracy of diagnosis, thus enabling timely interventions to prevent disastrous cardiac events (Wang et al., 2025). Recent improvements in ECG technology and analysis have made a significant impact on the accuracy of arrhythmia classification. Through the incorporation of deep learning algorithms in the interpretation of ECG, researchers are working on advanced methods that further improve the capacity to recognize arrhythmias from ECG signals automatically. The methods utilize intricate feature extraction processes to assess the data better, isolating the appropriate indicators that more conventional methods might miss. For instance, the double-channel feature fusion strategy demonstrated in the present study depicts how combining multiple transformation techniques can yield better classification results compared to conventional methods. This enhanced accuracy in ECG analysis not only guarantees better patient outcomes but also paves the way towards individualized care strategies aligned with a particular arrhythmic pattern (Vásquez-Iturralde et al., 2024). Additionally, literary research indicating the development of technologies for ECG evaluation reiterates the ongoing validity of investigation within this topic. Systematic reviews have documented the establishment of new detection and classification procedures pertaining to cardiac arrhythmias with a focus on the technological pace increase from 2017 to 2023. Through comprehensive bibliometric analysis, research indicates trends in the use of deep learning approaches and their performance in enhancing ECG interpretation. This is a critical understanding for clinicians and researchers alike, as they can use this to direct future research for the treatment of arrhythmia. Finally, the overlap of new ECG techniques only serves to reinforce the necessity for continued innovation in detecting cardiac arrhythmias so that healthcare practitioners are offered the most suitable means to treat patients (Vásquez-Iturralde et al., 2024) (Figure 3.13).

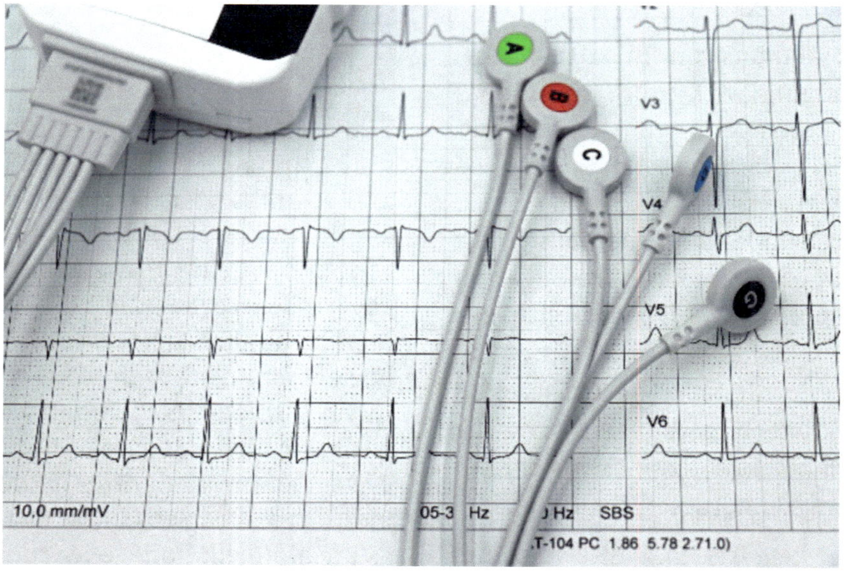

Figure 3.13. Electrocardiogram (ECG).

Source: https://heartrhythmcardiologist.com/wp-content/uploads/2024/12/pexels-martabranco-28585011-scaled.jpg.

3.5.2. Holter Monitoring

Holter monitoring is now an essential diagnostic test for the evaluation of cardiac arrhythmias, capable of capturing the complexities of cardiac rhythm over several hours. Unlike non-invasive ECGs that provide a snapshot of cardiac function, Holter monitors enable ongoing recording of the electrical activity of the heart for a mean of 24–48 hours. The prolonged monitoring is essential since most arrhythmias are transient and cannot be diagnosed within short clinic periods. The data obtained by Holter monitoring can provide valuable information about the variability of heart rate, rhythm abnormalities, and the detection of asymptomatic events, thereby providing valuable information to clinicians in diagnosing conditions not apparent on standard testing methods. Thus, Holter monitoring plays a significant role in the comprehensive evaluation of patients presenting to the clinic with arrhythmia-probability syndrome. Understanding Holter monitor data requires a broad understanding of its implications in the diagnosis of cardiac arrhythmias. Review of the recorded data can reveal arrhythmogenic rhythms such as atrial fibrillation, premature ventricular contractions, or other prominent electrical abnormalities. According to current guidelines, the integration of Holter monitoring data into clinical practice supports healthcare providers in developing tailored management strategies for patients' individualized arrhythmic settings. This is a practice that cannot be ignored, particularly when examining the mechanisms of the arrhythmias in question. The discovery of these mechanisms makes it easier to establish the most appropriate therapeutic interventions, ranging from lifestyle modifications to the initiation of advanced interventions such as catheter ablation or pharmacotherapy initiation, thereby maximizing patient outcomes. Furthermore, the use of Holter monitoring is not without its challenges. While improving diagnostic accuracy significantly, the technology also demands attention to a variety of factors influencing data reliability. Patient adherence and susceptibility to movement or interference artifacts may affect the reliability of the recordings. The ESC guidelines include consideration of clinical judgment in interpreting Holter data, but according to recommendations from relevant public health authorities. Health care professionals are thus called upon to integrate Holter monitoring findings with other testing, such as echocardiography and laboratory studies, to gain an integrated understanding of each patient's cardiac status. By understanding this complexity, clinicians can optimize treatment algorithms for patients undergoing testing for cardiac arrhythmias, underscoring the irreplaceable role of Holter monitoring in contemporary cardiology (Priori et al., 2015; Cosentino et al., 2019) (Figure 3.14).

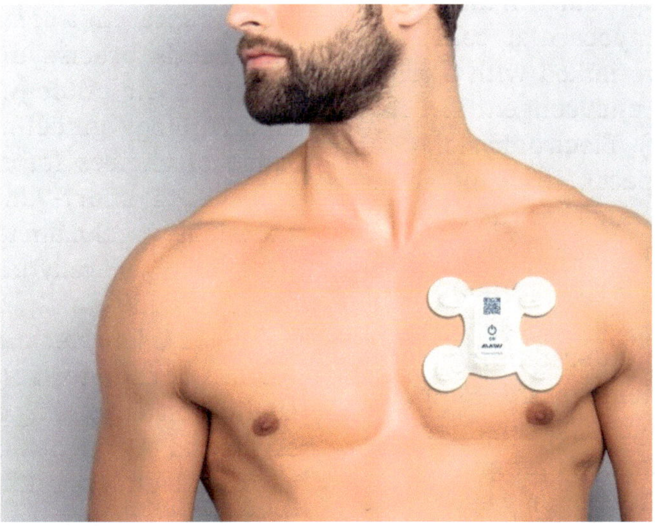

Figure 3.14. Holter monitoring.

Source: https://img1.wsimg.com/isteam/ip/d0573bb0-6d0b-4b25-973d-7bf7ee947dfb/F9258275-D6E4-49A4-A39D-BC11F6DB992B.jpeg/:/cr=t:0%25,l:0%25,w:100%25,h:100%25/rs=w:1280.

3.5.3. Electrophysiological Studies

Electrophysiological studies have a key place in the explanation of cardiac arrhythmias, and they are of significant concern in the knowledge of cardiac electrical activity. Using such techniques as intracardiac electrogram recordings and electrophysiological mapping non-invasively, investigators can identify aberrant electrical conduction pathways within the myocardium that result in arrhythmias. These experiments allow one to quantify conduction velocity, refractory periods, and autonomic modulation of cardiac rhythm, all relevant to understanding how dysregulation leads to arrhythmogenic foci. They also allow the quantification of both mechanical and electrical properties of cardiac tissue, reconciling structural abnormalities and functional disturbances. The complex analysis of electrophysiological properties eventually enhances the risk stratification of patients, guiding the selection of appropriate therapeutic interventions based on individual needs. Involvement of cellular mechanisms in arrhythmogenesis is also elucidated by electrophysiological studies with key proteins such as the Ryanodine receptor 2 (RyR2). This protein is of particular importance in the release of calcium ions from myocardial cells, and RYR2 gene mutations are linked with a range of cardiac arrhythmias and congenital heart disease (Lv et al., 2025). Electrophysiological studies can reveal the impact of these mutations on calcium handling, such as alterations in trigger mechanisms for arrhythmias such as catecholaminergic polymorphic ventricular tachycardia (CPVT) and long QT syndrome (LQTS). By understanding these molecular processes, scientists are equipping doctors with knowledge that enables the development of individualized therapies. Thus, electrophysiological studies not only educate us about arrhythmia mechanisms but also inspire new prevention and treatment approaches. In addition to elucidating genetic etiologies of cardiac arrhythmias, electrophysiological studies are instrumental in determining treatment possibilities. Various therapeutic modalities, including drug interventions and catheter ablation, are compared in terms of how they correct arrhythmias based on electrophysiological information (Nagpal et al., 2024). These studies allow real-time examination of arrhythmic events and thus promote refinement in ablation technique methods and patient results. They are also helpful in the identification of patients who would be candidates for devices such as pacemakers or defibrillators, particularly in the presence of autonomic dysregulation. As continuous advances in monitoring and imaging modalities improve, the role of electrophysiological studies in clinical practice remains of utmost significance in an effort to effectively handle cardiac arrhythmias and improve patient care.

3.6. Treatment Options

In approaching the treatment of cardiac arrhythmias, it is necessary to distinguish between various types of arrhythmias and mechanisms. Supraventricular tachycardias (SVTs) represent a common form of arrhythmia that needs precise diagnostic evaluation to identify their etiology. The European Society of Cardiology guidelines of 2019 highlight a range of choices for successful treatment of SVTs, both short- and long-term. In acute situations, vagal maneuvers or pharmacological agents are generally utilized to restore normal rhythm. Additionally, according to Sychov et al. (2022), long-term treatment may include the use of catheter ablation or antiarrhythmic medication, depending on the individual's illness status and overall health profile.. Consequently, a general understanding of the arrhythmia's mechanisms determines the selection of effective treatment. Management of arrhythmias caused by underlying conditions, particularly during the COVID-19 pandemic, has gained increased attention due to the complexity. Available evidences show that cardiac arrhythmias such as atrial fibrillation and ventricular tachycardia are prevalent among COVID-19 patients, with different management strategies based on severity and patient needs. Treatment in these instances typically consists of repletion of electrolytes, which remedies potential imbalances augmented by the viral infection, and discontinuation of medications that will contribute to arrhythmogenic risk. Additionally, preserving overall volume status and reducing catecholamine bursts are important interventions to manage heart rhythm changes in COVID-19 patients, as discussed in Mohamed et al. (2022). This interdisciplinary approach stresses the importance of positioning treatment options within the context of the patient's overall state of global health. Long-term management of cardiac arrhythmias might involve a course of lifestyle modification and therapeutic treatment to reduce recurrence risk and enhance patient quality of life. Regular monitoring and adjustment of treatment protocols are essential to the success of optimal outcomes in patients with chronic arrhythmias. Patient education for the recognition of arrhythmia symptoms can also empower the patient to report earlier for intervention, thus preventing potential complications. In patients who are resistant to pharmacologic management, electrophysiological studies can provide access to more advanced interventions like catheter ablation, which has become more effective in restoring sinus rhythm. Lastly, treatment protocol development, as embodied by existing guidelines, aims to tailor management strategies for varying patient populations, agreeing with the applicability of personalized strategies in cardiac arrhythmia treatment, as highlighted by Mohamed et al. (2022); Sychov et al. (2022) (Figure 3.15).

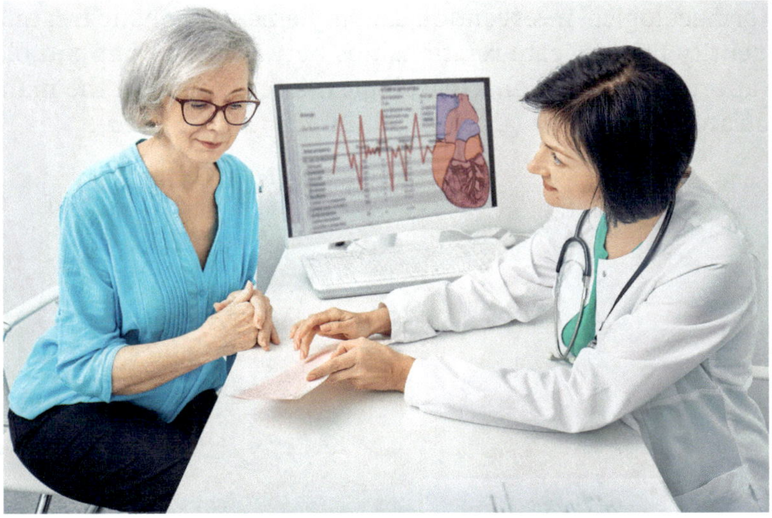

Figure 3.15. Treatment of cardiac arrhythmias.

Source: https://www.harleystreet.sg/img/arrhythmia.webp.

3.6.1. Pharmacological Interventions

Pharmacologic management is of vital significance in the management of cardiac arrhythmias, both the etiology and symptoms of these abnormal electrical heart rhythms. Anti-arrhythmic drug research has centered on the restoration of normal heart electrical conduction, and such drugs are usually categorized into several classes based on their mechanism of action. Class I agents, which block sodium channels, reduce depolarization rates and are also used routinely to treat conditions such as atrial fibrillation. Class II beta-blockers similarly inhibit adrenergic action and are protective against tachyarrhythmias. This multidimensional strategy highlights the need for individualized treatment protocols since a range of arrhythmias may be optimally treated by specific pharmacologic agents, particularly with respect to the complex interactions of pathologic factors that govern arrhythmic mechanisms. Emerging evidence has underlined the imperative to clarify cellular and molecular mechanisms underlying cardiac arrhythmias to optimize drug treatments. Age-related changes in cardiac function, including mitochondrial dysfunction, are increasingly recognized as contributory factors in the arrhythmogenicity of aging. Pharmacological therapies targeting the reversal of mitochondrial dysfunction hold potentially promising results in countering arrhythmic risk. For example, therapies that try to lower myocardial energetics and improve cellular calcium homeostasis might provide novel avenues for intervention. By targeting upstream mechanisms rather than merely downstream effects, such approaches have the potential to lead to more effective anti-arrhythmic therapy that addresses the etiology of arrhythmias rather than merely symptomatically treating them, thereby contributing to better patient outcomes and quality of life (Saadeh et al., 2021). In addition, the interaction between nonalcoholic fatty liver disease (NAFLD) and cardiovascular illness significantly hinders pharmacologic treatment of arrhythmias. NAFLD has been associated with a wide range of cardiovascular comorbidities, including arrhythmias, through the mediation of metabolic syndrome and cardiac remodeling. Due to this relationship, pharmacologic agents aimed at NAFLD also have a beneficial impact on the arrhythmic aftermath. Current research on potential drug targets against NAFLD and cardiovascular complications is crucial. A combination of lifestyle modification with pharmacological intervention can implement a holistic treatment paradigm. Thus, it becomes easy to identify the intricate relationships between different pathological conditions to adopt an integrated approach toward pharmacological intervention in the management of cardiac arrhythmia and associated conditions (Chen et al., 2022) (Figure 3.16).

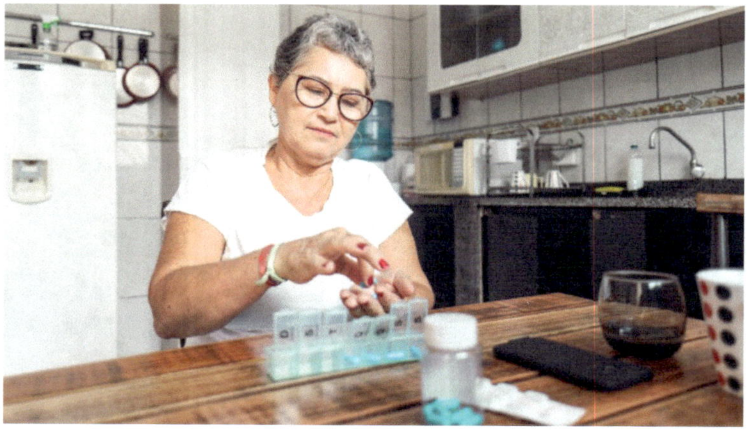

Figure 3.16. Arrhythmia drugs.

Source: https://post.healthline.com/wp-content/uploads/2021/02/Senior-woman-putting-medications-in-a-daily-pill-organize-1296x728-header.jpg.

3.6.2. Non-Pharmacological Therapies (e.g., Ablation)

Non-drug interventions have become indispensable components in the treatment of cardiac arrhythmias, particularly where traditional drug therapy fails or is unsuitable in patients. Among these interventions, catheter ablation stands out in its specialized approach to treating arrhythmias by stopping defective electrical pathways within the heart. The procedure typically involves the application of radiofrequency energy, generating heat, to destroy tissue responsible for abnormal electrical conduction. These focused interventions can significantly improve patient outcomes, decrease symptoms, and lower the demand for antiarrhythmic medication. Furthermore, the study indicates that success rates for procedures are often higher for conditions such as atrial fibrillation than with drug therapy alone, which helps to demonstrate its position as a key element of modern arrhythmia treatment pathways (Birză et al., 2025).

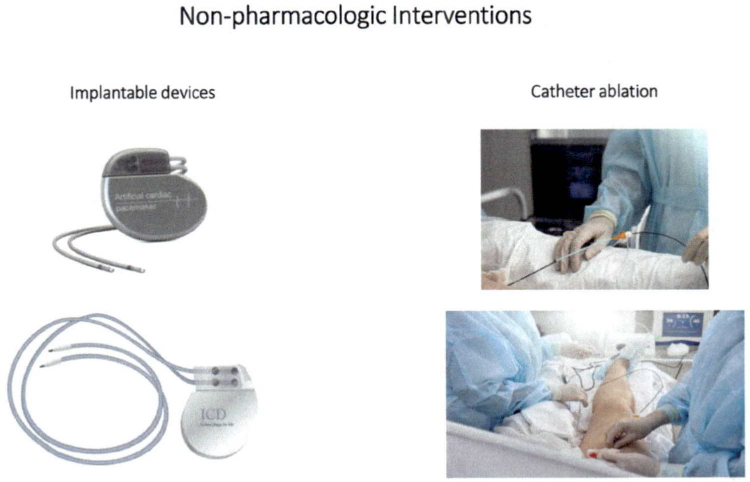

Figure 3.17. Non-pharmacologic interventions: implantable devices and catheter ablation.

Source: https://www.mdpi.com/pharmaceuticals/pharmaceuticals-16-00844/article_deploy/html/images/pharmaceuticals-16-00844-g001.png.

Incorporation of non-pharmacologic treatment modalities into cardiac arrhythmia management is further supported by evidence linking conditions such as obstructive sleep apnea (OSA) with increased arrhythmic events. OSA has the potential to induce sudden fluctuations in intrathoracic pressure as well as oxygenation aberrations, which directly lead to ventricular arrhythmias that make treatment a success (Nagpal et al., 2024). Therapy of OSA with CPAP therapy or changes in behavior also enhances the efficacy of other non-pharmacologic therapies, including catheter ablation. Emerging evidence indicates that patients with sleep apnea treated with CPAP could have improved maintenance of sinus rhythm following ablation, emphasizing the importance of a multi-treatment strategy that includes screening and comorbidity control for optimal arrhythmia therapy (Birză et al., 2025). Besides catheter ablation, emerging non-pharmacological therapies for cardiac arrhythmia are also under research to enhance patient outcomes. Transcatheter electrical cardioversion and the employment of implantable devices like leadless pacemakers and subcutaneous ICDs are key developments in this sector. These devices provide real-time monitoring and can deliver optimal therapies for arrhythmias detected, reducing the risk of complications from more invasive therapies. New therapies, including gene therapy and enhanced electrophysiological mapping, have the potential to further simplify treatment paradigms by making personalized, directed therapies available in the treatment of arrhythmia. Overall, non-pharmacological therapy development is significant in the management of the complex mechanisms of cardiac arrhythmias and improving patient outcomes (Nagpal et al., 2024) (Figure 3.17).

3.6.3. Lifestyle Modifications and Management

Adjustment and control of lifestyle are also significant in avoiding the risk of cardiac arrhythmias, which have a tendency to be provoked or aggravated by certain lifestyle factors. Dietary modification is part of these changes. Consumption of a diet that is heart-healthy with high fruit, vegetable, whole grain, and omega-3 fatty acid intake has been associated with a healthy cardiovascular profile and can reduce the frequency of arrhythmias. Moreover, a maintained healthy body weight also afforded by an equilibrated diet can eliminate obesity-related complications that predispose to cardiac conditions. Additionally, decreasing sodium intake will lower blood pressure levels and, thereby, reduce the heart's workload and the risk of arrhythmias.

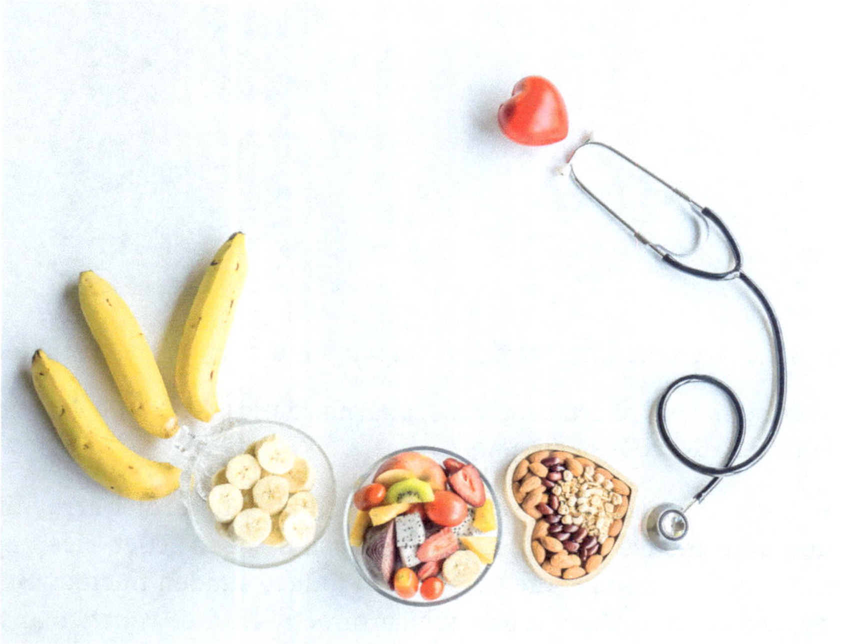

Figure 3.18. Lifestyle modifications for managing arrhythmia.

Source: https://www.harleystreet.sg/img/lifestyle-modifications-for-managing-arrhythmia.webp.

These dietary modifications underscore the importance of nutrition to cardiac health and are a central strategy for the management of arrhythmias. Regular exercise is another built-in way of life modification that can significantly impact the mechanisms of cardiac arrhythmia. Routine aerobic exercise benefits cardiovascular health, reduces stress, and improves overall heart function. Studies demonstrate that moderate exercise strengthens the heart's electrical conduction pathways and may reduce the incidence of atrial fibrillation, a common arrhythmia. Furthermore, exercise promotes weight control and helps with lower blood pressure levels and enhanced lipid profiles, all of which are closely associated with the risk of arrhythmia. It is essential, nonetheless, to personalize exercise programs for each patient, particularly those who have underlying cardiovascular disease. By encouraging patients to engage in physical exercise, healthcare providers can help patients become more active players in their management of arrhythmia as well as overall health. Stress reduction methods also play a significant role in lifestyle modification for reducing cardiac arrhythmias. Chronic stress has been identified as a risk factor for heart disease and can initiate deterioration of arrhythmias through mechanisms such as augmented adrenergic stimulation and inflammation. Therefore, implementation of stress reduction practices such as mindfulness, yoga, and cognitive-behavioral therapy may have beneficial effects on cardiac wellness. Further, having a consistent sleep pattern is critical, as disturbance in sleep has been implicated in arrhythmia development. By treating both psychological and physiological causes of stress, the cardiovascular system is enriched, building a strong foundation to handle cardiac arrhythmias effectively. An interdisciplinary strategy emphasizing lifestyle changes, such as diet, physical activity, and stress control, is essential in reducing the occurrence and severity of these frequently disabling conditions and ultimately improves patient outcomes (Figure 3.18).

SUMMARY

Finally, the intricate mechanisms of cardiac arrhythmias underscore the intricacies of cardiovascular pathophysiology. Various factors contribute to the development and evolution of these arrhythmias, including structural, electrical, and molecular changes in the heart. Significantly, the contribution of cardiac fibrosis to arrhythmias cannot be overstated. Evidence indicates that interstitial fibrosis is particularly prevalent in HFpEF patients, for whom it is a significant contributor to diastolic dysfunction and increased arrhythmic events. Therapeutic efforts to treat cardiac fibrosis have been successful, but the search for effective antifibrotic therapies has been an elusive challenge that has met with limited success in clinical trials (Sweeney et al., 2020). Secondarily, it is essential to realize that myocardial damage, more commonly from underlying cardiovascular disease, can increase the severity and incidence of arrhythmias. Recent studies confirm an in-depth relationship between myocardial damage, as evidenced by elevated troponin levels, and adverse outcomes in patients who have other cardiovascular comorbidities, particularly in contexts like COVID-19 (Guo et al., 2020). This foreboding correlation highlights the need for more sophisticated management strategies that remedy not only arrhythmias but also the prevention of myocardial damage and fibrosis. Therefore, enhancing our understanding of these complex processes can potentially provide a gateway to more effective therapeutic interventions and improved clinical outcomes. Lastly, the ongoing identification of new biomarkers and refinement of imaging modalities have the potential to identify and monitor cardiac arrhythmias and associated myocardial changes, for instance, fibrosis. Non-invasive methods, including advanced cardiac magnetic resonance imaging, have promising potential for tracking the extent of cardiac remodeling, culminating in risk stratification and individualized therapy. These developments in diagnostic modalities will have the potential to equip clinicians with the tools needed to detect arrhythmias early and modify interventions according to their reports. Improved insight into the mechanisms of cardiac arrhythmias, particularly the central roles played by fibrosis and myocardial injury, is paramount to improving patient prognosis and advancing the art of cardiovascular medicine.

The pathophysiologic pathways of cardiac arrhythmias are multifaceted and complex, both intrinsic and extrinsic, that interrupt the regular electrical activity of the heart. A central area of research is the role of potassium ATP (KATP) channels, whose activity has been shown to play a significant role in influencing arrhythmic events. It has been illustrated that low levels of openers of KATP channels, such as Ro 31–6930, have a protective effect during ischemia. This particular channel opener, administered at a comparatively low dose, can reduce the incidence and duration of reperfusion arrhythmias, documenting the fine line between clinical efficacy and side effects. High doses, however, have the paradoxical effect of shortening action potential further, thereby predisposing to pro-arrhythmic effects and demonstrating the subtle interaction between drug dosage and cardiac rhythm stability (MacKenzie et al., 2001). Intercellular electrical communication of cardiomyocytes also plays a pivotal role in the genesis and perpetuation of arrhythmias. Routine electrocardiographic methods rarely can capture the slight alterations in electrical communication under such conditions. Methods from information theory have enabled the development of measures quantitatively assessing these communicative processes within cardiac tissue in recent years. With the application of techniques such as Shannon entropy and mutual information, researchers can investigate how arrhythmic conditions such as anatomical and spiral reentry impact the information being communicated between cardiomyocytes. Not only does this method enlighten the issue of spatial heterogeneity of electrical communication in arrhythmias, but it also opens up new avenues for understanding the detection of effective therapeutic targets to administer (Aguilar-Rodríguez et al., 2014). These findings have clinical practice and future research implications. An understanding of the role of KATP channels in reperfusion arrhythmias can inform safer pharmacologic treatments, and the allowance of novel approaches like information theory metrics can continue to enhance our strengths in diagnosis. These developments can lead to more precise, rhythm-specific treatments that account for the limitations of traditional therapies for arrhythmias. Moreover, the growing understanding of the electrical landscape of the heart as a dynamic system rather than a reductionist syncytium justifies the need for ongoing research into cardiac arrhythmia processes. This knowledge will eventually result in the enhancement of therapeutic intervention aimed at optimizing patient outcomes in this challenging research field.

A CLOSER LOOK

TREATMENT DEVICES FOR HEART ARRHYTHMIA

A cardiologist may insert specific devices during a procedure in the electrophysiology lab. Devices to treat a heart arrhythmia include:

1. **Permanent Pacemaker:** This device sends small electrical impulses to your heart muscle to maintain a normal heart rate and keep your heart from beating too slowly.
2. **Implantable Cardioverter Defibrillator (ICD):** This device constantly monitors your heart rhythm. When it detects a swift, abnormal heart rhythm, it delivers energy to your heart muscle to make it beat in a regular rhythm. This device treats ventricular tachycardia and ventricular fibrillation, two life-threatening heart rhythms.
3. **Biventricular (B-V) Pacemakers and Defibrillators:** It is also called cardiac resynchronization therapy or CRT. These devices help to synchronize the contraction of your left ventricle. In addition to the leads that go to the right side of your heart, they have a lead that goes to your left ventricle. People with heart failure and uncoordinated left ventricular contractions may need this (Figure 3.19).

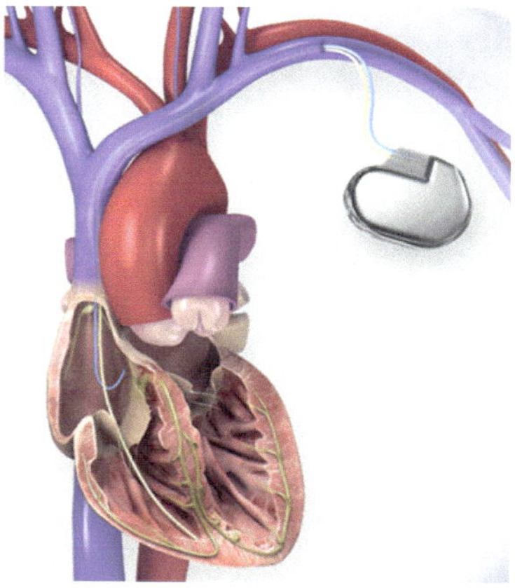

Figure 3.19. Implantable Cardioverter Defibrillator (ICD).

Source: https://www.heart.org/-/media/Images/Health-Topics/Arrhythmia/ICD-and-heart.jpg?sc_lang=en.

References

1. Abouzaid, A., Ali, K., Jatoi, S., Ahmed, M., Ahmad, G., Nazim, A., Mehmoodi, A., & Malik, J. (2024). Cardiac arrhythmias in pulmonary arterial hypertension and chronic thromboembolic pulmonary hypertension: Mechanistic insights, pathophysiology, and Outcomes. *Annals of Noninvasive Electrocardiology, 29*(5). https://doi.org/10.1111/anec.70010Agarwal, S., Mishra, A., & Katiyar, P. (2023). *Myocardial Infarction: A Comprehensive Review.* https://core.ac.uk/download/603896686.pdf (accessed on 29th May 2025).
2. Aguilar-Rodríguez, J., Ashikaga, H., Garland, J., Gorsky, A., et al. (2014). *Modeling the Heart as a Communication System.* http://arxiv.org/abs/1410.2169 (accessed on 29th May 2025).
3. Aitova, A., Berezhnoy, A., Tsvelaya, V., Gusev, O., Lyundup, A., Efimov, A., Agapov, I., et al. (2023). Biomimetic cardiac tissue models for *in vitro* arrhythmia studies. *Biomimetics, 8.* https://www.semanticscholar.org/paper/5c9c43a74e651cffb89c06c934ef7c93ed68f511 (accessed on 29th May 2025).
4. Alyari, M., Bakhtiarian, S., Gakharia, T., Nikandish, M., et al. (2020). *The Overview of the Management of Comorbid Cardiovascular Diseases and Diabetes During COVID-19.* https://core.ac.uk/download/493003542.pdf (accessed on 29th May 2025).
5. Birză, M. R., Negru, A., Frent, Ș., Florescu, A. R., Popa, A. M., Manzur, A. R., Lascu, A., et al. (2025). New insights of cardiac arrhythmias associated with sleep-disordered breathing: From mechanisms to clinical implications—A narrative review. *Journal of Clinical Medicine, 14.* https://www.semanticscholar.org/paper/19bb123029c1ed5d6e013083982716f376a95f4a (accessed on 29th May 2025).
6. Chen, B., Tang, W. W., Rodriguez, M., Corey, K., Sanyal, A., Kamath, P., Bozkurt, B., et al. (2022). NAFLD in cardiovascular diseases: A contributor or comorbidity? *Seminars in Liver Disease, 42*, 465–474. https://www.semanticscholar.org/paper/409dec7b908dae4007a1cb03bb06f46203eb08b4 (accessed on 29th May 2025).
7. Chen, Y., Lou, L., Zhang, X., Jin, L., Chen, Y., Chen, L., Li, Z. H., et al. (2023). Association between circulating leukocytes and arrhythmias: Mendelian randomization analysis in immuno-cardiac electrophysiology. *Frontiers in Immunology, 14.* https://www.semanticscholar.org/paper/affa5bf3724e4a7d0c1d32abfb6593b5eefe8bd9 (accessed on 29th May 2025).
8. Cosentino, F., Grant, P. J., Aboyans, V., Bailey, C. J., Ceriello, A., Delgado, V., Federici, M., et al. (2019). 2019 ESC guidelines on diabetes, pre-diabetes, and cardiovascular diseases developed in collaboration with the EASD. *European Heart Journal, 41*, 255–323. https://doi.org/10.1093/eurheartj/ehz486.
9. Daliento, L., & Folino, A. F. (2005). *Arrhythmias After Tetralogy of Fallot Repair.* https://core.ac.uk/download/pdf/86430.pdf (accessed on 29th May 2025).
10. De Neve, J., Demolder, A., Duytschaever, M., El Haddad, A., et al. (2019). *Directed Networks as a Novel Way to Describe and Analyze Cardiac Excitation: Directed Graph Mapping.* https://core.ac.uk/download/237011958.pdf (accessed on 29th May 2025).
11. De Ponti, R. (2005). *Cryothermal Energy Ablation of Cardiac Arrhythmias 2005: State of the Art.* https://core.ac.uk/download/pdf/86237.pdf (accessed on 29th May 2025).

12. Donahue, J. K., Chrispin, J., & Ajijola, O. (2024). Mechanism of ventricular tachycardia occurring in chronic myocardial infarction scar. *Circulation Research, 134*(3), 328–342. https://www.semanticscholar.org/paper/b519b4265499f1ac39245a237d35e73ba510e68a (accessed on 29th May 2025).

13. Duplaga, T. A., Krasnoborska, J., Samojedny, S., Superson, M., et al. (2024). *Revolutionizing Cardiovascular Treatments with the Use of AI: Current Status and Future Prospects.* https://core.ac.uk/download/620863037.pdf (accessed on 29th May 2025).

14. Gönczi, M., Kovács, M., Miskolczi, G., Végh, Á., et al. (2013). *Regulation of Gap Junction Function: The Role of Nitric Oxide.* https://core.ac.uk/download/16671971.pdf (accessed on 29th May 2025).

15. Guo, T., Fan, Y., Chen, M., Wu, X., Zhang, L., He, T., Wang, H., et al. (2020). Cardiovascular implications of fatal outcomes of patients with coronavirus disease 2019 (COVID-19). *JAMA Cardiology, 5*, 811–811. https://doi.org/10.1001/jamacardio.2020.1017.

16. Gutiérrez-Cuevas, J., López-Cifuentes, D., Sandoval-Rodríguez, A., García-Bañuelos, J., & Armendáriz-Borunda, J. (2024). Medicinal plant extracts against cardiometabolic risk factors associated with obesity: Molecular mechanisms and therapeutic targets. *Pharmaceuticals, 17.* https://www.semanticscholar.org/paper/a9e2311447209a03a30a85a9bda92997ee783a68 (accessed on 29th May 2025).

17. Haugsten, H. M., Sadredini, M., Hasic, A., Eriksen, M., & Stokke, M. (2023). Myocardial oxidative stress is increased in early reperfusion, but systemic antioxidative therapy does not prevent ischemia-reperfusion arrhythmias in pigs. *Frontiers in Cardiovascular Medicine, 10.* https://www.semanticscholar.org/paper/048346385305b1ebb1e77968e6e2e872eac7ec53 (accessed on 29th May 2025).

18. Houck, P. (2024). Pacemaker optimization mechanisms in the spectrum of cardiac disease: Rationale to protocol. *Hearts.* https://www.semanticscholar.org/paper/273755810f16705e989d1d4602a4109a4e606ce4 (accessed on 29th May 2025).

19. Jakovljević, M., Kozumplik, O., & Uzun, S. (2009*). Psychotic Disorders and Comorbidity: Somatic Illness vs. Side Effect.* https://core.ac.uk/download/14420499.pdf (accessed on 29th May 2025).

20. Ketkar, H., Tang, S., Rota, M., & Jain, S. (2021). Metabolic environment alters the transcriptomic landscape of the aged heart. *The FASEB Journal, 35.* https://www.semanticscholar.org/paper/463a3c8ea00f11882de21559ee1f05eb7b3d840e (accessed on 29th May 2025).

21. Kitsiou, A., Caforio, A. L. P., Porta-Sanchez, A., Vahanian, A., Iung, B., Carrera, C., Szymanski, C., et al. (2013). *ESC Core Curriculum for the General Cardiologist (2013).* https://core.ac.uk/download/55756305.pdf (accessed on 29th May 2025).

22. Krieger, E., Zeppenfeld, K., DeWitt, E., Duarte, V. E., Egbe, A., Haeffele, C., Lin, K. Y., et al. (2022). Arrhythmias in repaired Tetralogy of Fallot: A scientific statement from the American Heart Association. *Circulation: Arrhythmia and Electrophysiology, 15*, e000084. https://www.semanticscholar.org/paper/6a5131b1a304a25d18d4b29b67d5999c34d31d03 (accessed on 29th May 2025).

23. Lei, Q., Jiang, Z., Shao, Y., Liu, X., & Li, X. (2024). Stellate ganglion, inflammation, and arrhythmias: A new perspective on neuroimmune regulation. *Frontiers in Cardiovascular Medicine, 11.* https://www.semanticscholar.org/paper/24202f7a9b9c36b4a3c3598063e5de4a5651c1e2 (accessed on 29th May 2025).

24. Liu, J., Liu, X., Luo, Y., Huang, F., Xie, Y., Zheng, S., Jia, B., et al. (2023). Sphingolipids: Drivers of cardiac fibrosis and atrial fibrillation. *Journal of Molecular Medicine (Berlin, Germany), 102*, 149–165. https://www.semanticscholar.org/paper/f7ae9b078a1b047b05023413232e449543cff26e (accessed on 29th May 2025).

25. Lv, T., Li, S. Y., Li, Q., Meng, L., Yang, J., Liu, L., Lv, C., et al. (2025). The role of RyR2 mutations in congenital heart diseases: Insights into cardiac electrophysiological mechanisms. *Journal of Cardiovascular Electrophysiology*. https://www.semanticscholar.org/paper/7e988d12c0bc0bcc89cd02c471a2f3f48d3c78d3 (accessed on 29th May 2025).

26. MacKenzie, I., Northover, B. J., & Workman, A. J. (2001). *A KATP Channel Opener Inhibited Myocardial Reperfusion Action Potential Shortening and Arrhythmias*. https://core.ac.uk/download/1394939.pdf (accessed on 29th May 2025).

27. Mattioli, A. V. (2011). *Lifestyle and Atrial Fibrillation*. https://core.ac.uk/download/53989788.pdf (accessed on 29th May 2025).

28. Mohamed, H. A., El-Shaer, M., Al-Daydamony, M. M., & Hassan, M. (2022). Cardiac arrhythmia mechanisms in COVID-19: Review article. *The Egyptian Journal of Hospital Medicine*. https://www.semanticscholar.org/paper/fd87b8720b155aa203c24df7ce66b076a377dddf (accessed on 29th May 2025).

29. Mohamed, R., Almuhanna, A., Alajwad, H., Elshehawey, A., Almusaad, A., & AlTaweel, M. (2024). Unraveling the complexities of T wave alternans and QT prolongation in advanced chronic kidney disease: A case report and literature review. *International Journal of Clinical Science and Medical Research*. https://www.semanticscholar.org/paper/21390f0904bff8f968f3e6d8773560bb40905077 (accessed on 29th May 2025).

30. Muñoz, A., Baer, M., & Echebarría, D. B. (2016). *Nonlinear Physics of Electrical Wave Propagation in the Heart: A Review*. https://core.ac.uk/download/81580019.pdf (accessed on 29th May 2025).

31. Nagpal, A. K., Pundkar, A., Singh, A., & Gadkari, C. (2024). Cardiac arrhythmias and their management: An in-depth review of current practices and emerging therapies. *Cureus, 16*. https://www.semanticscholar.org/paper/f4b5121a1fe9853b93c41abb9650ecb9f92f14a9 (accessed on 29th May 2025).

32. Noyan, S., Öztemur, I. Y., & Akpınar, E. (2024). Novel role of the miR-568 through enhanced expression of NAPMT and TRMP7 in HL-1 cells. *Medical Records*. https://www.semanticscholar.org/paper/1d631bdfe7b2e1ec02c9a6eb847de20e789fb92e (accessed on 29th May 2025).

33. Pieroni, M., Zocchi, C., & Ciabatti, M. (2025). Cardiac involvement in Fabry disease: Recent advances, unresolved issues, and unmet needs. *European Heart Journal Supplements: Journal of the European Society of Cardiology, 27*, i51–i55. https://www.semanticscholar.org/paper/d07292da922e4bd5e2fa8cb6b2cc0260e553ef2e (accessed on 29th May 2025).

34. Ponikowski, P., Voors, A. A., Anker, S. D., Bueno, H., Cleland, J. G. F., Coats, A. J. S., Falk, V., et al. (2016). 2016 ESC Guidelines for the diagnosis and treatment of acute and chronic heart failure. *European Heart Journal, 37*, 2129–2200. https://doi.org/10.1093/eurheartj/ehw128 (accessed on 29th May 2025).

35. Postma, A., Christoffels, V., & Bezzina, C. (2011). Developmental aspects of cardiac arrhythmogenesis. *Cardiovascular Research, 91*(2), 243–251. https://www.semanticscholar.org/paper/fd326a049d4c26c0d4f8bd163ea10b97de26dadd (accessed on 29th May 2025).

36. Priori, S. G., Blomström-Lundqvist, C., Mazzanti, A., Blom, N., Borggrefe, M., Camm, A. J., Elliott, P., et al. (2015). 2015 ESC Guidelines for the management of patients with ventricular arrhythmias and the prevention of sudden cardiac death. *European Heart Journal, 36*, 2793–2867. https://doi.org/10.1093/eurheartj/ehv316 (accessed on 29th May 2025).

37. Qiao, Y. (2018). *Transcriptional Regulation of Arrhythmia: From Mouse to Human.* https://core.ac.uk/download/233214852.pdf (accessed on 29th May 2025).

38. Reemtsen, B., Finn, J. P., Alejos, J., Touma, M., Halnon, N., Nelson, S. F., et al. (2017). A path to implement precision child health cardiovascular medicine. https://core.ac.uk/download/323077346.pdf (accessed on 29th May 2025).

39. Rouhi, L. (2025). Cardiac phenotypes in LMNA mutations. *Current Opinion in Cardiology*. https://www.semanticscholar.org/paper/dc6d4620bdd6e32009b66a6b2d8b556470a4924f (accessed on 29th May 2025).

40. Saadeh, K., & Fazmin, I. T. (2021). Mitochondrial dysfunction increases arrhythmic triggers and substrates; potential anti-arrhythmic pharmacological targets. *Frontiers in Cardiovascular Medicine, 8*. https://www.semanticscholar.org/paper/f959299abd54e5fd748c066e210195f3a1f2315b (accessed on 29th May 2025).

41. Sampson, M. (2016). Understanding the ECG. Part 3: Arrhythmias. *British Journal of Cardiac Nursing, 11*, 15–20. https://www.semanticscholar.org/paper/064c1158b67d7aab82c78523be345758a2a68bed (accessed on 29th May 2025).

42. Shen, M. J., & Zipes, D. P. (2014). Role of the autonomic nervous system in modulating cardiac arrhythmias. *Circulation Research, 114*, 1004–1021. https://doi.org/10.1161/circresaha.113.302549 (accessed on 29th May 2025).

43. Shlobin, N., Thijs, R., Benditt, D., Zeppenfeld, K., & Sander, J. (2024). Sudden death in epilepsy: The overlap between cardiac and neurological factors. *Brain Communications, 6*. https://www.semanticscholar.org/paper/ae5ebc09a7fa4e6d20c9814d1fa55ef0377d6b5e (accessed on 29th May 2025).

44. Sweeney, M., Corden, B., & Cook, S. A. (2020). Targeting cardiac fibrosis in heart failure with preserved ejection fraction: Mirage or miracle? *EMBO Molecular Medicine, 12*. https://doi.org/10.15252/emmm.201910865 (accessed on 29th May 2025).

45. Sychov, O. S., Solovyan, G., Mikhalieva, T. V., & Lyzogub, S. V. (2022). Supraventricular tachycardias: The underlying mechanisms and the choice of treatment options. *Ukrainian Journal of Cardiology*. https://www.semanticscholar.org/paper/c69279e6638c944d2c565b6a6cc631e5cb490cf0 (accessed on 29th May 2025).

46. Tallo, F., Oliveira de, S. P., Gordinho, P. S. A., Yamaguti, L. R., Amarante de, A. E., Tavares, J., Pires-Oliveira, M., et al. (2023). Pharmacological modulation of the Ca^{2+}/cAMP/adenosine signaling in cardiac cells as a new cardioprotective strategy to reduce severe arrhythmias in myocardial infarction. *Pharmaceuticals, 16*. https://www.semanticscholar.org/paper/23c623d2be7e47a2fac90ff70f0dfb5a5f4bd5bd (accessed on 29th May 2025).

47. Vásquez-Iturralde, F., Flores-Calero, M., Grijalva, F., & Rosales-Acosta, A. (2024). Automatic classification of cardiac arrhythmias using deep learning techniques: A systematic review. *IEEE Access, 12*, 118467–118492. https://www.semanticscholar.org/paper/4b48b8ef3386da2fdfcceb7e79d98cf376d24573 (accessed on 29th May 2025).

48. Vlasova, V. P., Myshkina, N., & Fateeva, M. V. (2025). Cardiac arrhythmias and conduction disorders in geriatric patients with cardiovascular comorbidity. *Medicine and Biotechnology*. https://www.semanticscholar.org/paper/def463f077e86b7b8f99c7b176baedf18ceba30e (accessed on 29th May 2025).

49. Wang, C., Ma, J., Wei, G., & Sun, X. (2025). Analysis of cardiac arrhythmias based on ResNet-ICBAM-2DCNN dual-channel feature fusion. *Sensors (Basel, Switzerland), 25*. https://www.semanticscholar.org/paper/1f9b5b4b96dd662abdb7d76dc00909a4e10f11a7 (accessed on 29th May 2025).

50. Wang, M., & Tu, X. (2022). The genetics and epigenetics of ventricular arrhythmias in patients without structural heart disease. *Frontiers in Cardiovascular Medicine, 9*. https://www.semanticscholar.org/paper/c2d99bbae229c24d7ae9ff6352f60dd69779f789 (accessed on 29th May 2025).

51. Zhang, H., Qu, P., Liu, J., Cheng, P., & Lei, Q. (2025). Application of human cardiac organoids in cardiovascular disease research. *Frontiers in Cell and Developmental Biology, 13*. https://www.semanticscholar.org/paper/772ce19d07edd454b789ada672706eae9acbe25c (accessed on 29th May 2025).

52. Zhao, Y., Wan, J., Liao, B., & Qi, M. (2025). The neglected internodal tract—A cardiac conduction system structure homologous to the development and regulation of the sinoatrial node. *Reviews in Cardiovascular Medicine*. https://www.semanticscholar.org/paper/434f458898eecf2665b99d6610cd3b1065876aa9 (accessed on 29th May 2025).

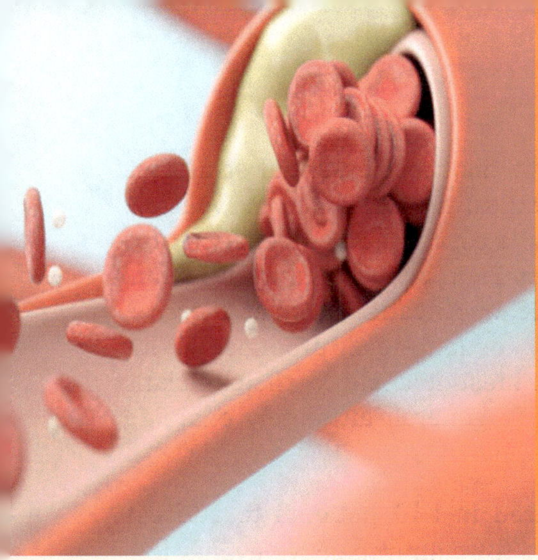

Chapter 4

ISCHEMIC HEART DISEASE

Contents

Introduction

Ischemic heart disease (IHD) is a leading global cause of morbidity and mortality and a critical contributor to the burden of cardiovascular disease. It can be defined as reduced blood supply to the heart muscle via constricted or blocked coronary arteries and is typically associated with angina, myocardial infarction, and heart failure, and thus has clinical importance. The multifactorial pathophysiology of IHD comprises many risk factors, which include hypertension, hyperlipidemia, diabetes, and habits such as smoking and physical inactivity. Thus, information regarding these risk factors becomes essential to develop logical prevention and therapeutic measures. In addition, earlier identification through advanced diagnosis can assist in taking appropriate interventions promptly, hopefully limiting cataclysmic effects such as myocardial infarction or sudden cardiac death. Hence, management of IHD becomes vital to improve cardiovascular health and reduce the healthcare cost for cardiovascular disease. Ischemic heart disease requires not only drug therapy but lifestyle modifications according to the individual's needs. New evidence has shown that the most essential strategies for enhancing patient outcomes are elucidated by emphasizing medical therapies and prevention. For instance, modern antihypertensive and lipid-lowering therapy is established as beneficial for the treatment of coronary heart disease and prevention of risk factors in endothelial dysfunction, which plays a key role in the causation of IHD. Furthermore, lifestyle modification, such as exercise, diet, and smoking cessation, is an addition to medication therapy for long-term prognosis. With the use of a multi-phased strategy combining drug treatment with lifestyle changes, the clinicians can enhance exponentially patient compliance and quality of life in general, ultimately enabling better management of ischemic heart disease and sequelae.

Individualized and multidisciplinary care treatment is required in IHD patients to address the complexity of the disease in each patient. This approach allows for comprehensive evaluation, considering not only clinical manifestations but also pathophysiologic alterations responsible for them. It has been found that patients with ischemic heart disease-induced heart failure are best treated by those evaluations that include assessment of left ventricular and right ventricular function and pulmonary function. This comprehensive evaluation allows for more individualized therapy plans tailored to specific heart failure and IHD requirements. By ensuring that such individualized plans are grounded in the most up-to-date guidelines of clinical practice, healthcare professionals can maximize monitoring protocols, reduce rehospitalization, and overall achieve better patient outcomes. Thus, it is of utmost significance to ensure well-organized management underpinnings to navigate the management pitfalls of IHD correctly, and as a result, get better health pathways among the afflicted (Figure 4.1).

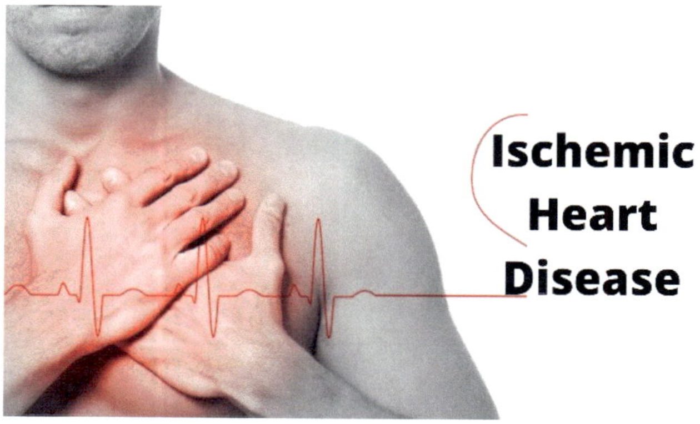

Figure 4.1. Understanding Ischemic Heart Disease.

Source: https://www.maxlab.co.in/categoryimage/1665660656.png.

Definition of Ischemic Heart Disease (IHD)

IHD, or coronary heart disease, is a highly prevalent form of cardiovascular disease characterized by a decrease in blood flow to the heart muscle due to the narrowing or blockage of the coronary arteries. IHD can affect the onset of severe complications like myocardial infarction or chronic heart failure. The pathogenesis of IHD is primarily because of atherosclerosis, a process where plaques build up in the arterial wall, reducing blood supply. The prevalence of IHD is rising internationally, emphasizing the need for effective prevention and control. Understanding this disease is not only important for doctors but also for at-risk patients because identification of symptoms and risk factors early on can lead to early treatment and significantly improve health outcomes, making studies of IHD increasingly relevant to contemporary medical discourse. The clinical presentation of Ischemic Heart Disease is very diverse, ranging from common features like chest pain to uncommon features like epigastric pain or even non-specific features like fatigue and fits. This heterogeneity usually leads to incorrect diagnoses; hence, the patients are subjected to severe delays in receiving appropriate treatment. Misdiagnosis leads to devastating consequences in the form of deterioration of the disease, along with high mortality. By widening the knowledge of atypical presentations, medical practitioners can improve the accuracy of diagnosis and institute timely intervention for affected people. Also, recognition of the risk factors of IHD, such as hypertension, diabetes, and hypercholesterolemia, is important in preventing the disease.

Multidimensional models of care that incorporate both typical and atypical presentations are needed in order to improve patient outcomes and reduce the burden of this increasingly common condition (Furia et al., 2024). The current evidence requires exercise-based cardiac rehabilitation as a core intervention in the treatment of Ischemic Heart Disease. Some systematic reviews have established that these interventions are successful in reducing the risk of non-fatal and fatal myocardial infarctions with subsequent enhanced survival and quality of life among IHD patients. Specifically, there was a robust evidence map indicating successful rehabilitation interventions with high levels of evidence for exercise therapy, which, aside from improving cardiovascular health, facilitates early return to work following cardiac events.

However, it should be noted that the level of proof for evidence can also vary significantly across various treatment comparisons, and some of them are underexplored. Therefore, while rehabilitation interventions are hopeful, more studies targeting primary end points, e.g., total mortality, are needed to validate the efficacy of such interventions and guide clinical practice in the management of IHD (Furia et al., 2024) (Figure 4.2).

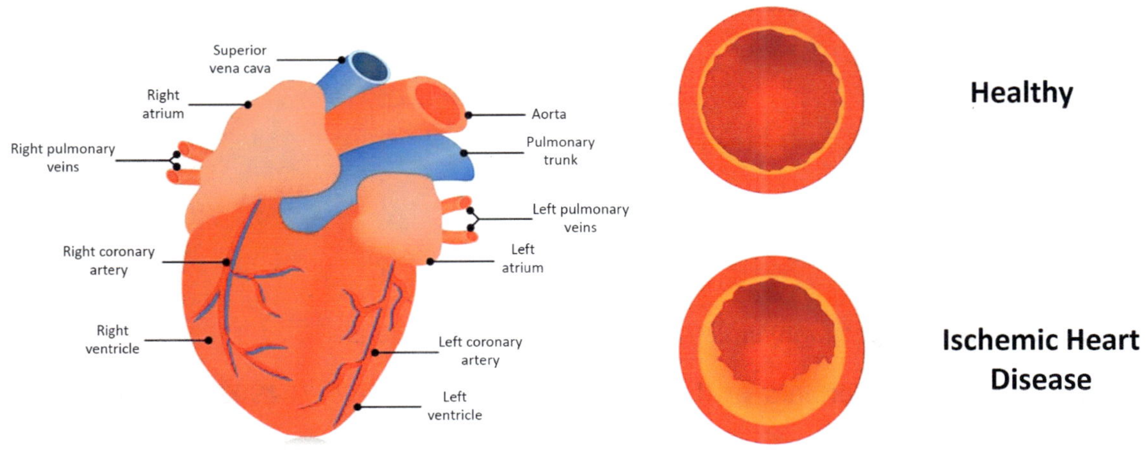

Figure 4.2. Ischemic heart diseases (IHD).

Source: https://drvaidji.com/cdn/shop/articles/heart_d.jpg?v=1710481948.

4.1. Pathophysiology of Ischemic Heart Disease (IHD)

The pathophysiology of IHD is a complex process with an interaction of many factors. Central to IHD pathogenesis is coronary artery atherosclerosis, which leads to the narrowing and occlusion of the coronary arteries. Atherosclerosis is due to the accumulation of lipids, inflammatory cells, and fibrous elements in the arterial wall, which renders the arteries stiff and less elastic. This impaired flexibility diminishes the ability of the arteries to expand with increasing myocardial oxygen demand, leading to ischemia, or insufficient blood flow to the muscle of the heart. In females, as well, there is growing evidence that coronary endothelial impairment and microvascular illness are more important than previously appreciated because they can involve less atherosclerotic burden but add significantly to the symptoms and progression of IHD (Seawright et al., 2019). Furthermore, the IHD expression varies among different populations, for example, due to the impact of comorbidities.

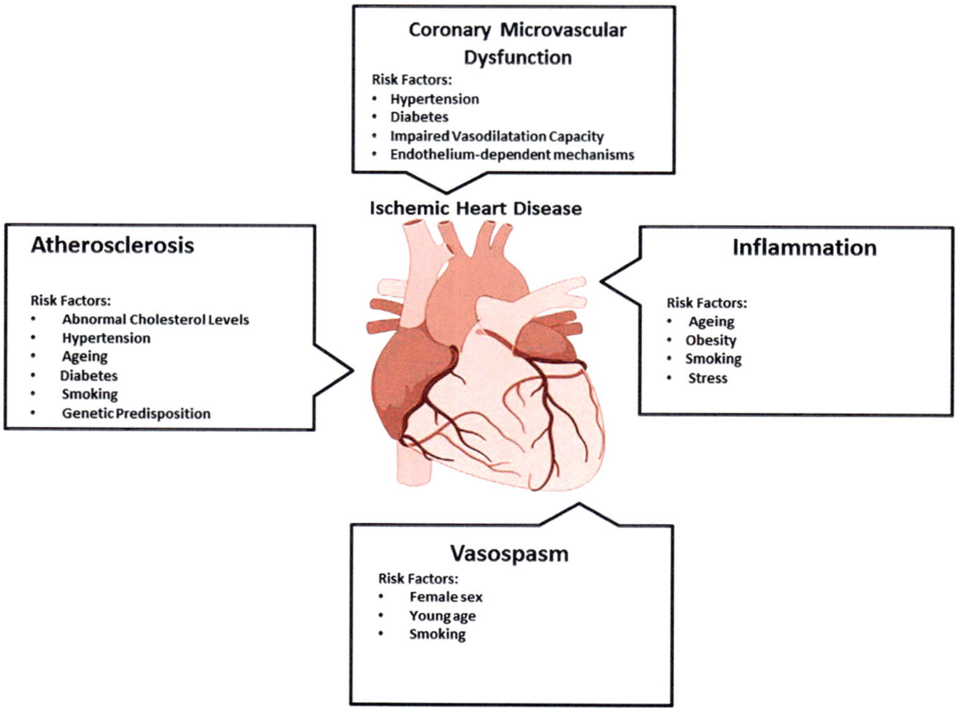

Figure 4.3. Multifaceted pathophysiology of ischemic heart disease.

Source: https://www.frontiersin.org/files/Articles/704903/fcell-09-704903-HTML-r1/image_m/fcell-09-704903-g001.jpg.

Diabetic patients, for instance, possess a particular pathophysiological pattern of macrovascular and microvascular disease. While in some patients, significant coronary stenosis exists, in others, coronary microvascular disease can occur with no obvious epicardial lesions. The disease is frequently challenging to diagnose and treat because usual cardiovascular assessment may fail to identify underlying microvascular disease. It has been demonstrated that genetic predispositions, particularly those affecting ATP-dependent potassium channels, may be involved in the IHD pathophysiology of diabetic patients and affect their ischemic response (Marchis et al., 2018). Such complexity requires personalized treatment strategies that consider such differences between patient groups. Pathophysiology of IHD should be understood to develop targeted therapeutic and prevention strategies. Appreciation of sex differences, for example, has caused reevaluation of screening and management plans, since women may present with atypical symptoms and prognostic factors other than those in men. Risk stratification must also consider the unconventional risk factors such as psychological distress and hormonal influences, particularly among young women. Increased understanding of the interaction of these biological and psychological factors will be essential in maximizing care. With constant research attempting to explain the pathways involved in IHD, it is also critical that health professionals adopt a holistic approach, considering the diverse factors contributing to this prevalent ailment in every sphere of life (Seawright et al., 2019) (Figure 4.3).

4.1.1. Mechanisms of Coronary Artery Obstruction

The pathophysiology of coronary artery blockage is multi-factorial, with morphological and physiological changes in the cardiovascular system. Atherosclerosis, or lipid, inflammatory cell, and fibrous tissue deposition, remains the most frequent cause of coronary artery blockage. Slow deposition leads to plaque formation that reduces the lumen of the artery and impedes blood flow to the myocardium. Additionally, certain risk factors, such as endothelial dysfunction, contribute to the pathogenic mechanism as well. Endothelium, when it is injured, acquires a loss of function in order to manage vascular tone and prevent thrombosis, causing acceleration of atheromatous lesion evolution. Above all, the enigma of coronary artery disease is exacerbated by the presence of coexistent non-obstructive pathophysiological conditions, such as microvascular dysfunction and coronary artery spasm, that may be capable of producing ischemic symptoms in the absence of significant obstruction of the coronary arteries, which echoes the heterogeneous pathophysiological substrate of ischemic heart disease. The overlap of structural and electrical myocardial changes represents the cornerstone of the augmentation of ischemic heart disease. A landmark article emphasizes that the evolution of myocardial ischemia may cause profound changes in cardiac tissue's electrical properties. With ischemia advancement, electrical heterogeneities within the heart amplify and have the potential to enhance arrhythmia risk. Disruption of electricity results from remodeling of ion channels, gap junctions, and impaired cellular metabolism due to inadequate oxygen supply. Moreover, these changes can result in impaired cardiac mechanics, which can negatively impact patient outcomes. The detection of the likely large effects of these electrical changes enables clinicians to organize effective therapeutic schedules that can eliminate arrhythmic risks due to coronary artery occlusion and are patient-specifically aimed at better regulation of ischemic heart disease. Recognition of the pleomorphic course of ischemic heart disease necessitates careful evaluation of patient phenotypes and stratification of risk. As highlighted, myocardial ischemia can escalate to myocardial infarction if the supply of blood is not reestablished within time. The chronic evolution of ischemic heart disease is typified by dramatic changes, including injurious structural remodeling and electrical alterations that have the potential to precipitate recurrent cycles of heart failure or sudden cardiac death. This dynamic progress highlights the importance of continuous management and assessment practices that are aware of the anatomical and functional characteristics of coronary artery obstruction. Further, advances in computational algorithms that account for patient-specific electrical and structural heterogeneity provide new avenues for basic and translational research. By illuminating the intricate expressions of ischemic heart disease, from inception to final complications, physicians can more accurately forecast outcomes and adapt treatment interventions for improved patient management and quality of life.

4.1.2. Role of Atherosclerosis in Disease Progression

Atherosclerosis is the primary driving force in the pathogenesis of ischemic heart disease, creating pathologic changes in the coronary arteries. The disease is characterized by the accumulation of lipids, inflammatory cells, and fibrous tissue in the wall of the artery to create plaques. The plaques are unstable and rupture, generating thrombosis that can severely restrict blood to the myocardium over time. This is exacerbated by endothelial dysfunction, which not only facilitates atherosclerosis initiation but also generates pro-inflammatory conditions that accelerate disease progression. The link between atherosclerosis and ischemic heart disease is thus heightened by the pathological effects of impaired endothelial function, predisposing to plaque formation and rupture and therefore rendering myocardial ischemia more likely. The other major factor in ischemic heart disease pathogenesis is the role of oxidative stress in atherosclerosis. Oxidative stress occurs due to an imbalance between the production of reactive oxygen species (ROS) and the body's antioxidant defenses. Elevated levels of ROS can induce endothelial dysfunction, a feature of early atherosclerotic lesions. Zheng et al. (2022) point out that oxidative stress may cause various forms of endothelial cell death, promoting vascular barrier dysfunctions and progression factors in escalating leukocyte adhesion and migration into the arterial wall. These are the prerequisites for an inflammatory cascade of actions that fuel atherosclerotic progression and eventually threaten ischemic events. Therefore, oxidative stress management is a key to preventing atherosclerosis and its complications, particularly in ischemic heart disease-susceptible patients. Additionally, the liaison between inflammation and atherosclerosis is the cornerstone of disease evolution in ischemic heart disease.

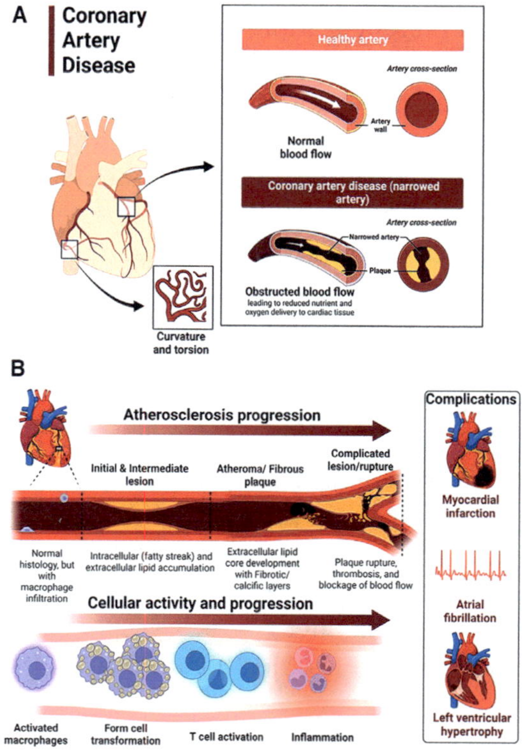

Figure 4.4. Atherosclerosis progression in coronary artery disease. (A) Coronary artery disease is characterized by narrowed coronary arteries due to advanced atherosclerotic fatty plaque. (B) Atherosclerosis in coronary artery disease and complications.

Source: https://www.researchgate.net/publication/371685758/figure/fig4/AS:11431281168881908@1687159242391/Atherosclerosis-progression-in-coronary-artery-disease-A-Coronary-artery-disease-is.tif.

Plaque inflammation is responsible for further instability and rupture and is involved in increasing ischemic events. As elaborated by Kibel et al. (2020), endothelial dysfunction is driven by chronic inflammation. It supports atherosclerosis in its advancement by various mechanisms, including inflammatory cell recruitment and the secretion of pro-inflammatory cytokines. This continuous chain of inflammation and oxidative stress establishes a vicious cycle that not only supports the formation of atherosclerotic plaques but also inclines the development of plaque instability and thrombosis. Thus, modulation of inflammatory pathways is a potential novel therapeutic strategy for the prevention of ischemic heart disease onset and in the attainment of maximum patient benefits. Understanding of such delicate interrelations is vital in developing more effective interventions in the control of cardiovascular diseases (Figure 4.4).

4.1.3. Impact of Ischemia on Myocardial Tissue

It is vital to understand the ischemia's impact on myocardial tissue in order to understand the whole spectrum of ischemic heart disease comprehensively. Ischemia, or a reduced supply of blood to the heart muscle, induces a chain of deleterious cellular changes. Insufficient oxygen supply induces metabolic stress and leads the myocytes to shift from aerobic to anaerobic metabolism. This process yields lactic acid, contributing to acidosis, which disrupts ion gradients and impairs cardiac function. Moreover, with the prolonged ischemic state, ROS accumulation causes oxidative stress, further aggravating cellular damage and inducing apoptosis. Thus, myocardial tissue structural organization is destroyed, resulting in reduced contractility and eventually heart failure. Hence, the effect of ischemia on myocardial tissue needs a detailed investigation to form effective therapeutic strategies. Apart from the acute cell response, ischemia triggers long-term adaptability that renders the health of myocardial tissue increasingly complex. Chronic ischemia can trigger a cascade of pathological remodeling processes by hypertrophy and fibrosis that lead to a detrimental effect on cardiac function. Studies have identified that ischemic states are capable of sensitizing the myocardium, making it susceptible to further ischemic injury, and thus, an unholy cycle of myocardial failure. Surprisingly, the connection between ischemia and psychological entities, i.e., major depressive disorder (MDD), is emerging as a significant area of research. MDD is associated with systemic processes like vascular dysfunction that predispose towards coronary heart disease and disrupt the protective mechanisms of the heart. The crosstalk between myocardial changes and psychological stress is a field worth investigating, as it can direct new interventions to limit ischemic damage and enhance cardiac resilience (Budiono et al., 2017). Novel evidence in the use of therapeutic drugs for ischemic heart disease points to potential cardioprotective therapies that can repress the adverse effects of ischemia on the myocardial tissue. Volatile anesthetics that are widely utilized during surgeries have been noted for their ability to alleviate ischemia and reperfusion injury. Experiments confirm that these anesthetics can activate cardioprotective pathways like potassium ATP (KATP) channel manipulation and regulation of the mitochondrial permeability transition pore (mPTP). These pathways allow for the attenuation of oxidative stress as well as cell survival following ischemic events. However, the efficacy of volatile anesthetics remains questionable because not all studies report uniformly positive outcomes. Those outcomes emphasize the necessity of balancing against risks of harmful hemodynamic effects and underscore the complexity of managing ischemic heart disease and preserving myocardial integrity (Applegate et al., 2012).

4.2. Risk Factors

The risk factors for IHD are multifactorial and can be classified into modifiable and non-modifiable risk factors. The non-modifiable risk factors include age, gender, race, and genetic factors. For instance, increased age is at a higher risk for the impact of cumulative exposure to cardiovascular stressors, while males will present with symptoms before females develop IHD following the menopause age. Genetic susceptibility factors such as specific single-nucleotide polymorphisms are involved in predisposing one to heart disease, pointing towards the complex interaction of determinants in IHD (Bulinski et al., 2011). While these predisposing factors are inherited, a wide array of lifestyle factors may impinge on the risk and thus relevance to comprehensive risk assessment for efficient management and preventive interventions. Factors for risk that can be modified include hyperlipidemia, hypertension, diabetes, smoking, and physical inactivity. These are the optimal targets for intervention, since their alteration can reduce the incidence and progression of IHD to a considerable extent. Hyperlipidemia and hypertension are the fundamental causes of the atherosclerotic process with subsequent coronary artery occlusion and resulting ischemia. Diabetes mellitus is also linked with endothelial dysfunction and increased inflammation, contributing to cardiovascular risk (De la Parte et al., 2021). Smoking remains one of the most significant preventable risk factors, with its damaging effects on vascular health well documented across all universes. Conversely, exercise and a healthy diet can minimize such risk factors, ranking lifestyle modification as an integral component of the prevention and management of IHD. Encouragement of awareness of the role played by such modifiable factors is a significant component of the war against ischemic heart disease. Rising data also suggests that psychosocial factors also contribute to an equally significant component of the risk profile of IHD patients. Depression, loneliness, and stress are connected to poorer cardiovascular outcomes, which suggests psychological well-being has tangible implications for heart function. Prolonged stress, for example, is found to elevate blood pressure and heart rate in the long term, ultimately causing the development of heart disease. Moreover, investigations employing advanced statistical models have also examined interactions among traditional risk factors and psychosocial factors that contribute to furthering our understanding of the multifactorial status of IHD (De la Parte et al., 2021). This global consideration of risk factors underscores the need for practices within healthcare settings that prioritize mental health care as equally vital as managing physiological risk factors, thereby opening avenues for improved control of ischemic heart disease (Figure 4.5).

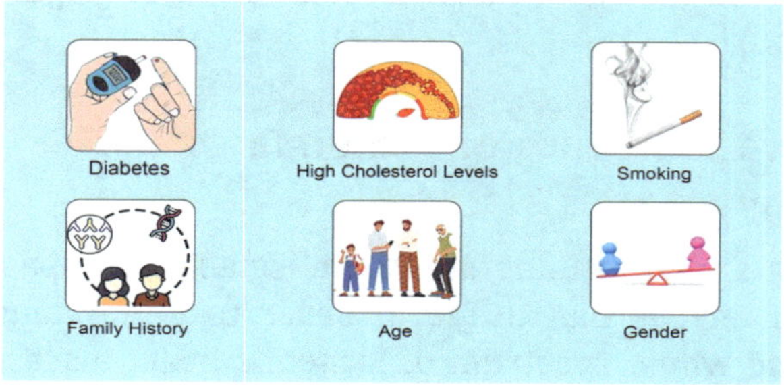

Figure 4.5. Risk Factors of Ischemic Heart Disease.

Source: https://cdn.hexahealth.com/Image/1726057539246-773896228.webp.

4.2.1. Modifiable Risk Factors (e.g., Smoking, Diet)

Modifiable risk factors play a very crucial role in the causation and development of IHD. Among these factors, smoking is one of the most powerful etiological factors for cardiovascular morbidity. The toxic substances in tobacco smoke induce endothelial injury, increased arterial stiffness, and the promotion of atherogenesis. In recent times, it has been evidenced that stopping smoking reduces the risk of IHD and other cardiovascular disorders significantly. This adaptation not only helps the cardiovascular system but also overall health. Community-level smoking awareness programs that sensitize individuals regarding the hazards of smoking can also considerably lower its prevalence, and consequently, the prevalence of IHD cases among high-risk populations. Public health interventions to quit smoking are hence essential to stop ischemic heart disease and promote long-term health outcomes (Rahimee et al., 2023). Dietary habit plays important role in the individual risk of developing IHD. A diet composed of high levels of saturated fats, trans fats, and sucrose can lead to dyslipidemia, which comprises elevated concentrations of LDL cholesterol and decreased concentrations of HDL cholesterol. This derangement predisposes to the formation of atherosclerotic plaques in the coronary arteries, which can produce occlusion of the blood supply and result in myocardial infarction. Conversely, a diet rich in fruits, vegetables, whole grains, and omega-3 fatty acids has been associated with better cardiovascular health results. The integration of nutrition education into community health initiatives can enable individuals to make nutritious food choices. Changing eating habits is feasible and can provide substantial reductions in the incidence of IHD and improve public health levels (Eram et al., 2023). Physical activity is another modifiable factor influencing ischemic heart disease risk. Regular physical exercise is beneficial in maintaining healthy body weight, lowering blood pressure, and regulating blood glucose levels—all crucial factors in reducing the chances of developing coronary artery disease. Sedentary lifestyle plays a significant role in causing obesity and secondary metabolic dysfunctions, both proven precursors for IHD. Encouraging populations to adopt active lifestyles through the availability of cost-friendly recreation centers or involvement in organized sports can facilitate environments where physical activity becomes integrated into daily routines. Furthermore, education campaigns that highlight the benefits of regular exercise can encourage people to take health matters seriously. By embracing widespread strategies that promote physical activity, communities can potentially observe reduced rates of IHD prevalence and increased overall health and longevity (Eram et al., 2023).

4.2.2. Non-Modifiable Risk Factors (e.g., Age, Genetics)

It is essential to identify the non-modifiable risk factors of IHD so that successful prevention strategies can be formulated. Age is one of the notable ones where the prevalence of IHD increases steadily with rising age. Older individuals, particularly those aged above 65 years, are more vulnerable due to natural loss of vascular function and an additive effect of years of exposure to modifiable risk factors. For instance, research identified that in IHD patients, the mean age was approximately 54.75 years with a very high proportion of the cases falling in the age group of 56–65 years. This suggests that vascular changes in shape and function with aging may be a significant factor in the causation and development of the disease, making continuous monitoring and early intervention in older populations even more necessary (Ali et al., 2025). Genetics also has a significant position to fulfill as an unalterable risk factor for IHD. A family history of heart disease can significantly predispose individuals towards such medical conditions, exhibiting the genetic component of cardiovascular health. It has been observed that almost 45.2% of patients suffering from IHD possess a positive family history of the illness, reflecting a genetically fixed susceptibility. Besides, there have been some specific genetic markers that may potentially influence cholesterol metabolism and inflammatory levels, hence increasing the risk to the disease (Ali et al., 2025).

These observations underscore the value of a multi-component strategy in the management of individual risk profiles, particularly in the presence of a hereditary risk of heart disease, hence influencing both public health policy and clinical practice (Ali et al., 2025). Apart from genetics and age, sex is another critical non-modifiable risk factor affecting the prevalence of IHD. Proof confirms that men are more susceptible than women, a distinction made by both biological and lifestyle determinants. In a survey of university students, it was observed that male students were less sensitive to cardiovascular risk factors than women, although they are more at risk. This observation suggests a need for targeted educational interventions to raise awareness and encourage lifestyle change among at-risk groups. The growing evidence of the interplay between sex, genes, and age paves the way for more tailored prevention strategies in the treatment of IHD. Uncovering these non-modifiable determinants is critical for establishing effective public health policies to stem the overall prevalence of ischemic heart disease (Figure 4.6).

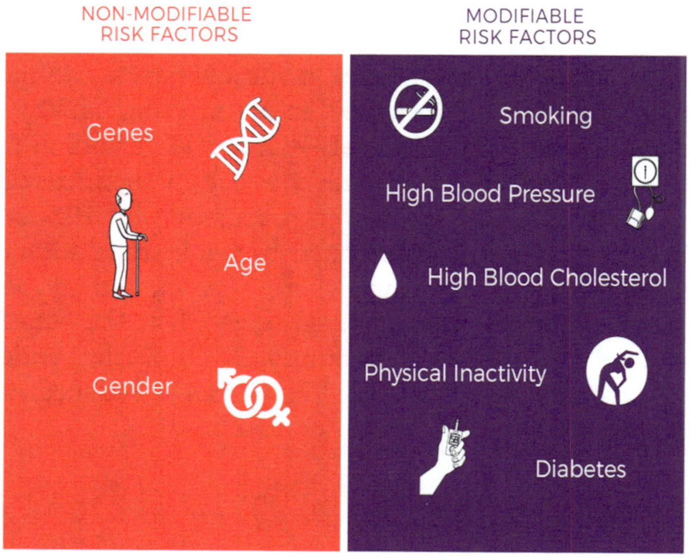

Figure 4.6. Non-modifiable risk factors versus modifiable risk factors.

Source: https://www.totalcardiaccare.com/wp-content/uploads/2018/09/RISK-FACTORS-OF-HAVING-A-HEART-DISEASE-Total-cardiac-care-_-Dr-mahadevan.png.

4.2.3. Psychological Factors and Their Influence on Heart Health

The relationship between psychological factors and heart health has been of specific interest in the case of IHD. MDD, in particular, has been identified as a crucial determinant of the incidence and outcomes of coronary heart disease (CHD). Evidence shows that MDD patients exhibit physiological alterations that make them more susceptible to ischemic episodes. For instance, the systemic disorders that are associated with depression, such as diabetes and obesity, contribute to vascular function impairment and atherosclerosis, both of which enhance heart disease risk. In addition, findings now suggest that MDD can impair the intrinsic protective mechanisms of the heart, thus leading to decreased infarct tolerance and cardioprotection. Characterization of these processes can provide an entry point for targeted therapeutic approaches, which are aimed at addressing the psychological factors that result in adverse cardiac outcomes (Budiono et al., 2017). Psychological distress has also been associated with increased risk for coronary heart disease in a variety of epidemiologic studies outside of MDD. A Glasgow cohort study of a large group documented that psychologically distressed men were at a 1.78-fold increased risk for the development of CHD compared to their non-distressed peers, even after adjusting for sociodemographic determinants and pre-existing illnesses. Specifically, the risk due to psychological distress was extremely high in men with co-morbid physical illnesses, suggesting an additive impact on cardiovascular disease. This emphasizes the importance of treating psychological problems in clinical practice, particularly for patients with comorbid mental illness and cardiovascular risk. Mental well-being intersecting with cardiac health emphasizes the importance of treating patients holistically, understanding the role played by psychological problems in shaping physical health status (Smith et al., 2005). Furthermore, understanding the relationship between psychological and cardiovascular status is not merely a matter of simple correlation. Instead, it is built on underlying physiological mechanisms that deserve to be studied further. In particular, states such as chronic stress, anxiety, and depression are believed to activate the sympathetic nervous system and interfere with the hypothalamic-pituitary-adrenal axis, producing adverse cardiac outcomes. These chronic physiological responses may also enhance inflammatory processes and vasculopathy, setting individuals at higher risk for the detrimental consequences of ischemic heart disease. Therefore, an understanding of the molecular and biological underpinnings of such connections is imperative to creating overall prevention strategies and treatment protocols. Emphasizing psychological factors in terms of ischemic heart disease not only elucidates the condition but also promotes healthier approaches towards cardiovascular health management (Budiono et al., 2017).

4.3. Symptoms and Diagnosis

Knowledge of IHD signs and symptoms is required for effective diagnosis and treatment. The most frequent presentation is pain over the chest, which is typically a pressure or squeezing sensation and radiates to the arms, back, neck, or jaw. Such pain, also called angina in a clinical environment, usually results from physical exertion or psychological stress and disappears with rest or nitroglycerin. Additionally, patients may manifest abnormal signs like fatigue, dyspnea, or palpitations, particularly in elderly or females. Clinicians cannot rely on classical signs due to their inconstant presentation; instead, an accurate assessment with a comprehensive patient history and physical examination is essential in establishing a working diagnosis of IHD. The diagnostic range of ischemic heart disease is an interdisciplinary one that applies a variety of techniques to determine both the presence and size of the disease. The noninvasive methods of myocardial perfusion imaging (MPI) have become increasingly visible, for their measurement of ischemic burden is better at predicting adverse outcomes than coronary anatomy. MPI determines myocardial blood flow and can risk stratify individuals based on their ischemic burden, providing prognostically helpful information. Standard MPI is consistent with an underlying risk of fewer than 1% for poor cardiac events such as myocardial infarction or cardiac death within a 12-month time frame, independent of any other factors such as age or gender. Therefore, MPI's role in the diagnostic process highlights the importance of assessing not just the disease state but also its overall impact on patient prognosis (Libhaber et al., 2017). Furthermore, echocardiography has emerged as a vital tool in diagnosing ischemic heart disease, particularly in its early stages. It offers insights into cardiac structure and function, detecting abnormalities at rest or under stress conditions. When performed on exercise or with drug stimulation, echocardiography can reveal subclinical myocardial dysfunction, which may be a manifestation of early ischemic alterations. It is this capability that allows the detection of patients destined to have heart failure, a condition that is typically related to chronic ischemic injury. Combining echocardiography with clinical findings enables clinicians to devise effective care plans on an individualized basis, optimizing therapeutic outcomes. Therefore, it not only serves as a diagnostic procedure but also as a prognostic marker that directs therapy in patients with ischemic heart disease symptoms (Benfari et al., 2024) (Figure 4.7).

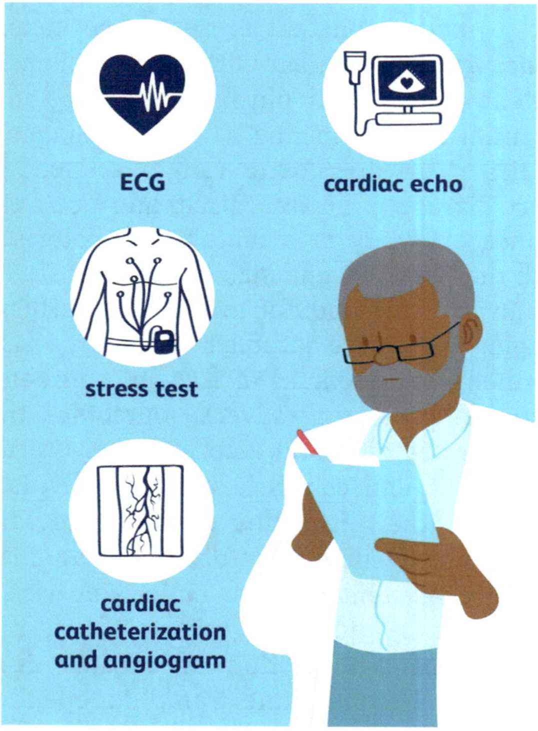

Figure 4.7. Ischemic heart disease diagnosis.

Source: https://www.verywellhealth.com/thmb/5MwW1Mf_koQxlsNd4A2ZBsuzeZ4=/750x0/filters:no_upscale():max_bytes(150000):strip_icc():format(webp)/coronary-artery-disease-diagnosis-5b2d5a7b3037130036f96c31.png.

4.3.1. Common Symptoms of Ischemic Heart Disease (IHD)

The presentation of IHD is predominantly characterized by angina pectoris, a pain or ache caused by the failure of the heart muscle to gain sufficient blood and therefore oxygen. The patients would describe the sensation as a tightening or pressure, typically in the chest area, but it might radiate to the shoulders, neck, arms, back, or jaw. This symptom tends to be exacerbated by exertion or emotional stress, situations that elevate cardiac demand and exacerbate the underlying myocardial ischemia. The severity and frequency of angina are highly variable between patients, sometimes occurring regularly as stable angina, and with other patients experiencing unstable angina, producing bouts of acute distress. An understanding of the nature of angina is crucial in the diagnosis and treatment of IHD symptoms. Another common symptom of ischemic heart disease is shortness of breath or dyspnea. This develops at rest or with exertion, reflecting the decreased pumping capability of the heart in response to reduced coronary blood flow. Of concern here is dyspnea because it is also a possible indicator of progression of IHD to more disastrous outcomes such as heart failure. A study that looked into the prevalence of heart failure in relation to ischemic heart disease finds that there is a deleterious interaction between the two, and thus having both necessitates urgent clinical evaluation (Zhou et al., 2025). Patients may describe their experience of dyspnea as windedness or inability to breathe in, which can significantly affect quality of life by limiting daily activities and social interactions. Patients may also present with additional symptoms such as fatigue, palpitations, and even nausea to make the classic presentation of IHD more challenging. Fatigue is frequently misleading as it may develop gradually, typically the consequence of age or physical inactivity. However, in patients with IHD, it might be a result of decreased cardiac function and insufficient oxygenation during stressful situations. Awareness of irregular or elevated heart rates may develop as a compensatory mechanism for ischemia, with further investigation into the heart's electrical stability being indicated. Nausea and sweating may accompany angina attacks, reflecting the body's autonomic response to ischemic attacks. Identification of these multifaceted symptoms is imperative for clinicians to develop a holistic perception of ischemic heart disease and provide integrated treatment (Dyankov et al., 2025) (Figure 4.8).

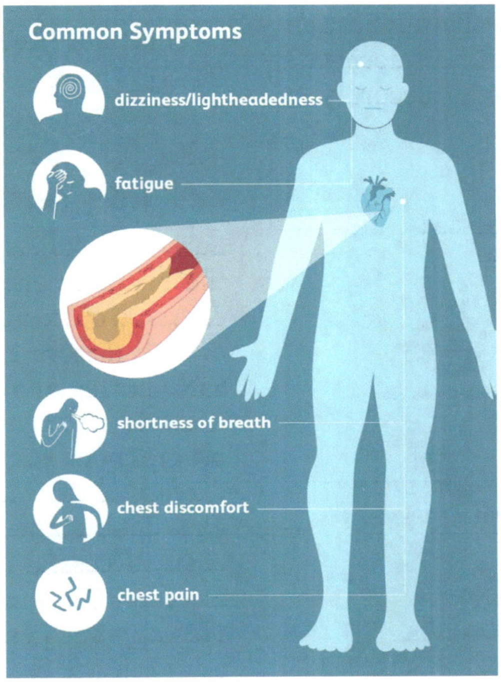

Figure 4.8. Symptoms of ischemic heart disease (IHD).

Source: https://www.verywellhealth.com/thmb/OklEMlAO5DhqvrlIAYW09c9fetY=/1001x0/filters:no_upscale():max_bytes(150000):strip_icc():format(webp)/coronary-artery-disease-symptoms-5b4f996646e0fb00376c3e90.png.

4.3.2. Diagnostic Tests (e.g., Electrocardiograms (ECG), Stress Testing)

The evaluation of IHD often involves the employment of diagnostic testing, of which most are ECGs and stress testing methods. An ECG is a simple device that may be utilized to identify electrical heart disorders that may signify ischemia. In a comparative study, researchers compared the efficiency of single-lead ECG versus bicycle ergometry. They found the single-lead ECG to have a greater area under the receiver operating characteristic curve of 67%, depicting greater diagnostic accuracy despite a statistically significant difference between the two tests not being found. These findings suggest that technological advancement of ECG can enhance the early diagnosis of IHD, potentially facilitating early intervention and improved outcomes in patients (Marzoog et al., 2025). Stress testing, particularly by methods like exercise or pharmacologic stress, provides a functional assessment of cardiac function under circumstances that cause ischemia. The use of stress ECG for the diagnosis of IHD is becoming increasingly common even among populations that have been deemed previously to be at low risk. Recent research has shown that ischemic ECG alterations in stress testing can reflect underlying abnormalities of wall motion, and some studies have suggested 33% of inducible regional wall motion abnormal patients had an ischemic ECG record. Even though sensitivity remains moderate, the relationship between stress-induced ECG alterations and critical ischemic conditions is an indication of the application of stress testing for guiding clinical decisions and the improvement of diagnostic accuracy in IHD (Kobal et al., 2024).

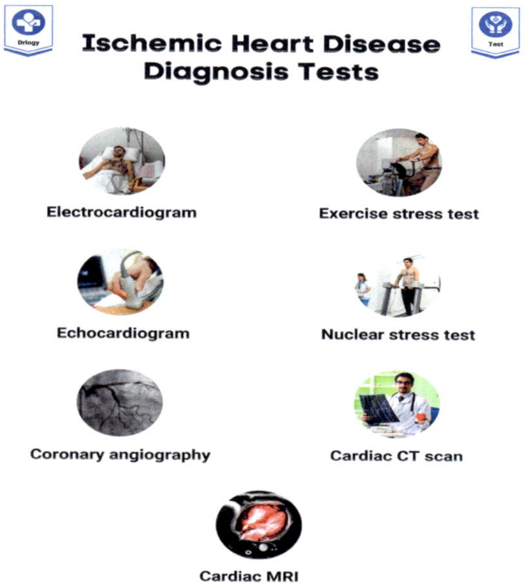

Figure 4.9. Ischemic heart disease (IHD) diagnosis tests.

Source: https://images.drlogy.com/assets/uploads/img/admin/health_blog/editor-img/ischemic_heart_disease_diagnosis_-_drlogy.webp.

Moreover, stress test report interpretation is based on advanced knowledge of several cardiac indices. Even where baseline ECG is devoid of ischemic changes, their appearance during stress testing can go a long way in deciding the course of treatment. Measurement of parameters such as left ventricular contractile reserve and coronary flow velocity reserve is related to the degree of ischemia, providing clinical value to the results of stress ECG. Therefore, the integration of diagnostic technology improvements, such as the single-lead ECG and enhanced stress imaging techniques, is expected to lead to improved diagnostic pathways for IHD, enabling better risk stratification and treatment optimization by clinicians (Kobal et al., 2024; Marzoog et al., 2025) (Figure 4.9).

4.3.3. Importance of Early Detection and Intervention

Early detection and treatment are significant in the management of IHD, having considerable effects on outcomes for the patients. Identification of risk factors and symptoms of IHD in the early stages allows for early intervention and lifestyle changes that can prevent disease progression. For instance, the use of modern diagnostic techniques, such as speckle tracking with dobutamine stress echocardiography, has been successful in diagnosing coronary artery disease (CAD) among patients at moderate risk. This approach enables healthcare providers to establish the presence of CAD more distinctly, which directly enhances the likelihood of early intervention and management methods that may potentially reduce morbidity and mortality associated with IHD (Kadhim et al., 2024). Emphasis on early detection is thus significant in precluding the disease's impact and promoting patients' long-term wellness. Moreover, public awareness of risk factors and warning signs of ischemic heart disease is vital for early detection. Evidence indicates wide knowledge gaps among older people about IHD, particularly among the poor population of Egypt, where evidence showed only a negligible percentage were aware of risk factors. The lack of awareness goes hand in hand with the urban-rural gap, demonstrating that rural population tends to have lower knowledge and, as a result, may have delayed medical visits (Rakab et al., 2024). This lack of awareness makes it imperative to implement educational measures promoting public knowledge regarding IHD. By increasing awareness and educating individuals about early symptoms of the disease, health systems can promote timely interventions, finally leading to improved health outcomes. Overall, it is crucial to strengthen the early detection and intervention patterns of ischemic heart disease for effective disease management. Implementing effective screening programs with innovative diagnostic techniques, along with mass educational campaigns in the population, can address the most critical areas of lost opportunity in treatment and diagnosis. These preventive measures not only reduce the IHD burden among high-risk populations, particularly the elderly, but also usher in a health-oriented culture promoting regular medical checkups and lifestyle changes. Through earlier detection and earlier interventions, healthcare providers are able to significantly enhance the quality of life of at-risk individuals for ischemic heart disease, ultimately translating into better health outcomes and reducing the overall prevalence of the disease.

4.4. Treatment Options

Management of IHD calls for a multidisciplinary strategy to successfully manage the condition due to its complexity. Lifestyle adjustments are the cornerstone of therapy, with initial strategies targeting the eradication of bad habits such as smoking. Abstinence has been demonstrated to significantly enhance patient results in research studies. Additionally, acceptance of a healthy life that includes a well-balanced diet, exercise, and weight control can reduce the risk factors against IHD. Patient education is a significant aspect of this phase, where patients learn to value the importance of remaining on prescribed medications and lifestyle modifications as a method of managing symptoms and decelerating the progression of the disease (Servito et al., 2023). Thus, these initial steps give rise to more specialized medical therapies. Drug therapy contributes towards lifestyle change and typically includes the co-administration of antiplatelet drugs, beta-blockers, and statins, which work towards stabilizing and improving cardiovascular health. Antiplatelet drugs such as aspirin reduce the risk of thrombus formation and resulting myocardial infarction, which is a common complication among IHD patients. Beta-blockers reduce myocardial oxygen demand by reducing heart rate and contractility, and therefore decreasing anginal symptoms. Statins are of special significance for their lipid-lowering effect as well as their capacity to stabilize plaques in coronary arteries.

In some patient groups, however, particularly more advanced presentations of ischemic heart disease, such as CADASIL patients, additional interventions could be warranted, including surgery aimed at improving coronary perfusion (Servito et al., 2023). In ischemic heart disease unresponsive to medical therapy, invasive therapies such as percutaneous coronary interventions (PCI) or coronary artery bypass grafting (CABG) may be necessary. These therapies aim to restore blood flow to ischemic myocardium via the recanalization of obstructed coronary vessels or via the creation of bypass loops. Despite their effectiveness, these treatments carry some risk; in the case of patients with conditions like CADASIL, the possibility of peri-procedure complications—most commonly stroke—needs to be addressed with appropriate consideration and a multidisciplinary approach. Cardiologists, surgeons, and neurologists need to work together to develop personalized treatment plans that balance the benefit of every revascularization with its risk in complex patients. Increased research into targeted therapies and clearer guidelines will continue to enhance strategic care management of ischemic heart disease in diverse populations of patients (Gore, 2012) (Figure 4.10).

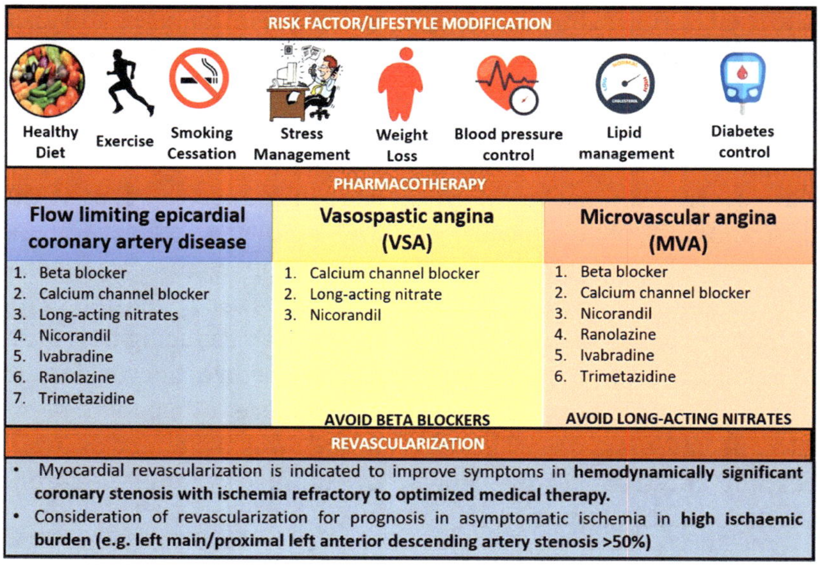

Figure 4.10. Management of ischemic heart disease (IHD).

Source: https://www.researchgate.net/publication/351525876/figure/fig3/AS:11431281086967309@1664417133412/Management-of-ischemic-heart-disease.png.

4.4.1. Lifestyle Modifications and Their Effectiveness

The relationship between IHD treatment and lifestyle modification is of ultimate importance in contemporary health care. Effective modification of lifestyle, such as dietetic modification, exercise, and smoking cessation, is of great potential for decreasing risk factors associated with IHD. The available evidence shows that a diet rich in fruits, vegetables, whole grains, and lean proteins may all be of benefit to lipid profiles and blood pressure levels. In contrast, consumption of saturated fats and refined carbohydrates has been linked to increased cardiovascular risk. In addition, frequent aerobic exercise can enhance cardiovascular fitness and aid in weight management, thereby diminishing the incidence of this long-term disease. These observations underscore the significance of lifestyle modification in improving worldwide heart health and its integration into patient care programs to ensure long-term adherence and better outcomes. MHealth technologies have played an increasingly prominent role over the last decade as a method for facilitating lifestyle change among patients with IHD.

As there is a convergence of mobile health applications and telehealth services, patients can potentially receive individualized guidance and counseling for healthy lifestyle adoption. These interventions have been shown to enhance patient adherence with lifestyle changes under recommendation with the provision of immediate feedback and reinforcement, especially with chronic conditions like IHD. Studies evaluating an mHealth-based disease management program identified substantial decreases in levels of low-density lipoprotein cholesterol among the individuals, demonstrating incredible improvement in cardiovascular risk profiles within six months. The ease and feasibility offered by these technologies allow patients to self-manage their health, making it simpler to follow lifestyle modifications and make them more efficient, thereby ensuring long-term cardiovascular wellness (Miki et al., 2024). The role of healthcare professionals in promoting lifestyle change cannot be overstated. They play a central role in educating patients on the likely benefits of lifestyle change and in developing an environment that supports health. Integrating lifestyle modification counseling into clinical practice provides patients with individualized tools and methods suitable for their circumstances. Moreover, research has also shown that continued observation and support by healthcare personnel can enhance the effectiveness of lifestyle change and yield maximum health benefits. For instance, a systematic review highlights that it is crucial to integrate pharmacological treatment with lifestyle modification to produce optimal results in patients with heart failure, which is a common consequence of undiagnosed IHD. With the delivery of interventions aimed at the multifactorial etiology of cardiovascular wellness, healthcare professionals can facilitate patients to engage in successful lifestyle changes that significantly reduce the risk for ischemic heart disease and promote improved quality of life (Elendu et al., 2024).

4.4.2. Pharmacological Treatments (e.g., Antiplatelets, Statins)

Management of IHD relies heavily on pharmacologic therapy with an intense focus on antiplatelets and statins. Antiplatelets such as aspirin and clopidogrel play a central role in avoiding the development of vascular events by avoiding platelet aggregation. They are particularly relevant to patients who have undergone coronary interventions since they avoid stent thrombosis and reinfarction. Furthermore, the adjunctive use of statins not only reduces cholesterol levels but also exerts anti-inflammatory action, which stabilizes atherosclerotic plaques. The synergistic action of antiplatelets and statins conforms to the basic principles of preventive cardiology to reduce cardiovascular morbidity and mortality from IHD. Understanding the pharmacodynamics and therapeutic action of these medications is key to optimizing treatment regimens in clinical practice. Adherence to prescribed pharmacologic therapy, however, is a significant issue with the management of ischemic heart disease. Research has shown that various psychosocial factors like depression and anxiety influence compliance with the medication regimen in patients.

Furthermore, beliefs regarding treatment efficacy significantly affect the degree of adherence, which is a key aspect in long-term control and prevention of rehospitalization. A study that had looked at these dynamics found that inhibitory control predicts pharmacological treatment adherence in patients with IHD directly, thereby supporting the role of psychological evaluations in clinical practice. A comprehensive strategy involving both the pharmacological and psychological determinants is therefore applied to enhance adherence, which in turn reduces the risk of ischemic heart disease-attributable poor outcomes (Flores-Mendoza et al., 2024). Besides, evidence-based pharmacologic management is limited by systemic barriers within healthcare systems. While recommendations are to employ lifestyle change and medications like antiplatelet and statins regularly for secondary prevention in atherosclerotic cardiovascular disease, their utilization differs between clinical practices (Laranjo et al., 2024). Barriers such as limited access to health care, clinical inertia, and absence of primary care infrastructure hamper management. These issues need to be resolved through integrated strategies, including improving health literacy and enhancing drug access at the national policy level. Promoting patient education along with institutional change, healthcare providers can facilitate enhanced compliance with pharmacological treatment and thereby improve total patient outcomes for ischemic heart disease. This integrative strategy is required to harmonize clinical guidelines and real-life practice (Figure 4.11).

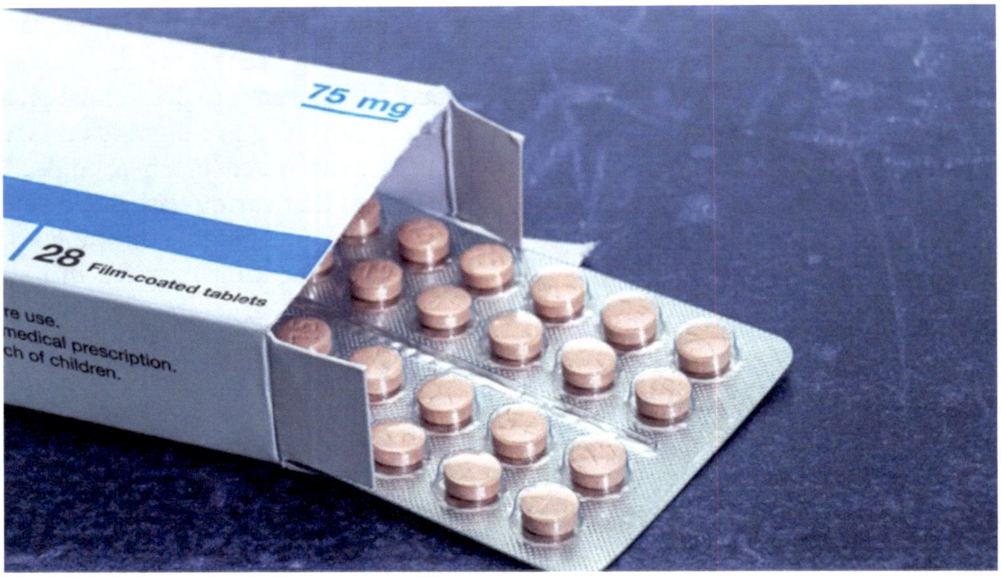

Figure 4.11. Statins for cardiovascular health.

Source: https://i0.wp.com/post.medicalnewstoday.com/wp-content/uploads/sites/3/2022/08/statin_cardiovascular_GettyImages1346002064_Header-1024x575.jpg?w=1155&h=1528.

4.4.3. Surgical Interventions (e.g., Angioplasty, Bypass Surgery)

Surgical intervention is a mainstay in the management of IHD, particularly in cases where patients present with severe coronary artery occlusion as well as other conditions that restrict the flow of blood to the heart muscle. Among the most commonly carried out operations are CABG and angioplasty. Angioplasty, such as the inflation of a balloon to compress plaque against the vessel wall and often the insertion of a stent, has been shown to improve blood flow and symptoms like angina. Being a minimally invasive procedure, it has quicker recovery times compared to more invasive surgery, and it is a beautiful first-line therapy for the majority of patients presenting with IHD. The choice between CABG and angioplasty typically lies in the site and extent of arterial occlusion, along with the overall health condition of the patients and some anatomical considerations. CABG is a more invasive surgery that creates a new pathway for blood to flow to the heart by bypassing blocked arteries with the use of grafts from the remainder of the body. Though CABG has traditionally been the preferred choice for multiple-vessel disease or left primary coronary disease, long-term benefits are reduction in symptoms and improved survival. It is evident that operative response in comorbid patients, such as type 2 diabetics, varies. For instance, bypass grafting in the coronary artery doesn't always preclude the risk of adverse outcomes among diabetic patients, as revealed by studies showing residual elevated mortality risk even when revascularization therapy was effective (Kotha et al., 2024). This underlines the necessity for tailored approaches to consider both the physiological and anatomical nuances of IHD within various patient populations. In addition, the role of surgery is not only in a successful procedure but also demands an in-depth understanding and command of post-operative care so that the best outcome is ensured. Research indicates that the patient who has undergone CABG with pre-existing comorbid conditions such as diabetes can have differential recovery patterns, namely in myocardial energetics and functional capacity (Kotha et al., 2024). The assessment of recovery will generally employ a variety of measures, including myocardial blood flow and exercise function testing. Surprisingly, studies have shown that despite having an initial disadvantage, diabetic patients can recover to a great extent following surgery, challenging earlier beliefs about surgical outcome among this group (Kotha et al., 2024). Therefore, continued investigation into the long-term effectiveness and modifications of surgical therapies is essential, especially in the high-risk population, to maximize treatment strategies and improve overall patient care for the treatment of ischemic heart disease (Figure 4.12).

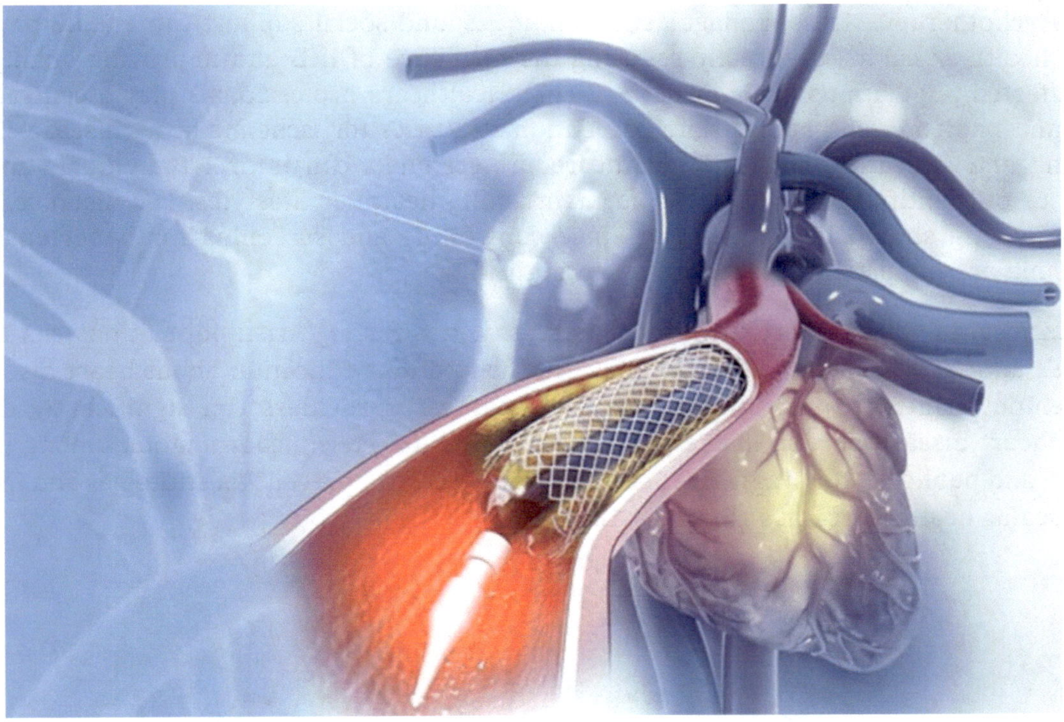

Figure 4.12. Angioplasty-and-Bypass-Surgery.

Source: https://www.metrohospitals.com/wp-content/uploads/2025/01/Choosing-Between-Angioplasty-and-Bypass-Surgery-A-Patients-Guide.jpg.

4.5. Prevention Strategies

Prevention of IHD is of utmost significance, as lifestyle components play a substantial role in developing and progressing IHD. Effective methods of prevention include diet modification, exercise, and weight management. A dietary intake pattern that promotes heart health, characterized by high consumption of fruits, vegetables, whole grains, and healthier fats, can decrease several risk factors like hypertension and diabetes. In addition, regular physical activity serves to not only sustain weight but also promote cardiovascular health through enhanced lipid profiles and blood pressure reduction. Evidence has ever shown that individuals who include regular exercise have reduced incidence of cardiac events, highlighting the utmost significance of the strategies of promoting health that support active living (Bondar et al., 2024). Targeting these preventive behaviors is a way that public health programs can successfully decrease the burden and incidence of IHD in various populations. Psychosocial determinants also have a role in determining prevention strategy effectiveness for IHD because mental illness, such as depression, can increase cardiovascular risks. Understanding the complex relationship between psychological well-being and cardiac health is key to developing prevention programs with widespread reach. IHD patients with depression typically have more severe problems, such as non-compliance with clinical recommendations and unhealthy coping mechanisms in the form of excessive food intake or smoking (Alazmi et al., 2024). Intervening in these psychosocial issues using collaborative care models can improve the overall health of patients by combining mental health and physical health treatment. Interventions that involve psychotherapy, stress management techniques, and social support can enable patients to embrace healthier habits, eventually reducing the incidence of IHD and improving quality of life among affected populations (Bondar et al., 2024). Healthcare professionals play a central role in crafting and implementing appropriate prevention strategies for ischemic heart disease. Through counseling and educating patients, healthcare professionals can inform individuals about the importance of identifying risk factors and maintaining healthier lifestyles. For instance, routine health screening should be encouraged since controlling and screening for hypertension and dyslipidemia are important aspects of preventing IHD

(Alazmi et al., 2024). Furthermore, contact activities for high-risk populations can enhance awareness and facilitate early interventions. Through patient education about heart disease and patient empowerment to control their health, healthcare providers can significantly decrease ischemic heart disease burden in the population. In the long term, coordination among patients, providers, and public health programs is essential for successful prevention strategies and improved cardiovascular health outcomes (Figure 4.13).

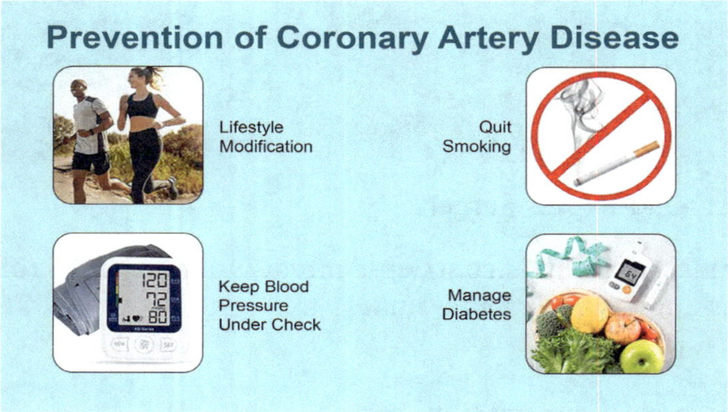

Figure 4.13. Prevention of coronary artery disease.

Source: https://cdn.hexahealth.com/Image/1726057592109-946310215.webp.

4.5.1. Importance of Public Health Initiatives

Public health interventions play a crucial role in IHD prevention by facilitating prevention and awareness strategies that help curb risk factors. By educating individuals on heart-healthy lifestyles, the interventions guide individuals toward healthy diets and physical activity, both of which are crucial in the minimization of cardiovascular diseases. Community health campaigns promoting the importance of nutrition and physical activity are vital, especially among disadvantaged populations where resources are minimal. The National Heart, Lung, and Blood Institute (NHLBI) has understood the importance of such educational campaigns by giving priority to research that identifies areas of health disparity and supports targeted interventions (Heart et al., 2002). Thus, encouraging public awareness through efficient health programs ultimately contributes to the decline of IHD rates and encouraging well-being in different communities. Moreover, public health programs not only target prevention but also facilitate early detection and control of ischemic heart disease. Risk factor screening programs that assess hypertension, diabetes, and high cholesterol can significantly contribute to the health outcome of individuals by facilitating timely interventions. Through increased availability of routine health checks, particularly among high-risk patients, public health programs are the first line of defense against the progression of heart disease. These programs play a crucial role in ensuring that those with greater risks are given adequate education and assistance to manage their conditions successfully. Involvement of research data in such initiatives, as emphasized by the NHLBI, also renders strategy responsive and evidence-based, meeting the particular needs of various populations (Heart et al., 2002). Effective public health action is, therefore, essential in an attempt to improve health equity when it comes to IHD. Beyond enhanced individual health, public health activities within the context of ischemic heart disease yield broader societal benefits. By decreasing IHD incidence, the programs lower the cost of healthcare expenditure, lost productivity, and premature mortality. Healthier people result in fewer hospitalizations and reduced demand for medical care, leading to significant cost savings in the healthcare system. The programs also encourage the creation of a culture of health that reinforces intersectoral cooperation among government and non-government agencies to create enabling environments for heart health. Involvement of the community in decision-making regarding health matters makes citizens more empowered and increases social cohesion. Persistent watchfulness and concentration on health inequities, as defined by thorough research studies, are significant to enhancing the overall efficiency of public health campaigns against ischemic heart disease. With all these collaborative efforts, society can aim towards a healthier future (Figure 4.14).

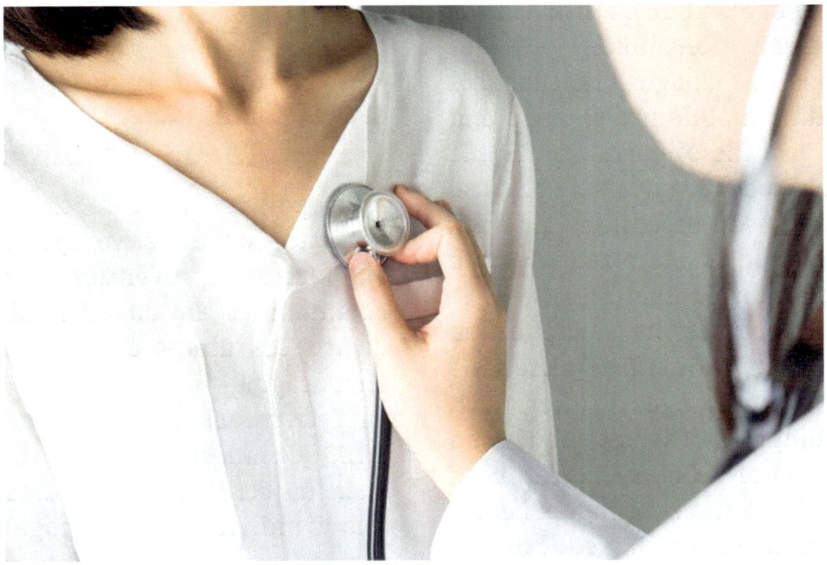

Figure 4.14. Importance of Public Health Initiatives.

Source: https://nutritionsource.hsph.harvard.edu/wp-content/uploads/2024/11/AdobeStock_189264942-1024x683.jpeg.

4.5.2. Role of Education in Risk Factor Management

The role education has to play in reducing IHD-related risk factors is central to fostering a healthier citizenry. Provision of information empowers the citizen to make informed lifestyle choices that minimize risk factors such as poor diet, increased blood pressure, and overweight or obesity. Educational interventions that address diet, exercise, and stress management are instrumental in modifying long-term patterns of behavior. For instance, community workshops highlighting the significance of an appropriate diet and regular physical activity can promote healthier habits among participants. Such initiatives are particularly vital in poor communities where access to health information could be substandard. With enhanced public awareness of diet risk consequences and metabolic determinants, evidence-based educational interventions can reduce the incidence of IHD considerably. Findings reveal that there is a potential for health education to revolutionize in offsetting the load of ischemic heart disease both on an individual scale and a social scale (Wang et al., 2025). Furthermore, health education through technology provides innovative solutions in managing risk factors. New media, including mobile health apps and eHealth websites, give the opportunity for the provision of personalized diet advice and physical exercise regimens. These interventions can track users' behavior, providing customized advice to encourage the adoption of healthier lifestyle options. For instance, studies have established that the application of mHealth applications can lead to significant changes in diet, such as increased consumption of whole grains and reduced consumption of processed meat, both critical in IHD risk prevention (Venugopal et al., 2024). Furthermore, incorporating educational content into routine healthcare interactions can enhance patients' understanding of their illnesses. With the easy integration of traditional education methods and technology, health professionals can establish a solid foundation for communicating crucial information about the disease risk factors of ischemic heart disease. Lastly, collaboration with community groups that involve stakeholders such as local organizations, schools, and healthcare centers can enhance educational outreach. Involvement with influencers and community leaders can reinforce health messages and travel more deeply into otherwise hard-to-reach populations. For example, initiatives encouraging schools to implement health education curricula not only benefit children but also extend their reach to parents and families, a ripple effect of awareness and behavior change. Interventions targeted to specific populations, such as those that address the particular issues of males who have been identified as being at higher risk for IHD, can make interventions more relevant and effective. It is only through such interventional approaches that health literacy disparities can be reduced and environments supportive of cardiovascular health can be created. Overall, an integrated approach involving education, technology, and community engagement is required for effective management of the risk factors causing ischemic heart disease (Wang et al., 2025).

4.5.3. Community Support and Resources for Prevention

A proper response to the problems of IHD demands an effective system of community support and prevention services. Grassroots communities play an essential role in promoting awareness about cardiovascular health and encouraging people to make lifestyle changes that decrease risk factors associated with IHD. Community-based health programs such as screening programs and workshops allow individuals to recognize symptoms of cardiovascular disease and learn about their risk factors. Enlisting the support of local health workers, schools, and institutions to promote healthy diets, physical activity, and cessation of smoking can significantly reduce the rate of IHD.

Moreover, collective action by community leaders and health professionals can develop tailored resources for specific demographic needs, ultimately leading to better health outcomes among the population. In addition, community programs organized on a broad scale may enhance access to preventive care that is central to controlling ischemic heart disease. Regionally directed programs can provide residents with low-cost or no-cost health screening, dietary instruction, and physical exercise training. Facilitating group participation, such programs also build social support, which is integral to sustaining a healthy lifestyle. For instance, walking groups within neighborhoods can offer safe havens and encourage people to persist with physical activity, thereby promoting healthy lifestyles. The programs not only motivate people to participate but also help them better understand and manage their personal health, while also teaching them how to share common knowledge with others who have similar health conditions within their neighborhoods. Support from international organizations doubles the strength of the community resources for ischemic heart disease prevention and offers a comprehensive strategy for risk reduction. For instance, capacity-building opportunities provided by programs organized by institutions like the International Atomic Energy Agency (IAEA) introduce local healthcare professionals to the most recent diagnostic techniques and treatment modalities specific to IHD. With a focus on gender-based risk factors, such programs attend to vulnerability in women, leveraging community resources to address the special needs of all groups. A case in point from Latin America and the Caribbean's development of diagnostic centers and training programs is leveraging international aid in developing a system of knowledge sharing that facilitates innovation in preventative healthcare strategies (Peix et al., 2024). Lastly, the combination of neighborhood participation and global collaboration significantly enhances the community's authority in combating ischemic heart disease effectively (Zhang et al., 2024) (Figure 4.15).

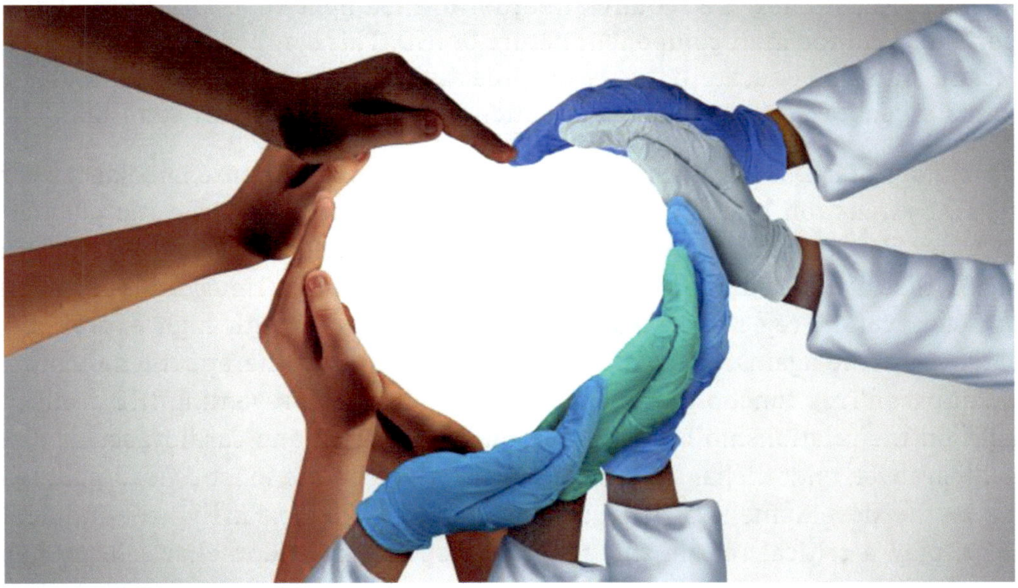

Figure 4.15. Community Support.

Source: https://www.nhlbi.nih.gov/sites/default/files/styles/16x9_crop/public/2024-02/shutterstock_1722577084.jpg?h=b6102556&itok=MSwsaDRE.

SUMMARY

In summarizing a review of IHD, there should be the integration of the vast evidence for the multi-factorial etiology of cardiovascular disease. Clinical studies demonstrate that lifestyle factors like exercise, diet, and consumption patterns largely contribute to the risk of developing IHD. For instance, recent genetic studies have pointed to a protective interaction between tea drinking and cardiovascular risk, where increased tea consumption is linked with decreased hypertension rates and stroke risks involved in heart disease (Gao et al., 2022). This points to the importance of diet in the treatment of IHD, noting that preventive measures can significantly affect the occurrence of the disease. Therefore, an understanding of the causal associations can help with more effective public health and patient interventions to reduce the burden of IHD. The qualitative nature of experience, particularly for women with IHD, is also central to a complete understanding of the disease. Utilizing methodologies such as Colaizzi's phenomenological approach allows researchers to capture the lived experiences of patients, shedding light on emotional and psychological dimensions that accompany chronic illnesses like IHD. Through thematic analysis, significant insights emerge regarding how women perceive their interactions with health care systems, their symptoms, and the emotional weight of managing a chronic disease (Praveena et al., 2021). These qualitative results not only serve to enrich the IHD theoretical model but also inform clinical practices attuned to the needs and circumstances of the patients. Overall, the complexity of Ischemic Heart Disease necessitates synthesizing quantitative and qualitative research evidence to better comprehend and manage the disease. From further research into associations of lifestyle change, emotional experience, and disease outcome, it is evident that effective management strategies need to encompass a broad spectrum of patient experiences. Ongoing research studies, including randomized controlled trials and phenomenological studies, are required in order to shed light on associations of diet patterns, patient experience, and the multicomponent nature of IHD. This synthesis of evidence will not only enable clinicians but also educate patients on proactive care for their cardiovascular well-being with the ultimate goal of better outcomes in patients with this prevalent condition.

Pathophysiology of IHD is significantly influenced by immune response imbalances of regulatory T cells (Tregs). Dysfunction of Tregs leads to the formation of atherosclerotic plaques and thus worsens IHD risk. Mendelian randomization analysis identified a set of 197 single-nucleotide polymorphisms that are instrumental variables associated with various subtypes of Tregs. This study identified several Treg subpopulations, specifically those with high expression levels of CD28, as potentially safe against IHD risk. According to the study, therapeutic modalities directed to the modulation of Treg function can be a novel approach to preventing IHD from developing, shedding light on the relationship between immune modulation and cardiovascular disease (Hou et al., 2024). Moreover, endothelial dysfunction is shown to be the most crucial pathogenic factor contributing to the development of IHD, usually caused by hypoxia. Hypoxia-inducible factors, namely HIF2α, play a critical role in the adaptive response of endothelial cells to hypoxia. The management of inflammation and vascular integrity processes depends on the interaction between HIF2α and its dimerization partner, ARNT. Upon adaptation of endothelial cells to environmental stress, disruption of HIF signaling makes cardiovascular pathologies more susceptible, and these eventually progress to IHD. Therefore, the targeting of these pathways is a therapeutic promise for the improvement of vascular wellness and overall cardiac performance in patients predisposed to IHD (Ullah et al., 2023). Lastly, the intricate relationship between immune responses and endothelial pathologies defines the intricacy in IHD pathogenesis. Current evidence indicates that Treg function as well as endothelial signaling play pivotal roles in the induction of the diseases. Through studying these mechanisms, researchers can identify prospective therapeutic targets that can enhance cardiovascular resilience. With improved knowledge of Treg involvement and endothelial cell function, there is hope for new treatments attacking the underlying causes of IHD. It is this multidisciplinary strategy that lays stress on conducting continuous research in IHD molecular and cellular interactions, thereby exploring new opportunities for better management in clinical practice (Ullah et al., 2023; Hou et al., 2024).

A CLOSER LOOK

COMPLICATIONS OF ISCHEMIC HEART DISEASE (IHD)

IHD can lead to a variety of complications affecting patient outcomes and quality of life significantly. The most obvious complication is myocardial infarction (MI) or heart attack, whereby blood supply to a portion of the heart is stopped, and the heart tissue is damaged. Research has also indicated that the therapeutic modalities, such as the glucagon-like peptide-1 (GLP-1) receptor agonists, can significantly reduce myocardial infarction risk among patients. In the Harmony Outcomes trial, the GLP-1 agonist albiglutide demonstrated a 25% relative risk reduction in MI events, thus bringing into evidence its effectiveness in preventing ischemic events among high-risk patients with type 2 diabetes and established cardiovascular disease (Krychtiuk et al., 2024). Hence, the management of IHD not only involves management of the disease process but also interventions to prevent the onset of MI. Ischaemic heart disease, along with myocardial infarction, typically leads to other conditions such as heart failure, arrhythmias, and restenosis of the coronary arteries. Heart failure develops when the heart's volume of blood pumping is compromised, and the body attempts to compensate through various physiological pathways, which ultimately lead to progressive cardiac failure. The IHD patients are also at higher risk of arrhythmias, which have a significant effect on cardiac function and mortality.

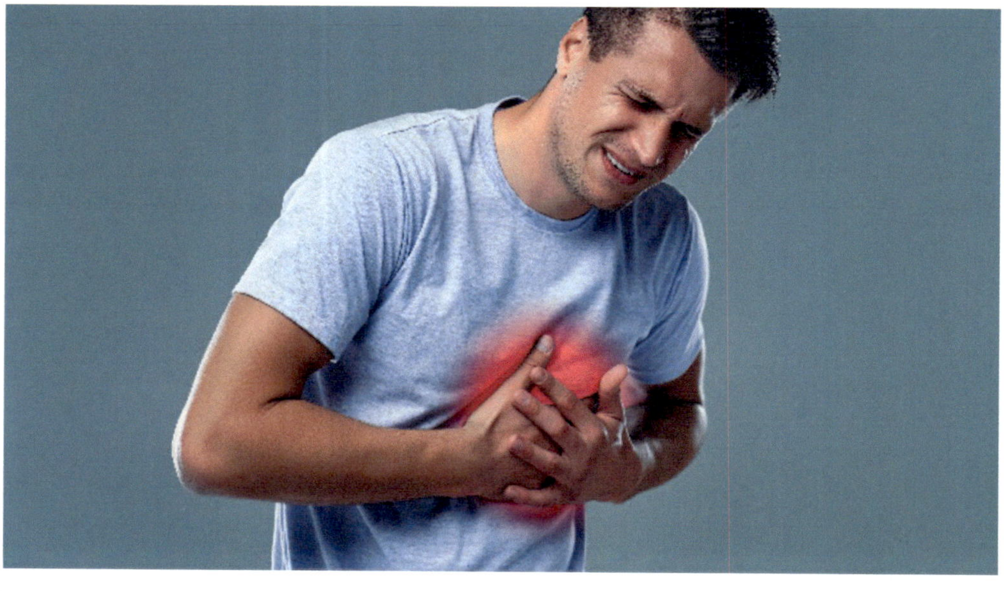

Figure 4.16. Complications of Ischemic Heart Disease.

Source: https://d35oenyzp35321.cloudfront.net/Heart_Failure_In_Youngsters_498e3b1f38.jpg.

There is a reason to believe that mental health intervention, particularly for depression and anxiety, can play a substantial role in cardiovascular status in this population. IHD patients who undergo the proper treatment of mental health report lower rehospitalization and overall mortality, which speaks to the interdependence of physical and psychological well-being (Carmin et al., 2024).

This speaks to the need to take a holistic approach in the treatment of ischemic heart disease complications. Lastly, the complications of ischemic heart disease can also express themselves as socioeconomic factors, complicating treatment and recovery. The economic burden of repeated admissions, medications, and lost time from work can be heavy on patients and healthcare systems. Therefore, the control of IHD should not only include drug therapies but also strategies to reduce socioeconomic inequalities that may limit access to care. For example, interventions that improve mental health management and adaptation to chronic stressors of having heart disease can significantly contribute to patient outcomes. By integrating care programs such as medical and psychosocial management, healthcare providers are better positioned to help patients adapt to the intricate landscape of IHD complications, eventually improving their overall quality of life and mortality rates (Figure 4.16).

References

1. Alazmi, A. H. S., Khiriy, S. A., Khiriy, M. A., Alabdulaal, F. A., Aldossry, K. M. H., ALshammari, K. R., Otaibi, R. H. S. A., Alrowaily, M. J., Sawadi, H. a. M., Al-Shahrani, S. N., Alanzei, N. a. S., Aldossri, B. M. M., Alruwaily, K. M. a. A., Aldosari, H. N. F., Anzi, A. S. A., & Al-Moshawwh, M. A. (2024). Comprehensive Nursing Care in Coronary Heart Disease: Biochemical Markers, Strategies, Challenges, and Evidence-Based Approaches for Effective Patient Management and Outcomes. *Egyptian Journal of Chemistry*, *67*(13), 1449–1463. https://doi.org/10.21608/ejchem.2024.335773.10782Ali, A., Khan, M. U., Hussain, S., & Ali, S. (2025). Trends and demographic patterns of ischemic heart disease risk factors in patients at a tertiary care cardiology department. *Insights-Journal of Health and Rehabilitation*. https://www.semanticscholar.org/paper/97a4858adf8698f9e7ecb08a253225dca1fe26d7 (accessed on 29th May 2025).
2. Applegate, R. L., Krafft, P. R., Leitzke, A. S., Tang, et al. (2012). *The Role of Volatile Anesthetics in Cardio Protection: A Systematic Review.* https://core.ac.uk/download/323068253.pdf (accessed on 29th May 2025).
3. Benfari, G., Cameli, M., Campora, A., D'Andrea, et al. (2024). *Stress Echocardiography in Heart Failure Patients: Additive Value and Caveats.* https://core.ac.uk/download/618720427.pdf (accessed on 29th May 2025).
4. Bondar, L. I., Osser, B., Osser, G., Mariş, M. A., Piroş, L. E., Almăşan, R., Toth, C., et al. (2024). The connection between depression and ischemic heart disease: Analyzing demographic characteristics, risk factors, symptoms, and treatment approaches to identify their relationship. *Clinics and Practice, 14*, 2166–2186. https://www.semanticscholar.org/paper/b2bb4338115a5bb86ee586e1f88446f52a3d02f8 (accessed on 29th May 2025).
5. Budiono, B. P., Headrick, J. P., Neumann, D. L., Peart, et al. (2017). *The Heartbreak of Depression: 'Psycho-Cardiac' Coupling in Myocardial Infarction.* https://core.ac.uk/download/196605092.pdf (accessed on 29th May 2025).
6. Bulinski, A., Butkovsky, O., Shashkin, A., Yaskov, et al. (2011). *Statistical Methods of SNP Data Analysis with Applications.* https://core.ac.uk/download/47106312.pdf (accessed on 29th May 2025).
7. Carmin, C. N., Ownby, R. L., Fontanella, C. A., Steelesmith, D. L., & Binkley, P. F. (2024). Impact of mental health treatment on outcomes in patients with heart failure and ischemic heart disease. *Journal of the American Heart Association: Cardiovascular and Cerebrovascular Disease, 13.* https://www.semanticscholar.org/paper/6a06ca60a357235bac09e87d3269f32eca15cd05 (accessed on 29th May 2025).
8. Ciucă-Pană, M., Boulmpou, A., Ileri, C., Manzi, G., Golino, M., Ostojic, M., Galimzhanov, A., et al. (2025). Chronic heart failure and coronary artery disease: Pharmacological treatment and cardiac rehabilitation. *Medicina, 61.* https://www.semanticscholar.org/paper/308d3ae19050cd5654730e0f697e2d4bb81e0c77 (accessed on 29th May 2025).
9. De La Sen. P. M., Ghosh, S., Samanta, G. (2021). *Bayesian Analysis for Cardiovascular Risk Factors in Ischemic Heart Disease.* https://core.ac.uk/download/547400844.pdf (accessed on 29th May 2025).

10. De Marchis, M., D'Amato, A., Fedele, F., Mancone, et al. (2018). *Diabetes Mellitus and Ischemic Heart Disease: The Role of Ion Channels*. https://core.ac.uk/download/159269109.pdf (accessed on 29th May 2025).

11. Del Furia, M. J., Arienti, C., Cattadori, G., Di Marco, S., & Kiekens, C. (2024). Overview of Cochrane systematic reviews on interventions for rehabilitation in people with ischemic heart disease: A mapping synthesis. *Journal of Clinical Medicine, 13*. https://www.semanticscholar.org/paper/41da34acf05036ae86fa031c1b7ceba1ea160c27 (accessed on 29th May 2025).

12. Dyankov, K., Dimitrova, V., Radkova, M., & Karamfiloff, K. (2025). Real-life data and the utility of echocardiography in young patients under 45 years with ischemic heart disease: A single-centered retrospective analysis. *European Heart Journal – Cardiovascular Imaging*. https://www.semanticscholar.org/paper/429668794947ac63fd5eda34d754d693c0d8f001 (accessed on 29th May 2025).

13. Elendu, C., Amaechi, D. C., Elendu, T. C., Fiemotonghan, B., Okoye, O. K., Agu-Ben, C. M., Onyekweli, S. O., et al. (2024). A comprehensive review of heart failure: Unraveling the etiology, decoding pathophysiological mechanisms, navigating diagnostic modalities, exploring pharmacological interventions, advocating lifestyle modifications, and charting the horizon of emerging therapies in the complex landscape of chronic. *Medicine, 103*. https://www.semanticscholar.org/paper/c43f3b6c7ad03ee3fe4bb548340fee6319b2fd81 (accessed on 29th May 2025).

14. Eram, F., Quamri, M. A., Bhat, M. D. A., Siddiqui, U., Nida, S. (2023). Perspective of ischemic heart disease (Iqfari Marad-i-Qalb) with reference to Unani medicine. *Bangladesh Journal of Medical Science*. https://www.semanticscholar.org/paper/cef32e3ad843c9fd9e44f0233920e21436aaed8e (accessed on 29th May 2025).

15. Flores-Mendoza, J. B., Salvador-Cruz, J., Robles-Garcia, R., Aceves, C. J. L., & Diaz-Loving, R. (2024). Development of a predictive model for adherence to pharmacological treatment in ischemic heart disease: Consideration of psychosociocultural, neuropsychological, and mental health variables. *European Heart Journal*. https://www.semanticscholar.org/paper/96308971094a3994f9e24599f4f7145a4af3e932 (accessed on 29th May 2025).

16. Franczyk, B., Rysz, J., Olszewski, R., & Gluba-Sagr, A. (2024). Do implantable cardioverter-defibrillators prevent sudden cardiac death in end-stage renal disease patients on dialysis? *Journal of Clinical Medicine, 13*. https://www.semanticscholar.org/paper/6196b16bbe08fd1d0a78eb889fecf5525c399aad (accessed on 29th May 2025).

17. Gao, N., Ni, M., Song, J., Kong, M., Wei, D., & Dong, A. (2022). Causal relationship between tea intake and cardiovascular diseases: A Mendelian randomization study. *Frontiers in Nutrition, 9*. https://www.semanticscholar.org/paper/6676ae5e366bf6b067398dbd1e4e2f44311b4248 (accessed on 29th May 2025).

18. Gore, J. (2012). Guidelines for the management of stable ischemic heart disease. *NEJM Journal Watch, 2012*. https://www.semanticscholar.org/paper/06d156caa3ccd303134e19142808d1cf41430389 (accessed on 29th May 2025).

19. Hermans, S., Lemmens, R., Nuyens, D., Thijs, et al. (2011). *Genetics of Atrial Fibrillation and pOssible Implications for Ischemic Stroke*. https://core.ac.uk/download/pdf/8602293.pdf (accessed on 29th May 2025).

20. Hou, Y., Si, K., Yang, J., Liu, T., Abdelazeem, B., Theerasuwipakorn, N., Zhao, J., et al. (2024). Association between regulatory T cells and ischemic heart disease: A Mendelian randomization study. *Journal of Thoracic Disease, 16*, 564–572. https://www.semanticscholar.org/paper/0d651a2cfc9552a239b1c65827acfe40a7469c82 (accessed on 29th May 2025).

21. Kadhim, M. M., Al-Saad, S. F., Al-Jumaily, H. S., & Hassan, Z. F. (2024). Role of dobutamine stress test and speckle tracking in ischemic heart disease, comparative study. *Medical Journal of Babylon*. https://www.semanticscholar.org/paper/1507b79aa54737479a5ed594e951f42f9c92f138 (accessed on 29th May 2025).

22. Khakuasheva, I. A., Umetov, M. A., Kuzhonova, M. Z., Gataova, I. M., & Abazova, D. Z. (2025). Optimization of treatment of endothelial dysfunction and arterial stiffness in patients with arterial hypertension and ischemic heart disease. *Medical Alphabet*. https://www.semanticscholar.org/paper/a980f355450354a3d43bfb0827f80e665d06fe56 (accessed on 29th May 2025).

23. Kibel, A., Lukinac, A. M., Đambić, V., Jurić, I., & Selthofer-Relatić, K. (2020). Oxidative stress in ischemic heart disease. *Oxidative Medicine and Cellular Longevity, 2020*, 1–30. https://doi.org/10.1155/2020/6627144 (accessed on 29th May 2025).

24. Kızılaslan, S., & Samancı Tekin, Ç. (2024). Risk factors of ischemic heart disease and risk-related awareness in university students. *STED / Sürekli Tıp Eğitimi Dergisi*. https://www.semanticscholar.org/paper/1233ade427d608977ee419ee95a007bd2b7fee23 (accessed on 29th May 2025).

25. Kobal, S., Arbucci, R., Zagatina, A., Padang, R., Peteiro, V. J. P., Boshchenko, A., Čelutkienė, J., et al. (2024). Functional correlates of ischemic electrocardiographic changes during stress echocardiography: Data from Stress Echo 2030 Survey. *European Heart Journal*. https://www.semanticscholar.org/paper/49a96c3cd7d672df6ac8d6673b38a680f6828dd4 (accessed on 29th May 2025).

26. Kotha, S., Giannoudi, M., Procter, H., Jex, N., Chowdhary, A., Thirunavukarasu, S., Swoboda, P., et al. (2024). The impact of type 2 diabetes on short term myocardial morphological, functional, and energetic recovery post coronary artery bypass surgery in patients with ischemic heart disease. *European Heart Journal*. https://www.semanticscholar.org/paper/21f21dabb3d3e42f7a2b58a401cb8385be54d983 (accessed on 29th May 2025).

27. Krychtiuk, K., Marquis-Gravel, G., Murphy, S., Alexander, K. P., Chiswell, K., Green, J. B., Leiter, L. A., et al. (2024). Effects of albiglutide on myocardial infarction and ischemic heart disease outcomes in patients with type 2 diabetes and cardiovascular disease in the Harmony Outcomes trial. *European Heart Journal. Cardiovascular Pharmacotherapy*. https://www.semanticscholar.org/paper/26298b8aa3d8a0cef93d61b2efd17658fbf1a34d (accessed on 29th May 2025).

28. Laranjo, L., Lanas, F., Chan. S. M. F., Chen, D. A., Hynes, L., Imran, T. F., Kazi, D. S., et al. (2024). World Heart Federation roadmap for secondary prevention of cardiovascular disease: 2023 update. *Global Heart, 19*. https://www.semanticscholar.org/paper/0aa4c11cb2d2fa923dbd9c23091b3fc3757e2e1b (accessed on 29th May 2025).

29. Libhaber, C. D., & Vangu, M. D. T. W. H. (2017). *Value of Nuclear Cardiology for the Diagnosis and Risk Stratification of Coronary Artery Disease*. https://core.ac.uk/download/268426649.pdf (accessed on 29th May 2025).

30. Makubi, A. (2016). *Heart Failure and Anemia in Sub-Saharan Africa: Etiology, Characterization, Prognosis and the Role of Oral Iron – Experiences from Tanzania*. https://core.ac.uk/download/70344051.pdf (accessed on 29th May 2025).

31. Marder, E., DeLong, M. R., Gazzaniga, M. S., Wichmann, T. (2008). *2008 Progress Report on Brain Research*. https://core.ac.uk/download/71349141.pdf (accessed on 29th May 2025).

32. Martinez-Navarro, H., Zhou, X., & Rodriguez, B. (2024). Mechanisms and implications of electrical heterogeneity in cardiac function in ischemic heart disease. *Annual Review of Physiology*. https://www.semanticscholar.org/paper/e742cb16af148096e973a7bc50af868ab4e4544d (accessed on 29th May 2025).

33. Marzoog, B., Chomakhidze, P., Gognieva, D., Silantyev, A., Suvorov, A., Abdullaev, M., Mozzhukhina, N., et al. (2025). Development and validation of a machine learning model for diagnosis of ischemic heart disease using single-lead electrocardiogram parameters. *World Journal of Cardiology, 17*. https://www.semanticscholar.org/paper/bde8ee3046c12162869b54df935494b8ac8a3946 (accessed on 29th May 2025).

34. Miki, T., Yamada, J., Ishida, S., Sakui, D., Kanai, M., & Hagiwara, Y. (2024). Exploring the feasibility and initial impact of an mHealth-based disease management program for chronic ischemic heart disease: Formative study. *JMIR Formative Research, 8*. https://www.semanticscholar.org/paper/22dd16949e664fb5a121c5686e4acbda7ffe0854 (accessed on 29th May 2025).

35. Mokhaberi, N., Schneider, E. P., Aftzoglou, M., Hüners, I., Körner, M., Armbrust, L., Biermann, D., et al. (2024). Risk factors and surgical outcomes in pediatric patients with congenital heart disease and ischemic colitis. *Pediatric Surgery International, 41*. https://www.semanticscholar.org/paper/a2b87b266426c067a3bf0a96df087f8f0cd8c52a (accessed on 29th May 2025).

36. National Heart, Lung, and Blood Institute. (2002). *National Heart, Lung, and Blood Institute (NHLBI) Strategy for Addressing Health Disparities*. https://core.ac.uk/download/pdf/11540991.pdf (accessed on 29th May 2025).

37. Nawwai, A. B. M. (2024). Ischemic heart disease; an overview of atypical presentation & misdiagnosis. *Clinical Research and Clinical Trials*. https://www.semanticscholar.org/paper/e6574c3ed2a75b8b2c587576037d4e4efb24bfa7 (accessed on 29th May 2025).

38. Peix, A., Mesquita, C. T., Massardo, T., Gutierrez-Villamil, C., Berrocal, I., Puente, A., Astesiano, A., et al. (2024). How International Atomic Energy Agency can support the management of ischemic heart disease in women. *European Heart Journal – Cardiovascular Imaging*. https://www.semanticscholar.org/paper/343d5585b676d6ecf58b49473a3dd5e346763c05 (accessed on 29th May 2025).

39. Praveena, K. R., & Sasikumar, S. (2021). Application of Colaizzi's Method of Data Analysis in Phenomenological Research. *Medico Legal Update*. https://www.semanticscholar.org/paper/d128d49e665e4da227d8adaf92af1641a5c9155a (accessed on 29th May 2025).

40. Rahimee, Q., Behsoodwal, K. A., & Azemi, M. A. (2023). Assessing Community Awareness of Ischemic Heart Disease Risk Factors in Nangarhar: A Comprehensive Study. *Nangarhar University International Journal of Biosciences*. https://www.semanticscholar.org/paper/2f77f92d1ad81c6170a32f78f0d66d16d69acdbe (accessed on 29th May 2025).

41. Rakab, M., Baklola, M., Elsalakawi, B. H., Zaki, M. M., Elsaeidi, M. E., Fouad, H., Walid, B., et al. (2024). Ischemic heart disease awareness in Egypt's aging population: Findings from a

national cross-sectional study. *The Egyptian Heart Journal, 76.* https://www.semanticscholar.org/paper/e2d284bfb8ea2710f701bc0b6d761f189e117cc2 (accessed on 29th May 2025).

42. Rzyman, K. (2024). Myocardial ischemic syndrome: A necessary nomenclature update of coronary artery disease. *Science Insights.* https://www.semanticscholar.org/paper/b035894e35d556e2cf7c0cbff871163167c35e57 (accessed on 29th May 2025).
43. Safiri, S., Karamzad, N., Singh, K., Carson-Chahhoud, K. V., Adams, C., Nejadghaderi, S. A., Almasi-Hashiani, A., et al. (2021). Burden of ischemic heart disease and its attributable risk factors in 204 countries and territories, 1990–2019. *European Journal of Preventive Cardiology.* https://www.semanticscholar.org/paper/1a17ac2a794d26e2beefcc71821dfdb02df64a98 (accessed on 29th May 2025).
44. Seawright, J., Park, K., Kaufman, N., & Waheed, N. (2019). *Ischemic Heart Disease in Women.* https://core.ac.uk/download/570893543.pdf (accessed on 29th May 2025).
45. Servito, M., Gill, I., Durbin, J., Ghasemlou, N., Popov, A. F., Stephen, C., & El-Diasty, M. (2023). Management of coronary artery disease in CADASIL patients: Review of current literature. *Medicina, 59.* https://www.semanticscholar.org/paper/2cbd2d88f73f0ed92d9f019ab139dfd78c09e109 (accessed on 29th May 2025).
46. Smith, D. G., Hart, C. L., Rasul, F., Stansfeld, et al. (2005). *Psychological Distress, Physical Illness, and Risk of Coronary Heart Disease.* https://core.ac.uk/download/1393698.pdf (accessed on 29th May 2025).
47. Sun, Z., Yun, Z., Lin, J. S., Sun, X., Wang, Q., Duan, J., Li, C., et al. (2024). Comprehensive Mendelian randomization analysis of plasma proteomics to identify new therapeutic targets for the treatment of coronary heart disease and myocardial infarction. *Journal of Translational Medicine, 22.* https://www.semanticscholar.org/paper/1a271a47daed90560bcb1ff07f2b20f82c7ab49b (accessed on 29th May 2025).
48. Ullah, K., Ai, L., Humayun, Z., & Wu, R. (2023). Targeting endothelial HIF2α/ARNT expression for ischemic heart disease therapy. *Biology, 12.* https://www.semanticscholar.org/paper/9e5b1d5560511375723c5ab42fadc15d8b4dd325 (accessed on 29th May 2025).
49. Venugopal, D., Amin, V. P., Shandilya, A. V., Jonnavithula, S., Irfan, A., Syed, S., Bhalodia, P., et al. (2024). Abstract 4146029: State-wide burden of ischemic heart disease attributable to dietary risk factors in the United States from 1990–2021: A benchmarking systematic analysis. *Circulation.* https://www.semanticscholar.org/paper/a9908a6b084041b0274354beefbab65eace87aed (accessed on 29th May 2025).
50. Wang, Y., Li, Q., Bi, L., Wang, B., Lv, T., & Zhang, P. (2025). Global trends in the burden of ischemic heart disease based on the Global Burden of Disease Study 2021: The role of metabolic risk factors. *BMC Public Health, 25.* https://www.semanticscholar.org/paper/a0854da35a4d38b0f4da0693b7609fcae0422d66 (accessed on 29th May 2025).
51. Zhang, H., Zheng, X., Huang, P., Guo, L., Zheng, Y., Zhang, D., Ma, X. (2024). The burden and trends of heart failure caused by ischemic heart disease at the global, regional, and national levels from 1990 to 2021. *European Heart Journal. Quality of Care & Clinical Outcomes.* https://www.semanticscholar.org/paper/20bfbca8f86b5c6305e12f8673e272e4441b402a (accessed on 29th May 2025).

52. Zheng, D., Liu, J., Piao, H., Zhu, Z., Wei, R., Liu, K. (2022). ROS-triggered endothelial cell death mechanisms: Focus on pyroptosis, parthanatos, and ferroptosis. *Frontiers in Immunology, 13.* https://doi.org/10.3389/fimmu.2022.1039241 (accessed on 29th May 2025).

53. Zhou, M., Xu, Y., Zhang, L., Yang, Y., & Zheng, J. (2025). Comprehensive bioinformatics analysis of hub genes in ischemic heart failure and atrial fibrillation. *Frontiers in Cardiovascular Medicine, 12.* https://www.semanticscholar.org/paper/8211b7d1f9ee8ccffc4db01e6a1baba8cd084813 (accessed on 29th May 2025).

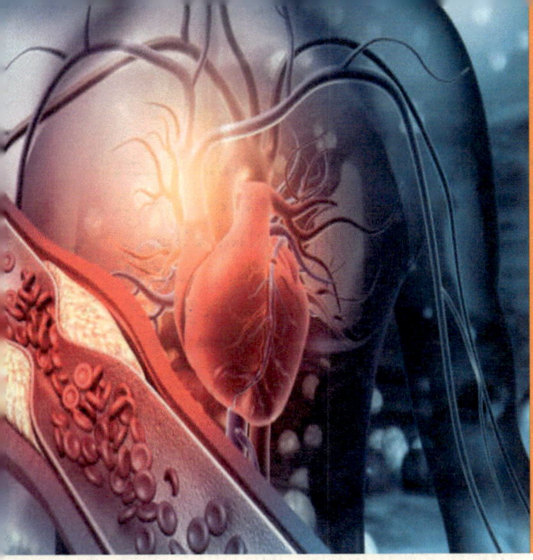

Chapter 5
CARDIAC ATHEROSCLEROSIS

Contents

Introduction

The cardiac atherosclerosis chapter is preceded by laying the groundwork for an in-depth study of this disabling cardiovascular disease. Atherosclerosis, as reflected by the growth of plaques within arterial walls, slowly evolves to reduce artery diameter, leading to extreme reduction in blood flow and ultimately leading to severe complications such as acute coronary syndrome (ACS). The illness remains an important worldwide cause of morbidity and mortality, necessitating comprehensive knowledge about its pathophysiology, risk factors, and treatment strategies. As pointed out in the current literature, lifestyle modification and increased prevalence of risk factors such as obesity and physical inactivity are major contributing factors to the increased atherosclerotic disease burden, particularly among developing nations experiencing rapid economic development (Parvez et al., 2024). A robust introduction, besides providing the required definitions, situates cardiac atherosclerosis in the overall context of cardiovascular issues at stake. The multifaceted nature of cardiac atherosclerosis necessitates rigorous examination of its etiologic processes and risk factors. Several factors, such as hypertension, hyperlipidemia, smoking, and diabetes, are extensively reported as risk factors in the course of the disease. Further, recent research has underscored the role of hormonal effects, particularly in specific populations, such as in several reports of spontaneous coronary artery dissection (SCAD). A woman in her early years of life who had been taking hormonal contraceptives, for instance, developed SCAD, which raised even more questions about the potential link between estrogen exposure and vascular stability (Parvez et al., 2024). It is critical to acknowledge these interrelationships in developing preventive regimes and effective treatment modalities since this underlines the importance of an integrative research and clinical practice approach in the management of cardiac atherosclerosis. The introduction not only serves as an introduction to the topic but also as a launching ground for more detailed elaboration in the course of the chapter. A full understanding of cardiac atherosclerosis depends upon examining not only past perspectives but also modern research findings in vascular medicine. Doctors and researchers must recognize the evolution of the atherosclerosis knowledge base, which has been shaped by key milestones, including the establishment of specialized societies in response to the growing burden of cardiovascular disease (Kong et al., 2017). Throughout this chapter, it will discuss the relevance of atherosclerosis within diverse populations as it discusses novel therapeutic strategies. Through the incorporation of evidence from diverse lines of research, the introduction offers the venue for an analytic examination of the complexity and challenges that cardiac atherosclerosis presents within the context of modern medicine (Figure 5.1).

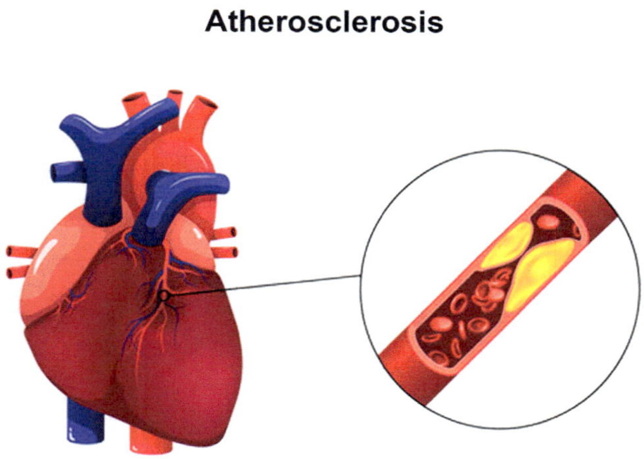

Figure 5.1. Atherosclerosis.

Source: https://www.aapc.com/codes/webroot/upload/articles_pdf/2022/cca/2022-08-24_13-59-26.webp.

Definition of Cardiac Atherosclerosis

Cardiac atherosclerosis is a cumulative disease that entails the accumulation of fibrous and lipidic components within arterial walls, particularly of the coronary arteries supplying the heart muscle. Endothelial damage is the beginning of the pathological process and is often brought about by such causes as hypertension, smoking, and hypercholesterolemia. As the endothelium is compromised, it allows the entry of low-density lipoprotein (LDL) cholesterol, which oxidizes and plays a role in the formation of fatty streaks. These early lesions evolve into mature plaques, which subsequently possibly rupture and risk leading to impairment of blood flow and culminating in acute cardiovascular events like myocardial infarctions. Consequently, understanding the mechanism of cardiac atherosclerosis and its process is essential for organizing effective prevention and treatment, and thus requires ongoing research in this area. Clinical implications of cardiac atherosclerosis extend beyond mere plaque formation since the disease induces severe hemodynamic alterations in the coronary circulation.

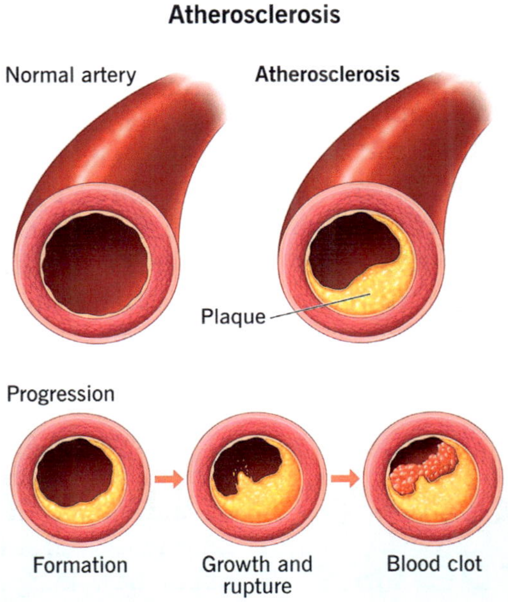

Figure 5.2. Atherosclerosis involves gradual plaque buildup inside your artery.

Source: https://my.clevelandclinic.org/-/scassets/images/org/health/articles/16753-atherosclerosis-illustration?io=transform:fit,width:780.

As the atheroma progresses to occlude and narrow the arteries, the patients are likely to present with angina or the more severe forms of acute coronary syndrome. The spectrum of the disease emphasizes the importance of accurate diagnostic tools, such as coronary angiography and multi-detector row computed tomography (MDCT), which assist in establishing the severity and extent of the atherosclerotic changes. Furthermore, advances in imaging technology enabled us to comprehend better the pathophysiology of coronary artery anomalies and how variations of these structures may be involved in atherosclerosis. To this end, the interaction between arterial anomalies and disturbed blood flow represents merely an example of how other factors increase the clinical situation encompassing cardiac atherosclerosis, with early detection and treatment required in as many people as possible, especially if they are asymptomatic (Markovic et al., 2025). There is also increasing evidence of a causative relationship between cardiac atherosclerosis and other cardiovascular events, for example, strokes due to thromboembolism. Atrial fibrillation

(AF) is one such case, the most common cause of cardioembolic stroke, and it represents a significant public health concern. The literature indicates that AF-related thrombus formation frequently occurs in the left atrial appendage and that its occurrence raises the risk of future thromboembolic events. Interestingly, cardiac atherosclerosis is a cause of the pathologic milieu within the cardiovascular system, perhaps increasing the incidence of AF. Thus, an improved understanding of atrial cardiopathy and its relationship to atherosclerotic change can possibly elucidate potential mechanisms for stroke prevention in patients without manifest AF (Ko et al., 2022). As the literature matures, it is increasingly clear that the relationship between cardiac atherosclerosis and other cardiovascular illnesses necessitates treatment and prevention from a combined approach, underscoring the complexity of cardiovascular disease (Figure 5.2).

5.1. Pathophysiology of Cardiac Atherosclerosis

The pathophysiologic process of atherosclerosis of the heart is inexorably linked with the interplay between lipid deposition, endothelial dysfunction, and persistent inflammation. The process is initiated by the deposition of low-density lipoproteins (LDLs) in the intima of the arterial wall, thus triggering an inflammatory process. This LDL oxidation attracts monocytes that are transformed to macrophages and ingest oxidized LDL to form foam cells, the hallmark feature of early atherosclerotic lesions. Damage to the endothelial cells, often augmented by risk factors such as diabetes and hypertension, allows for increased permeability and further invasion of inflammatory cells. Through this continuous process, it creates a path for plaque development and maturation, finally resulting in involvement of the arterial lumen, thus leading to ischemic events in the heart. Understanding these processes will be necessary to develop prevention and treatment strategies tailored to cardiac atherosclerosis. As the atherosclerotic plaque evolves, it is a multicellular complex composed of lipids, inflammatory cells, and fibrous tissue. Cell proliferation and apoptosis, particularly in smooth muscle cells, have a great influence on the stability of plaque. Chronic inflammation not only causes the development of atherosclerosis but also significantly contributes to plaque rupture—a prevalent cause of acute coronary syndromes. It has been shown through research that myeloproliferative neoplasms (MPNs), characterized by clonal hematopoiesis in the absence of the Philadelphia chromosome, increase thrombotic risk associated with atherosclerosis via cytokine release and vascular remodeling. The long-term inflammatory state related to MPNs could amplify cardiovascular morbidity and mortality, demonstrating how underlying hematologic disorders can amplify atherosclerotic processes and complicate patient prognoses (Todor et al., 2024). Recent advancements in our knowledge of signaling pathways, such as the Wnt pathway have brought about new insights into the pathophysiology of atherosclerosis. Three key processes in the development and evolution of plaque include endothelial dysfunction, monocyte penetration, and smooth muscle cell response, all of which are influenced by the Wnt pathway. Inhibition of Wnt signaling has been viewed as a viable therapeutic strategy to decrease atherosclerosis, as it is capable of inhibiting the inflammatory process and improving plaque stability. By blocking several components of the Wnt pathway, researchers aim to develop more effective therapies for vulnerable patients at risk of atherosclerotic cardiovascular disease. The involvement of chronic inflammation and specified signaling pathways illustrates the multifactorial nature of cardiac atherosclerosis and underlines the need for new approaches in prevention and treatment (Afroz et al., 2024) (Figure 5.3).

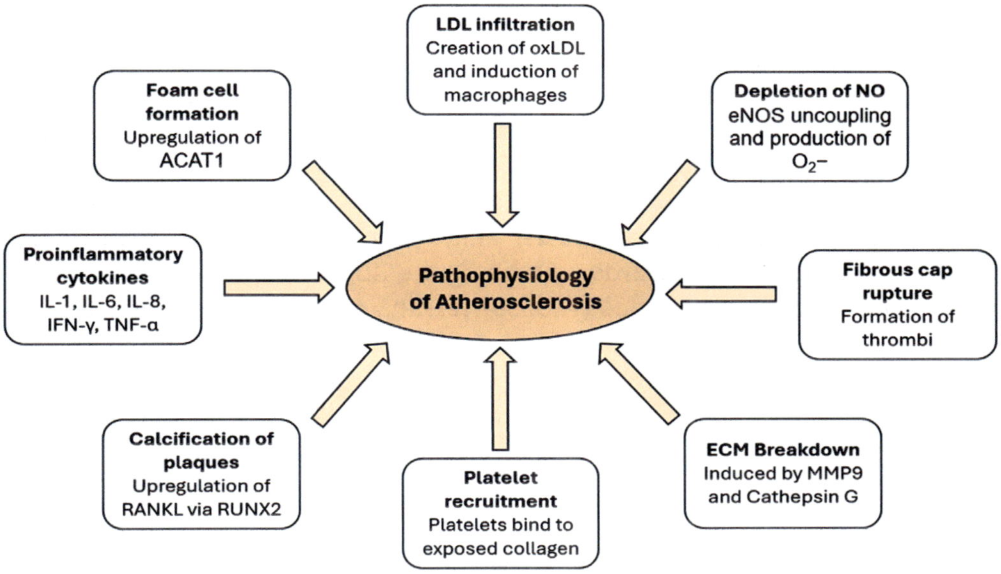

Figure 5.3. Figure summarizing the pathophysiology of atherosclerosis. From the infiltration of LDLs to the creation of a calcified fibrous cap and its rupture, multiple factors contribute to the initiation and progression of atherosclerosis.

Source: https://www.mdpi.com/ijms/ijms-26-01364/article_deploy/html/images/ijms-26-01364-g002.png.

5.1.1. Mechanisms of Plaque Formation

The mechanisms of plaque formation in cardiac atherosclerosis are multifactorial and involve the interaction of cellular changes, lipid accumulation, and inflammatory changes. At the core of all these is the penetration into the intima of the arteries of LDL that becomes oxidized, causing inflammation. This response is characterized by the deposition of immune cells, predominantly macrophages, which phagocytose the oxidized LDL and transform into foam cells, characteristic of early atherosclerotic lesions. They mature to produce a fatty streak, which will subsequently result in more serious atherosclerotic plaques. This initial step highlights the central role of inflammation in atherosclerosis development and underscores the requirement for robust inflammatory signaling to promote plaque growth and stability. The association between serotonin receptors, or the 5-HT2B receptor, and atherosclerosis provides a new insight into plaque formation. Elevated levels of serotonin have been associated with coronary artery disease, which suggests its involvement in the process of atherosclerosis. Atherosclerosis-susceptible apolipoprotein E-deficient (ApoE-/-) mice were employed in research to demonstrate that atherogenic plaque dimension was decreased significantly following pharmacological inhibition and genetic lack of the 5-HT2B receptor. Furthermore, these therapies induced decreased macrophage invasion, along with decreased inflammatory signaling cascades, including NLRP3 inflammasome stimulation. This evidence implicates the 5-HT2B receptors' critical function in the modulation of the atherosclerotic plaque inflammatory microenvironment, proposing possible therapeutic targets for the management of cardiovascular diseases (Liu et al., 2024). Structural stability of the atherosclerotic plaques is vital to their stability and the prevention of acute cardiovascular events. The fibrous cap, which is composed mainly of smooth muscle cells and extracellular matrix material, represents a critical barrier to plaque rupture. Cap development involves regulation by cellular recruitment, clonal growth, and interaction among various molecular signaling pathways. It is essential to understand how the fibrous cap is developed, because cap rupture is one of the major causes of coronary thrombosis that may lead to myocardial infarction and sudden death. It is demonstrated through studies how crucial it is to view the fibrous cap as a neo-media that replaces the original media, which becomes compromised in atherogenesis. This perspective has treatment implications for anti-atherosclerosis, and it points towards stabilizing the fibrous caps to enhance their protective role against cardiovascular complications (Alonso-Herranz et al., 2023) (Figure 5.4).

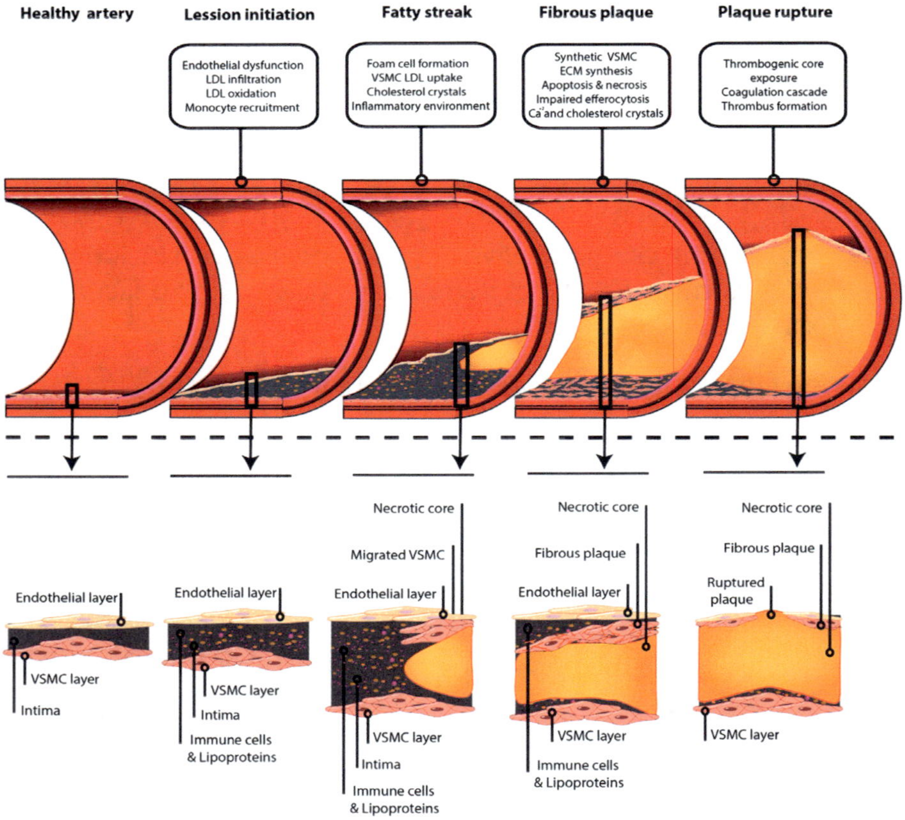

Figure 5.4. Schematic representation of atheroma plaque formation from a healthy artery to plaque rupture underlying the most important events that contribute to its development in each stage.

Source: https://www.mdpi.com/ijms/ijms-23-03346/article_deploy/html/images/ijms-23-03346-g003.png.

5.1.2. Role of Inflammation in Atherosclerosis

The role of inflammation in the development and progression of atherosclerosis has been of immense interest over the past decade, transforming the concept of cardiovascular disease. Atherosclerosis is characterized by the accumulation of lipids, inflammatory cells, and fibrous elements within the walls of arteries, leading to plaque deposition. This chronic inflammatory response is the result of various factors, including endothelial injury, oxidative stress, and dyslipidemia, which provide a favorable setting for atherogenic processes. The interplay among these factors not only accelerates plaque development but also causes plaque instability and initiates acute cardiovascular events. It is through an understanding of inflammation-mediated pathologic change that investigators can investigate potential targets of therapy for limiting atherosclerosis progression and improving outcomes for patients. Moreover, clinical uses of inflammation in atherosclerosis extend to cardiovascular diagnostic and therapeutic strategies. The standard diagnosis of atherosclerosis focuses at the expense of the etiological inflammatory disease processes on architectural changes within the arteries. Here, the new imaging modalities, e.g., 18-Fluoro-Deoxyglucose-Positron Emission Tomography (FDG-PET), have emerged as useful for their capability to depict inflammation in cardiovascular tissue.

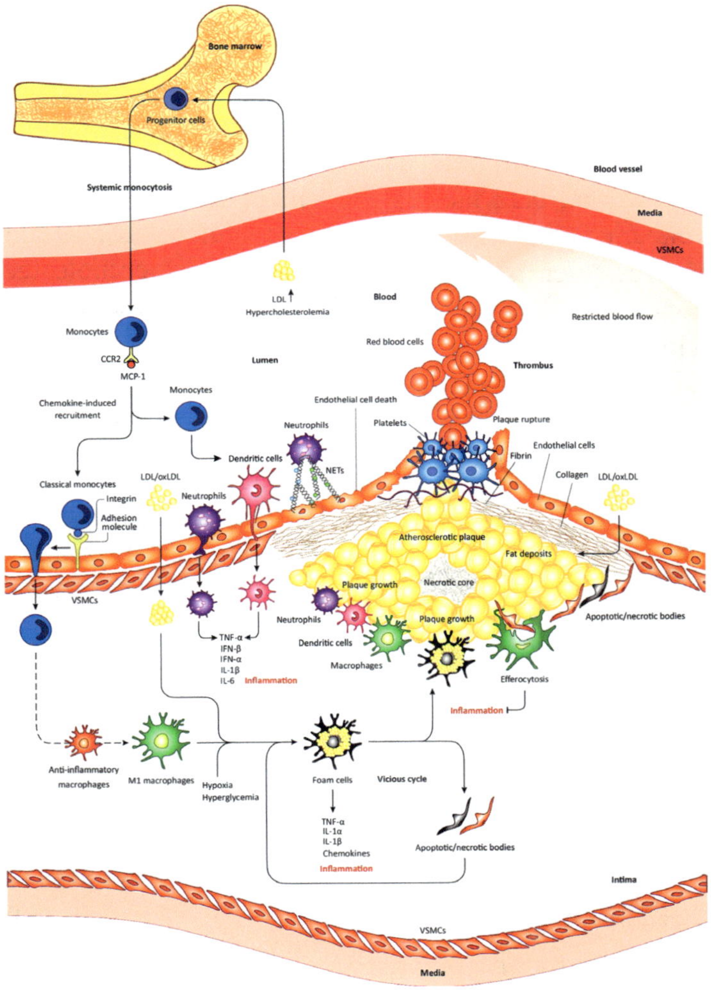

Figure 5.5. Atherosclerotic plaque, the infiltration of inflammatory cells, and inflammation.

Source: https://media.springernature.com/full/springer-static/image/art%3A10.1038%2Fs41419-024-07166-8/MediaObjects/41419_2024_7166_Fig1_HTML.png?as=webp.

With advances in identifying inflammatory processes engaged in atherosclerosis, these imaging modalities provide valuable information on disease status and course. Furthermore, integrating radiomics into FDG-PET imaging would enhance diagnostic precision by leveraging machine learning to identify quantitative features predictive of inflammation levels. Such advances will revolutionize the approach to how cardiovascular inflammation is addressed, and the call for greater complexity of understanding its role in atherosclerosis (Almuqbil, 2024). With the mounting evidence that inflammation is a key driver of atherosclerosis, regulation of this inflammatory process holds out great therapeutic promise. Recent evidence suggests that the modulation of inflammation is as crucial as regulating traditional risk factors, such as cholesterol levels and blood pressure. Anti-inflammatory measures, such as the use of specific pharmacologic agents, have also proved to be effective in lowering cardiovascular events by stabilizing atherosclerotic plaques and avoiding rupture. Also, lifestyle changes that minimize systemic inflammation, including diet and exercise, further lower risk. As studies of the pathophysiology of atherosclerotic inflammation advance, so too does it become increasingly clear that examining cardiovascular health from an integrated standpoint—one focused on inflammatory mechanisms—could lead to enhanced prevention and therapeutic approaches for individuals at risk for cardiac atherosclerosis (Khattab et al., 2025) (Figure 5.5).

5.1.3. Impact on Coronary Arteries

The impact of cardiac atherosclerosis on coronary arteries significantly influences overall cardiovascular well-being, particularly through mechanisms of blood flow dynamics and endothelial function. Atherosclerosis, or the buildup of plaques within the walls of the arteries, narrows and hardens the arteries. This pathologic process compromises the ability of the arteries to buffer blood flow, leading to altered patterns of shear stress. Low and oscillatory wall shear stress (WSS), in specific, has been shown to induce endothelial dysfunction, contributing to downstream vascular disease as well as to the progression of atherosclerosis itself (Haverstaad et al., 2010). Accordingly, coronary artery disease patients are apt to manifest greater risk for cardiovascular adverse events through the reduced adaptability of their coronary arteries, immediately linking structural changes of atherosclerosis to its key functional impairments. Apart from the immediate outcome of plaque buildup, the interaction of dyslipidemia with coronary artery health is also a significant determinant in the role of cardiac atherosclerosis. Various types of dyslipidemia, such as combined hyperlipidemia or simple hypercholesterolemia, are associated with the increased prevalence of multivessel coronary artery disease. Research confirms that such conditions raise the risk of coronary artery calcium (CAC) deposition, a sign of atherosclerotic burden and cardiovascular morbidity (Alamir et al., 2018). The higher the degree of involvement in various coronary arteries, the higher the risk of major cardiovascular events. Thus, such an understanding is crucial in the development of targeted prevention mechanisms to reverse the implications of atherosclerosis on coronary arteries. Besides, the importance of various levels of competitive flow within the coronary arteries highlights the complexity that accompanies cardiac atherosclerosis. Competitive flow from indigenous coronary arteries impacts graft patency in coronary artery bypass grafting, where shear stress dynamics are of utmost relevance. Highly competitive flow conditions, typically observed in low lesioned individuals, can lead to adverse WSS patterns that trigger endothelial damage and graft failure (Haverstaad et al., 2010). Moderate flow conditions, on the other hand, represent a better effect with similarities to the absence of competitive flow, thus informing surgical planning as well as patient management. Understanding these interactions not only underscores the multifaceted influence of atherosclerosis on coronary artery health but also guides clinical decision-making at the time of intervention to optimize patient outcomes.

5.2. Risk Factors

The interaction among numerous risk factors and the development of cardiac atherosclerosis is intricate and profound. Atherosclerosis typically entails the development of lipid-rich plaques in arterial walls, instigated by a range of risk factors including hypertension, diabetes, and obesity. Such factors also significantly contribute to endothelial dysfunction that precedes alterations in atherosclerosis. For example, hypertension imposes excessive stress on arterial walls, leading to micro-injuries that invite inflammatory processes and plaque formation. Similarly, diabetes mellitus is associated with dyslipidemia and hyperglycemia, which provide a background for plaque formation.

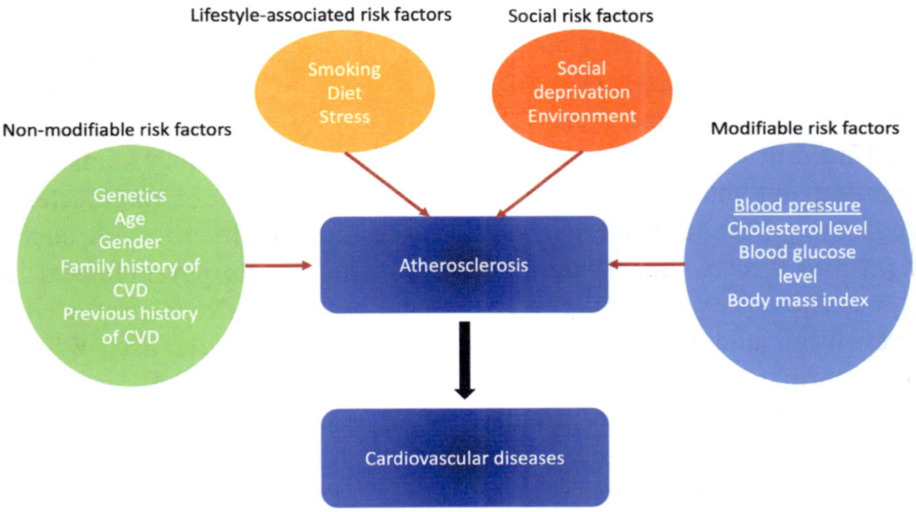

Figure 5.6. Risk factors for atherosclerosis development.

Source: https://www.researchgate.net/publication/362839883/figure/fig1/AS:11431281187276672@1694172043511/Risk-factors-for-atherosclerosis-development.tif.

The multifactorial etiology of these risk factors necessitates specific prevention strategies that consider not only individual determinants but also their interactions, thereby possibly reducing the burden of cardiac-associated morbidity and mortality in atherosclerosis. Furthermore, the increasing occurrence of cardiovascular diseases among cancer patients undergoing immune checkpoint inhibitor (ICI) therapy suggests that it is essential to value cardiovascular risk factors in different contexts. Evidence indicates that patients treated with ICIs may experience metabolic abnormalities that exacerbate pre-existing cardiovascular disorders and elevate the risk of cardiac hospitalization. Among such patients, a history of cardiovascular disease, diabetes, and chronic kidney disease (CKD) is an established predictor of cardiac adverse effects during ICI therapy (Bennetts et al., 2024). These cases highlight the need for clinicians to monitor cardiovascular status closely, particularly in patients with pre-existing risk factors. They also pose questions about the long-term cardiovascular effects of treatments that are mainly designed to treat cancer, necessitating comprehensive care strategies that include cardiovascular risk management. In light of these confounding variables, it is essential to recognize the distinctive patterns of dysfunction characteristic of heart failure (HF) risk factors if the clinical intervention is to prove efficacious. It has been shown that specific cardiovascular risk factors correlate with various preclinical cardiac dysfunctions. For instance, atherosclerotic cardiovascular disease (ASCVD) has been traditionally associated with left ventricular systolic dysfunction. At the same time, hypertension was seen to be related to diastolic dysfunction and increased filling pressures (Grant et al., 2025). Such risk factor discrimination not only augments the information regarding pathophysiology but also offers insight into directed screening and preventive interventions. By an integrated approach of prevention and management of the risk factors of cardiac atherosclerosis, the patient outcomes can be optimized, and even the incidence of HF and associated complications could be minimized in the high-risk group (Figure 5.6).

5.2.1. Modifiable Risk Factors

The concept of modifiable risk factors is core to the comprehension and avoidance of atherosclerosis of the heart, as they are related to an increased propensity towards the manifestation of cardiovascular diseases. Foremost among these are lifestyle choices such as diet, physical activity, smoking, and alcohol consumption. Repeatedly, research has discovered that poor dietary habits, especially those rich in saturated fats and sugar, are a robust reason for the development of atherosclerosis. Moreover, physical inactivity exacerbates this condition by causing obesity and metabolic syndromes. Smoking, a documented risk factor, raises endothelial injury and inflammation in vascular beds, directly leading to plaque formation. By the identification and management of these modifiable risk factors, health promotion interventions are capable of significantly lowering cardiac atherosclerosis prevalence rates and overall cardiovascular wellness (Jones et al., 2024).

Psychiatric status, or depression and anxiety, has been a significant modifiable risk factor for heart atherosclerosis. Psychological distress can lead to unfavorable lifestyle habits such as poor dietary intake, low physical activity, and cigarette smoking, all contributing to an aggravation of the cardiovascular state. In addition, depressed patients can acquire elevated inflammatory biomarkers, which aid in the enhancement of atherosclerosis. Treatment of mental health through such interventions not only boosts psychological health but also acts as a significant protective agent against cardiovascular disease. Educational public health programs that integrate mental care with cardiovascular disease education have the potential to offer an integrated method for reducing modifiable risk factors and enhancing overall patient' outcomes (Anand et al., 2024). Another very much-needed area of modifiable risk factors is the chronic disease management of diabetes, hypertension, and dyslipidemia. These disorders can further add to atherosclerosis by having an impact on the lipid deposition process and inflammatory processes of the vasculature. Proper management of these disorders is generally synonymous with educating the patient about compliance with drugs, dietary modification, and exercise regimes. Further, monitoring blood pressure and cholesterol levels plays a significant role in preventing the progression of atherosclerosis. It is recommended that healthcare professionals adopt a multidisciplinary approach, emphasizing a drug-free lifestyle change over a drug treatment regimen to empower patients to actively manage their cardiac health. Thus, management of these risk factors that can be modified therefore has not only advantages of health in the short term but can also yield long-term reductions in the occurrence of cardiac atherosclerosis (Jones et al., 2024).

5.2.2. Non-Modifiable Risk Factors

It is crucial to understand the non-modifiable risk factors of cardiac atherosclerosis since they form the core of the etiology of cardiovascular disease. Age is one of the most significant non-modifiable risk factors for the development of cardiovascular disease; the older he/she gets, he/she develops physiological changes that increasingly compromise vascular wellbeing. The blood vessels become less flexible, and lipids are permitted to settle, encouraging atherosclerosis. Moreover, gender also influences the risk distribution, and males are prone to developing coronary artery disease at a younger age than females.

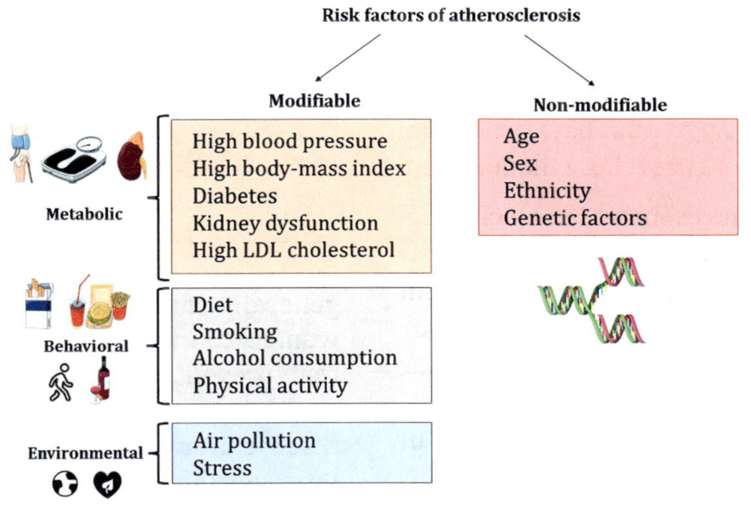

Figure 5.7. Modifiable and non-modifiable risk factors of atherosclerosis.

Source: https://pressbooks.bccampus.ca/pathology/wp-content/uploads/sites/1260/2022/08/Risk-factors-1.png.

This is primarily because of the hormonal effect since premenopausal women have protection by estrogen that alters lipid profiles and enhances vascular function. When individuals move forward in life and age, the increasing incidence of heart disease is an irreversible fact, directing attention towards the necessity of identifying such irrevocable risk factors in the management of cardiovascular health. Susceptibility to an inherited predisposition is also a prevalent non-modifiable risk factor for cardiac atherosclerosis. The genetic predisposition in an individual largely influences the likelihood of cardiovascular diseases. It has been established that individuals whose first-degree relatives died because of heart disease are susceptible to such diseases and that there is a genetic and not a lifestyle factor. The genetic predisposition may influence a number of the physiological determinants involved, including lipid metabolism, blood pressure, and inflammation. Apart from this, there are some specific genetic mutations that have been identified as raising atherosclerosis risk even higher, for which overall information regarding family medical history is needed during risk assessment. Detection of the genetic etiology of cardiac atherosclerosis can thus direct early intervention strategies and treatment regimens as per individual requirements, eventually leading to better health outcomes in high-risk populations. Finally, the impact of unmodifiable risk factors is also transferred to certain medical conditions, which are themselves associated with the causation of cardiac atherosclerosis. Diabetes mellitus and high blood pressure, for instance, are conditions that, although they are usually linked with lifestyle aspects, may also be a result of genetic factors that render a person more vulnerable to their influence. Diabetes, on the other hand, triggers atherosclerotic changes by uncontrolled hyperglycemia that later affects endothelial function and provokes inflammation.

Hypertension induces increased mechanical stress on the vessel wall, leading to endothelial damage and plaque formation. Low vitamin D status has been identified as a major unmodifiable determinant of cardiovascular condition, with patients suffering from advanced coronary atherosclerosis having lower levels of vitamin D than patients without (Dziedzic et al., 2019). This intersection of chronic illness and unchangeable risk factors underscores the complexity of cardiac atherosclerosis and requires targeted medical treatment and optimization of life in high-risk populations (Tambo et al., 2016) (Figure 5.7).

5.2.3. Lifestyle Choices and Their Impact

Lifestyle factors are the primary explanation for the causation and development of cardiac atherosclerosis, an illness defined by the deposition of plaques within the arteries. These include dietary habits, physical exercise, and other activities that influence the cardiovascular system directly. For instance, high intake of saturated fat, refined sugar, and processed food has the potential to cause obesity and dyslipidemia, which are among the most significant risk factors for atherosclerosis. Moreover, inactivity is exacerbated by these risks because a passive lifestyle constrains worldwide cardiovascular fitness and metabolism. Such determinants of lifestyle that are interconnected accentuate the importance of adopting improved habits to prevent the incidence of atherosclerosis and consequent cardiovascular diseases. In some populations, for instance, like in Saudi Arabia, lifestyle factors arise uniquely and may play an essential role in the incidence of cardiovascular diseases. There is evidence indicating that CVD is prevalent among Saudi nationals, and the aetiology within the country is in line with Western countries due to shared risk factors such as obesity and smoking (Clark et al., 2012). Cultural origin plays a significant role in determining these lifestyle options, and gender differences contribute to challenges of a distinctive nature. Whereas men are generally involved in more physical activity, women can be faced with cultural constraints that prevent them from accessing preventive health interventions. It is crucial to understand these cultural subtleties to effectively design interventions that support healthy lifestyle decisions within such populations. In addition, lifestyle decision-making among particular groups, like Saudi women, needs to be addressed through culturally nuanced interventions that take into account the specific issues they encounter. The limited focus on cardiovascular health in such settings, especially for women, can lead to a lack of action towards improving awareness regarding the risks of unhealthy lifestyles. By promoting community programs, empowering women and educating them, along with providing them with access to resources promoting physical activity and nutritional consumption, there can be a dramatic decrease in cardiovascular well-being. The strategy must be focused on reducing the burden of cardiac atherosclerosis through designing environments supportive of healthier lifestyles (Brooks et al., 2002). Therefore, culturally appropriate strategies must be accorded their utmost priority for effective secondary prevention and general health in risk groups.

5.3. Symptoms and Diagnosis

The clinical syndrome of cardiac atherosclerosis can vary significantly in different patients, depending primarily on the amount and location of arterial obstruction. Angina pectoris is usually the presenting symptom, a pain or pressure in the chest that can radiate to the arms, neck, jaw, or back. The pain worsens with activity or emotional tension and is relieved by rest. Additionally. Some people may experience palpitations, exhaustion, or shortness of breath. With rapid and severe symptoms including persistent chest pain and possibly lethal arrhythmias, advanced instances might even result in myocardial infarction. Since atherosclerosis is a disease that worsens over time, lowering quality of life and raising the risk of death, it is crucial to identify these signs early in order to diagnose the condition. Cardiac atherosclerosis diagnosis relies on an abundance of imaging techniques and diagnostic tests allowing physicians to assess the extent of the occlusion of arteries and the heart condition. Most commonly employed are coronary angiography, which provides a direct visualization of coronary arteries, and non-invasive tests such as cardiac magnetic resonance (CMR) and coronary computed tomography angiography (CCTA). CMR can determine myocardial viability and potential thrombus formation, while CCTA offers high-resolution anatomical information about the degree of atherosclerosis (Mousa et al., 2025). Coupled with patient history and physical examination, these modalities facilitate accurate diagnosis and risk stratification, enabling clinicians to tailor treatment approaches effectively. Under certain circumstances, such as pregnancy or unusual clinical presentation, there is potential for unusual symptoms, which may lead to potential misdiagnosis or delayed treatment. For instance, spontaneous coronary artery dissection related to pregnancy (P-SCAD) may have non-typical symptoms that are not initially recognized as cardiac in origin, like nausea or dyspnea (Haris et al., 2025). This highlights the need for increased clinical suspicion of non-typical presentations, especially among younger patients or those with non-typical cardiovascular risk factors. Utilization of intensive diagnostic approaches, taking into account multiple patterns of symptoms, is required to detect cardiac atherosclerosis in its initial phase and perform timely intervention techniques for improved patient outcomes (Figure 5.8).

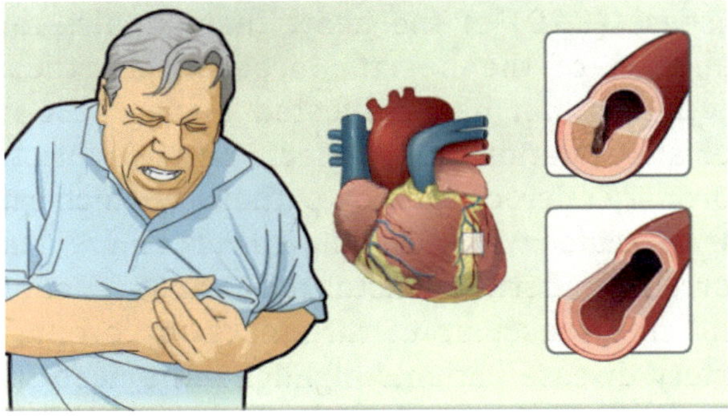

Figure 5.8. Angina symptom of atherosclerosis.

Source: https://en.benhvienthucuc.vn/wp-content/uploads/2024/01/angina-symptom-of-atherosclerosis-e1704467150581.jpg.

5.3.1. Common Symptoms of Cardiac Atherosclerosis

Cardiac atherosclerosis, one of the progressive arterial disease types, is characterized by a vast spectrum of symptoms that can be highly impactful on a patient's quality of life. Angina, the most prevalent of these, is chest pain or discomfort caused by an insufficiency in blood supply to the heart muscle. Angina is experienced as pressure, squeezing, or heaviness over the chest and is most frequently induced by exertion or emotional stress. There are also patients with recurrent angina attacks that are relieved by rest. These fleeting symptoms signify an impending risk of hazardous cardiovascular occurrences such as heart attacks. One needs to recognize the delicacy of angina since it often warrants prompt medical evaluation and treatment in a bid to arrest further progression and prevent associated risks inherent in cardiac atherosclerosis. Breathlessness is another common manifestation of cardiac atherosclerosis that arises when the heart cannot maintain enough blood supply relative to the body's workload during exercise. It may be felt when one needs to walk up stairs or climb uphill, resulting in effortless fatigue while performing routine activities. This is a significant symptom since it is a sign of impending coronary artery disease (CAD) of the heart that impairs the function of the heart. Moreover, shortness of breath can be manifested during rest in certain situations and reflects an appropriate coronary microcirculation pathology, which can be associated with ischemia or heart failure. The correlation between disturbed cardiac function and microvascular disturbances in coronary artery disease patients highlights the need for thorough clinical evaluation. The presentation of symptoms suggests underlying pathology that requires early treatment to prevent cardiac status compromise. Even heart atherosclerosis patients can present with non-specific symptoms like weakness and fatigue, which may pose difficulties in diagnosis. Although most of these have historically been explained by numerous innocent processes or even aging, in some instances, they could be a sign of more sinister cardiac failure. Fatigue usually occurs as a result of the heart's compromised ability to function maximally through its critical functions, yielding suboptimal oxygen delivery to peripheral tissues. Besides, iron deficiency, typically unrecognized in heart disease patients, exacerbates fatigue and is prevalent in chronic heart disease, including heart failure (HFrEF) (Savarese et al., 2022). The symptom, particularly in females, can occur before a bad outcome and signifies the importance of elaborate examinations, including diagnosis for underlying iron deficiency and its potential implications (Vancheri et al., 2020). Recognition of these common symptoms is essential part of early treatment and control of cardiac atherosclerosis and thereby improving patient outcomes (Figure 5.9).

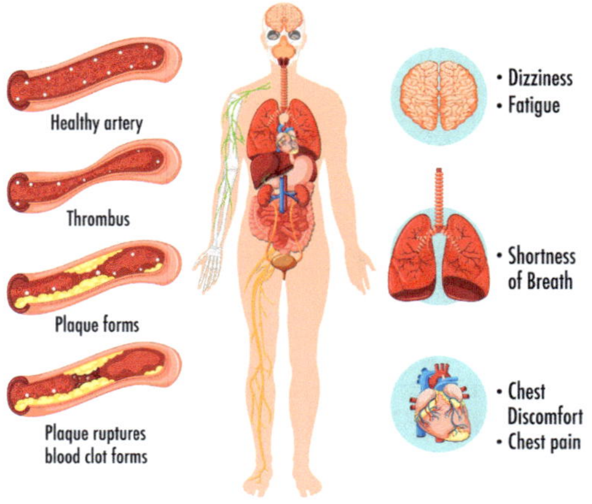

Figure 5.9. Symptoms of atherosclerosis.

Source: https://ealabs.co.in/wp-content/uploads/2022/02/11575413_51623-620x577.jpg.

5.3.2. Diagnostic Tests and Procedures

Early identification of atherosclerosis of the heart is crucial for effective treatment and management, requiring an aggressive armamentarium of diagnostic testing and tools. These tools allow clinicians to assess the severity of stenosis of the arteries and associated cardiovascular risk. Techniques most frequently employed include non-invasive imaging techniques such as echocardiography, stress testing, and coronary artery calcium scoring. Each test varies in its capability to uncover pathological changes in arterial configuration. For instance, echocardiography provides valuable information related to cardiac function, while stress testing might visualize the action of the heart during exertion, perhaps demonstrating ischemic conditions. Because the 2021 Price Transparency Rule aims to enhance health care price competition, the pricing of such diagnostic tests and procedures is increasingly relevant to consider in different settings, as variation can impact accessibility and patient outcomes, particularly across insurance status groups (Reddy et al., 2025). The price variation for diagnostic tests and procedures has a direct impact on patient care for cardiac atherosclerosis. Research has shown significant inter- and intrahospital price variations, with identical tests having vastly different prices depending on institution and patient insurance. Analysis revealed that the median ratio of highest to lowest commercial hospital prices could be greater than threefold for some cardiac interventions (Reddy et al., 2025). This difference exacerbates disparities in access to care because people with Medicaid receive fewer diagnostic tests than their privately insured counterparts. Differential pricing structures can also have a significant impact on how frequently patients undergo essential cardiac procedures, which can postpone required interventions and impair health outcomes. An understanding of such dynamics brings into perspective the need for healthcare reform to regulate costs incurred through diagnostic procedures and tests. Additionally, insurance status and its relationship to the predictability of access to diagnostic tests form the linchpin of understanding the cardiac care environment for atherosclerosis. Studies indicate that commercially insured patients are more likely than Medicaid beneficiaries to receive cardiac procedures and tests like echocardiograms and cardiac catheterizations. This disparity can not only be the result of economic incentives for medical providers but also of other facets of society, including socioeconomic status and access to quality care. Diagnostic equity among different insurance schemes underscores the necessity for healthcare policies that maximize access to required tests and ensure all patients receive the correct treatment, regardless of coverage. Resolution of such disparities is critical in the promotion of effective early detection and treatment of cardiac atherosclerosis, and ultimately, ideal cardiovascular health outcomes in diverse patient populations (Figure 5.10).

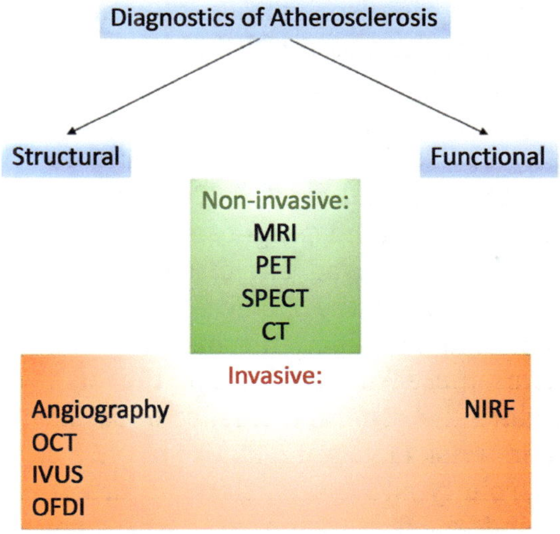

Figure 5.10. The variety of methods in diagnostics of atherosclerosis.

Source: https://www.frontiersin.org/files/Articles/1134097/fcvm-10-1134097-HTML/image_m/fcvm-10-1134097-g001.jpg.

5.3.3. Importance of Early Detection

The early detection of cardiac atherosclerosis is essential, particularly in light of its position as the major cause of morbidity and death worldwide. Atherosclerosis usually presents insidiously over years, and patients may have no evidence of disease until a critical event, e.g., myocardial infarction or stroke. Delayed presentation may have disastrous implications because the period for successful intervention can be lost. Broad and preventive screening interventions, from highly specialized imaging modalities, can identify patients at risk much earlier in the disease course. For instance, imaging modalities such as MDCT coronary angiography have emerged as reliable interventions for the imaging of coronary anatomy, allowing for the detection of anatomical abnormality or high-grade stenosis that would lead to severe cardiovascular events (Markovic et al., 2025). Early detection enables the administration of preventive interventions by medical professionals, which have the potential to alter the path of the disease. Early detection also helps in personalizing treatment algorithms in patients with cardiac atherosclerosis. Clinicians can use more than one therapeutic intervention at a time, from lifestyle interventions such as diet and exercise to pharmacotherapy such as statins and antihypertensives, if the disease is diagnosed in the initial phase. The earlier the administration of these therapies, the more they not only stabilize the disease by managing risk factors but can also significantly reduce the risk of adverse cardiovascular events. Clinically, case series have demonstrated that patients who have atypical symptoms, such as exertional angina, still retain significant CAD even though initial diagnostic workup is unremarkable. These instances emphasize the necessity of heightened clinical suspicion and complete follow-up, especially with strategies like CTCA that were pivotal in revealing subclinical CAD in patients previously deemed asymptomatic (Gill et al., 2024). In general, early detection of cardiac atherosclerosis is the key to improved patient prognosis and avoidance of the dangerous complications of this widespread disease. With the advent of sophisticated diagnostic tools and understanding of the disease's pathophysiology, the medical community today is better placed than ever to detect vulnerable groups and treat patients before the development of deadly events. With evolving healthcare systems, there will be a focus on the inclusion of routine screening and health awareness campaigns to reduce the general incidence of cardiac conditions. Vigilance by both patients and clinicians on potential risk factors might also instill a culture of early detection, leading to a significant reduction in morbidity and mortality from cardiac atherosclerosis. Lastly, emphasizing early diagnosis can help shift the narrative from reactive management to proactive health promotion in cardiovascular care (Figure 5.11).

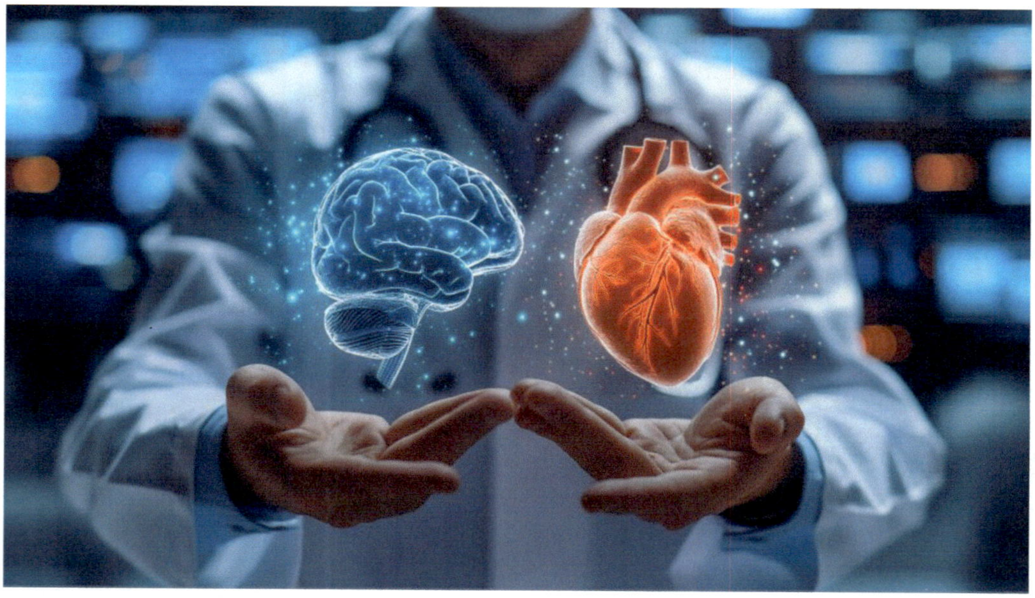

Figure 5.11. Early detection of atherosclerosis.

Source: https://cvrti.utah.edu/wp-content/uploads/2024/06/07-12-26.jpg.

5.4. Treatment Options

Cardiac atherosclerosis is managed mainly by a multi-component approach aimed at pharmacologic treatment and lifestyle modification. The initial management includes drugs such as statins that are the foundation for lowering LDL cholesterol levels, thus inhibiting plaque formation in arteries. Angiotensin-converting enzyme (ACE) inhibitors and diuretics are also often used medications to manage blood pressure and reduce the workload on the heart. These medications have been found to be beneficial in improving cardiovascular outcomes, especially in patients with risk factors of heart disease, diabetes, and obesity (Gour, 2023). Nevertheless, the ground of treatment in the management of atherosclerosis is through lifestyle adaptation, which involves diet change, exercise, and smoking cessation, among others, that all contribute to the overall improvement of the cardiovascular status of the patient. In case initial treatment fails, practitioners can study second-line treatment to curb cardiovascular risk and acute cardiac events further. It can involve the use of more potent drugs such as beta blockers and anti-thrombotics, together with surgical procedures such as CABG or PCI. The procedures are very beneficial for patients with evident symptoms of coronary vascular disease. They are generally most frequently designed to reinstate the circulation of blood towards the heart, thus reducing ischemia and risk of myocardial infarction. Treatment option typically involves consideration of the particular patient's overall clinical presentation and risk stratification (Gour, 2023). Both clinicians and patients should practice shared decision-making for them to receive optimal treatment plans. Recent research indicates that the consideration of the influence of the gut microbiota on cardiovascular health can offer novel therapeutic prospects for cardiac atherosclerosis treatment. Present research hypothesizes that the gut microbiome is not only involved in metabolic health but also takes part in the pathogenesis of a wide range of cardiovascular disorders, such as atherosclerosis. This association highlights the potential significance of considering gut health in the overall treatment approach. Although therapeutic options for current treatments of cardiovascular health disorders, such as myocarditis, are scarce, manipulation of the gut microbiota is promising for future treatments. With a focus on this gut-heart axis, future treatments can enhance current approaches, offering a more inclusive management protocol to individuals with greater atherosclerosis risk. With growing research, the incorporation of gut microbiome aspects into prevention and treatment protocols can improve patient outcomes for cardiovascular disease management (Figure 5.12).

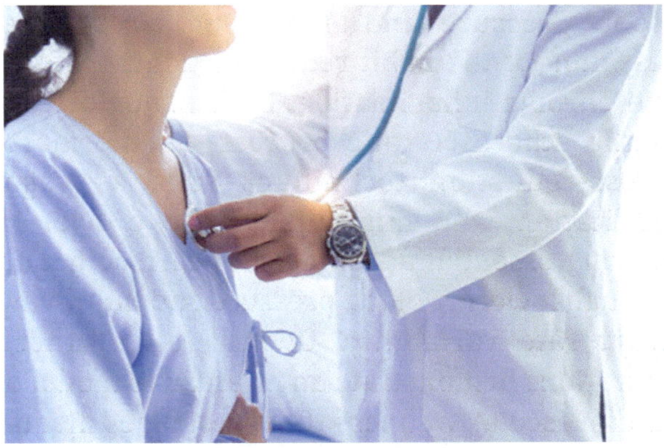

Figure 5.12. Treatment of cardiac atherosclerosis.

Source: https://www.aapc.com/codes/webroot/upload/articles_pdf/2022/cca/2022-08-24_13-59-43.webp.

5.4.1. Lifestyle Modifications

Lifestyle changes are the very core of preventing and controlling cardiac atherosclerosis, a disease so irretrievably intertwined with the lifestyle factors themselves. Incorporating physical activity is the most beneficial aspect of life modification, as exercise has been shown to improve cardiovascular function significantly. Aerobic exercise at low- to moderate-intensity levels not only improves endothelial function but also causes weight loss, which lowers obesity-related risk factors for atherosclerosis. Moreover, nutritional intake significantly impacts cardiovascular health; intake of whole foods, fruits, vegetables, and lean proteins can potentially decrease blood cholesterol levels and inflammation. The adoption of dietary and physical changes reflects the need for preemptive action against diet-related heart diseases, reflecting the interlinking of lifestyle and overall cardiovascular health (Rajpurohit et al., 2025). Similarly significant is the reduction of risk factors involved in causing atherosclerosis to begin. The most potent lifestyle modification is cessation of cigarette smoking, since cigarette smoking is a proven major cause of cardiovascular disease. In addition to reducing blood pressure and improving circulation, cessation of the habit reduces oxidative stress and chronic inflammation, both major drivers of the atherosclerotic process. Furthermore, stress-reduction techniques such as yoga, meditation, and mindfulness are crucial in offering essential advantages of cardiac health through lowering blood pressure and improving heart rate variability. Overall, all of these alterations demonstrate an integrative model of cardiovascular wellness that recognizes mental well-being significantly impacts physical health status (Li et al., 2025). Finally, compliance with lifestyle alteration can improve cardiovascular health as well as lifespan. The process of aging has been involved in the etiopathogenesis of most chronic diseases, including atherosclerosis and its consequences. Therefore, the use of anti-aging interventions along with lifestyle modification has a significant role to play in determining an individual's risk profile. As an example, frequent aerobic exercise and proper diet may prevent age-related impairment of cardiac function. Besides, scientific proof shows caloric limitation and diets rich in nutrients contain inherent anti-aging properties, thus an inherent means of resisting cardiovascular disease threats (Li et al., 2025). This highlights how these dietary habits and lifestyle choices can be a revolution that drives individuals towards selfcare among the elderly (Li et al., 2025).

5.4.2. Pharmacological Interventions

Pharmacotherapy plays a pivotal role in the management of cardiac atherosclerosis, primarily through modulation of lipoprotein levels and inflammation. Among the most common pharmacologic agents employed for this are statins, a class of medications that lower the levels of LDL cholesterol. Statins function by inhibiting the enzyme HMG-CoA reductase and thereby effectively decrease the synthesis of cholesterol in the liver, resulting in plaque stabilization within the arterial wall. The ESC Guidelines in prescribing the use of statins highlight that healthcare providers should consider every patient's unique context while deciding on treatment regimens (Visseren et al., 2021). Personalization of this kind maximizes therapeutic effect with minimized side effects, calling to the forefront the importance of personalized medicine in cardiovascular disease management, including atherosclerosis. Other than statins, novel pharmacologic treatments, such as proprotein convertase subtilisin/kexin type 9 (PCSK9) inhibitors, are now also valuable adjuncts in the battle against atherosclerosis. The monoclonal antibodies decrease significantly the levels of LDL cholesterol by blocking the binding of PCSK9 with LDL receptors, promoting receptor recycling and the removal of cholesterol from the circulation. Therefore, statin-resistant patients who are unable to achieve target levels of LDL with medication alone consistently benefit from this new therapy. Moreover, the recent evidence points towards them as having the potential to provide cardiovascular protection beyond lipid lowering, and hence with a larger therapeutic potential in the treatment of cardiac atherosclerosis. PCSK9 inhibitors need to be studied in terms of long-term effects to more accurately assess their effectiveness and safety in different patient populations, warranting their introduction into ongoing treatment models. Another problem that emphasizes the necessity of integrated pharmaceutical therapies is the relationship between phosphate and cardiovascular disease. Elevated serum phosphate has been associated with an elevated risk of cardiac atherosclerosis, particularly among those with chronic kidney disease. With deteriorating renal function, serum phosphate remains elevated, promoting pathologic processes such as vascular calcification and left ventricular hypertrophy (Zhou et al., 2021). Management of hyperphosphatemia through dietary modification and phosphate binder therapy is an exciting method of lowering cardiovascular risk and enhancing overall outcomes. Future research efforts will need large-scale, randomized controlled trials to establish a causality argument between phosphate control and cardiovascular benefit, ultimately integrating these findings into the clinic to better manage the subtleties of cardiac atherosclerosis treatment (Figure 5.13).

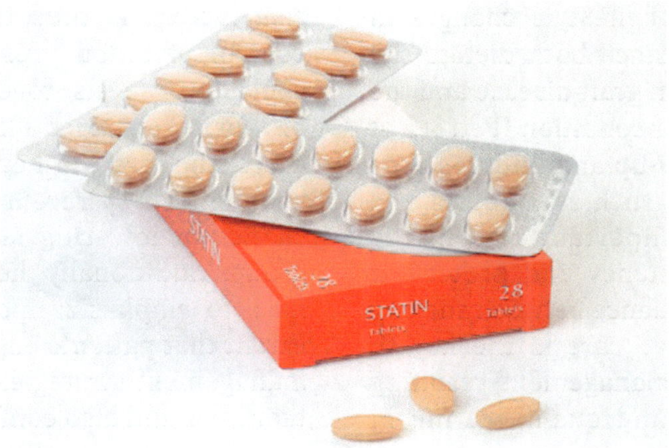

Figure 5.13. HPE statins.

Source: https://hospitalpharmacyeurope.com/wp-content/uploads/2016/11/HPE-statins.jpg.

5.4.3. Surgical Procedures

Treatment of cardiac atherosclerosis by surgery usually involves procedures aimed at restoring normal circulation to the affected heart muscle as a result of plaque buildup in the coronary arteries. Surgical procedures are often definitive in managing end-stage coronary artery disease, where non-surgical measures have been ineffective. Among the most widely used surgical interventions are CABG and PCI, which are meant to mitigate symptoms and lower the risk of myocardial infarction. An optimally coordinated surgical strategy improves patient outcomes, especially when coupled with extensive pre-operative evaluation and postoperative treatment aimed at reducing complications and maximizing recovery. CABG is a frequent operative procedure in patients with severe occlusion of coronary arteries giving an alternative pathway of blood supply that avoids the occlusions. It is typically done with saphenous veins or arterial grafts, and surely enough, arterial grafting has the upper hand over venous, mainly because the long-term patency rate of the arterial grafts is clearly greater than that of the veins, and the surgical result largely relies on this choice. Studies indicate that while the saphenous vein grafts (SVG) are employed in over 90% of CABG procedures, these have a higher rate of failure in the first year following surgery, mainly due to reasons such as thrombosis and intimal hyperplasia (Sandner et al., 2022). Consequently, the selection of graft types and compliance with optimal surgical techniques constitute the cornerstone to obtaining maximum long-term results in the treatment of coronary artery atherosclerotic lesions. Effective postoperative care following surgery for cardiac atherosclerosis plays a great role in bringing about an optimum long-term result. It is by rigorous secondary prevention measures, beginning with statin treatment and antiplatelet medication, that the incidence of graft loss and repeat MI. More recent investigations highlight monitoring and follow-up of lipid levels and persistence of lifestyle changes in CABG and PCI patients since both dictate the rate of progression of vein graft disease and the cumulative cardiovascular condition (Petrova et al., 2024). Further, follow-up and interventions for comorbid conditions such as diabetes and hypertension play an important role in the maintenance of graft patency and protection against adverse events. Balance between surgery and careful postoperative care is the key to effective atherosclerosis management, resulting in improved outcomes and quality of life in patients.

5.5. Prevention Strategies

Effective prevention therapies for atherosclerosis of the heart are essential in mitigating the disease prevalence and complications. Worth noting is risk stratification by coronary artery calcium scoring, which assists healthcare providers in identifying patients at risk of adverse cardiac outcomes. This advanced imaging technology enables clinicians to diagnose subclinical coronary atherosclerosis, effectively guiding intervention planning. For example, adding low-dose aspirin for patients found to be high-risk will lead to a considerable reduction in the incidence of heart attacks, as evidenced by a 44% decrease observed in a cohort of middle-aged men who were part of the Physicians' Health Study. If effectively applied, such prevention is likely to provide an active approach towards combating cardiac events, bridging knowledge and action gaps for high-risk populations in clinical settings (Siegel, 2025). Under diabetes, where individuals are at elevated risk of myocardial infarction, special precautions are also equally significant. Epidemiologic data indicate that diabetic patients have a two-fold increased risk of MI compared to their non-diabetic counterparts, with the risk in women even more marked. Controlling modifiable risk factors is thus the way forward. Tight control of blood pressure, blood sugar, and cholesterol levels, together with the adoption of lifestyle changes like quitting smoking and exercising, are the key interventions that has been shown by recent studies to have a good chance of lowering MI risk in this high-risk group. Additionally, health care professionals have to emphasize individualized care to the extent that patients engage in appropriate self-management strategies that complement drug therapies and also confer better cardiovascular health outcomes (Dr. Susmitha, 2025). In addition, heightened awareness and education on prevention of cardiac atherosclerosis can confer healthier public health outcomes. Programs initiated within the community to raise awareness among individuals regarding the necessity of developing heart-healthy habits, such as regular nutrition and physical activity, can provide patients with the capability of controlling their cardiovascular health. Habits such as increased physical activity and dietary modification are essential components in reducing the risk variables of atherosclerosis. Moreover, the use of technology, such as telehealth and mobile health technology, can enable regular monitoring and treatment of at-risk individuals. Collectively, these strong, multi-spectrum preventative strategies can bring about a culture of cardiovascular well-being, which substantially reduces the disease burden of cardiac atherosclerosis within different populations (Siegel, 2025) (Figure 5.14).

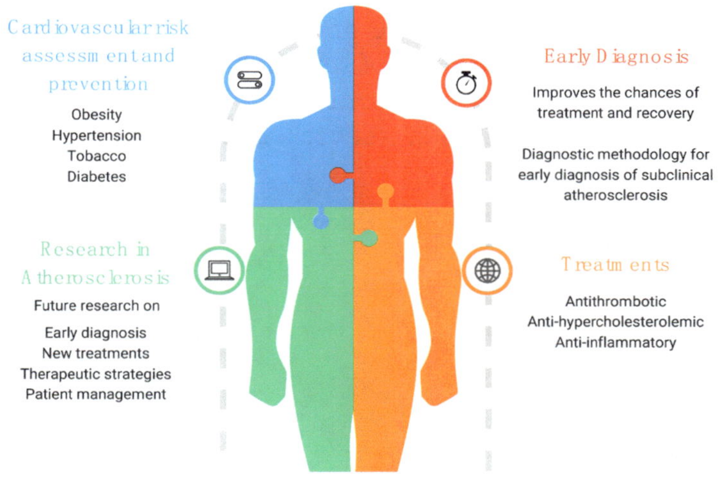

Figure 5.14. Prevention strategies in the context of atherosclerosis.

Source: https://www.mdpi.com/ijms/ijms-25-06016/article_deploy/html/images/ijms-25-06016-g002.png.

5.5.1. Importance of Regular Health Screenings

Regular health screenings play a critical role in early detection and treatment of cardiac atherosclerosis, a disease that can lead to fatal cardiovascular events such as heart attack and stroke. Detection of factors such as elevated cholesterol levels, elevated blood pressure, and other metabolic parameters at an early stage enables healthcare workers to initiate preventive measures and lifestyle changes tailored to individual patients' needs. This proactive approach not only provides patient information on their cardiovascular status but also allows them to make smarter decisions about treatment and lifestyle. Lastly, regular screenings are a part of cardiovascular care that bridges gaps between patient awareness and physician intervention. Implementation of screening schedules into routine health care can significantly reduce the prevalence of advanced heart disease and improve overall patient outcome for individuals at risk for cardiac atherosclerosis. Adherence to accepted screening guidelines cannot be overemphasized. For instance, the National Cholesterol Education Program Adult Treatment Panel III guidelines recommend that individuals older than 20 years should undergo screening for cholesterol every five years. Still, the majority of primary care providers do not do it regularly. According to studies, over 71 million Americans report that they have high blood cholesterol, but not many of them manage it effectively (Mattina et al., 1990). This conflict highlights the urgent need for health practitioners to prioritize regular cholesterol screening as a crucial tool for identifying individuals at risk of cardiac atherosclerosis. Regular screening allows health experts to intervene in a timely manner, lessening the cumulative impact of cardiovascular disease due to unprotected risk factors. Regular health screenings also establish broad awareness of cardiovascular disease among susceptible groups. By offering opportunities for patient education, healthcare providers can dispel myths regarding cardiac health and the importance of preventive measures. Patient adherence to screening procedures and lifestyle changes that prevent the risks associated with cardiac atherosclerosis is reinforced by effective communication strategies. For example, information gleaned through screening can initiate discussions on changes in diet, physical exercise, and the abandonment of harmful habits such as cigarette smoking. When patients are proactive in their health care, the likelihood of developing serious cardiovascular diseases is significantly lowered. As we cultivate a culture of supporting regular health screening, we are not only able to reduce the incidence of atherosclerosis, but we can also promote healthier lifestyles among our populations (Lehigh Valley Health Network, 2002) (Figure 5.15).

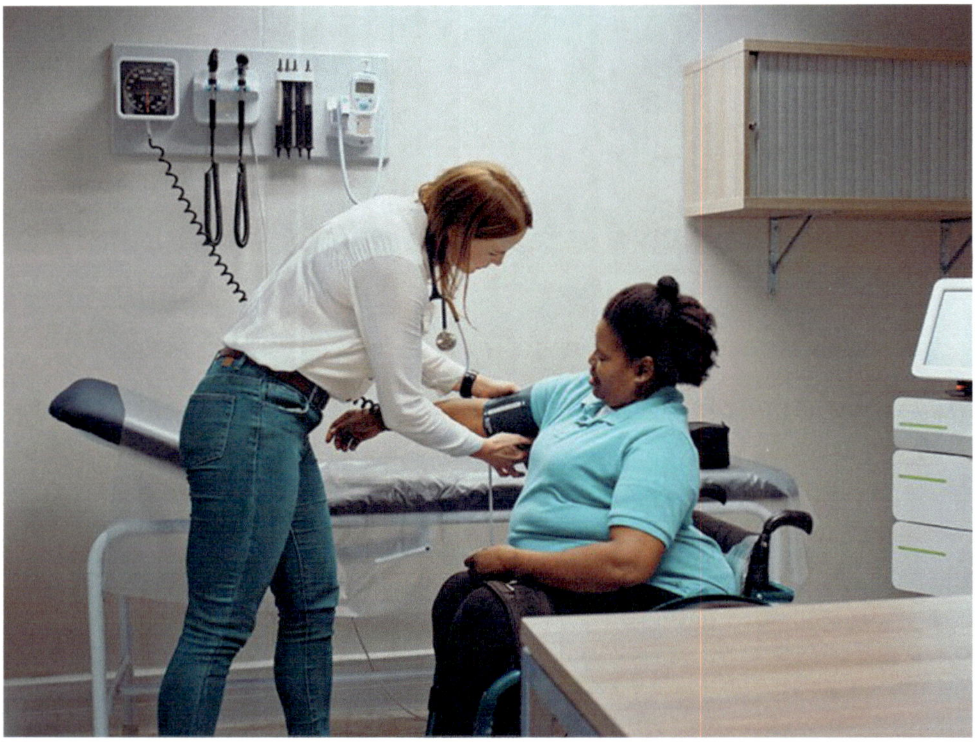

Figure 5.15. Preventing heart disease with checkups and routine screens.

Source: https://media.post.rvohealth.io/wp-content/uploads/2023/02/woman-doctor-taking-patient-blood-pressure-exam-wheelchair-disabled-disability-732x549-thumbnail.jpg.

5.5.2. Dietary Recommendations

Dietary recommendations are crucial in the treatment of cardiac atherosclerosis towards a heart-specific, multifaceted nutrition. A framework for nutrient intake involves increased plant food consumption, including whole grains, fruits, vegetables, legumes, and nuts. These foods are linked with reduced atherosclerosis risk, forming a facilitating environment for cardiovascular well-being. Substituting unhealthy fats, such as butter and other animal fats, with healthier fats like olive oil and other unsaturated fats is essential. According to the available evidence, such substitution is inversely associated with decreased CVD risk and is of a crucial part of dietary treatments that are aimed at counteracting the deleterious effects of atherosclerosis on cardiovascular health. Further, differentiation between various food sources of dietary protein in the context of cardiac atherosclerosis should be made. Present evidence suggests that red meat and processed meat are associated with greater CVD risk, but moderate consumption of poultry is not associated with the same deleterious effects (Moz et al., 2023). Such a detailed understanding allows health care practitioners to recommend food patterns that reduce risky foods while maintaining nutritional sufficiency. Further, consumption of dairy deserves special attention; moderate full-fat and reduced-fat dairy food intake is not observed to elevate CVD risk. Additionally, serving sizes of cheese and daily consumption of yogurt have shown potential protective effects, reinforcing the necessity of tailored dietary recommendations in conformity with patient-specific needs. Sophisticated dietary advice systems, particularly machine learning-based ones, form a breakthrough approach in the management of cardiac atherosclerosis. These models capitalize on extensive databases to calculate optimal dietary choices for risk group members to enhance both practitioner and patient decision-making capacity (Moz et al., 2023). With the inclusion of foods that are marked as heart-healthy, these recommendations can assist patients in making effective dietary adjustments to decrease their cardiovascular risks. Moreover, the study of intricate food interactions, i.e., the effect of interaction between various components of food, develops a greater understanding regarding the contribution of some arrangement towards the health and well-being of the heart. Lastly, the use of evidence-based nutritional methods combined with advanced tools has the potential to reduce the economically and socially expensive burden of cardiac disease, placing evidence-based nutrition as an active factor in cardiovascular therapy.

5.5.3. Exercise and Physical Activity

An increasing number of studies emphasize the role of exercise and physical activity in determining cardiovascular health, particularly in cardiac atherosclerosis. Regular physical activity has been linked to significant advantage to lipid profiles, reducing hypertension, and enhancing endothelial function, all of which are crucial determinants of atherosclerosis development. As prescribed in a range of clinical studies, exercise is both a preventive action and a part of rehabilitation for those who have cardiovascular disease. The promise of formal physical training, particularly in the setting of rehabilitation therapy, to increase survival rates and functional capacity reinforces the argument to embrace an active role for exercise as a life choice among individuals with risk for cardiac disease (Kasiakogias et al., 2020). These results reinforce the demand for health professionals to advocate for regular physical training as a measure against the formation and progression of cardiac atherosclerosis. In addition, exercise has been shown to improve the inflammatory mechanisms behind cardiovascular disease. Inflammatory processes constitute a significant factor in promoting and advancing atherosclerosis, and this observation has prompted researchers to look towards regular exercise's anti-inflammatory action. Studies demonstrate how moderate exercise efficiently suppresses systemic inflammation, while immune function as a whole is improved, potentially negating the harmful actions of atherosclerosis. This interaction between inflammation and exercise is critical to an understanding of how physical exercise may serve as a therapeutic intervention. Notably, clinicians have to take the patient's individual health status into account when they prescribe exercise programs, and thereby individualize interventions to create maximal effect (François Mach et al., 2019). Individualizing interventions in this way not only maximizes adherence to physical exercise but also maximizes its protective effects against cardiac atherosclerosis. Finally, the encouragement of exercise as a public health measure offers an opportunity to address the increasing disease burden of cardiovascular diseases. Given the substantial evidence of physical inactivity and its associated risks of atherosclerosis, policies promoting exercise should be prioritized. Community intervention that fosters access to safety zones for exercise, and sensitization regarding the advantages of exercise, can shape a culture of health and a preventive environment. Interestingly, clinicians also play a significant role in counseling patients about the required types and intensities of exercise to match their health condition. Ensuring that the patients are adequately educated about exercise benefits not only promotes a proactive healthy mindset but also aids in realizing the necessity for cardiovascular care throughout their lives. Thus, the inclusion of physical exercise in everyday discourse about cardiac health is crucial in reducing atherosclerosis's impact on public health (Kasiakogias et al., 2020) (Figure 5.16).

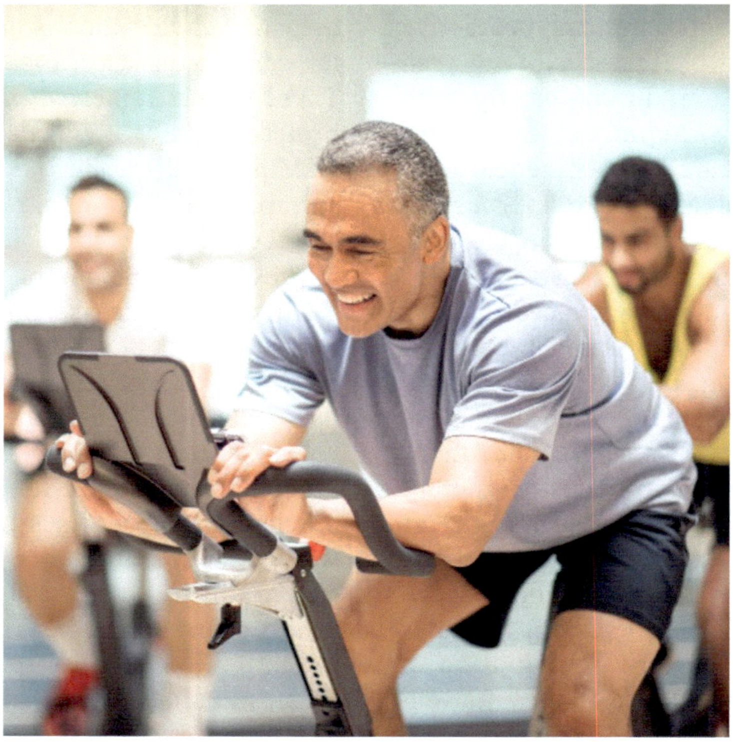

Figure 5.16. Exercise and Physical Activity.

Source: https://ysm-res.cloudinary.com/image/upload/ar_1:1,c_fill,dpr_3.0,f_auto,g_faces:auto,q_auto:eco,w_500/v1/yms/prod/52f484b6-dbe4-4715-87b2-b8e6e05ca421.

SUMMARY

This review is a significant milestone in the understanding of cardiac atherosclerosis, summarizing the large body of evidence that has been accrued on its pathogenesis and clinical impact. The heterogeneity of the disease process is characterized by the accumulation of lipids and inflammatory cells within the walls of arteries, leading to the formation of plaques that impair normal circulation. Recent studies have unraveled genetic risk factors that predispose an individual to atherosclerosis, emphasizing the need for personalized prevention tactics. Integrating data from genome-wide association studies, researchers have begun unveiling the links between metabolic disease states, such as hypercholesterolemia, and cardiovascular disease development, emphasizing the need for a multi-factorial treatment and prevention approach in practice (Li et al., 2019). Moreover, the role of serum urate levels has fallen under the spotlight as it relates to cardiac atherosclerosis, showing a strong association with adverse cardiovascular outcomes. Elevated urate levels have been implicated in both essential hypertension and gout as well as coronary atherosclerosis, suggesting an overlapping pathophysiological mechanism is engaged. The observation suggests the potential benefit of modulating urate as therapy for a healthier cardiovascular status. However, investigators need to unravel the complex interplay of genetic factors on urate levels and cardiovascular risk, as observed from the existence of pleiotropic influences in observational studies. It is critical to grasp the intricacies of the relationships for the establishment of successful therapeutic interventions (François Mach et al., 2019). In summary, cardiac atherosclerosis management requires an all-encompassing understanding of its causes and consequences based on genetics, biochemistry, and clinical practices. The integration of advanced investigation with conventional clinical practice holds the promise of enhancing patient management. As scientific knowledge continues to shed light on mechanisms of this multifactorial disease, healthcare professionals must remain vigilant about applying evidence-based methods sensitive to individual patients' conditions and emerging data on risk factors. More collaboration between scientists, clinicians, and public health organizations can give rise to innovative prevention programs directed towards the prevention of the growing cardiovascular disease burden due to atherosclerosis (François Mach et al., 2019; Li et al., 2019).

Cardiac atherosclerosis, a prevalent cardiovascular disease, is defined by the accumulation of lipids, inflammatory cells, and fibrous elements within the arterial vessel wall, leading to plaque development. The pathologic process has significant effects on myocardial ischemia and ultimate clinical ramifications. The key risk factors for atherosclerosis include dyslipidemia, hypertension, smoking, and diabetes. Understanding the multifactorial etiology of this disease helps health professionals develop individualized preventive and therapeutic management plans. Emphasis on lifestyle modification, including dietary change and increased physical activity, is necessary to manage these risk factors effectively and to avoid further disease progression. Compliance of the patients with pharmacologic therapy prescribed could also optimize overall treatment efficacy, which is linked with a reduction in adverse cardiovascular events. Current guidelines in managing cardiac atherosclerosis have stressed the importance of early detection and intervention. Application of screening instrumentation and diagnostic studies, such as coronary angiography and non-invasive imaging techniques, allows identification of atherosclerotic changes before the occurrence of clinically relevant manifestations. Continuous advances in technology enable early detection and direct management. Detailed guidelines from both the European Society of Cardiology and the

European Atherosclerosis Society encourage healthcare professionals to consider patient-specific variables when creating management plans. In addition, these guidelines aim to bridge the gaps between clinical practice and evidence-based guidelines, emphasizing the need for individualized therapy in cardiac atherosclerosis to improve long-term patient outcomes. Cardiac atherosclerosis also requires multidisciplinary care. There has to be collaboration between healthcare professionals such as cardiologists, dieticians, and nurse practitioners to create an integrated treatment model that includes the medical, social, and psychological determinants of treatment. Educational activity to raise awareness of cardiac health is a central component of effective disease management initiatives. Regular updating of treatment guidelines against emerging research also guarantees that an evidence-based approach culture continues to dominate. Practitioners need to be attentive and responsive to new research and guidelines, incorporating them into practice. Lastly, by adhering to established guidelines while being responsive to the unique challenges each patient presents, healthcare professionals can provide the optimal care and improve the quality of life in patients affected by cardiac atherosclerosis (François Mach et al., 2019; Vahanian et al., 2021).

A CLOSER LOOK

COMPLICATIONS OF CARDIAC ATHEROSCLEROSIS

Cardiac atherosclerosis is the leading cause of a variety of cardiovascular complications with severe consequences for the patient's health. The dynamic nature of atherosclerosis leads to the formation of plaques in the coronary arteries, eventually leading to reduced flow of blood to the myocardium. Consequently, the reduction in oxygen and nutrient supply tends to manifest as angina or chest pain. Secondly, plaque instability under severe conditions can lead to rupture, triggering acute coronary syndromes such as myocardial infarction. Ischemia and subsequent tissue necrosis not only enhance the risk of heart failure but also hasten the development of arrhythmias, which subsequently may complicate patient management. These clinical presentations need to be appreciated in the setting of cardiac atherosclerosis since early intervention can prevent severe outcomes that can jeopardize long-term health.

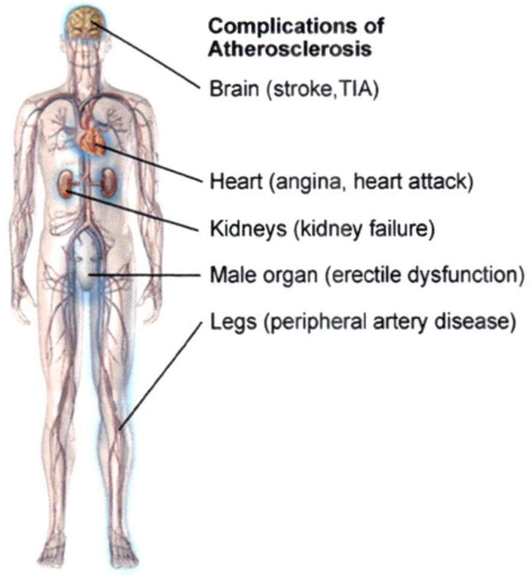

Figure 5.17. Atherosclerosis complications.

Source: https://medmovie.com/_uploads/ahaw_0200i_640x480.png.

Moreover, the cardiac atherosclerosis complications are not only confined to coronary artery disease but also include other vital organs and systems. Among them is the heightened frequency of systemic hypertension as a result of the vascular atherosclerotic alterations that would lead to heightened arterial stiffness and resistance. This, subsequently, elevates the work burden on the heart and aggravates existing cardiac conditions, as well as triggering heart failure. In addition, atherosclerosis plays a role in the increased risk of cerebrovascular accidents, or stroke, since emboli can result in the deprivation of blood in the brain. The interrelatedness of these systemic complications and heart disease highlights the importance of a multifaceted multidisciplinary approach to the management of patients with atherosclerosis, not only treating cardiac function but also addressing broader vascular health to reduce overall risks. Further, immune mechanisms have also become important in the generation of cardiac atherosclerosis, precipitating complications. Immune checkpoint pathways, that is, PD-1 and CTLA-4, are responsible for regulating immune mechanisms that protect cardiac tissue from damage. The mechanisms have been reported to be dysregulated, and this causes heightened inflammation, accelerating the development of atherosclerotic plaques as well as the risk of resulting heart failure. For instance, the induction of T lymphocyte invasion and the liberation of pro-inflammatory cytokines have been linked with increased myocardial damage in atherosclerosis. These findings indicate a relationship between immune processes and cardiac health and suggest that therapy against immune checkpoints could represent a novel approach to the management of atherosclerosis complications of the heart. It is an essential understanding for formulating effective strategies to manage the multiple complexities of this common cardiovascular condition (Figure 5.17).

References

1. Afroz, R., & Goodwin, J. E. (2024). WNT signaling in Atherosclerosis: Mechanisms to therapeutic implications. *Biomedicines, 12*(2), 276. https://doi.org/10.3390/biomedicines12020276Alamir, A., Brown, A., Budoff, M., Chaus, et al. (2018). *The Correlation of Dyslipidemia with the Extent of Coronary Artery Disease in the Multiethnic Study of Atherosclerosis.* https://core.ac.uk/download/323077693.pdf (accessed on 29th May 2025).
2. Almuqbil, N. (2024). Role of FDG-PET radiomics in the diagnosis of cardiovascular inflammation: A narrative review. *Journal of Clinical and Diagnostic Research.* https://www.semanticscholar.org/paper/6d91c97c69b3a43e1c3bf943fd7f457840e37103 (accessed on 29th May 2025).
3. Alonso-Herranz, L., Albarrán-Juárez, J., & Bentzon, J. (2023). Mechanisms of fibrous cap formation in atherosclerosis. *Frontiers in Cardiovascular Medicine, 10.* https://www.semanticscholar.org/paper/b34774223d1dcb75e66c05c2f8a0c9a54d50b06f (accessed on 29th May 2025).
4. Ambale-Venkatesh, B., Bahrami, H., Bakhshi, H., Bluemke, et al. (2017). *Progression of Coronary Artery Calcium and Incident Heart Failure: The Multi-Ethnic Study of Atherosclerosis.* https://core.ac.uk/download/323077092.pdf (accessed on 29th May 2025).
5. Anand, V. V., Mahesh, R., Lim, J. S., Chong, B., Kong, G., Lee, E., Tan, B., et al. (2024). Unique regional risk profiles and cardiovascular outcomes of patients with acute coronary syndrome in the absence of standard modifiable risk factors: A systematic review and meta-analysis. *European Heart Journal.* https://www.semanticscholar.org/paper/7d7b5dbf2ce4a64723f7d1c80190be03a416fd0d (accessed on 29th May 2025).
6. Bennetts, J., Walker, R., Williams, T., Sverdlov, A., & Ngo, D. (2024). Abstract 4117414: Risk factors associated with cardiac hospital admissions in cancer patients treated with immune checkpoint inhibitors. *Circulation.* https://www.semanticscholar.org/paper/2f9bfa2d69fd5329135e30f74c792f15c6d3d83b (accessed on 29th May 2025).
7. Brooks, L. L. (2002). *The Effects of After-School Physical Activity and Adult Encouragement on Adolescents.* https://core.ac.uk/download/5066041.pdf (accessed on 29th May 2025).
8. Cavarretta, E., Dal Sasso, E., Forte, M., Frati, et al. (2017). *The Light and Shadow of Senescence and Inflammation in Cardiovascular Pathology and Regenerative Medicine.* https://core.ac.uk/download/141694265.pdf (accessed on 29th May 2025).
9. Clark, R., Rawas, H., Windsor, C., Yates, et al. (2012). *Cultural Challenges to Secondary Prevention: Implications for Saudi Women.* https://core.ac.uk/download/10909715.pdf (accessed on 29th May 2025).
10. Dawi, J., Affa, S., Misakyan, Y., Fardeheb, S., Kades, S., Kiriaki, A., Mohan, A. S., et al. (2024). Exploring cardiovascular implications in systemic lupus erythematosus: A holistic analysis of complications, diagnostic criteria, and therapeutic modalities, encompassing pharmacological and adjuvant approaches. *Biomolecular Concepts, 15*(1). https://www.semanticscholar.org/paper/795051584767223854dbf9bdc086bc01352e5b7b (accessed on 29th May 2025).
11. Dziedzic, E. A., Gąsior, J., Pawłowski, M., Wodejko-Kucharska, B., Saniewski, T., Marcisz, A., & Dąbrowski, M. J. (2019). Vitamin D level is associated with severity of coronary artery atherosclerosis and incidence of acute coronary syndromes in non-diabetic cardiac patients.

Archives of Medical Science: AMS, 15, 359–368. https://www.semanticscholar.org/paper/fa269f88756a1e50cdd722c4e26bbee4b3d5ea08 (accessed on 29th May 2025).

12. Ellenbogen, M., Marine, J. E., Arbab-Zadeh, A., Pathiravasan, C., Swann, J., & Brotman, D. J. (2024). Relationship between insurance status and receipt of cardiac tests and procedures during hospitalization: A cross-sectional study. *Journal of the American Heart Association: Cardiovascular and Cerebrovascular Disease, 13.* https://www.semanticscholar.org/paper/8d5cea089ff7f7fdc5d811a5c7cb91bacab1c7a7 (accessed on 29th May 2025).
13. Evans, P. C., Rainger, G. E., Mason, J. C., Guzik, T. J., Osto, E., Stamataki, Z., Neil, D., et al. (2020). Endothelial dysfunction in COVID-19: A position paper of the ESC Working Group for Atherosclerosis and Vascular Biology, and the ESC Council of Basic Cardiovascular Science. *Cardiovascular Research, 116*, 2177–2184. https://doi.org/10.1093/cvr/cvaa230 (accessed on 29th May 2025).
14. Gill, S., Emblin, K., Daniels, R., & Mokbel, K. (2024). Chest pain at rest with unremarkable ECG and cardiac enzymes: Case study emphasizing the importance of clinical suspicion in the diagnosis of coronary artery disease. *In Vivo, 39*, 524–531. https://www.semanticscholar.org/paper/1691311d654402f0d5d5eb8615bb4e6c4cb006c9 (accessed on 29th May 2025).
15. Gour, T. (2023). Treatment options for high cardiometabolic risk patients with atherosclerosis. *Journal of Student Research.* https://www.semanticscholar.org/paper/0de94c86199ed70d1183c56a19742e88898085b4 (accessed on 29th May 2025).
16. Grant, J., Zhang, S., Wallace, A. S., Nambi, V., Echouffo, J. B., Minhas, A. A., Matsushita, K., et al. (2025). Abstract P1155: Different heart failure risk factors have distinct patterns of preclinical cardiac dysfunction: The Atherosclerosis Risk in Communities (ARIC) Study. *Circulation.* https://www.semanticscholar.org/paper/bacd55547c5c160dabe9f44f7460b0a7def34b71 (accessed on 29th May 2025).
17. Gulomitdinov, S. N. (2025). Assessment of neurological risk factors in patients undergoing cardiac surgery with cardiopulmonary bypass (CPB). *International Journal of Medical Sciences and Clinical Research.* https://www.semanticscholar.org/paper/c5bb3d28b4518a51f279fc9b246b26bcf8d63bb5 (accessed on 29th May 2025).
18. Haris, M., Hammad, A., & Kumar, V. (2025). Pregnancy-associated coronary artery dissection (P-SCAD): A crucial differential diagnosis for chest pain during pregnancy. *Brain & Heart.* https://www.semanticscholar.org/paper/5e3692ce798a308167eaf3a2b55f9af082d53f60 (accessed on 29th May 2025).
19. Haverstaad, R., Kirkeby-Garstad, I., Lovstakken, L., Nordgaard, et al. (2010). *Impact of Competitive Flow on Wall Shear Stress in Coronary Surgery: Computational Fluid Dynamics of a LIMA-LAD Model.* https://core.ac.uk/download/55842550.pdf (accessed on 29th May 2025).
20. Huang, S., Kang, Y., Liu, T., Xiong, Y., Yang, Z. X., & Zhang, Q. (2025). The role of immune checkpoints PD-1 and CTLA-4 in cardiovascular complications leading to heart failure. *Frontiers in Immunology, 16.* https://www.semanticscholar.org/paper/c17ee09d4ab1a06dd04609a752149d0dbe4cca59 (accessed on 29th May 2025).
21. Jones, A., Ali, M. U., Kenny, M., Mayhew, A., Mokashi, V., He, H., Lin, S., et al. (2024). Potentially modifiable risk factors for dementia and mild cognitive impairment: An umbrella review and meta-analysis. *Dementia and Geriatric Cognitive Disorders, 53*, 91–106. https://www.

semanticscholar.org/paper/c388f9316ec76db1c747d4aeccdaff4f10f78659 (accessed on 29th May 2025).

22. Kasiakogias, A., & Sharma, S. (2020). Exercise: The ultimate treatment to all ailments? *Clinical Cardiology, 43*, 817–826. https://doi.org/10.1002/clc.23369 (accessed on 29th May 2025).
23. Khattab, M., Baig, M., El Zarif, T., Barac, A., Ferencik, M., Henry, M. L., Lopez-Mattei, J., et al. (2025). How to use imaging: Complex cases of atherosclerosis, myocardial inflammation, and cardiomyopathy in cardio-oncology. *Circulation: Cardiovascular Imaging.* https://www.semanticscholar.org/paper/dd56f15a616ae3db299d47e5df605f336e8f8f8f (accessed on 29th May 2025).
24. Ko, D., & Benjamin, E. (2022). Atrial cardiopathy and cardioembolic stroke. *Annals of Internal Medicine, 176*, 131, 132. https://www.semanticscholar.org/paper/21e804b9e4237c47de6cf3b2876b77c5dfd3dac2 (accessed on 29th May 2025).
25. Kong, W., Du, J., Zhu, Y., & Dong, E. (2017). Basic and translational vascular research in China: Past, present, and future. *Circulation Research, 121*(4), 335–337. https://www.semanticscholar.org/paper/25b31d373270ade17de79213c2f0f055d5211a13 (accessed on 29th May 2025).
26. Lehigh Valley Health Network. (2002). *Healthy You.* https://core.ac.uk/download/267869835.pdf (accessed on 29th May 2025).
27. Li, Q., Zhang, H., Xiao, N., Liang, G., Lin, Y., Yang, X., Yang, J., et al. (2025). Aging and lifestyle modifications for preventing aging-related diseases. *FASEB Journal: Official Publication of the Federation of American Societies for Experimental Biology, 39*(9), e70575. https://www.semanticscholar.org/paper/88824116cc0ccc3370bbfd5797218ab6302270a3 (accessed on 29th May 2025).
28. Mach, F., Baigent, C., Catapano, A. L., Koskinas, K. C., Casula, M., Badimón, L., Chapman, M. J., et al. (2019). 2019 ESC/EAS Guidelines for the management of dyslipidemias: Lipid modification to reduce cardiovascular risk. *European Heart Journal, 41*, 111–188. https://doi.org/10.1093/eurheartj/ehz455 (accessed on 29th May 2025).
29. Markovic, A. M., Tomić, A., Nisevic, M., Parapid, B., Boskovic, N., Vitas, M., Jevtovic, M., et al. (2025). The role of MDCT coronary angiography in the detection of benign varieties and anomalies of coronary blood vessels—A narrative review. *Medicina, 61*. https://www.semanticscholar.org/paper/26b13730d1ab519e5256f3f2eec330c3a4a126a6 (accessed on 29th May 2025).
30. Mattina, J. (1990). *Analysis of Cholesterol Screening Practices.* https://core.ac.uk/download/480740846.pdf (accessed on 29th May 2025).
31. Mousa, M., Mahmoud, I. Z., Elkammash, T. H., Gad, A., & Noureldin, R. (2025). Cardiac magnetic resonance in association with coronary CT angiography in the assessment of right coronary artery aneurysm with atrial fistula causing myocardial ischemia. *Cureus, 17.* https://www.semanticscholar.org/paper/370fa91104dc9cf0983a1abb453f64c0c5074a8e (accessed on 29th May 2025).
32. Moz, S. H., Hosen, M. A., Santo, M. N. S., Kabir, S., Adnan, M. N., & Galib, S. M. (2023). Precision cardio diet: Transforming cardiac care with artificial intelligence-driven dietary recommendations. *Radioelectronic and Computer Systems.* https://www.semanticscholar.org/paper/046a7301127bcdecd3c2f43f0457ff15d0f1006e (accessed on 29th May 2025).

33. Padró, T., Manfrini, O., Bugiardini, R., Canty, J. M., Cenko, E., De Luca, G., Duncker, D. J., et al. (2020). ESC Working Group on Coronary Pathophysiology and Microcirculation position paper on 'coronary microvascular dysfunction in cardiovascular disease'. *Cardiovascular Research, 116*, 741–755. https://doi.org/10.1093/cvr/cvaa003 (accessed on 29th May 2025).

34. Parvez, M., Khattak, T., Kavarthapu, A., & Pulivarthi, K. (2024). 8416 Spontaneous coronary artery dissection due to estrogen containing oral contraceptive pills: A case report. *Journal of the Endocrine Society, 8.* https://www.semanticscholar.org/paper/3c4082372df2b1b040c7f50f7d098602ed46cea4 (accessed on 29th May 2025).

35. Petrova, E. B., Shishko, O. N., Grigorenko, E. A., Statkevich, T. V., Pleshko, A. A., Chernyak, S. V., Kozich, I. A., et al. (2024). Noninvasive diagnosis of preclinical stages of coronary and precerebral atherosclerosis in patients with newly diagnosed hypo- and hyperthyroidism. *Emergency Cardiology and Cardiovascular Risks.* https://www.semanticscholar.org/paper/78cde4c6c7f3466e2b80fb64158d183eaa9c0258 (accessed on 29th May 2025).

36. Pichandi, S., Pasupathi, P., Rao, Y. Y., Farook, J., Ambika, A., Ponnusha, B. S., Subramaniyam, S., et al. (2011). *The Role of Statin Drugs in Combating Cardiovascular Diseases – A Review.* https://core.ac.uk/download/pdf/14696.pdf (accessed on 29th May 2025).

37. Rajpurohit, R., Joshi, G., Srivastava, A. K., & Angmo, D. (2025). Optimizing heart health through Ayurveda: A detailed focus on the prevention and treatment of Hridroga. *International Ayurvedic Medical Journal.* https://www.semanticscholar.org/paper/cab10a33b5bb334924744c2e8173dfd4738b059f (accessed on 29th May 2025).

38. Reddy, K. P., Mehta, S., Eberly, L. A., Khatana, S., Chatterjee, P., Fanaroff, A. C., Groeneveld, P. W., et al. (2025). Inter- and intrahospital price variation for common cardiovascular admission diagnoses, diagnostic tests, and therapeutic procedures. *Journal of the American Heart Association, 14*(6), e038660. https://www.semanticscholar.org/paper/cb3bc8c7798d7a4d04c5cb2439e27b634670ab32 (accessed on 29th May 2025).

39. Riccardi, G., Giosuè, A., Calabrese, I., & Vaccaro, O. (2021). Dietary recommendations for prevention of atherosclerosis. *Cardiovascular Research.* https://www.semanticscholar.org/paper/ca23dd510d6886e7d00c4a3892197f1c886990cf (accessed on 29th May 2025).

40. Sandner, S. E., & Ruel, M. (2022). Secondary prevention is as important as surgical technique. *Journal of Cardiac Surgery, 37*, 3673, 3674. https://www.semanticscholar.org/paper/fe852067b3065bb7a22ea4e24d78cd5b66f1a5cb (accessed on 29th May 2025).

41. Savarese, G., von Haehling, S., Butler, J., Cleland, J. G. F., Ponikowski, P., & Anker, S. D. (2022). Iron deficiency and cardiovascular disease. *European Heart Journal, 44*, 14–27. https://doi.org/10.1093/eurheartj/ehac569 (accessed on 29th May 2025).

42. Siegel, A. (2025). Aspirin guided by coronary artery calcium scoring for primary prevention in persons with subclinical coronary atherosclerosis. *Medical Research Archives.* https://www.semanticscholar.org/paper/31e60632bccc5b65c09358dae99373ee52efdd6a (accessed on 29th May 2025).

43. Susmitha, G. (2025). Assessing the increased risk of myocardial infarction in diabetes mellitus patients and strategies for prevention. *International Journal of Scientific Research in Engineering and Management.* https://www.semanticscholar.org/paper/404dddd05a32b9742458ea422b32f56984c66a17 (accessed on 29th May 2025).

44. Tambo, A., Roshan, M. H. K., & Pace, N. (2016). Testosterone and cardiovascular disease. *The Open Cardiovascular Medicine Journal, 10*, 1–10. https://www.semanticscholar.org/paper/3356de7a8c35c4bd23fd7418fbdca0622a8ce136 (accessed on 29th May 2025).

45. Todor, S. B., Ichim, C., Boicean, A., & Mihaila, R. (2024). Cardiovascular risk in Philadelphia-negative myeloproliferative neoplasms: Mechanisms and implications—A narrative review. *Current Issues in Molecular Biology, 46*, 8407–8423. https://www.semanticscholar.org/paper/b6027d536ec0c9abb3c41fdb30573d4737df243e (accessed on 29th May 2025).

46. Uchiyama, S., Hoshino, T., Minematsu, K., Meledje, M. L., Charles, H., Albers, G. W., Caplan, L. R., et al. (2024). Risk of major vascular events in patients without traditional risk factors after transient ischemic attack or minor ischemic stroke: An international prospective cohort. *European Stroke Journal.* https://www.semanticscholar.org/paper/b2660b12b6483324dffc00bfe45b4a4e70ff5f05 (accessed on 29th May 2025).

47. Vahanian, A., Beyersdorf, F., Praz, F., Milojevic, M., Baldus, S., Bauersachs, J., Capodanno, D., et al. (2021). 2021 ESC/EACTS guidelines for the management of valvular heart disease. *European Heart Journal, 43*, 561–632. https://doi.org/10.1093/eurheartj/ehab395 (accessed on 29th May 2025).

48. Vancheri, F., Longo, G., Vancheri, S., & Henein, M. Y. (2020). Coronary microvascular dysfunction. *Journal of Clinical Medicine, 9*, 2880. https://doi.org/10.3390/jcm9092880 (accessed on 29th May 2025).

49. Visseren, F. L. J., Mach, F., Smulders, Y. M., Carballo, D., Koskinas, K. C., Bäck, M., Bénétos, A., et al. (2021). 2021 ESC Guidelines on cardiovascular disease prevention in clinical practice. *European Heart Journal, 42*, 3227–3337. https://doi.org/10.1093/eurheartj/ehab484 (accessed on 29th May 2025).

50. Wang, J., Zhang, X., Yang, X., Yu, H., Bu, M., Fu, J., Zhang, Z., et al. (2023). Revitalizing myocarditis treatment through gut microbiota modulation: Unveiling a promising therapeutic avenue. *Frontiers in Cellular and Infection Microbiology, 13.* https://www.semanticscholar.org/paper/b5ff6ad62e1c4705c05d6912417df5c541d37b18 (accessed on 29th May 2025).

51. Xue, L., Xiangrui, M., Yazhou, H., Athina, S., Maria, T., Wei-Qi, W., Aliya, G., et al. (2019) Genetically determined serum urate levels and cardiovascular and other diseases in UK Biobank cohort: A phenome-wide mendelian randomization study. *PLoS Medicine, 16*, e1002937–e1002937. doi: https://doi.org/10.1371/journal.pmed.1002937.

52. Yahan, L., Zhipeng, W., Li, F., Yaohua, X., Beilei, Z., Xuya, K., Yanqing, Z., et al. (2024) Deficiency of 5-HT2B receptors alleviates atherosclerosis by regulating macrophage phenotype through inhibiting interferon signaling. *British Journal of Pharmacology*. doi: https://www.semanticscholar.org/paper/7a138526f22a75612da7783246d9f85a23a566d5 (accessed on 29th May 2025).

53. Zhou, C., Shi, Z., Ouyang, N., & Ruan, X. (2021). Hyperphosphatemia and cardiovascular disease. *Frontiers in Cell and Developmental Biology, 9.* https://doi.org/10.3389/fcell.2021.644363.

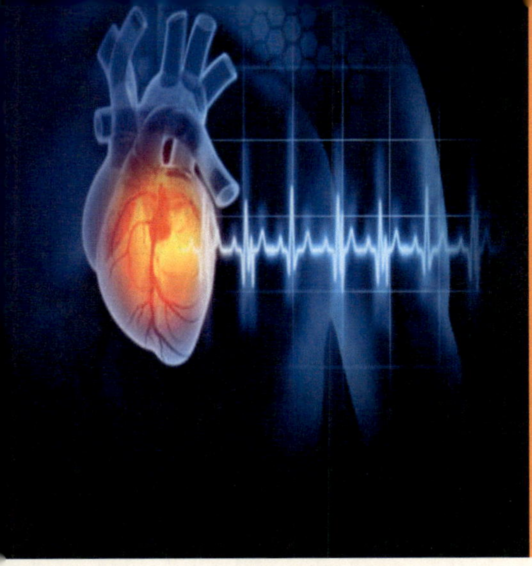

Chapter 6
HEART FAILURE

Contents

Introduction

Heart failure (HF) is a significant public health concern, affecting millions of individuals worldwide and characterized by the inability of the heart to pump blood effectively. HF can result from various cardiac conditions, including coronary heart disease, hypertension, and cardiomyopathy, that lead to a variety of disabling signs such as fatigue, shortness of breath, and edema. Fluid overload, or congestion, is particularly a leading cause of decreased quality of life in HF patients, profoundly impairing their daily functioning and well-being. Despite progress in pharmacological treatments to alter the disease process, therapy for congestion mainly depends on loop diuretics, which have experienced little innovation over the last half-century. This reliance on existing therapies underscores the absolute necessity of better insight into the management of heart failure and new therapeutic agents (Cuthbert et al., 2024). Heart failure is now being classified, with increasing emphasis on subtypes such as heart failure with preserved ejection fraction (HFpEF) and heart failure with reduced ejection fraction (HFrEF). Of these, HFpEF is of particular concern, often linked with obesity and metabolic syndromes. Obese patients with HFpEF have more pronounced symptoms, poorer hemodynamics, and worse prognosis in the long term than non-obese individuals. This category of patients should be paid special attention as weight reduction methods employed to date may exacerbate the underlying pathologies, leading to undue loss of skeletal muscle mass along with fat. This combined loss is crucial since decreased skeletal muscle function is associated with frailty, again making the clinical situation complex for patients with HFpEF (Kitzman et al., 2024). Therefore, understanding the interaction among heart failure, obesity, and potential novel treatments is crucial for effective management. Novel research strategies and clinical trials are essential in countering the complex situation of heart failure. An attractive area of research includes the study of mitochondrial uncoupling agents, which possess new mechanisms for weight loss with maintenance of skeletal muscle mass. New medications, such as HU6, aim to enhance metabolic function by increasing fat oxidation without caloric deprivation, thereby preventing frailty.

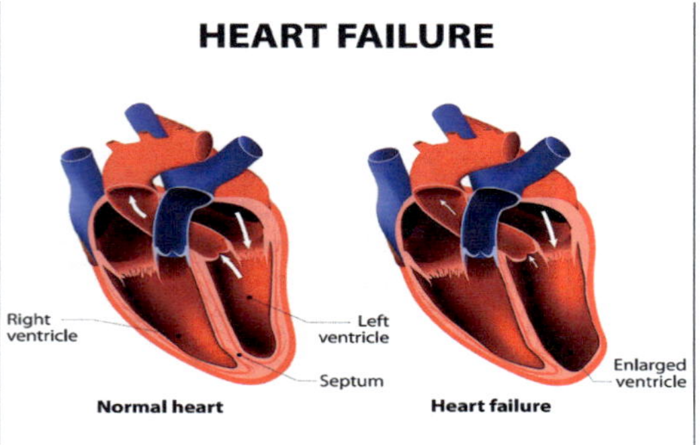

Figure 6.1. Heart failure (HF).

Source: https://continentalhospitals.com/uploads/mceu_22197202211699430774969.jpg.

The initiation of trials like HuMAIN-HFpEF is a milestone step toward the assessment of novel agents that can address the pressing demands of HFpEF patients with obesity. By studying the effects of these agents on weight reduction, body composition, inflammation, and exercise tolerance, researchers maximize the chances of improved outcomes for patients. This strategy not only identifies the necessity for new treatments but also emphasizes an integrated approach to the treatment of heart failure, maximizing overall health benefit (Kitzman et al., 2024) (Figure 6.1).

Definition of Heart Failure (HF)

HF is a complex clinical syndrome that occurs when the ability of the heart to pump blood is compromised, resulting in an insufficient blood supply to the body to meet metabolic needs. It is characterized by varied symptoms, including dyspnea, fatigue, and edema, which lead to impairments in exercise tolerance and quality of life. The disease has varied presentations in different individuals and presents in types such as HFrEF and HFpEF. All the subtypes are reflective of distinct underlying pathophysiologies and thus need distinct therapeutic interventions. Effective management depends on a good understanding of HF's complex nature and determinants of its development, which involves an interplay between cardiac, neurohormonal, and hemodynamic factors, revealing the urgency of addressing heart failure as an urgent public health challenge. Worsening heart failure (WHF) is a critical component of the heart failure continuum and a state of acute deterioration with a requirement for management adjustments.

This event is not only an indication of the dynamic nature of heart failure but also an indicator of disease progression. An episode of WHF is both discernible and quantifiable by an increase in HF symptoms that is typically witnessed with an increased requirement for medical intervention involving a change in diuretic therapy. Prevalence of WHF is very high and its impact on prognosis is unparalleled, highlighting the need for integrative approaches towards early detection and treatment of such attacks, ideally before they necessitate hospitalization (Manca et al., 2025). Present definitions and management protocols of WHF are often divergent, particularly in outpatient settings, highlighting a research and clinical area that remains to be studied to enhance patient outcomes. The association of heart failure with comorbidities such as atrial fibrillation (AF) must also be kept in mind while establishing the scope of heart failure. AF can directly affect the prognosis in the context of patients with mildly reduced ejection fraction (HFmrEF). Research shows that AF appears in around 43% of HFmrEF patients, and its presence is linked with a significant risk for bad events, such as increased rates of all-cause mortality and hospital readmission (Schupp et al., 2024). These associations are crucial for designing comprehensive treatment programs, as the treatment for heart failure must consider its interconnections with other cardiovascular disorders. Rhythm and rate control strategies in the management of AF may prove crucial to maximizing long-term prognosis for this patient population, illustrating the interaction between heart failure and co-morbidities that add complexity to the disease state.

6.1. Types of Heart Failure

It is important to understand the different types of heart failure to facilitate effective intervention and management. Heart failure may be generally divided into two types: heart failure with preserved ejection fraction (HFpEF) and heart failure with reduced ejection fraction (HFrEF). HFpEF is characterized by the failure of the heart to fill with sufficient blood during diastole, typically due to diseases like hypertension or obesity. On the other hand, HFrEF is a condition where the pumping function of the heart is weakened, typically due to ischemic heart disease or cardiomyopathy etiology. Such designations provide varying amounts of information about the pathophysiologic processes involved and allow clinicians to formulate individualized treatment strategies. Recognizing the difference between these types is significant since they respond differently to therapies, and hence, can yield better patient outcomes and more effective utilization of healthcare resources (Siopi et al., 2024). A significant difference within the categories of heart failure is acute and chronic heart failure. Acute heart failure occurs abruptly and typically with acute, severe symptoms that may be life-threatening and require immediate medical treatment. They may either present with constrictive symptoms such as edema or breathlessness, necessitating urgent interventions like vasodilators or diuretics. Or, chronic heart failure develops insidiously over several years, with an stable symptom pattern that can unpredictably shift to deteriorate. This variation is essential not only for acute management but also for long-term care plans because patients with chronic heart failure may require constant observation and consequent adjustment of care to manage their condition effectively. Understanding these dynamics allows the adaptation of interventions by health workers as well as effective patient education and caregiver education (Alimadadi et al., 2020). Aside from the acute and chronic differences, heart failure is also classified based on its etiology, which includes ischemic heart disease, dilated cardiomyopathy, and hypertrophic cardiomyopathy, among others. Ischemic heart disease typically underlies HFrEF due to myocardial injury caused by reduced perfusion, most often caused by atherosclerosis. Dilated cardiomyopathy (DCM) and ischemic cardiomyopathy (ICM) are prevalent types that lead to heart failure with distinct pathophysiological mechanisms. Determining the underlying etiology is most crucial for management, since this will immediately dictate treatment and prognostic implications. For instance, treatments can include pharmacologic interventions, lifestyle modifications, and potentially more invasive procedures such as implantable devices. New testing techniques, including machine learning analysis of cardiac data, also have the potential to improve these classifications further and better help treat patients, which makes research in the area of cardiovascular health a priority (Alimadadi et al., 2020) (Figure 6.2).

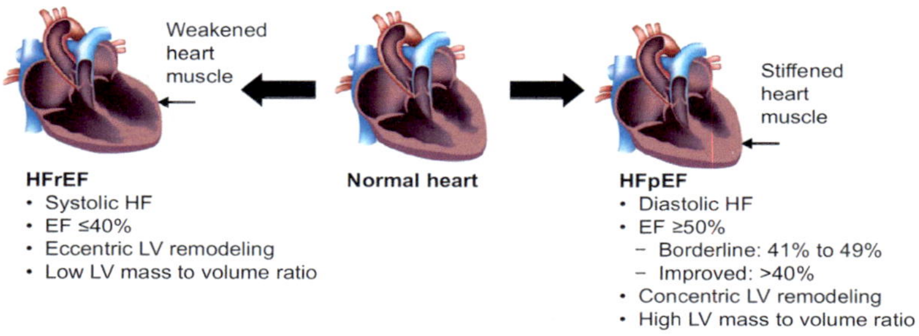

Figure 6.2. Heart failure with preserved ejection fraction (HFpEF) and heart failure with reduced ejection fraction (HFrEF).

Source: https://www.researchgate.net/publication/347488009/figure/fig1/AS:1024487977918465@1621268376661/Key-Differences-Between-HFpEF-and-HFrEF-1-10-HF-heart-failure-HFpEF-heart-failure.png.

6.1.1. Systolic Heart Failure

Systolic heart failure, which is the inability of the heart to eject blood during the contract phase, is a significant cause of patient morbidity and mortality. Systolic heart failure commonly manifests by way of left ventricular dysfunction and can be caused by a variety of etiologies, including coronary artery disease, systemic hypertension, and dilated cardiomyopathy. Since the left ventricles have decreased ejection fraction, the patients may be presented with fatigue, dyspnea, and edema. The impact of systolic heart failure is more than just clinical presentation, as it can lead to reduced exercise tolerance and lower quality of life. Consequently, early diagnosis and multimodal treatment measures are needed to maximize the patient's outcomes, as inappropriate or delayed therapy may potentially worsen the condition to a more severe heart failure status, leading to hospitalization and increased healthcare costs. Improvements in technology have enhanced patient care for systolic heart failure. Present developments involve implantable cardiac defibrillators and cardiac resynchronization therapy with significant enhancements in survival and quality of life. New telemonitoring algorithms are also being developed, which present the potential for earlier intervention and reduction of acute decompensation risk. These systems keep patient hemodynamics under surveillance through technologies like HeartLogic™, HeartInsight, and TriageHF that provide multiparametric scores based on variations in cardiac function even during asymptomatic phases. This prophylactic care through remote monitoring develops an integrated strategy between hospital therapy and territorial networks of cardiology for remaining within homogeneous diagnostic and therapeutic requirements. This model enables timely medication and lifestyle adjustment, which ultimately yields improved health outcomes for patients with systolic heart failure (Carriere et al., 2025). Another key aspect of systolic heart failure is its possibility of being associated with diseases such as preeclampsia, which manifests as systolic or diastolic dysfunction during pregnancy. These examples highlight the complexity of heart failure presentations and necessitate particular management methods taken within the scenario of the patient's physiological status. If heart failure results due to preeclampsia, treatment can include diet modification, diuretic therapy, and careful utilization of beta-blockers and vasodilators. Given the resulting complications for the condition, adopting a multidisciplinary approach by healthcare professionals for effective peripartum management is crucial. Close observation and teamwork between cardiologists, obstetricians, and anesthesiologists are crucial to reduce risks for maternal and neonatal morbidity and mortality during childbirth (Bandyopadhyay et al., 2024). Treating systolic heart failure among these high-risk groups emphasizes the need to identify various underlying causes of heart failure, which will allow individualized interventions that meet specific patient needs (Figure 6.3).

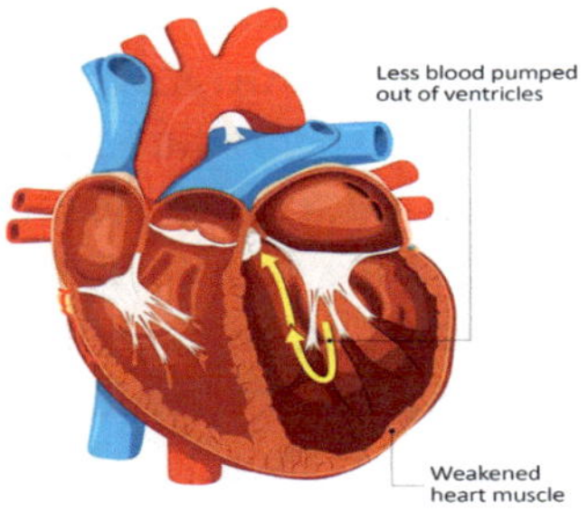

Figure 6.3. Systolic heart failure.

Source: https://drraghu.com/wp-content/uploads/2022/09/Systolic-heart-failure-img.jpg.

6.1.2. Diastolic Heart Failure

Increased prevalence of diastolic heart failure (HFpEF) is a significant public health problem, particularly as the aging population grows. With rigid ventricles, this complication is represented by failure of the heart to fill up in diastole. The complication primarily occurs with comorbid conditions including hypertension, coronary artery disease, and diabetes. As the term suggests, the prevalence of diastolic heart failure is increasing, which creates management and treatment challenges in healthcare systems. Also, an aging population exacerbates this condition since elderly patients tend to develop this form of heart failure more easily. Proper identification of the etiology and clinical presentation is important so that appropriate treatment modalities and preventive strategies can be devised. Thus, a focus on diastolic heart failure becomes an imperative to improve patient outcomes in this burgeoning population. Diastolic heart failure diagnosis relies on several clinical assessments and imaging techniques. An essential part of diagnosis is assessing the E/A ratio, which measures the flow pattern through the mitral valve. A 95.2% sensitivity indicates its effectiveness in detecting diastolic dysfunction. Concentrations of Blood for Brain Natriuretic Peptide (BNP) are also found to be a useful biomarker, with a sensitivity of 88.3% in making heart failure diagnoses. Such diagnostic tests not only confirm the condition but also distinguish it from other types of heart failure. Accurate diagnosis is essential given the complications implicated in diastolic heart failure and its tendency to overlap with various comorbid conditions. Improved diagnostic accuracy will translate into more tailored treatment approaches that, by extension, will help patients and reduce the burden on public health facilities. Diastolic heart failure must be treated multi-facetedly, including both pharmacological and non-pharmacological measures in an attempt to optimize patient outcomes. Dual treatment measures are more effective than monotherapy, affirming the value of integrated treatment plans. Diabetic individuals, for instance, are more likely to develop heart failure, suggesting tight blood sugar control is necessary in managing both diseases concurrently. Lifestyle modifications such as physical training and dietary adjustment were shown to enhance symptomatology and quality of life of patients with asymptomatic diastolic dysfunction. As practice progresses, preventive interventions and public health initiatives aimed at preventing the development of diastolic heart failure and addressing the increasing health problems that accompany it will be crucial. This anticipatory strategy is central to developing a healthier population and reducing the long-term impact of heart failure in general (Figure 6.4).

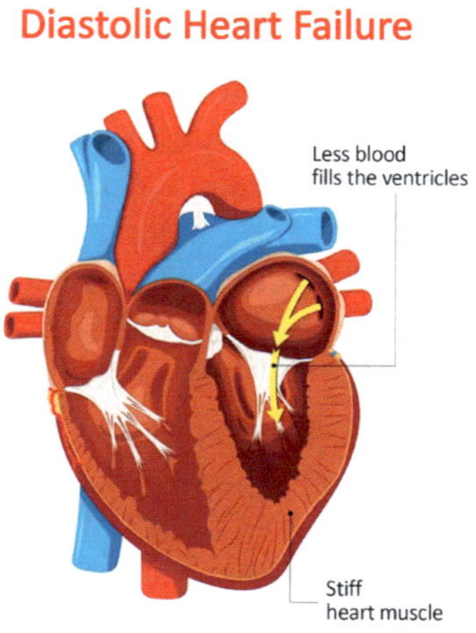

Figure 6.4. Diastolic heart failure.

Source: https://drraghu.com/wp-content/uploads/2022/09/Diastolic-heart-failure-img.jpg.

6.1.3. Right-Sided Versus Left-Sided Heart Failure

Right-sided and left-sided heart failure differ primarily in the chambers of the heart affected and their resultant physiological consequences. Left-sided heart failure, the more common form, occurs when the left ventricle becomes unable to pump oxygen-rich blood into the body efficiently. This dysfunction leads to the pooling of blood within the lungs, with associated pulmonary congestion, along with shortness of breath and tiredness. On the contrary, right-sided heart failure is typically caused by left-sided heart failure or lung disease, where the right ventricle is unable to pump blood to the lungs for oxygenation. Systemic venous congestion resulting from backward blood flow in right-sided heart failure may be manifested as edema of the extremities and a bloated abdomen. Understanding these variations is essential in the diagnosis, treatment, and management of heart failure so that patients receive individualized interventions based on their specific heart dysfunction. Right-sided versus left-sided heart failure symptoms exhibit the various impacts each situation has on the quality of life of a patient. Left-sided heart failure patients typically present with symptoms related to decreased cardiac output, including exertional dyspnea and orthopnea, that lead to significant impairment of physical activity and overall well-being. Right-sided heart failure is typically supported by signs of fluid retention, manifested in peripheral edema and jugular venous distension. These symptoms may be painful and distressing, altering lifestyles and impacting mental well-being. Furthermore, interaction between the two can further deteriorate patient conditions, with left-sided congestion leading to right-sided complications. Identification of these signs is essential to health practitioners because it informs appropriate diagnostic pathways and management strategies, offering a comprehensive approach towards the management of heart failure (Kirchhof et al., 2016). Management of right-sided and left-sided heart failure involves a variety of therapeutic measures, particular to the causative etiologies and clinical presentations of such individuals. Left-sided heart failure may be treated with the administration of diuretics to relieve congestion, angiotensin-converting enzyme (ACE) inhibitors to improve ventricular function, and beta-blockers to modulate heart rate and rhythm. Conversely, treatment for right-sided heart failure often involves consideration of the underlying etiology, such as pulmonary hypertension or left-sided failure. Medications aimed at both illnesses in certain situations may be necessary. Lifestyle modifications, including diet and exercise, are also central to successful treatment regimens. This complex strategy not only addresses the clinical aspects but also meets the psychosocial needs of the patients, ultimately enhancing their quality of life and outcomes for treating heart failure (Kirchhof et al., 2016) (Figure 6.5).

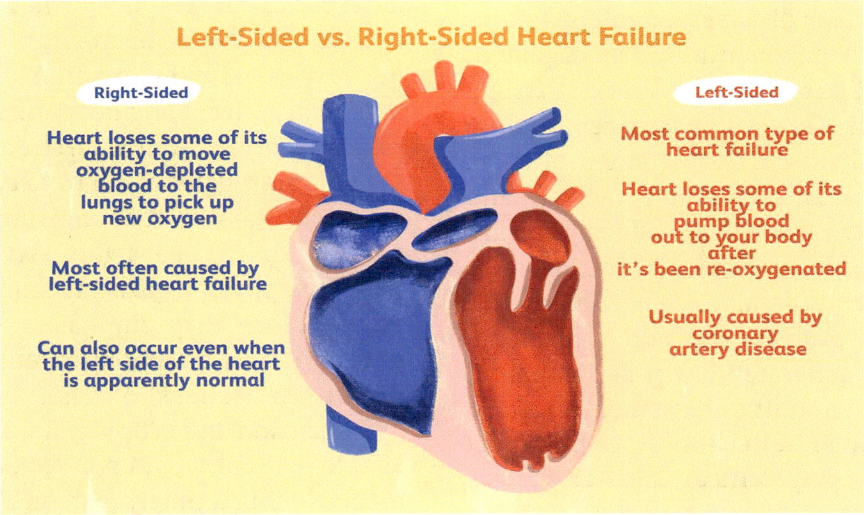

Figure 6.5. Left- versus right-sided heart failure.

Source: https://www.verywellhealth.com/thmb/7n_JqokNrTf9sph5vk4PmiYu-zw=/1500x0/filters:no_upscale():max_bytes(150000):strip_icc()/VWH-JessicaOlah-LeftvsRightSidedHeartFailure-Standard-33b2b8e3250644d9a5d61024b8144c18.jpeg.

6.2. Causes of Heart Failure

Identifying the etiology of heart failure involves the study of several pathophysiologic pathways responsible for cardiac dysfunction. Myocardial remodeling is one of the leading causative factors in heart failure as a complex process involving changes in the form and function of the heart. The process begins with pathophysiologic stimuli such as pressure overload with hypertension or volume overload due to valvular heart disease, which can start at compensatory alterations. But these adaptations inevitably bring about changes in cardiac myocyte structure and function, ultimately leading to disruption of the delicate balance of myocardial tissue. This remodeling, while adaptive at first, tends to progress towards a maladaptive situation, resulting in further progression of heart failure, highlighting the critical importance of early intervention and recognition of such transition phases and their impact on patient outcomes. Assessment of biomarkers is an essential part of the evaluation of the risk for cardiovascular disease, particularly in heart failure prognosis. N-terminal-pro-B-type natriuretic peptide (NT-proBNP) is a vital biomarker here as its elevated levels indicate increased cardiac stress and dysfunction. In a systematic population-based analysis from multiple prospective studies with over 95,000 patients with no prior cardiovascular history, the associations between NT-proBNP levels and various outcomes were determined. The results showed that patients in the top third of NT-proBNP levels had a significantly increased likelihood of developing heart failure, coronary heart disease, and stroke, an increase in risk ratio by 2.00 for these combined outcomes. This evidence favors the consideration of NT-proBNP measurement along with standard risk factors to enhance the prediction and prevention of heart failure and other cardiovascular diseases, enabling a more holistic strategy for patient care and management (Adam et al., 2016). Furthermore, various molecular processes of cardiac remodeling culminate directly in the development of heart failure. Myocyte loss, cardiac hypertrophy, and extracellular matrix homeostasis disruption are central processes driving this pathophysiologic process. Chronic inflammation, particularly in the setting of myocardial infarction, augments these changes to generate fibrosis and impaired cardiac function. In addition to structural effect, metabolic derangement and mitochondrial dysfunction also play critical roles as factors impeding the heart's ability to maintain adequate performance during stress. Greater insight into such molecular mechanisms is needed, as this opens up approaches to therapy that could bypass adverse remodelling and the subsequent onset of heart failure. Gene therapy advances provide new prospects for potential intervention centered on modifying central regulators of this remodelling process and hence greater optimism concerning the therapy of heart failure and restricting cardiac complications (Angelini et al., 2017) (Figure 6.6).

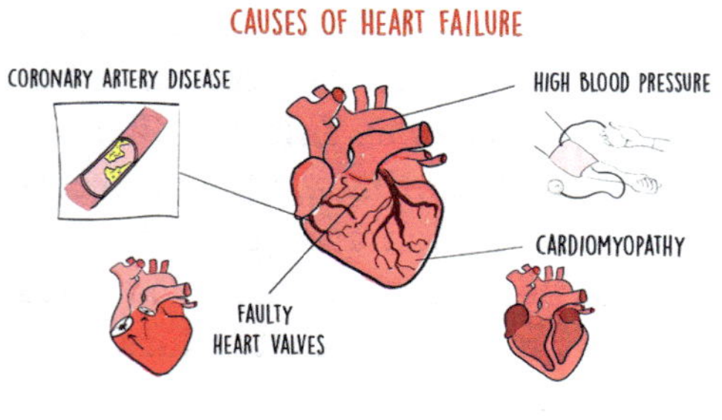

Figure 6.6. Causes of heart failure.

Source: https://i.ytimg.com/vi/zmq_qQ2tCoQ/maxresdefault.jpg.

6.2.1. Coronary Artery Disease (CAD)

CAD is an essential precursor to heart failure, with vascular health making an important contribution to cardiac function. CAD results from atherosclerotic plaque formation in coronary vessels and vessel narrowing to reduce blood delivery to the myocardium. Poor perfusion may lead to ischemic heart disease, which can result in myocardial infarction. Over time, as the heart struggles to adapt to oxygen demands, it adapts its structure and function, typically ending up in heart failure. Understanding the pathophysiological mechanisms of CAD is critical since they emphasize the importance of early detection and intervention treatments. Raised awareness of risk factors such as hypertension, hyperlipidemia, and diabetes can enable preventive intervention and therapeutic maneuvers in a timely fashion and thus prevent the process of progression to heart failure and improve outcomes in patients. The relationship between CAD and heart failure is greater than stepwise; it is multifactorial and complex. CAD patients often present with symptoms of heart failure due to the decreased efficiency of the heart due to ischemic events. During angina or myocardial infarction attacks, the myocardial cells get injured and may suffer loss of contractile function, decreasing the global cardiac function of the heart. Also, the ensuing structural remodeling of the heart muscle—existing in the form of hypertrophy and fibrosis—tends to enhance heart failure. The interaction between CAD and heart failure enhances healthcare system burden, bearing in mind that these comorbidities are normally to blame for poor clinical outcomes. It requires an integrated care process involving cardiovascular specialists and general practitioners in cross-professional planning and management. Recent evidence manifests that the efficient management of coronary artery disease is paramount to the prevention of the development of heart failure, as well as improving the prognosis for patients. New therapies, ranging from lifestyle changes to drug treatment, are significant in the management of CAD risk factors. Therapeutic regimens of statin treatment, antihypertensives, and antiplatelet drugs have been crucial in reducing cardiovascular events in CAD patients. Additional research also emphasizes the significance of multidisciplinary management that entails dietary changes, exercise, and psychological counseling in CAD patients. The combination of these treatments aims at optimizing cardiac health, reducing the onset of heart failure, and enhancing the quality of life in at-risk subjects. Lastly, the recognition of coronary artery disease as a prime element in heart failure pathogenesis calls for forward-looking strategies that target cardiovascular health, in essence, bridging gaps between prevention, cure, and chronic care (Cruz et al., 2024; Katic et al., 2024) (Figure 6.7).

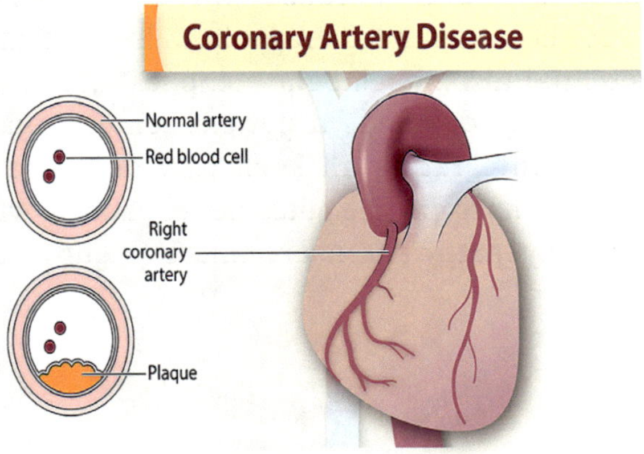

Figure 6.7. Coronary artery disease. (CAD)

Source: https://www.cdc.gov/heart-disease/media/images/coronary-artery-disease.jpg.

6.2.2. Hypertension

The link between hypertension and heart failure is established, with chronic high blood pressure significantly increasing the risk of cardiac dysfunction. Hypertension increases the workload of the heart by augmenting systemic vascular resistance, thereby speeding left ventricular hypertrophy. This adaptive thickening of the structure of the heart initially benefits the heart in accommodating increased demand but, with time, becomes maladaptive and contributes to cardiac dysfunction. As hypertrophy progresses, it might lead to HFpEF, a condition that is notoriously difficult to treat owing to its multifactorial pathophysiology. Furthermore, the frequency of hypertension in the population emphasizes the possible role that effective management of blood pressure can play in the prevention of heart failure development and emphasizes the importance of early detection and treatment strategies that can control hypertensive states. Management of hypertension is crucial in the prevention of heart failure development and in overall cardiovascular wellness. Current guidelines, such as those from the European Society of Cardiology (ESC) and European Society of Hypertension (ESH), position lifestyle modification and pharmacologic therapy as key components of hypertension management. Lifestyle modifications, including dietary modification, exercise regularly, and weight loss, significantly contribute to lowering blood pressure. These therapies, in combination with adequate antihypertensive medications, not only manage hypertension but also reduce the incidence of heart failure (Lees et al., 2020). Patient education is also critical in ensuring compliance. Recognition of the link between uncontrolled hypertension and heart failure can induce behavior change, with attendant better health outcomes. Although much has been achieved in managing hypertension, there remain challenges in achieving maximum control across various populations. Variations in access to medical treatment, differing responses to antihypertensive therapy, and lack of adherence to prescribed regimens are some of the factors accounting for the chronic issue of uncontrolled hypertension. Prioritization of individualized treatment approaches, including ongoing monitoring and adjustment of medications based on individual responsiveness, is vital in such cases. In addition, ongoing research into the pathophysiology that underlies the association between hypertension and heart failure can guide more effective interventions and therapeutic choices (Lees et al., 2020). Since the prevalence of heart failure is expanding globally, it is imperative to treat and understand hypertension to reduce its effects on public health and enhance quality of life in those with heart failure.

6.2.3. Cardiomyopathy

Cardiomyopathy is a notable condition that has a direct bearing on heart failure, with the progressive weakening of heart muscle function. Cardiomyopathy is categorized into many types, such as dilated, hypertrophic, and restrictive cardiomyopathy, each with distinct pathophysiological features but with the same result: the loss of the heart's ability to pump efficiently. The development of cardiomyopathy can be traced to an array of causative factors such as genetic susceptibilities, derangements in metabolism, and exposure to toxins. Notably, impairments frequently advance to heart failure when the heart can no longer maintain adequate circulation to overcome the demands of the body and therefore necessitates a better comprehension of the interrelationship between cardiomyopathy and heart failure in clinical practice.

The clinical manifestations of cardiomyopathy are not just decreased cardiac output, as they can make the patient susceptible to various complications, including arrhythmias. Atrial fibrillation (AF) is explicitly a frequent finding in patients with cardiomyopathy due to the structural and electrical remodeling of the cardiac muscle. AF not only aggravates the presentation of heart failure but also poses a risk for thromboembolic complications. There is evidence that diabetes, systemic arterial hypertension, and obesity are significant risk factors for both cardiomyopathy and AF onset. Moreover, anxiety disorders also interplay with these conditions, which indicates a potential mechanism by which anxiety can be an independent AF risk factor, enhancing the arrhythmogenic substrate caused by cardiomyopathy (Ceccacci et al., 2019). This intricate notion points to the importance of targeted intervention strategies to neutralize the risks. In the context of heart failure management, understanding the importance of low ejection fraction (EF) in cardiomyopathy is vital. Although lower EF (<50%) has been linked with an increased risk of stroke, data are quite confusing among clinical populations. Some studies indicate that extremely low EF may raise stroke risk, particularly in patients with additional vascular risk factors (Pullicino et al., 2013). Practitioners should thus closely assess the severity of EF in patients with cardiomyopathy because not only does it direct heart failure therapy, but also indicates potential thromboembolic complications. Such complexity demands a patient-centered care model, integrating all such risk factors and thereby improving the outcomes of patients with cardiomyopathy and heart failure (Figure 6.8).

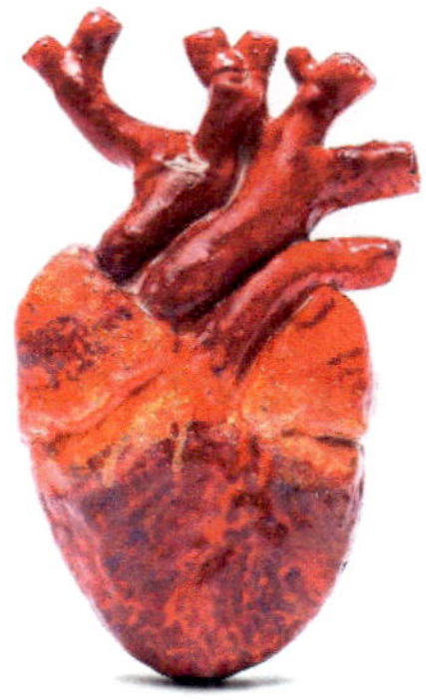

Figure 6.8. Cardiomyopathy.

Source: https://www.aopa.org/-/media/Images/AOPA-Main/Go-Fly/Medical/Health-Conditions/Heart-and-Circulatory-System/Cardiomopathy.jpg.

6.3. Symptoms of Heart Failure (HF)

HF is defined by a broad range of signs that may significantly influence the quality of life and overall health of a patient. Among the reported signs are dyspnea, fatigue, and edema. Dyspnea, or breathlessness, even in the absence of pulmonary disease, is familiar with exertion or when lying down and significantly compromises daily activities and mood. There is also the possibility of fatigue, which can be incapacitating and result from reduced cardiac output or fluid overload. Edema manifested as swelling in the abdomen, legs, and ankles is due to fluid retention, worsening the patient's physical status. It is crucial to identify these symptoms early since timely intervention will improve patient outcomes and reduce the morbidities of heart failure. With myocardial infarction (MI), this knowledge is crucial to identify the predictors of the signs of heart failure so that it can be managed accordingly. Recent studies have also found some indicators, such as rising dyspnea and a reduced left ventricular ejection fraction, to be predictive of higher rehospitalization risk for heart failure (Hwang et al., 2025). In one post-MI cohort, individuals with these symptoms were found to have a strong correlation with poorer outcomes and high levels of healthcare utilization. To identify high-risk patients who may require early intervention techniques or escalated therapy, their surveillance is essential for out-of-hospital follow-up. Such prevention can prevent the late stage of heart failure and enhance the overall care plan. Self-care activities and risk factor identification are also essential in understanding heart failure symptoms and their significance. Markers such as the ELAN-HF score are developed to predict the risk of readmission and death in patients with acute decompensated heart failure (ADHF) (Vinck et al., 2022). The score takes into account multiple clinical and laboratory parameters and gives a stratified picture of patient risk. Of specific note, those presenting with more severe symptoms, such as those in functional classes III and IV of the NYHA, are more likely to experience adverse outcomes, such as mortality and readmission (Vinck et al., 2022). Education and self-management of the patient may enable the patient to manage their symptoms better, take appropriate lifestyle changes, and adhere to treatment protocols, thereby ensuring more positive health outcomes for heart failure patients (Figure 6.9).

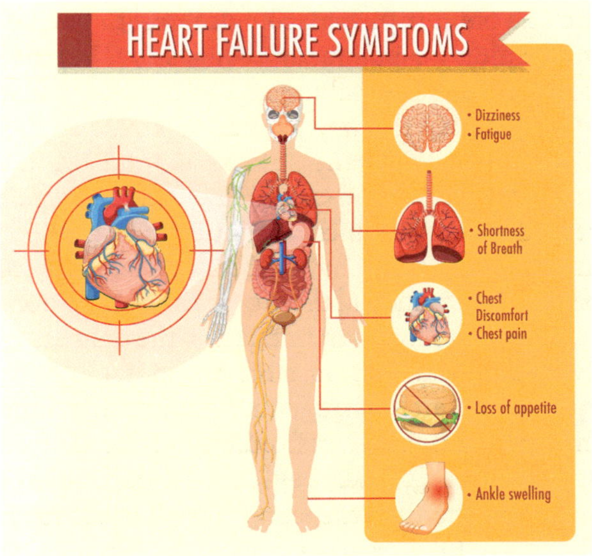

Figure 6.9. Symptoms of heart failure (HF).

Source: https://drraghu.com/wp-content/uploads/2022/10/symptom-heart-faliure-1.jpg.

6.3.1. Shortness of Breath

Shortness of breath, or dyspnea, is quite possibly the most disabling symptom of heart failure. The ailment is acquired due to inefficient pumping of the heart, leading to inadequate circulation of blood, lack of oxygen, and lung congestion with fluid. Therefore, patients typically struggle to breathe, particularly while engaging in exercises or when they lie down, a state known as orthopnea. This only worsens as the disease advances, significantly affecting the patient's quality of life. Clarifying the mechanisms behind dyspnea during heart failure is valuable for the creation of effective interventions capable of alleviating this distressing symptom and enhancing patient well-being, since untreated dyspnea has been shown to lead to increased anxiety and decline in overall health status, contributing to the severity of these patients. Proper management of breathlessness is central in the case of heart failure treatment. Add-on application of comprehensive palliative care interventions can be beneficial. These interventions will often include not just pharmacological treatment, i.e., medication for pulmonary congestion, but also non-pharmacological management in the guise of respiratory therapy as well as stress coping mechanisms. Current studies emphasize the imperative of person-centered treatment in this regard, through which practitioners can tailor interventions to the individualized needs of each patient. Integration of these types of interventions is required to assist in mitigating the distress of dyspnea, making it possible for individuals to more completely engage in daily activities and thereby increase overall quality of life as well as sustain a greater degree of independence while controlling the condition (Shevcova et al., 2024). New treatment candidates are being studied to further manage shortness of breath in individuals with heart failure. Empagliflozin represents a significant advancement in drug development, demonstrating a potential to reduce hospitalizations due to heart failure and improve outcomes for individuals with preserved and reduced ejection fractions. Data from trials, including the EMPEROR-Preserved trial, indicate that this medication not only controls the underlying causes of heart failure but also directly addresses symptoms such as dyspnea. Thus it is a valuable addition to treatment regimens (Zannad et al., 2023). By targeting both symptom reduction and improved cardiac function, novel therapies like empagliflozin represent a significant advance in worldwide heart failure treatment, eventually transforming the patient experience and curing the pervasive issue of shortness of breath (Figure 6.10).

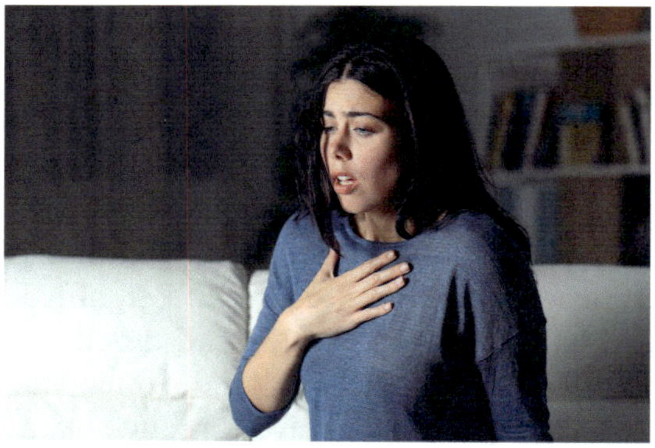

Figure 6.10. Shortness of breath.

Source: https://sa1s3optim.patientpop.com/assets/images/provider/photos/2312977.jpeg.

6.3.2. Fatigue and Weakness

The combination of weakness and fatigue is the basis of heart failure's clinical presentation, significantly impacting patients' quality of life and daily activities. Heart failure patients have traditionally described fatigue as an overwhelming feeling of exhaustion that is disproportionate to their level of activity. The symptom is understandable by the decreased ability of the heart to maintain blood flow, causing inadequate delivery of oxygen to tissues. As the heart struggles to provide sufficient circulation, the energy requirements of the body overwhelm its capacity to deliver, leading to increasing fatigue. Additionally, the psychological effects of chronic illness can exacerbate the sense of fatigue, creating a self-reinforcing cycle that further limits activity and further compounds patients' status. Weakness, which can also occur with fatigue, further confounds the clinical syndrome of heart failure. Patients frequently report severe pain in muscles, which can make them susceptible to a combination of disuse atrophy due to reduced physical activity and metabolic derangement secondary to heart failure per se. In diseases such as Becker muscular dystrophy (BMD), where cardiac involvement is not uncommon, symptoms such as weakness and generalized muscular weakness can become predominant, as in the case of a recent study on a patient with BMD who presented very severe symptoms before treatment (Gishto et al., 2024). Such findings highlight the need for detailed assessments considering physical as well as neuromuscular causes of weakness among heart failure patients. Interplay of weakness, fatigue, and heart failure necessitates a multidisciplinary management and treatment strategy. Interventions can be necessary for patients who not only tackle the root cardiac dysfunction but also its accompanying symptoms that prevent recovery. Strategies used in the clinic can include guideline-directed medical therapy (GDMT), exercise rehabilitation, and counseling to gain physical as well as emotional strength. Through comprehension of the multifaceted nature of diseases like Heyde's syndrome, in which weakness and fatigue are merely manifestations of more pervasive systemic problems, medical practitioners can apply entireistic treatment protocols to drive maximum patient results (Abouzid et al., 2024). This is essential in improving the quality of life of patients navigating the multidimensionality of heart failure (Figure 6.11).

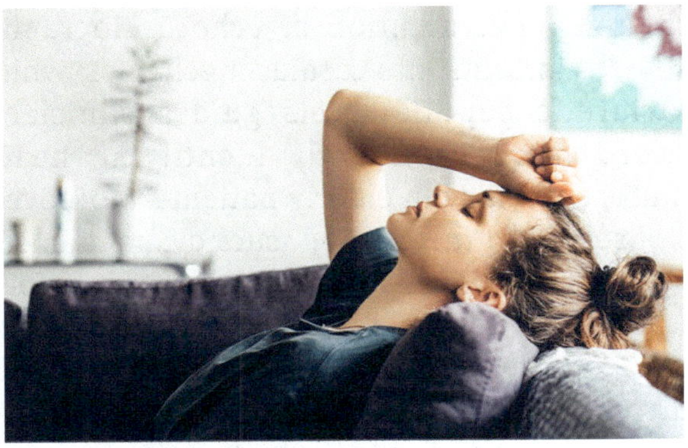

Figure 6.11. Fatigue.

Source: https://emi.parkview.com/media/Image/Dashboard_835_fatigue_6_23.jpg.

6.3.3. Swelling in the Legs and Ankles

With congestive heart failure, the swelling in the ankles and legs, also known medically as peripheral edema, is a key clinical indicator of the development of the disease. Peripheral edema results from the decreased ability of the heart to circulate blood, with the effect of fluid accumulation in peripheral tissues. When the heart is no longer able to circulate blood well, increased pressure in the blood vessels forces fluid into interstitial spaces and causes swelling. Severe as this condition is, the fact that approximately 5 million Americans are afflicted with congestive heart failure attests to the pressing need for more research to discover effective remedies that will alleviate symptoms and enhance patients' outcomes (Fackelmann, 1998). Furthermore, the presence of edema of the lower extremities is not only a reflection of the severity of heart failure but also a significant part of patient assessment. Clinicians often measure the degree of swelling as a means of quantifying the effectiveness of treatment programs and adjusting therapy accordingly. The reduction in the status of edema can be linked directly with drug therapy, i.e., diuretics that reduce excess fluid by enhancing renal excretion. In addition, lifestyle modification, such as sodium restriction through diet and exercise, can help prevent swelling by improving cardiovascular health and enhancing venous return. This interplay between clinical management and evaluation points out that the effective management of ankle and leg edema enhances the quality of life among heart failure patients (Blumgart et al., 1928). Notably, while peripheral edema is a common symptom of advanced heart failure, it also points to underlying health status demanding careful assessment. For instance, rheumatic heart disease patients may have similar edema despite the apparent lack of circulatory failure. Health workers' awareness of edema's multifactorial etiology will enable them to differentiate between conditions that mask, and not solely result from, cardiac insufficiency. This is a more nuanced approach that will allow clinicians to provide targeted and effective intervention for reducing morbidity rates due to heart failure. In this context of intricacies, further research into leg and ankle swelling pathophysiology is promising new therapeutic avenues, paving the way towards more effective patient management for heart failure therapy (Fackelmann, 1998) (Figure 6.12).

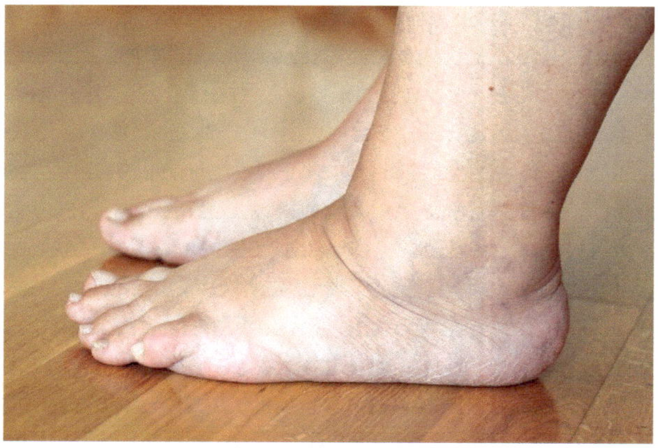

Figure 6.12. Leg swelling.

Source: https://coastalvascular.net/wp-content/uploads/2024/11/iStock-1406909750.jpg.

6.4. Diagnosis of Heart Failure (HF)

Diagnosis of HF is a complex process that frequently poses difficulty owing to its heterogeneity and the diversity of the underlying disorders that may cause its development. Clinical assessments most often start with a complete patient history and physical examination, with attention to such symptoms as dyspnea, fatigue, and edema. But these symptoms by themselves are not pathognomonic for HF, and further diagnostic tests are needed. Advanced imaging techniques, particularly echocardiography, play a crucial role in the assessment of cardiac structure and function to enable the detection of structural and functional abnormalities by clinicians. Recent studies demonstrate that a high percentage of hemodialysis patients, for example, have HF diagnostic criteria according to both structural and functional measurements, underlining the importance of comprehensive evaluations in multispectrum patient groups (Kim et al., 2024). Natriuretic peptides, especially BNP and N-terminal pro-B-type natriuretic peptide (NT-proBNP), are also central components of the heart failure diagnostic algorithm. These biomarkers are released secondary to myocardial wall tension and volume overload, and thus their measurement is a valuable adjunct to clinical experience. In elderly patients, the diagnostic utility of natriuretic peptides is further augmented by the common co-occurrence of other conditions, such as COPD and renal insufficiency. Research has established specific NT-proBNP thresholds that correspond to a positive predictive value for the diagnosis of acute heart failure, particularly in elderly patients and those with known comorbid conditions (Berthelot et al., 2024). These differences in interpreting NT-proBNP levels are essential in an effort to improve diagnostic specificity within this at-risk group further. Overall, heart failure diagnosis relies significantly on the integration of clinical assessments, imaging studies, and biomarker screening. The addition of echocardiography provides insights into cardiac mechanics, while natriuretic peptide levels guides clinicians toward more confidently identifying heart failure, especially in elderly patients. Moreover, as observed in the case of acute dyspnea onset in patients with end-stage renal disease, proper diagnosis is essential in the management of heart failure and the optimization of patient outcomes (Figure 6.13). Lastly, enhancing our understanding of diagnostic tools and the criteria continues to be essential in the management of the increasing incidence of heart failure and improved prognostic evaluation (Berthelot et al., 2024; Kim et al., 2024).

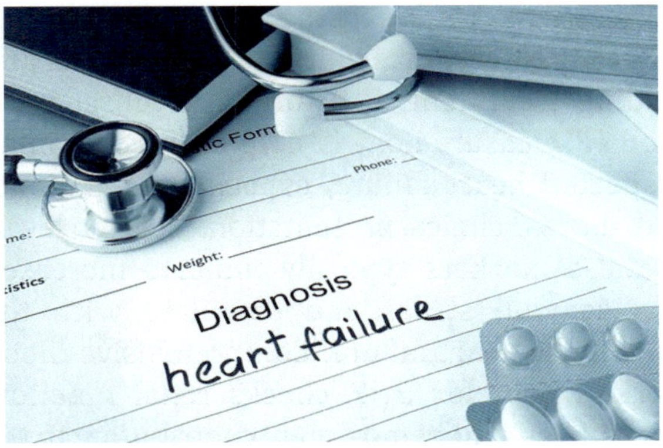

Figure 6.13. Diagnosis of heart failure (HF).

Source: https://web-ih-sc-prd-hdl-wus2.azurewebsites.net/_next/image?url=%2Fsc10media%2Fimages%2Fintermountain-health%2Fblogs%2Fblog%2Fposts%2F2017%2F02%2Fheart-failure-diagnosis.ashx%3Fh%3D461%26iar%3D0%26w%3D700%26hash%3D0B4D5EDD33D532E90591F2D24D5B58A3&w=1920&q=75.

6.4.1. Medical History and Physical Examination

Thorough medical history and thorough physical examination are the foundation of the appropriate diagnosis of HF. During medical history, the clinician collects information on symptoms such as dyspnea, weakness, and peripheral edema, which are symptomatic of HFs presence and severity. Evaluation of the patient's risk factors, including ischemic heart disease, hypertension, or diabetes, enables clinicians to determine the cause of heart failure.

Moreover, classification systems like the New York Heart Association (NYHA) functional classification are beneficial in the provision of information about the limitation and prognosis of the patient. For instance, a patient with NYHA Class III would have extreme limitations in activity, which would determine the treatment option. Improved diagnostic accuracy relies heavily on the initial collection of this information; thus, it is a crucial step in effectively managing heart failure (Kwast et al., 2025). Physical examination is also essential in diagnosing and managing heart failure. Providers usually take blood pressure and heart rate to determine hemodynamic stability. Jugular venous distension, pulmonary crackles, or peripheral edema is clinical proof of fluid overload, one of the common complications of heart failure. Additionally, auscultation of heart sounds may identify gallops or murmurs that are evidence of left ventricular failure. On assessing such physical signs, physicians can and locate compensatory mechanisms and the severity of cardiac impairment.

Physical examination becomes essential not only for diagnosis but also to monitor the course of heart failure over time. Research indicates that patients with chronic heart failure present with subtle signs and symptoms that are easily overlooked, thereby highlighting the importance of careful examination in clinical practice (Duca et al., 2024). In addition, laboratory studies and imaging studies add to the information obtained from the physical examination and history. Determination of biomarkers such as BNP levels can make the diagnosis of heart failure, with echocardiography giving insight into cardiac function and structure. These investigations together enable adequate staging of heart failure, determining appropriate treatment for a specific patient. For instance, an echocardiogram can ascertain EF, which informs decisions on pharmacologic treatment and possible referral for advanced therapy. Integrating history, exam, and diagnostic results eventually optimizes the clinician's ability to arrive at an accurate diagnosis and formulate a general management plan for heart failure patients, eventually minimizing patient outcomes and quality of life (Duca et al., 2024; Kwast et al., 2025) (Figure 6.14).

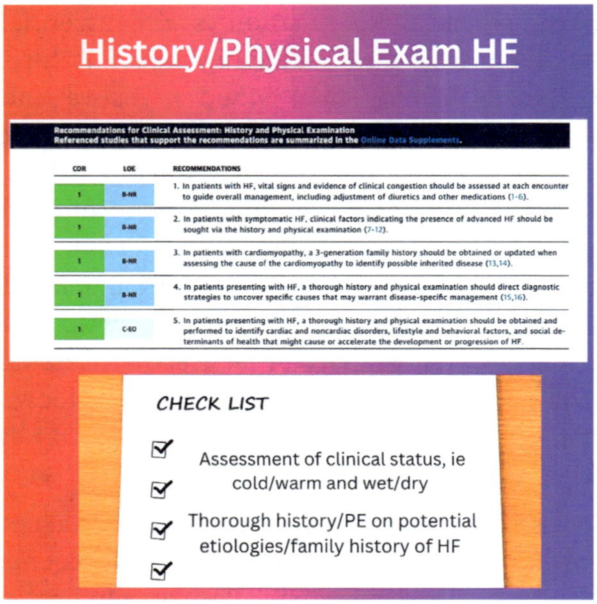

Figure 6.14. Medical history and physical examination of heart failure (HF).

Source: https://encrypted-tbn0.gstatic.com/images?q=tbn:ANd9GcQhoTE0eWd5L8hYdQOtRtja2CG0SdQXcDcrg&s.

6.4.2. Diagnostic Tests (e.g., Echocardiogram, Blood Tests)

Diagnostic tests are crucial in the assessment and management of heart failure. Among some of the most significant tests are the echocardiogram, an imaging test that is not invasive and provides valuable information on cardiac structure and function. By this test, doctors can measure left ventricular ejection fraction (LVEF), which is a very critical parameter for diagnosing HFrEF. Moreover, echocardiography aids in identifying structural abnormalities such as valvular disease or myocardial hypertrophy that are causal to heart failure. The accuracy of echocardiograms enhances the clinicians ability to classify heart failure and initiate interventions promptly accurately. Therefore, echocardiography remains a cornerstone diagnostic modality for the management of heart failure, and its findings have a direct correlation with patient outcome and prognosis (Atherton et al., 2018). Blood work is also critical in the diagnostic workup for heart failure, providing prognostic data and guiding treatment. BNP or its precursor NT-proBNP measurement is helpful in confirming suspected heart failure, especially in patients with unclear clinical presentation. Elevated levels of these markers typically indicate increased cardiac wall stress and correlate with the severity of heart failure. Comprehensive blood work, except for BNP, checks renal function, electrolytes, and hemoglobin, contributing to the extensive patient assessment. The combination of biomarker analysis with non-invasive imaging, therefore, provides a robust diagnostic profile that facilitates proper diagnosis as well as proper heart failure management (Kirchhof et al., 2016). Invasive diagnostic tests such as coronary angiography may also be justified in carefully chosen cases where heart failure is suspected to be due to an ischemic cause. In refractory or high-risk feature-positive patients for coronary artery disease, invasive assessment may yield invaluable data on whether revascularization or additional interventions are required. Imaging modalities such as CT coronary angiography provide additional non-invasive imaging modalities to distinguish ischemic and non-ischemic etiologies for heart failure. Particular diagnostic modalities need to be chosen to tailor management strategies to individual patient profiles, enhancing the overall efficacy of treatment and optimizing outcomes. Lastly, an integrative diagnostic testing strategy is part of the holistic evaluation of heart failure patients (Atherton et al., 2018).

6.4.3. Importance of Early Detection

The importance of the early detection of HF cannot be overstated, especially considering the high mortality and morbidity of the condition. Early proper diagnosis is critical for enabling early interventions that can successfully salvage patient outcomes and restrict healthcare costs. Natriuretic peptides (NPs), particularly N-terminal pro-B-type NP, are now crucial biomarkers for the early diagnosis and therapy of HF according to guidelines prepared by the Eurasian Society of HF and Turkish Association of Family Medicine. These guidelines endorse the assessment of NP level for screening at risk or diagnosis in symptomatic individuals in primary care. By applying NP testing in routine clinical practice, providers can make timely referrals for patients to receive necessary treatment interventions in a timely fashion, which ultimately enhances health-related quality of life in HF patients (Çelik et al., 2025). Aside from the diagnosis of HF, early detection serves to monitor disease progression and evaluate response to therapy. NP level/outcome correlation is an indicator of the necessity to implement biomarker testing during routine management of HF patients. Elevated values of BNP or N-terminus-proBNP are an indicator of the need for early clinical intervention, allowing for early revision of management strategies that can prevent adverse outcomes. Active application of biomarkers not only allows for more personalized treatment but also maximizes treatment strategies, which have the potential to reduce hospitalization and associated healthcare costs. Therefore, early diagnosis provided by early detection methods serves both clinical functions, maximizing individual patient care as well as augmenting broader benefits for public health (Kayani et al., 2024). Moreover, the evolving environment of HF treatment emphasizes incorporating new biomarkers with traditional methods to enhance early detection methodologies. New biomarkers like galectin-3 and soluble suppression of tumorigenicity 2 are being investigated for their potential in conferring enhanced sensitivity and specificity in diagnosing and treating HF. These advances emphasize the ongoing need for research and adaptation in clinical practice so that doctors and medical providers may effectively deal with the nuances of the disease. Through comprehensive evaluations and applications of both established and emerging biomarkers, clinicians can gain a complete understanding of the person-specific manifestation of HF in any given patient. Early identification thus puts emphasis on the capacity of healthcare systems to address the rising prevalence of heart failure and ensure that patients receive personalized care in order to optimize results and improve quality of life (Kayani et al., 2024; Çelik et al., 2025) (Figure 6.15).

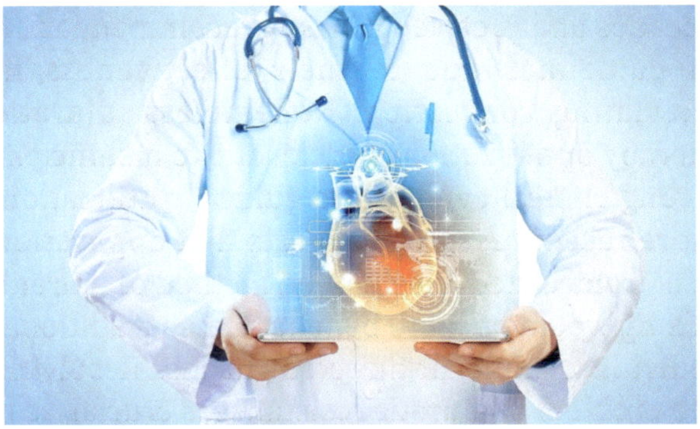

Figure 6.15. Importance of early detection of heart disease.

Source: https://www.biospectrumasia.com/uploads/articles/ai_in_healthcare-14585.jpg.

6.5. Treatment Options

Effective treatment of heart failure requires a thorough understanding of the various available therapies, particularly HFpEF. As an entity of disease, HFpEF represents a significant percentage of the population with severe heart failure, and its prevalence dramatically increases in elderly individuals and patients with cardio-metabolic comorbid conditions. Although in the past, few therapeutic choices for HFpEF existed, recent randomized controlled trials have opened new pharmacological avenues to achieve improved patient outcomes. The complexity of HFpEF, with its multifaceted clinical phenotype and evolving diagnostic criteria, emphasizes the necessity for evidence-based management approaches to address the specific needs of each patient. A thorough analysis of the latest clinical data and guideline publications is essential to guide clinicians regarding the best treatment approaches to manage HFpEF (Peikert et al., 2024). Among the medications for the treatment of heart failure, diuretics, particularly loop diuretics, play a key role in the alleviation of symptoms of fluid congestion. Congestion is one of the hallmarks of decompensated heart failure and frequently leads to hospitalization. Loop diuretics have been the pillars of treatment for decades and received a class I recommendation in guidelines due to their effectiveness in alleviating congestion. Nonetheless, diuretic therapy optimization is tricky due to insufficient strong clinical evidence to guide its utilization. More recent research suggests that application of a protocolized and stepped method of diuretic dosing would be more beneficial than traditional individual clinician-directed means. Resolving the problem of diuretic resistance is crucial, as it is linked with unfavorable clinical prognosis and the necessity of seeking additional treatments and their clinical effectiveness (Wu et al., 2024). The introduction of novel treatment modalities in the treatment of heart failure is followed by research aimed at overcoming inherent drawbacks, such as diuretic resistance and the heterogeneity of pathophysiologic mechanisms in heart failure. Emerging drug therapy strategies are continuing, expanding the HFpEF therapeutic armamentarium and optimizing symptom control. Lifestyle modification, including diet and exercise, is increasingly becoming accepted as an essential component of a worldwide treatment plan. Combining non-pharmacological intervention with drug therapy enables clinicians to optimize patient quality of life and improve clinical outcomes. As our understanding of heart failure evolves, it remains incumbent on us to stay abreast of the latest research and clinical practice guidelines to deliver the most optimal, tailored therapy regimens to patients with this complex disease (Peikert et al., 2024; Wu et al., 2024) (Figure 6.16).

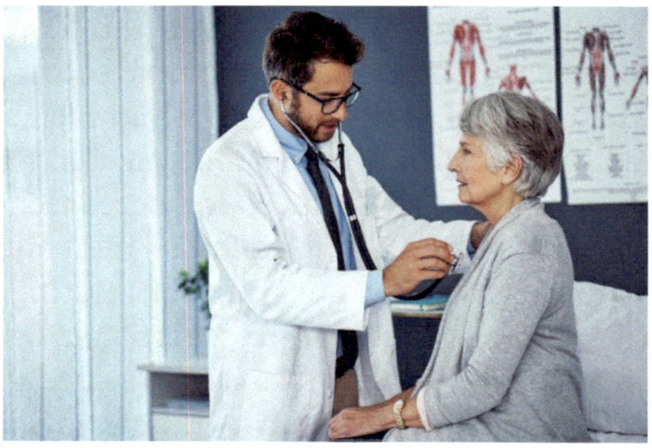

Figure 6.16. Expanding treatment options for heart failure through clinical trials.

Source: https://www.mainlinehealth.org/-/media/images/blog/2024/05/heart-failure-clinical-trials.jpg?h=836&w=1254&la=en&hash=111220E42843286BBC03DC452627BC2B.

6.5.1. Lifestyle Changes

Heart failure, a multifactorial condition afflicted by numerous people worldwide, demands radical lifestyle alteration to manage symptoms and prevent disease development. One of the initial steps towards management success is adherence to a heart-healthy diet based on fruit, vegetables, whole grains, lean protein, and healthy fat intake, along with reduced sodium intake. Such a dietary approach lowers blood pressure, stabilizes weight, and reduces fluid buildup. Further, there is evidence that suggests that by educating patients about sustainable eating based on their cultural food diets, healthcare providers can achieve better compliance with such modifications (N/A, 2020). Implementing such modifications in diet not only may enhance the quality of life of those patients with heart failure but may also contribute to reduced overall healthcare costs associated with hospitalization and treatment of severe complications. In addition to nutritional supplementation, exercise is crucial to the management of heart failure. Exercise enhances cardiovascular function, reduces fatigue, and enhances fitness, which is critical for maintaining independence, particularly in the elderly. Structured exercise, such as walking, swimming, or cycling, can be tailored to one's capability in a way that avoids exacerbating symptoms. Moreover, evidence suggests that integrating motivational interviewing techniques can encourage patients to overcome exercise obstacles by tapping into their intrinsic motivation (N/A, 2020). These kinds of interactions enable healthcare professionals to address patients' concerns, improve self-management of their health, and create tangible plans that emphasize physical activity. Thus, incorporating regular exercise as part of an overall lifestyle change strategy has the potential to significantly improve the health outcome of patients with heart failure. Lastly, the psychological aspect of the management of heart failure is often overlooked but no less crucial. Most patients suffer from concomitant anxiety and depression, which makes the enforcement of ordered lifestyle adjustments challenging. Psychosocial care, like counseling or support groups, provides a life-altering input by enabling the patient to overcome the emotional issues while establishing a support system of encouragement. By addressing such psychosocial elements, health workers facilitate the patients in establishing supportive relationships that help patients adopt lifestyle changes. In addition, the engagement of community stakeholders in the establishment of resource networks guarantees a support system within access, thus enhancing patients' abilities to achieve sustainable changes (N/A, 2020). Appreciation of this interaction between lifestyle and mental health is an important and essential part in the holistic management of heart failure and in the final outcome and quality of life.

6.5.2. Medications

HF treatment includes a heterogeneous approach that is heavily reliant on the effective use of drugs. Some pillar treatments include beta-blockers, angiotensin-converting enzyme inhibitors (ACEi), and mineralocorticoid receptor antagonists (MRA), which contribute to improving hemodynamics, reducing morbidity, and decreasing mortality. These medications are determined by clinical algorithms as well as evidence-based recommendations. But most importantly, underutilization of these therapies is an essential challenge because medication adherence barriers typically stem from a fear of side effects. Patient unwillingness to adhere to their prescribed therapy can also be further deterred by limited dialogue between patients and healthcare professionals, emphasizing the imperative for improved dialogue and education on these invaluable drugs (Mangal et al., 2024). Thus, effective bridging of these communication gaps is crucial in enhancing adherence and optimizing outcomes in treatment for patients with heart failure. Determinants of patient compliance in the consumption of medication regimens in heart failure are multifarious, and the weight of co-morbid diseases, especially chronic kidney disease (CKD), is of particular concern. CKD complicates the medication regimen in nature, so it tends to create increased susceptibility to side effects such as renal impairment or hyperkalemia. Of note, historic clinical trials have excluded patients with advanced CKD, and hence the extensibility of results to this group has been compromised. Clinicians are thus faced with significant challenges in prescribing guideline-concordant medical therapies because they must tread a thin line between maximizing therapeutic benefits and minimizing potential harm due to polypharmacy (Tumelty et al., 2024). This intricacy warrants an individualized strategy to drug management, taking into account the patient's personal health picture and specific needs of heart failure patients with concurrent CKD. Navigating medication complexities in heart failure patients requires adherence to a stepwise approach to best deal with and evaluate drug-related problems. Physicians must devise methods to elicit and address side effects from medications, possibly through intensive analysis of the medication regimen for all patients and engaging in discussions about their grievances. This can involve the application of technology and processes that streamline documentation and communication of side effects, ultimately allowing for timely adjustments to medication regimens. Once side effects are identified and attributed to specific drugs, measures like dose reduction or drug substitution can lead to a more optimized treatment plan. Part of the pursuit of improved patient outcomes is that physicians must establish an environment conducive to open discussion and shared decision-making between providers and patients (Mangal et al., 2024). By embracing these principles, overall management of medicine in heart failure can be significantly enhanced (Figure 6.17).

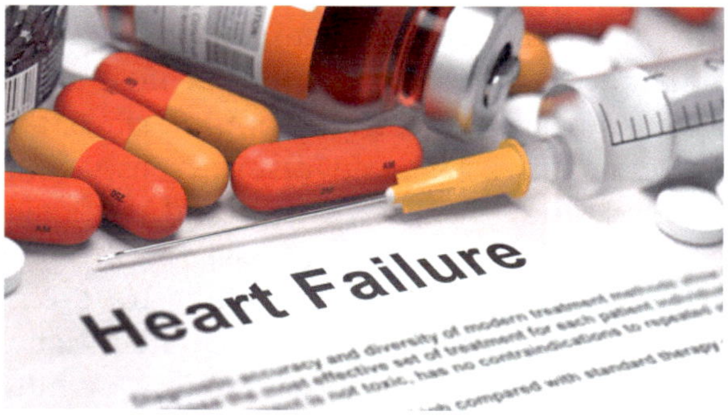

Figure 6.17. Medications.

Source: https://www.worldwide.com/wp-content/uploads/2017/03/Whats-Next-in-Heart-Failure-Therapy.jpg.

6.5.3. Surgical Interventions

Surgical procedures play a key role in the treatment of heart failure, particularly in patients where conventional medical therapies fall short. One of the most common procedures is cardiac resynchronization therapy (CRT), which involves the implantation of a device that synchronizes the ventricles' contraction. This therapy is particularly beneficial in patients with heart failure with reduced ejection fraction, as it can improve heart function and, in the long term, enhance clinical outcomes. Additionally, surgical treatments such as mitral valve repair or replacement directly treat valvular deficiencies that produce heart failure symptoms. Surgical treatments not only remove symptoms but also aim to enhance quality of life and promote survival by directly addressing underlying cardiovascular conditions that contribute to the advancement of heart failure. The introduction of less invasive surgical techniques has further augmented heart failure patient treatment. Procedures such as transcatheter aortic valve replacement (TAVR) are groundbreaking for those patients who are high-risk for undergoing traditional surgical methods. TAVR has been incredibly beneficial in treating aortic stenosis of the valve, an illness that is highly related to heart failure. New surgical strategies reduce recovery time and the general surgical burden on patients, making them more comfortable for frail patients or those with numerous comorbidities. Significantly, with a growing population of the elderly and higher rates of heart failure, such less-invasive options are bound to become a standard component of global heart failure management, demonstrating how surgery can maintain congruence with evolving clinical practice in a manner that benefits patients. Comorbid conditions secondary to heart failure have also been treated with bariatric surgery, particularly where obesity is involved as a component in the patient's condition. Bariatric surgical weight loss treatments have been found to improve cardiac function, reduce the weight of symptoms, and, in some studies, enhance survival rates in patients with heart failure. The overlap between heart failure and obesity highlights the need for individualized planning for treatment, considering the specificity of each patient. Lifestyle change and pharmacologic interventions are also required to augment surgical care to optimize patient outcomes. The increasing use of surgical treatments for heart failure illustrates the interplay between innovation in therapy and individualized care, highlighted by the need to modify interventions to treat both primary cardiac disease and associated health conditions, as illustrated in recent evidence on comorbid obesity and heart failure management (Ibrahim et al., 2024) (Figure 6.18).

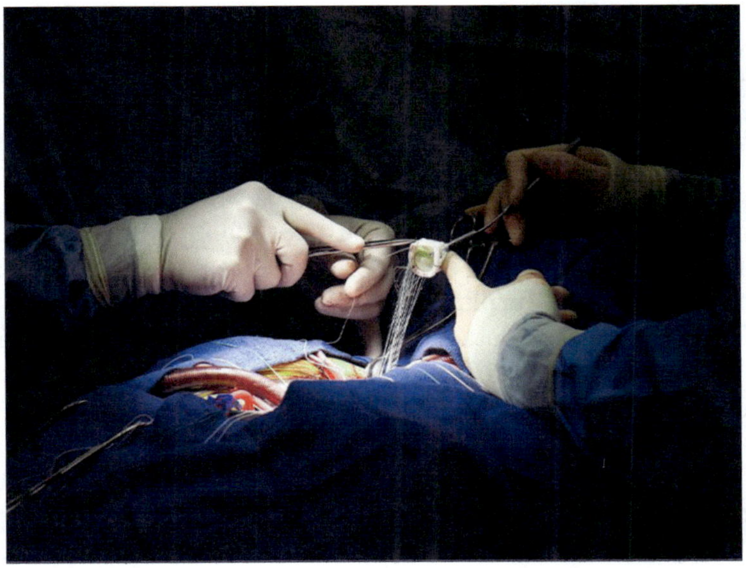

Figure 6.18. Heart Surgery.

Source: https://media.post.rvohealth.io/wp-content/uploads/sites/3/2024/03/Heart-Surgery-Aortic-Valve-Replacemen-thumbnail.jpg.

SUMMARY

The overview of a chapter on heart failure encapsulates the key takeaways from the analysis of its complexities. Heart failure remains a complicated syndrome that requires a comprehensive approach to management that goes beyond the acute care situation. The high-risk period after an acute cardiac event is particularly salient, as it is one of heightened vulnerability for patients. As highlighted in recent literature, optimizing treatment early at this juncture is critical to improving long-term outcomes, avoiding readmissions, and providing quality of life enhancement for patients. In managing this vulnerable period through an organized process, improved care can result and ultimately mitigate mortality risks associated with heart failure (Magaña Serrano et al., 2024). This highlights the necessity of ongoing research and agreement on therapeutic guidelines as per individual patient needs. The interplay among various parts of the heart, particularly when treating right heart failure (RHF), is another important aspect of heart failure management. With interventions like left ventricular assist device (LVAD) implantation, the risk of progression to RHF can have a significant impact on patient outcomes. Precise prediction and control of RHF are essential because they could complicate the post-surgical recovery and adaptation process. Clinical assessment should incorporate both hemodynamic and organ function assessments to predict any problems that could arise in the right ventricle, particularly in patients undergoing LVAD therapy. Continuing observation and a personalized plan can optimize the treatment of heart failure patients, aligning the treatment regimens with the individual situation to improve the patient's postoperative recovery and in the long run (Adamopoulos et al., 2024). Overall, the recapitulation of a discussion of heart failure highlights the importance of a holistic, patient-centered approach to treatment. This not only entails the care of acute courses and short-term sequelae but also emphasizes the significance of long-term follow-up and educating patients about lifestyle modification. Because heart failure is a chronic condition that needs ongoing treatment, doctors need to embrace a multidisciplinary approach in promoting cooperation between specialties. This interprofessional team working together can maximally improve the quality of care and clinical outcomes to address both the physical and psychosocial needs of patients. The consideration of the management of heart failure then follows the importance of treatment innovation in approach and commitment to continuous improvement in cardiac care (Adamopoulos et al., 2024; Magaña Serrano et al., 2024).

Grasping the intricate interaction between sarcopenia and heart failure is critical to progressing patient care. Sarcopenia, which is the depletion of skeletal muscle mass and function, is highly associated with increased levels of BNP and NT-proBNP in patients with heart failure. Patients with sarcopenia have been found to have very significantly elevated levels of BNP (MD: 87.76, 95% CI 20.74 – 154.78, I2 = 61%, P = 0.01) and NT-proBNP (MD: 947.45, 95% CI 98.97 – 1795.93, I2 = 35%, P = 0.03) compared to patients without muscle wasting. Further, decreased appendicular skeletal muscle mass is also linked with elevated levels of these natriuretic peptides (MD: 118.95, 95% CI 46.91 – 191.00, I2 = 93%, P < 0.01) and (MD: 672.01, 95% CI 383.72 – 960.30, I2 = 2%, P < 0.01). These findings underscore the imperative to conduct more studies to investigate the potential role of sarcopenia in modulating plasma natriuretic peptide levels in heart failure patients (Prokopidis et al., 2024). Aside from muscle mass pathology, the testing modalities utilized to predict adverse outcomes in patients with heart failure have recently been put under the microscope. The SARC-F questionnaire and Hand Grip Strength (HGS) are now key metrics for the prediction of short-term mortality risk in hospitalized elderly patients with acute heart failure. Results provide evidence of a strong correlation between the performance of these measures and 30-day all-cause post-discharge mortality in this high-risk population. Using the SARC-F and HGS, clinicians can identify more vulnerable patients and apply targeted interventions to improve outcomes. This simultaneous focus on muscle bulk and functional strength testing presents a holistic approach to the management of heart failure, highlighting the relevance of both physical status and symptomatic presentation as determinants of prognosis (Okoye et al., 2024). Integration of the results of both the sarcopenia and mortality prediction tool studies presents a composite perspective of the management of heart failure. Skeletal muscle mass and body strength measurement not only establishes a baseline for patient condition risk assessment but also allows for risk stratification of adverse outcomes. In addition, recognizing the physiological effects of muscle deterioration in heart failure patients could lead to more personalized therapy focused on both cardiac function and reserves. Such a comprehensive approach could enhance patient management by early detection of high-risk patients as well as by promoting interventions such as rehabilitation with exercise and diet. Ultimately, an interactive implementation of sarcopenia research and functional assessment tools will lay the foundation for improved clinical outcomes in heart failure management (Okoye et al., 2024; Prokopidis et al., 2024).

A CLOSER LOOK

LIVING WITH HEART FAILURE (HF)

Living with congestive heart failure means coping with an intricate balance of physical symptoms, affective disturbances, and lifestyle adjustments. The chronicity of this condition has a significant effect on the daily life of most patients. Patients often complain about numerous different symptoms, like fatigue, shortness of breath, and emotional distress, which may result in decreased quality of life. While they deal with such expressions, frustration and despair are common because of the volatility of the condition. The cyclical pattern of relative wellness punctuated by flare-ups that require hospitalization makes it even harder for them to adapt. A study examining patients with heart failure's cognitive representation and emotional experiences highlights their struggle to recognize and manage symptoms. It postulates a short-term need for improved patient education and support systems to promote improved self-management activities (Koontalay et al., 2024). Effective self-care behavior is highly crucial in the case of patients who are fighting heart failure, and such behavior has an imperative role to play in symptom management as well as in quality of life. Self-care management and maintenance have been shown to encourage resilience during the disabling effects of this condition. By engaging in active self-care interventions, such as symptom monitoring on a consistent basis and adherence to dietary limitations, patients can decrease the effect of clusters of various symptoms, including emotional and breathing distress. This relationship emphasizes providing patients with means to improve their self-efficacy and to use tools with which to manage their conditions effectively.

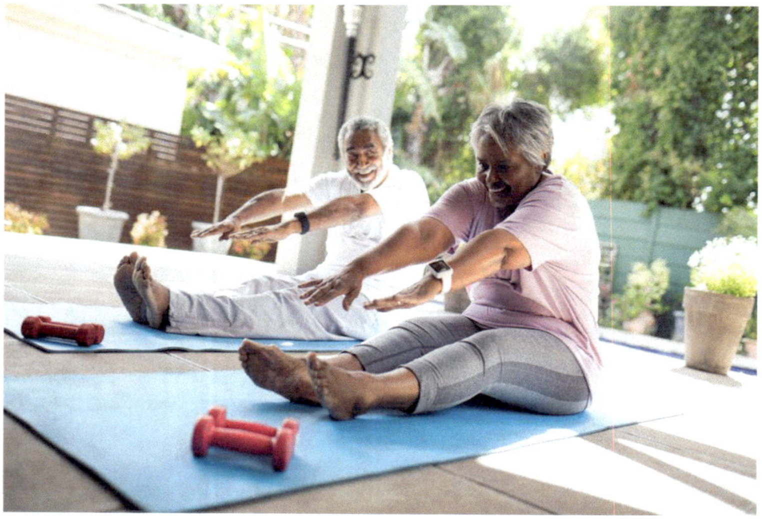

Figure 6.19. Living with heart failure.

Source: https://www.mcmasteroptimalaging.org/images/default-source/blog-post-images/exercise-for-chronic-heart-failure.tmb-blogpost.jpg?Culture=en&sfvrsn=34bf01d6_4.

With improved self-care activities, patients with heart failure can minimize its adverse effects on daily activity and overall quality of life (Yao et al., 2024). The psychological climate of living with heart failure is typically associated with adversity, the overriding experience being loss of normality and independence. Patients often struggle with the limitations of their condition, which can impact their relationships and community involvement. The emotional burden of the sense of being stuck in a perpetual cycle of hospital visits and treatments tries to get into perspective the psychological impact of this chronic disease. While the patients try to maintain the illusion of normalcy, the sense of loneliness can increase fear and misery. To overcome these emotional complications, healthcare providers must not only treat the physiological conditions of heart failure but also integrate supportive psychosocial interventions. It can empower patients to be well in control of their lives once again and facilitate improved emotional resilience against chronic illness (Koontalay et al., 2024) (Figure 6.19).

References

1. Abouzid, M., Abdelhakeem, A., Elshafie, S., & Ghorab, A. (2024). Heyde's syndrome: a challenging case of severe aortic stenosis and gastrointestinal bleeding. *BMJ Case Reports*, *17*(4), e258316. https://doi.org/10.1136/bcr-2023-258316Adam, S., Butterworth, A., Luchner, A., Wood, A. M., Brendan, B., et al. (2016). Natriuretic peptides and integrated risk assessment for cardiovascular disease: An individual-participant-data meta-analysis. https://core.ac.uk/download/74324877.pdf (accessed on 29th May 2025).

2. Adamopoulos, S., Bonios, M., Ben, G. T., Gustafsson, F., Abdelhamid, M., Adamo, M., Bayés-Genís, A., et al. (2024). Right heart failure with left ventricular assist devices: Preoperative, perioperative and postoperative management strategies. A clinical consensus statement of the Heart Failure Association (HFA) of the ESC. *European Journal of Heart Failure*. https://www.semanticscholar.org/paper/9b7d79d65ffd0d25b4334c224a563c67742ad1bf (accessed on 29th May 2025).

3. Agarwal, M., & Pakhare, S. N. (2024). Emerging therapeutic strategies in heart failure management: A narrative review of current evidence and future directions. *International Journal of Cardiology Sciences*. https://www.semanticscholar.org/paper/fb9eed11754f3f020edd629a942e2be6995c7f81 (accessed on 29th May 2025).

4. Alimadadi, A., Manandhar, I., Aryal, S., Munroe, P., Joe, B., & Cheng, X. (2020). Machine learning based classification and diagnosis of clinical cardiomyopathies. *Physiological Genomics*. https://www.semanticscholar.org/paper/b3bffa2c372e908e4ebad116b1c8b33685b293fd (accessed on 29th May 2025).

5. Amun, A. (2022). *Reducing Readmission (and Mortality) for Older Patients & Survivors of Life-Threatening Conditions: A Study Using the STAARR Protocol*. https://core.ac.uk/download/548485676.pdf (accessed on 29th May 2025).

6. Angelini, F., Bordin, A., Carrizzo, A., Chimenti, A., et al. (2017). *A Review of the Molecular Mechanisms Underlying the Development and Progression of Cardiac Remodeling*. https://core.ac.uk/download/98346388.pdf (accessed on 29th May 2025).

7. Atherton, J., Sindone, A., De Pasquale, C. G., Driscoll, A., Macdonald, P. S., Hopper, I., Kistler, P. M., et al. (2018). National Heart Foundation of Australia and Cardiac Society of Australia and New Zealand: Guidelines for the prevention, detection, and management of heart failure in Australia 2018. *Heart Lung and Circulation, 27*, 1123–1208. https://doi.org/10.1016/j.hlc.2018.06.1042 (accessed on 29th May 2025).

8. Bandyopadhyay, A., Puri, S., Samra, T., & Ashok, V. (2024). Preeclamptic heart failure — perioperative concerns and management: A narrative review. *Perioperative Medicine, 13*. https://www.semanticscholar.org/paper/e73840767c2adbd8055e87107f849ec58bada272 (accessed on 29th May 2025).

9. Berthelot, E., Bailly, M. T., Cerchez, L., X., El Blidi, R. M., Bounab, R., Mewton, N., Dobbs, J. E., et al. (2024). Setting the optimal threshold of NT-proBNP and BNP for the diagnosis of heart failure in patients over 75 years. *ESC Heart Failure, 11*, 3232–3241. https://www.semanticscholar.org/paper/23faf7f6a2dbe6155471ec68fdf9ad0382768385 (accessed on 29th May 2025).

10. Biggins, S. W., Angeli, P., García-Tsao, G., Ginés, P., Ling, S. C., Nadim, M. K., Wong, F., et al. (2021). Diagnosis, evaluation, and management of ascites, spontaneous bacterial peritonitis and hepatorenal syndrome: 2021 practice guidance by the American Association for the Study of Liver Diseases. *Hepatology, 74*, 1014–1048. https://doi.org/10.1002/hep.31884 (accessed on 29th May 2025).

11. Blumgart, H. L., & Weiss, S. (1928). Clinical studies on the velocity of blood flow: IX. The pulmonary circulation time, the velocity of venous blood flow to the heart, and related aspects of the circulation in patients with cardiovascular disease. *The Journal of Clinical Investigation, 5*(2), 343–377. https://www.semanticscholar.org/paper/c394311f9e1a1749075d1a71cfff1c70fa279527 (accessed on 29th May 2025).

12. Brennan, P. F., Burke, L., Casper, G., Kossman, D., et al. (2006). *Creating Technology-Enhanced Practice: A University-Home Care-Corporate Alliance.* https://core.ac.uk/download/213077394.pdf (accessed on 29th May 2025).

13. Carriere, C., Guarnaccia, A., Del Mestre, E., Lo Casto, M., Maione, D., Piccinin, F., Zecchin, M., et al. (2025). Remote monitoring in patients with heart failure and ventricular dysfunction: Operating protocol of Trieste cardiology. *Giornale Italiano di Cardiologia, 26*(2), 90–99. https://www.semanticscholar.org/paper/e8674f43019f511e9ca4901b25e3027dd7a6a99b (accessed on 29th May 2025).

14. Ceccacci, A., Fedele, F., Lavalle, C., Maestrini, V., et al. (2019). *Triggers for Atrial Fibrillation: The Role of Anxiety*. https://core.ac.uk/download/188833222.pdf (accessed on 29th May 2025).

15. Çelik, A., Öztürk, G., Cavusoglu, Y., Ardic, C., Nalbantgil, S., Arıca, S., Temizhan, A., et al. (2025). Guideline for the use of natriuretic peptides in the early diagnosis and management of heart failure in primary care (Joint Consensus Report by the Eurasian Society of Heart Failure and the Turkish Association of Family Medicine). *Balkan Medical Journal, 42*, 94–107. https://www.semanticscholar.org/paper/ae27050f71d9114797806faa01f567ed918a890d (accessed on 29th May 2025).

16. Coats, A. (2017). *The Management of Co-morbidities in Patients with Heart Failure – Obstructive Sleep Apnea, 10*. https://www.semanticscholar.org/paper/6ac100ac8e99228f7c4b971b60b648ffe075e71b (accessed on 29th May 2025).

17. Cuthbert, J., & Clark, A. L. (2024). Diuretic treatment in patients with heart failure: Current evidence and future directions – Part I: Loop diuretics. *Current Heart Failure Reports, 21*, 101–114. https://www.semanticscholar.org/paper/100dc31a131f65a35915055e9467a52f4379105c (accessed on 29th May 2025).

18. Duca, S., Tudorancea, I., Haba, M., Costache, A., Şerban, I., Pavăl, D. R., Loghin, C., et al. (2024). Enhancing comprehensive assessments in chronic heart failure caused by ischemic heart disease: The diagnostic utility of Holter ECG parameters. *Medicina, 60*. https://www.semanticscholar.org/paper/59a3bd3fce6fd7c07b42757a0700ce45ee6208b6 (accessed on 29th May 2025).

19. Fackelmann, K. (1998). *The Overworked Heart: Research Suggests Molecular Mechanisms for Heart Failure.* https://www.semanticscholar.org/paper/9a91f37880ec6419dc71934b626e58a9843ac411 (accessed on 29th May 2025).

20. Ghany, M. G., & Morgan, T. R. (2019). Hepatitis C guidance 2019 update: American Association for the Study of Liver Diseases–Infectious Diseases Society of America recommendations for

testing, managing, and treating hepatitis C virus infection. *Hepatology, 71*, 686–721. https://doi.org/10.1002/hep.31060 (accessed on 29th May 2025).

21. Gishto, T., Methoxha, S., Shuka, N., Preci, R., & Simoni, L. (2024). Management of cardiac involvement in Becker muscular dystrophy: A case report. *Cureus, 16*. https://www.semanticscholar.org/paper/888f67543222d825a4670a6572f16fb8bda20181 (accessed on 29th May 2025).
22. Hwang, S. Y., Uhm, I. A., Kim, S. H., Kim, J., & Jeong, M. H. (2025). Atypical symptoms on admission predict progression to heart failure in patients with first-time myocardial infarction: Using data from the Korean Multicenter Cohort Registry. *The Journal of Cardiovascular Nursing*. https://www.semanticscholar.org/paper/39702182935a09e8de1263c6f8cad713e7f4a3af (accessed on 29th May 2025).
23. Ibrahim, R., Pham, H. N., Vest, A. R., & William, P. (2024). Managing obesity in heart failure: Latest evidence and knowledge gaps. *Current Treatment Options in Cardiovascular Medicine*. https://www.semanticscholar.org/paper/91bf837f3c0ad12671fa0c84b08c7d7c848b9b7d (accessed on 29th May 2025).
24. Jayte, M., Mohamud, A., & Dubad, F. (2024). Postpartum cardiomyopathy with congestive heart failure: A case report. *SAGE Open Medical Case Reports, 12*. https://www.semanticscholar.org/paper/07703d90b08debeadbdbafe9f37ee335124cbdfe (accessed on 29th May 2025).
25. Kang, S. (2024). Diagnosis and treatment strategies for diastolic heart failure. *MEDS Public Health and Preventive Medicine*. https://www.semanticscholar.org/paper/e2450cb31810f92a7e443a2f2a40578a83fb0d4d (accessed on 29th May 2025).
26. Katic, L., Choi, J., Diaz Saravia, S., Silverman, A., Nagourney, A., Torelli, V. A., Gupta, S., et al. (2024). The interplay between cardiovascular disease and lung cancer. *Cureus, 16*. https://www.semanticscholar.org/paper/9dec88ca7fd7aa60220195bca2d4da9b9896d597 (accessed on 29th May 2025).
27. Kayani, M., Fatima, N., Yarra, P. C., Almansouri, N., Deepshikha, K., Balasubramanian, A., Parvathaneni, N., et al. (2024). Novel biomarkers in early detection of heart failure: A narrative review. *Cureus, 16*. https://www.semanticscholar.org/paper/623d8c916f46624e594d6c74b6a9cb0e7cb7a8f8 (accessed on 29th May 2025).
28. Kim, B., Bae, S. H., Kim, S., Im, S., Kim, H., Heo, J. H., Shin, H., et al. (2024). Pre- and post-hemodialysis differences in heart failure diagnosis by current heart failure guidelines in patients with end-stage renal disease. *Journal of Cardiovascular Imaging, 32*. https://www.semanticscholar.org/paper/c6cf29c9508ca8d6f12ff0106eff87c8d290d08a (accessed on 29th May 2025).
29. Kirchhof, P., Benussi, S., Kotecha, D., Ahlsson, A., Atar, D., Casadei, B., Castellá, M., et al. (2016). 2016 ESC guidelines for the management of atrial fibrillation developed in collaboration with EACTS. *European Heart Journal, 37*, 2893–2962. https://doi.org/10.1093/eurheartj/ehw210 (accessed on 29th May 2025).
30. Kitsiou, A., Caforio, A. L. P., Porta-Sanchez, A., Vahanian, A., Iung, B., Carrera, C., Szymanski, C., et al. (2013). *ESC Core Curriculum for the General Cardiologist (2013)*. https://core.ac.uk/download/55756305.pdf (accessed on 29th May 2025).
31. Kitzman, D., Lewis, G. D., Pandey, A., Borlaug, B. A., Sauer, A. J., Litwin, S. E., Sharma, K., et al. (2024). A novel controlled metabolic accelerator for the treatment of obesity-related heart

failure with preserved ejection fraction: Rationale and design of the Phase 2a HuMAIN trial. *European Journal of Heart Failure*. https://www.semanticscholar.org/paper/2ce5472dc16d546b281d615bd4a4be931d2ce8ed (accessed on 29th May 2025).

32. Koontalay, A., Botti, M., & Hutchinson, A. (2024). Illness perceptions of people living with chronic heart failure and limited community disease management. *Journal of Clinical Nursing*. https://www.semanticscholar.org/paper/284c6742b8e1ee28c56ccb3cf12e8869d666c00c (accessed on 29th May 2025).

33. Kwast, S., Hoffmann, J., Pökel, C., Falz, R., Schulze, A., Schröter, T., Borger, M. A., et al. (2025). Cardiopulmonary exercise capacity markers and their link to symptom burden in patients at risk for heart failure with non-reduced ejection fraction. *Scientific Reports, 15*. https://www.semanticscholar.org/paper/f0eb0ff1cd38928d924faa11d1339aa08d98e372 (accessed on 29th May 2025).

34. Lees, C., Stampalija, T., Baschat, A., da Silva, C. F., Ferrazzi, E., Figueras, F., Hecher, K., et al. (2020). ISUOG practice guidelines: Diagnosis and management of small-for-gestational-age fetus and fetal growth restriction. *Ultrasound in Obstetrics and Gynecology, 56*, 298–312. https://doi.org/10.1002/uog.22134 (accessed on 29th May 2025).

35. Lin, V., Hutchinson, P. J. A., Kolias, A., Robba, C., & Wahlster, S. (2025). Timing of neurosurgical interventions for intracranial hypertension: The intensivists' and neurosurgeons' view. *Current Opinion in Critical Care*. https://www.semanticscholar.org/paper/61dc0b0db5515b770505223606341efa82162920 (accessed on 29th May 2025).

36. Magaña, S. J. M., Cigarroa, L. J. A., Chávez, M. A., Ivey-Miranda, J. B., Mendoza, Z. G. H., Olmos, D. L., Chávez, L. S. A., et al. (2024). Vulnerable period in heart failure: A window of opportunity for the optimization of treatment – A statement by Mexican experts. *Drugs in Context, 13*. https://www.semanticscholar.org/paper/fec11d9e6727af3a01c65c2228aa297d116a3c19 (accessed on 29th May 2025).

37. Manca, P., Limonta, R., Marini, M., Orso, F., Carigi, S., De Gennaro, L., Tinti, M. D., et al. (2025). [Worsening heart failure: Definition, management and treatment]. *Giornale Italiano di Cardiologia, 26*(3), 173–184. https://www.semanticscholar.org/paper/411a7541dbf0b7f3a2e0be7f709bff7c4c4d1093 (accessed on 29th May 2025).

38. Mangal, S., Hyder, M. A., Mancini, J., Zarzuela, K., McDonald, W., Safford, M., Lachs, M., et al. (2024). Physician-reported facilitators and barriers for side effect management of heart failure medications. *Journal of the American Heart Association: Cardiovascular and Cerebrovascular Disease, 13*. https://www.semanticscholar.org/paper/a5a35ff265149c479262bcf414a222abd9685f2e (accessed on 29th May 2025).

39. N/A. (2020). *Motivational Interviewing Impact on Cardiovascular Disease*. https://core.ac.uk/download/322838243.pdf (accessed on 29th May 2025).

40. Okoye, C., Morelli, V., Franchi, R., Mazzarone, T., Guarino, D., Maccioni, L., Cargiolli, C., et al. (2024). Usefulness of the SARC-F questionnaire and the measurement of the hand grip strength in predicting short-term mortality in older patients hospitalized for acute heart failure. *European Geriatric Medicine, 15*, 1839–1847. https://www.semanticscholar.org/paper/6b2fa98692e0714261aef27c03d0dedf8326663a (accessed on 29th May 2025).

41. Peikert, A., & Solomon, S. D. (2024). Contemporary treatment options in heart failure with preserved ejection fraction. *European Heart Journal. Cardiovascular Imaging*. https://www.

semanticscholar.org/paper/1e7260d275be149cc92b23d0ddf47211fc3d591f (accessed on 29th May 2025).

42. Prokopidis, K., Morwani-Mangnani, J., McDowell, G., Lip, G. Y. H., Venturelli, M., Sankaranarayanan, R., & Isanejad, M. (2024). Sarcopenia is linked to higher levels of B-type natriuretic peptide and its N-terminal fragment in heart failure: A systematic review and meta-analysis. *European Geriatric Medicine, 15*, 893–901. https://www.semanticscholar.org/paper/3b6372b50c59ff079fd9cd2a51f9fb905b8f23b1 (accessed on 29th May 2025).

43. Pullicino, P., & Raynor, S. (2013). *Is Low Cardiac Ejection Fraction a Risk Factor for Stroke?* https://core.ac.uk/download/46602443.pdf (accessed on 29th May 2025).

44. Sanchez, C. C., Rojas, H. A., Lima, B. J., Rodriguez, C., Devani, A., Boosahda, V., Mareddy, N. S. R., et al. (2024). Inflammatory bowel disease and cardiovascular disease: An integrative review with a focus on the gut microbiome. *Cureus, 16*. https://www.semanticscholar.org/paper/359d86369c3adacaa47fbf1b2681d2c5fd7429d9 (accessed on 29th May 2025).

45. Schupp, T., Schmitt, A., Reinhardt, M., Abel, N., Lau, F., Abumayyaleh, M., Dudda, J., et al. (2024). Prognosis and treatment strategies for atrial fibrillation in heart failure with mildly reduced ejection fraction. *European Journal of Preventive Cardiology*. https://www.semanticscholar.org/paper/7fd2ea3f6ef4f0ba54efdacc017b4eb912aac586 (accessed on 29th May 2025).

46. Shevcova, V. I., Pashkova, A. A., Kolpacheva, M. G., & Salamatova, V. N. (2024). Palliative care for chronic heart failure: Non-pharmacological methods of relieving the main symptoms. *Meditsinskiy Sovet = Medical Council*. https://www.semanticscholar.org/paper/855ea3b62a0755e588dcb2b36b0454a0d2c247bb (accessed on 29th May 2025).

47. Siopi, S. A., Antonitsis, P., Karapanagiotidis, G., Tagarakis, G., Voucharas, C., & Anastasiadis, K. (2024). Cardiac failure and cardiogenic shock: Insights into pathophysiology, classification, and hemodynamic assessment. *Cureus, 16*. https://www.semanticscholar.org/paper/d7186d00765939a8dee82f4beb66daed105661e5 (accessed on 29th May 2025).

48. Tumelty, E., Chung, I., Hussain, S., Ali, M., Addada, H., & Banerjee, D. (2024). An updated review of the management of chronic heart failure in patients with chronic kidney disease. *Reviews in Cardiovascular Medicine, 25*. https://www.semanticscholar.org/paper/4420d909cc66e0b4a1e53a365fcd576d663c0d35 (accessed on 29th May 2025).

49. Vinck, T. A. M., Deneer, R., Verstappen, C. C. A. G., Kok, W., Salah, K., Scharnhorst, V., Otterspoor, L., et al. (2022). Validation of the ELAN-HF score and self-care behavior on the nurse-led heart failure clinic after admission for heart failure. *BMC Nursing, 21*. https://www.semanticscholar.org/paper/95650b0db5004a88cfca25467c0820d3b7894d0b (accessed on 29th May 2025).

50. Williams, B., Mancia, G., Spiering, W., Agabiti, R. E., Azizi, M., Burnier, M., Clement, D. L., et al. (2018). 2018 ESC/ESH guidelines for the management of arterial hypertension. *European Heart Journal, 39*, 3021–3104. https://doi.org/10.1093/eurheartj/ehy339 (accessed on 29th May 2025).

51. Wu, L., Rodriguez, M., El Hachem, K., & Krittanawong, C. (2024). Diuretic treatment in heart failure: A practical guide for clinicians. *Journal of Clinical Medicine, 13*. https://www.semanticscholar.org/paper/6103230da591a8975769197478d2baad5ff8534b (accessed on 29th May 2025).

52. Xu, Y. (2024). Heart failure in diabetes mellitus: The pathogenesis and treatment. *Theoretical and Natural Science*. https://www.semanticscholar.org/paper/a8bc8da4933a704aec6a4b45301a0c53dbb8a95b (accessed on 29th May 2025).

53. Yao, Q., Luo, J., Song, B., Yang, J., Yuan, X., Li, X., Tian, W., et al. (2024). The effect of heart failure symptom clusters on quality of life: The moderating effect of self-care behaviors. *Journal of Clinical Nursing*. https://www.semanticscholar.org/paper/5eb543d5bebffad6825e36cc1d1d47f3a5bf0c2a (accessed on 29th May 2025).

54. Zannad, F., & Macari, S. (2023). Drug treatment with empagliflozin was beneficial in people with heart failure with preserved ejection fraction: Plain language summary of the EMPEROR-Preserved study. *Future Cardiology*. https://www.semanticscholar.org/paper/9176dc1af02bbdcac864979772b57d073dab335a (accessed on 29th May 2025).

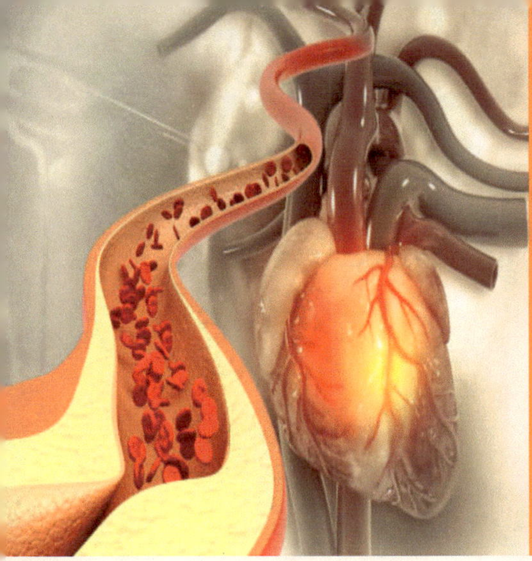

Chapter 7

HYPERTENSION AND HYPERTENSIVE HEART DISEASE

Contents

Introduction

Hypertension is a significant public health problem worldwide as it often leads to serious cardiovascular complications like hypertensive heart disease (HHD). Hypertension is an abnormal level of blood pressure that can cause damage to several organ systems, especially the cardiovascular system. Hypertension has been noted to be widespread in prevalence, with estimates suggesting that it reaches over 1 billion individuals globally. Though common, a significant number of patients remain undiagnosed or are under-treated for hypertension, which enhances the risk for HHD development. The new guidelines set by the European Society of Hypertension and the European Society of Cardiology emphasize an active approach in diagnosing increased blood pressure by applying stricter blood pressure values for better effect and preventing developments into more complicated cardiovascular diseases. The integration of these updated clinical guidelines offers an algorithm to enhance patient outcomes and helps to close some gaps in hypertension management strategies (Wang, 2025). Hypertensive heart disease is a cluster of cardiovascular complications that arise as a consequence of chronically elevated blood pressure. The relationship of hypertension to heart disease is confirmed, as long-term exposure to elevated blood pressure can lead to left ventricular hypertrophy, heart failure, and increased morbidity and mortality. This multifaceted disorder not only reflects the severity of hypertension but also highlights the importance of early detection and treatment. A notable shift in more recent guidelines is the inclusion of an elevated BP category with emphasis on the identification of individuals at risk at an earlier stage of their disease process. Furthermore, variations between guidelines' classification of raised blood pressure underpin the need for tailored approaches in clinical practice. By emphasizing the subtle differentiations designed to enhance the care of high-risk patients, clinicians can make a substantial difference in the prognosis of people with hypertension (Wang, 2025). The advent of novel therapeutic strategies has also changed the face of hypertension treatment. Specifically, newer technology in interventional therapies, like renal denervation, holds hope for resistant hypertensive patients, a notoriously difficult-to-treat subgroup. The evolution of such treatment follows shifting guidelines that not only promote stricter blood pressure control but also recommend integrating new modalities. The complicated nature of hypertension is increased by the knowledge that HDP can be a manifestation of underlying cardiovascular illness as well as a risk factor in and of itself. Those with worse pre-pregnancy cardiovascular status are substantially more likely to develop HDP, which testifies to the merit of comprehensive cardiovascular assessment in childbearing women. Collectively, these results indicate a burgeoning future of more aggressive and individualized hypertension treatment, ultimately in a bid to minimize the risks of hypertensive heart disease (Figure 7.1).

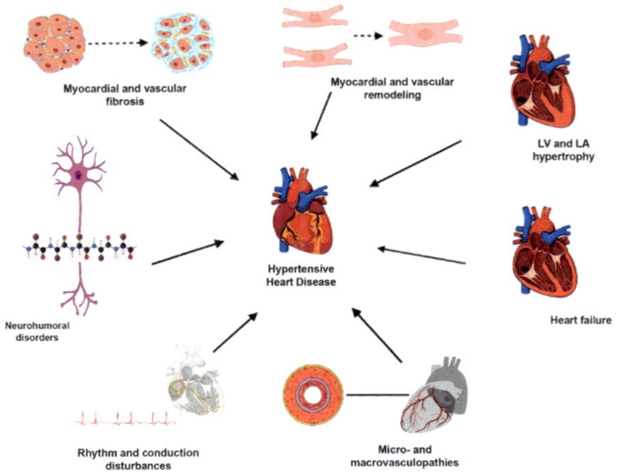

Figure 7.1. Pathomorphological, pathophysiological, and clinical patterns of hypertensive heart disease.

Source: https://www.mdpi.com/jcm/jcm-12-02606/article_deploy/html/images/jcm-12-02606-g001.png.

Definition of Hypertension

High blood pressure, also known as hypertension, is a chronic health condition characterized by constantly elevated arterial blood pressure. The condition can be measured by two readings: systolic pressure, the level of pressure in the arteries during heartbeats, and diastolic pressure, which is the pressure during heart muscle relaxation. Hypertension is a reading of 130 mm Hg or greater systolic and/or 80 mm Hg or greater diastolic, as defined by the American Heart Association. It is not an isolated physiological measurement; it is also itself a significant risk to cardiovascular health and produces all forms of heart disease and other systemic pathology. Because hypertension is most of the time asymptomatic, it is oftentimes called a silent killer, and it must be monitored all the time to prevent the development of associated complications (Laukkanen et al., 2021). Lastly, categorizing hypertension as a serious disease condition plays a critical role in disseminating information and control practices aimed at decreasing its prevalence in diverse populations. A vast number of variables, including lifestyle, genetics, and comorbidities propels the progression of hypertension. A few of these risk factors can be modified, including obesity, physical inactivity, excessive salt intake, and alcohol consumption, which can increase blood pressure. The genetic predisposition of hypertension further shows a multifactorial interaction between environmental and genetic predispositions (Xu et al., 2019). For instance, familial history of hypertension can increase the risk of an individual such that genetics plays a very significant role besides lifestyle. The importance of physical fitness in the management of hypertension cannot be overestimated, as physical exercise is a valuable strategy for lowering blood pressure (Laukkanen et al., 2021). Understanding these multifactorial determinants is crucial in designing effective public health strategies and interventions for prevention and treatment. The implications of uncontrolled hypertension cannot be overstressed, as it is a significant predictor of hypertensive heart disease. This condition is characterized by a range of cardiovascular complications, including left ventricular hypertrophy, heart failure, and ischemic heart disease. Chronic pressure overload of the heart due to elevated blood pressure can lead to structural and functional alterations, ultimately impairing cardiovascular efficiency and increasing the risk of cardiac events. The severity of this risk is a basis for the necessity of early detection and control of hypertension (Xu et al., 2019). Health care professionals must emphasize the significance of outpatient follow-up and patient education in ensuring the best blood pressure control. Creating awareness of the burden of hypertension and lifestyle modifications can play a key role in reducing the burden of hypertensive heart disease and enhancing the overall health outcome in the affected individuals (Figure 7.2).

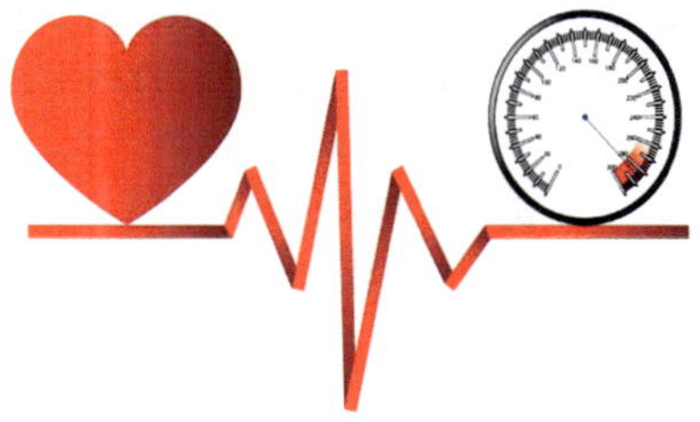

Figure 7.2. Hypertension.

Source: https://ijcscardiol.org/wp-content/uploads/2021/02/shutterstock_411862570-1024x737.x61798.jpg.

Importance of Understanding Hypertensive Heart Disease (HHD)

It makes sense only to an understanding of the pathophysiology of hypertension and its impact on the cardiovascular system, which is HHD. Hypertension, a chronic disease characterized by elevated blood pressure that is long-standing, imposes excessive tension on the heart. Over time, this chronic pressure leads to structural and functional alterations in the heart, ultimately leading to hypertensive heart disease. Understanding such dynamics is essential to prevention and treatment, given that hypertension has been established as the most important risk factor for heart failure and other cardiovascular diseases. This further emphasizes the need for combined public health interventions aimed at educating populations on how best to manage hypertension in a bid to avert HHD risk development. By correcting this disease in its early stages, medical practitioners are in a position to reduce the resultant morbidity and mortality rates associated with hypertensive heart disease. The different impacts of hypertensive heart disease involve more than the straightforward cardiovascular complications; it encompasses undertones of general health outcomes as well. Patients with HHD are usually at higher risk for comorbidities such as diabetes and chronic kidney disease, which complicate treatment and lead to poorer outcomes. Furthermore, the interrelationship of hypertension with other organs suggests that the disease is systemic, particularly in light of existing evidence showing a relationship between HHD and a higher risk for severe illness with conditions such as COVID-19. As cardiovascular health is the prime requisite of a person's well-being, adequate information on HHD becomes essential.

The significance of an interdisciplinary association with cardiologists, primary care providers, and public health professionals becomes key as they converge to solve the intricacies of hypertensive heart disease and encourage complete management regimens. Incorporation of evidence-based practice into the management of hypertensive heart disease will most probably improve the outcome of patients and reduce healthcare costs. Knowledge of the current guidelines, such as those published by prominent health organizations, will remind clinicians to apply uniform treatments according to unique patient characteristics. As several of these hypertensive patients may be taking agents on the renin-angiotensin-aldosterone system, such as ACE inhibitors and ARBs, their effects must be known to reduce adverse effects. In addition, regular monitoring for cardiac injury and other complications, particularly in high-risk groups, should receive full attention. With the progression of understanding disease pathophysiology and possible therapeutic modalities, including the role of such factors as diabetes and inflammation, the healthcare community must be sensitive to modifying their strategies. In the end, this dedication to learning about and treating hypertensive heart disease can translate to better methodologies for prevention and improved quality of life for patients (Figure 7.3).

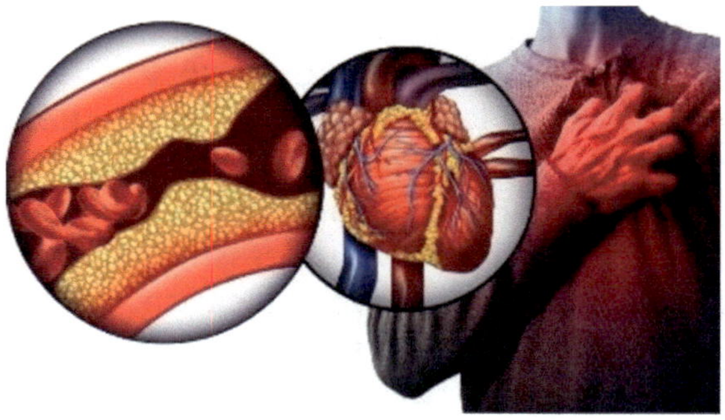

Figure 7.3. Hypertensive heart disease (HHD).

Source: https://www.hindustantimes.com/ht-img/img/2024/05/16/1600x900/Cardiovascular_Disease_1715869475281_1715869495041.jpg.

7.1. Causes of Hypertension

The multifactorial pathogenesis of hypertension reveals a mutually intricate interrelation between genetic predisposition, lifestyle determinants, and environmental factors. Genetic factors engaged in the pathogenesis of hypertension include variations in genes concerned with blood pressure regulation, e.g., sodium retention and vascular tone. Family history of hypertension increases one's susceptibility immensely, suggesting that genetic attributes predispose to elevated blood pressure. In addition, lifestyle risk factors such as excessive sodium intake, lack of exercise, and obesity also raise this condition. Diets rich in salt can lead to increased fluid retention that results in high blood pressure. Additionally, obesity is associated with increased vascular resistance and cardiovascular system stress. Therefore, it is crucial to determine the specific mechanisms involved in these associations to develop effective prevention and treatment interventions for hypertensive heart disease (Lees et al., 2020). Additionally, psychological and environmental determinants significantly contribute to the pathogenesis of hypertension.

Chronic stress is one such psych factor, which can lead to raised blood pressure levels through autonomic nervous system dysregulation and increased catecholamine release. Interpersonal conflict and socio-economic stressors also influence unhealthy coping behaviors such as smoking and poor diet, thereby perpetuating cumulative physiological impacts. Environmental factors like air pollution and exposure to some chemicals also contribute to an increased risk of developing hypertension. For instance, studies have demonstrated that exposure to heavy metals and endocrine-disrupting chemicals impairs vascular function and blood pressure regulation.

The inclusion of psychological and environmental factors in the study of hypertension highlights the need for a complete understanding and treatment of the condition (Williams et al., 2018). Underlying illnesses also make a significant contribution to the etiology of hypertension. Diabetes mellitus, chronic kidney disease, and sleep apnea are associated with the development of high blood pressure. Diabetes, characterized by insulin resistance and hyperglycemia, can lead to hypertension and vascular damage via increased arterial stiffness and inflammation. End-stage renal disease disrupts the regulation of electrolyte and fluid balance, causing fluid overload and high blood pressure. Sleep apnea, characterized by recurring suspension of breathing during sleep, can lead to increases in blood pressure due to repeated intermittent hypoxemia and increased sympathetic nervous system activity. Identification of such comorbidities is crucial in developing effective management strategies for hypertension and hypertensive heart disease patients, and it emphasizes the necessity of targeted interventions and multi-disciplinary patient management (Lees et al., 2020) (Figure 7.4).

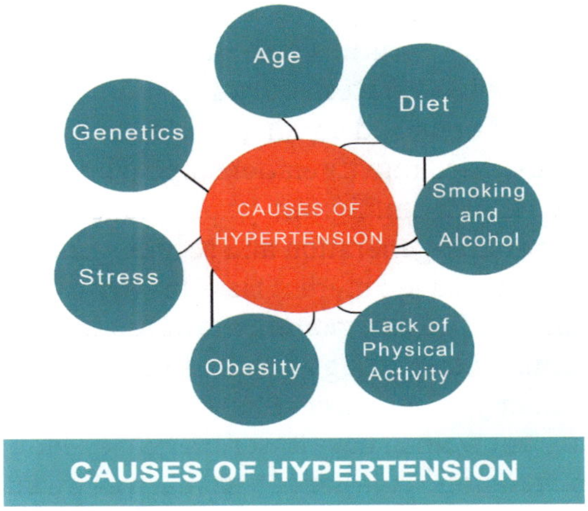

Figure 7.4. Causes of hypertension.

Source: https://encrypted-tbn0.gstatic.com/images?q=tbn:ANd9GcT1gFCxb0EHraT9SzH5teiUuJwjECMoSqTOdQ&s.

7.1.1. Genetic Factors

In the investigation of the genetic etiology of hypertension and hypertensive heart disease, one must pay attention to the complicated interplay between hereditary susceptibility and environmental factors. Genetic variation can have an enormous impact on an individual's susceptibility to hypertension, regulating physiological mechanisms such as vascular function and blood pressure control. Studies have revealed that specific populations, particularly African Americans, have a genetic tendency to develop hypertension due to distinctive genetic traits that make them susceptible to the disease. These genetic traits include gene variations of genes involved in the renin-angiotensin-aldosterone system (RAAS) and sodium transporters, which control water retention and vasoconstriction. Understanding such determinants of genetics not only directs the evaluation of risk but also paves the way for the implementation of personalized medical approaches in treating hypertension and other diseases since specific interventions would be designed based on the genetic composition of the individual (Arendshorst et al., 2024). Additionally, studies of genes underlying hypertensive states surpass just familial predispositions and entail a whole-course study of gene-environment relationships. The findings of studies on immigrant populations indicate that both first-generation and second-generation immigrants have different risks for hypertensive conditions, possibly pointing towards the role of environmental setting as well as genetic factors. For example, research has noted that while immigrant women have lower pregnancy-induced hypertension compared to native Swedish women, the risk in the second-generation immigrants is found to increase, suggesting an adjustment to environmental factors. This shifting pattern emphasizes the importance of exploring how genetic factors can possibly interact with social determinants and lifestyle to diminish or enhance the risk of hypertensive heart disease and hypertension (Wändell et al., 2024). Finally, expanding understanding of the genes involved in hypertension emphasizes the potential of novel therapeutic targets to transform clinical practice. Genetic research has now identified central pathways in which oxidative stress and inflammation overlap to affect renal function and blood pressure regulation. These results have occasioned a focus on interventions that can interrupt such harmful processes. Therapies targeted at blocking reactive oxygen species (ROS) production and the renin-angiotensin system, for instance, have emerged as intriguing options for treating hypertension. By illuminating the specific genetic factors at play, healthcare professionals can better predict the onset of disease, tailor therapies, and participate in preventive interventions based on both the genetic and environmental contexts that shape an individual's health pathway (Arendshorst et al., 2024).

7.1.2. Lifestyle Choices

Lifestyle plays a vital role in preventing and controlling hypertension and hypertensive heart disease. Dietary habits are of key importance, with high consumption of sodium linked to raised blood pressure levels. On the other hand, consumption of fruit, vegetables, whole grain foods, and low-fat dairy products, which are typical of the DASH diet, has been proven to lower blood pressure. This dietary strategy involves reduced sodium intake and increased potassium, calcium, and magnesium ingestion. By adopting healthy feeding practices, hypertensive heart disease can be prevented or avoided through a reduction in the risk of hypertension. Education about dietary practices for the population enhances adherence to these practices, leading to healthier populations and reduced healthcare costs. Physical activity is another essential element of a healthy life that can help manage hypertension. Regular aerobic exercise, like walking, jogging, and swimming, has proven to lower systolic as well as diastolic blood pressure. Physical activity also enables a person to maintain a healthy weight, which is essential because overweight is a significant risk factor for hypertension and heart disease. Furthermore, lifestyle modification involving mind-body therapies such as Yoga can provide additional benefits. Yoga per se, and especially Yoga Nidra, has been associated with blood pressure decreases through mechanisms such as increased heart rate variability. The practice can foster relaxation and stress reduction, essential components for the maintenance of optimal cardiovascular health. Thus, incorporating regular exercise and mind-body treatments into daily life can significantly improve personal efforts to manage hypertension and overall cardiac health. Mental health is often overlooked in the management of lifestyle choices regarding hypertension. Stress, being chronic, leads to elevated levels of anxiety, which in turn increases blood pressure. Stress management is thus crucial in the prevention of hypertensive heart disease. Mindfulness practices such as meditation and slow breathing practices have been found to significantly lower stress levels and improve overall emotional resilience.

Furthermore, studies show changes in heart rate variability following mindfulness interventions, indicating the possible helpful influence on blood pressure regulation. Incorporating stress management into life changes provides a general approach to combating hypertension. With lifestyle being addressed by health care providers, interventions and assistance with mental health become essential to holistic hypertension management plans. Merging the physical and mental aspects of well-being, individuals are more capable of achieving improved cardiovascular well-being as well as overall quality of life, ultimately reducing hypertension's burden and hypertensive heart disease (Figure 7.5).

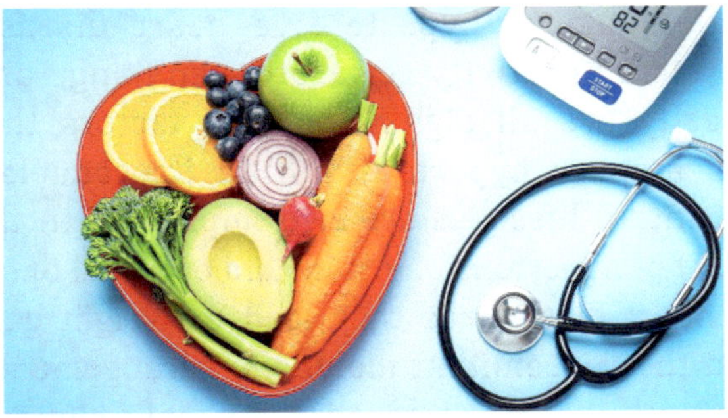

Figure 7.5. Role lifestyle choices in preventing and controlling hypertension and hypertensive heart disease.

Source: https://www.pcrm.org/sites/default/files/2021-09/healthy-blood-pressure.jpg.

7.1.3. Environmental Influences

Understanding the environmental determinants of hypertension and hypertensive heart disease is essential to developing effective prevention and treatment plans. Many ecological determinants, such as pollution, socioeconomic status, and lifestyle, play an vital role in cardiovascular health. For instance, exposure to air pollutants has been linked to elevated blood pressure and to aggravating a pre-existing hypertensive condition. Furthermore, low socioeconomic status is known to be related to poor health care access, which results in delayed diagnosis and inadequate control of hypertension. Such a twinned relationship will necessitate the consideration of environmental determinants in public health interventions aimed at the prevention of hypertension and its complications. This is evident in the research on hypertensive heart disease (Masenga et al., 2023). Food habits cannot be disregarded in determining the outcome of hypertension. Elevated sodium intake, typically of processed foods, is a significant environmental risk factor for elevated blood pressure. Repeated experiments have shown that excessive salt intake is linked with water retention and, as a result, increased vascular resistance and heart rate. Limited potassium intake can also enhance these results, showing the large role diet has in the risks of hypertension. Public awareness campaigns to educate individuals on healthy eating habits have been promising to mitigate these dietary hazards. Promoting lower levels of salt intake and consumption of foods rich in potassium enables populations to develop environments that, besides reducing the level of blood pressure, enhance overall cardiovascular health, as suggested by the many-sided interactions discussed in research on hypertensive heart disease (Zhao et al., 2023). Additionally, social behaviors such as lack of physical activity and cigarette smoking significantly determine the development of hypertension. Places that discourage physical activity—most typically explained in terms of urbanization and limited access to recreational space—cause sedentary lifestyles with the effect of raising blood pressure. Likewise, smoking remains one of the most significant risk factors for hypertension as well as hypertensive heart disease, where environmental determinants significantly play a role in smoking behavior. The prevalence of smoking is often higher among socioeconomically disadvantaged groups, in whom stressors and stigma may propel individuals toward tobacco use as a coping mechanism. To this degree, the reduction of such environmental determinants through targeted interventions can foster healthier lifestyle practices and enhance cardiovascular well-being. The integration of these determinants is central to developing an all-encompassing understanding of hypertension and hypertensive heart disease (Masenga et al., 2023; Zhao et al., 2023) (Figure 7.6).

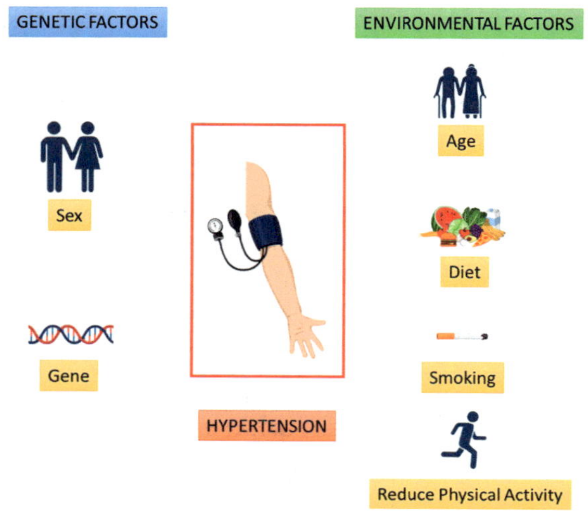

Figure 7.6. Overview of the main genetic and environmental factors involved in hypertension.

Source: https://www.mdpi.com/jcdd/jcdd-11-00154/article_deploy/html/images/jcdd-11-00154-g001.png.

7.2. Risk Factors for Hypertensive Heart Disease (HHD)

The development of HHD has a close connection with both modifiable and unmodifiable risk factors. In the most vulnerable patients, unremitting uncontrolled hypertension, characterized by long-standing elevated blood pressure, predisposes individuals to severe cardiovascular morbidity. The disease causes structural remodeling of the heart, particularly the left ventricle, which typically becomes hypertrophied as it strives to deal with augmented workload. It is of prime importance to comprehend these structural remodeling, as they progress to the impairment of function with time. Other conditions, such as a high-sodium intake diet and inherited tendencies, further worsen the effects of hypertension, thus becoming more likely to acquire HHD (hypertensive heart disease). Thus, controlling these factors through clinical measures and lifestyle adjustment continues to be central in preventing HHD and its complications as recorded in recent literature (Masenga et al., 2023).

In addition to dietary influences, lifestyle factors also play a key role in predisposing individuals to hypertensive heart disease. Physical inactivity, cigarette smoking, and obesity are all significant risk factors that can amplify hypertension and its sequelae. Sedentary lifestyles are also implicated in the onset of hypertension per se and eventual onset of heart disease, as they lead to weight gain and the concomitant metabolic derangements. Moreover, smoking tobacco not only elevates blood pressure but also accelerates arterial degradation, putting individuals at a greater risk for all cardiovascular diseases. Effective management of cardiovascular risk must therefore place priority on exercise and smoking cessation as part of patient treatment and education programs. As emphasized in analyses of the hypertensive population, synergistic control measures of these risk factors are required to reduce overall cardiovascular risk and improve patient outcomes in hypertension (Pinto et al., 2023). Psychological stress and its interaction with hypertensive heart disease must also be closely examined. Chronic stress has been known to be a significant cause of hypertension, most likely because it provokes physiological responses that elevate blood pressure levels, such as heightened heart rate and vascular resistance. Stress-led behaviors, such as unhealthy food choices and reduced physical activity, can also amplify existing hypertension and its effects on the heart. In addition, the relationship between mental illnesses such as depression and anxiety and hypertension further supports the requirement for a multidisciplinary treatment approach. Stress and mental status control should therefore be integrated into interventions stopping hypertensive heart disease before it occurs. By acknowledging the multi-dimensional nature of hypertensive risk factors, health care providers are able to modify interventions that interrupt the body as well as the mind's end of patient care when it comes to hypertension (Masenga et al., 2023; Pinto et al., 2023).

7.2.1. Age and Gender

The interaction of age and gender exerts a significant influence on the presentation and prevalence of hypertension as well as hypertensive heart disease. Epidemiologically, hypertension increases with age, especially after the age of 50 years, which indicates that the elderly are at an increased risk of cardiovascular complications. Studies have proven that men tend to have greater blood pressure levels than women until the age of menopause, when women's risk increases tremendously to bring their level closer to men. The disparity may be due to hormonal adaptation to menopause, resulting in increased arterial stiffness and greater blood pressure. As such, the age- and gender-specific patterns of hypertension are often such as to necessitate age- and gender-differentiated screening and treatment approaches, such that individualized interventions may be applied in preventing hypertensive heart disease in different populations. Furthermore, cardiovascular responses to physical stressors such as exercise are represented differently in various age and gender groups, highlighting salient features of hypertension management. It has been established by research that hypertensive patients are likely to experience augmented blood pressure reactions to physical exercise, and sex differences emerge as age increases. Interestingly, the male and female subjects had different hemodynamic patterns during stress. Specifically, younger patients with hypertension had much larger decreases in metabolic equivalents under exercise compared to their older counterparts.

These variations underscore the need to customize exercise prescriptions and monitor cardiovascular responses across various demographic groups to regulate hypertension and prevent hypertensive heart disease more effectively. The clinical practice significance of these findings is paramount, as age and gender stratifications could inform differential treatment strategies that enhance patient outcomes. Study findings inevitably underscore gender and age as significant predictors of hypertension disorders. For instance, high-risk individuals in terms of age, obesity, and hypertension must be closely followed to prevent the onset of hypertensive heart disease. This also puts more weight on the risk stratification by gender since males are more prone to developing cardiovascular complications at younger ages than females, however, with women going through hormonal changes in midlife, particularly after post-menopause because of the shifts in estrogen levels, their risk for the development of hypertension increases. Therefore, screening protocols should consider risk factors specific to age and gender and include lifestyle modification to address this growing point of discussion in public health. The insidious way in which age and gender combine to affect hypertension calls for a holistic approach to both treatment and prevention protocols, ultimately maximizing patient care and outcomes regarding hypertensive heart disease (Figure 7.7).

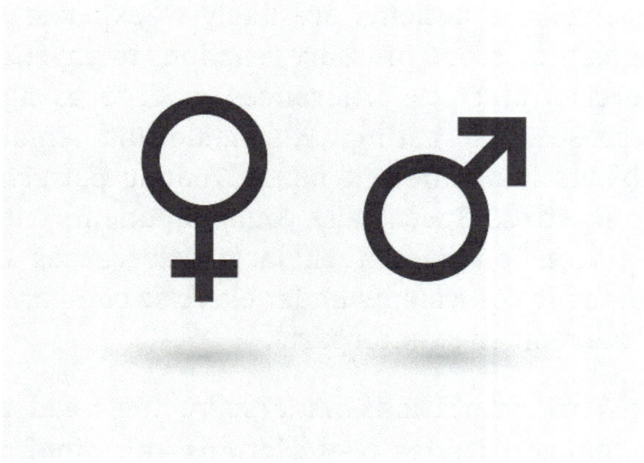

Figure 7.7. Age and Gender.

Source: https://www.recoveryconnection.com/wp-content/uploads/2017/02/Fotolia_74023011_Subscription_Monthly_M.jpg.

7.2.2. Comorbid Conditions

Comorbidities significantly enhance the burden of hypertension and hypertensive heart disease and complicate their diagnosis and treatment. Hypertensive patients often have multiple chronic diseases, with CKD and diabetes mellitus being the most prevalent of them. The association of these conditions can create a vicious circle, as hypertension exacerbates the progression of kidney failure, and vice versa. For example, when a study was conducted on geriatric patients admitted to the hospital, 86.7% of the patients with an estimated glomerular filtration rate below the normal value had two or more comorbidities since the diseases interrelate with one another (Nastasa, 2023). Healthcare professionals need to be aware of these interconnections since this highlights the application of a holistic approach to the management of all health conditions co-present in the patient at the same time. The management of hypertension can also be complex with comorbid diseases, particularly in older patients. A study revealed that approximately 55% of the hypertensive patients had other chronic diseases, which indicates the prevalence and complexity of comorbidities in this population (Sharma et al., 2022). The comorbid disease conditions not only influence the drug compliance but also the effectiveness of antihypertensive drugs. For instance, patients with coronary artery disease may require some treatment regimens that are different from those for patients having blood pressure management as the primary aim. Therefore, practitioners must assess all the conditions carefully before the treatment is prescribed, as divergent reactions to medication rely significantly on the general state of health in the patient. Comorbidities not only complicate treatment but also add to the overall risk of adverse health outcomes. This is particularly notable in an expanding population of elderly individuals where the prevalence of both hypertension and its related comorbidities continues to rise. The high nonadherence to antihypertensive drugs at a reported 23.8% for severe cases highlights the challenge of patients with multiple chronic diseases co-occurring (Sharma et al., 2022). This nonadherence can be expected to raise hypertension and ensuing heart disease, creating a cycle of worsening health. Therefore, a preventive strategy must be implemented by healthcare systems in the form of tailored educational documents and support groups to improve patient adherence and self-management of patients with comorbid hypertension (Figure 7.8).

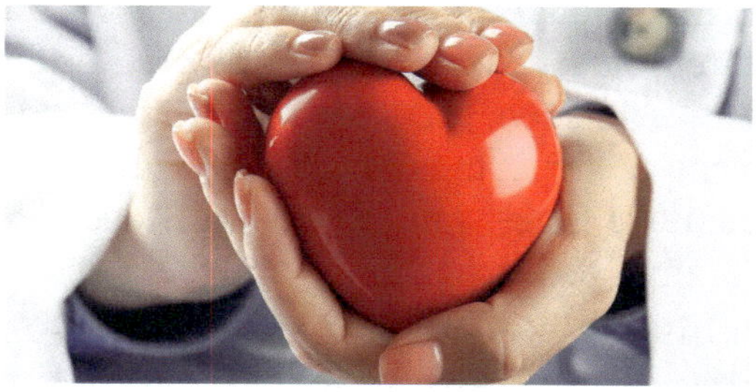

Figure 7.8. Hypertension and comorbidities.

Source: https://casanacare.com/wp-content/uploads/2023/06/Hypertension-and-Comorbidities-A-common-and-dangerous-combination-scaled.webp.

7.2.3. Socioeconomic Status

Socioeconomic status (SES) has a significant impact on hypertension and hypertensive heart disease incidence and control. Lower socioeconomic classes are more likely to be exposed to high blood pressure risk factors. Exposure may be in the form of decreased access to care, poor nutrition, and increased stress levels. Moreover, low SES comes with decreased health literacy that limits an individual's level of engagement in preventive health activities and compliance with treatment protocols. According to the literature, the combination of socioeconomic risk factors and health outcomes is central to the healthcare burden of chronic diseases such as hypertension. Eradication of these disparities demands an intervention that is multicomponent in nature, consisting of community-based interventions to promote access to care, education, and healthier living environments. The influences of SES on hypertension are also compounded by systemic mechanisms such as neighborhood environments and social support networks. Residents of low-income communities frequently live under challenging conditions, including limited access to recreational areas and healthy foods, which result in physical inactivity and unhealthy diets. Additionally, these communities contain poor healthcare facilities, which enhance the latencies in identifying and managing hypertension. There is emerging evidence to show that the development of heart failure syndromes may be influenced by such socioeconomic disparities, particularly as populations experience increasing rates of obesity and their related comorbidities. With growing awareness of heart failure with preserved ejection fraction, it is imperative to know how SES influences such trends to develop efficient public health interventions for populations at risk, particularly in low-income nations, where the healthcare burden remains high (Groenewegen et al., 2020). Additionally, effective policies for the management of heart disease and hypertension rely on socioeconomic status awareness of patient adherence and response to treatment. Social determinants of health can create challenges to optimal care, disrupting adherence to medication treatment and lifestyle modifications that are essential in the treatment of hypertension. For example, economic limitations can lead to an inability to buy prescribed antihypertensive medications or adhere to a heart-healthy diet. A vicious cycle of bad health outcomes can also be created by the emotional turmoil that comes with financial instability, which can worsen preexisting health conditions. Thus, public health policy must prioritize care approaches that are combined and address the unique problems of those with lower SES so that clinical guidelines, such as those from the European Society of Cardiology (Visseren et al., 2021), can usefully target these important social determinants of health.

7.3. Pathophysiology of Hypertension

The pathophysiology of hypertension is a multifactorial interaction between genetic, environmental, and physiological factors in causing an increase in blood pressure. At the core of this process is the abnormality of RAAS, which is responsible for maintaining blood pressure equilibrium by regulating fluid state and vascular tone. During states of increased RAAS activity, there are increased levels of angiotensin II, leading to arteriolar constriction and sodium retention and further sustaining hypertensive states. Chronic hypertension, which is defined by persistent systemic vascular resistance elevations, results in vascular remodeling and heightened blood vessel stiffness. This remodeling not only impacts blood flow but also further taxes the heart, with the potential of leading to hypertensive heart disease, which is a formidable long-term health concern. Effective management and prevention of hypertension-related complications, therefore, depend on a proper comprehension of these underlying mechanisms. In delineating the contribution of endothelial dysfunction to hypertension, one must appreciate the function of nitric oxide (NO) in vascular homeostasis. NO functions as a vasodilator under normal circumstances, but in patients with hypertension, the balance is upset, which results in less NO being available. One possible explanation for this is oxidative stress, which produces reactive oxygen species that scavenge NO and prevent it from having its vasodilatory effects. When endothelial cells become impaired in their capacity for NO production, vasoconstriction becomes dominant, further raising blood pressure. Furthermore, this impairment has an intimate relationship with inflammatory processes, where cytokines and other biomolecules are involved in vascular injury and increased resistance. The intricate interplay between endothelial health and hypertension emphasizes the need for appropriately guided therapy capable of reversing the endothelial dysfunction to dampen hypertensive growth and its resulting cardiovascular complications, such as left ventricular hypertrophy and heart failure. The pathophysiology of hypertension might also be influenced by extrinsic factors, such as pregnancy complications that can significantly alter cardiovascular physiology. During pregnancy, a woman's body undergoes sudden physiological alterations that predispose it to hypertensive complications, including gestational hypertension and preeclampsia. Besides bringing short-term health problems, both conditions also have long-term implications on heart function as they can lead to cardiac metabolic dysfunction and cardiac structural remodeling. Pregnancy maladaptations have been shown to impose an increased risk of future cardiovascular disease and heart failure, as noted in studies. Understanding the mechanisms by which hypertension develops and is sustained in pregnancy yields essential information regarding its pathophysiology. It highlights the necessity of attentive monitoring and management of cardiovascular health in women throughout and after pregnancy, with attention to both short- and long-term cardiovascular risk (Cameron et al., 2018; Aryan et al., 2020) (Figure 7.9).

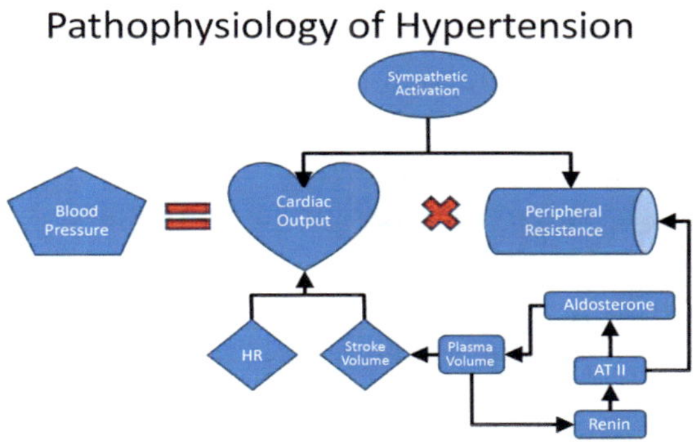

Figure 7.9. Pathophysiology of hypertension.

Source: https://www.researchgate.net/profile/Shrikrushna-Unhale/publication/340579663/figure/fig2/AS:879144158101507@1586615709384/Fig-Pathophysiology-of-Hypertension.jpg.

7.3.1. Mechanisms of Blood Pressure Regulation

Blood pressure (BP) control is a multifaceted process that relies on several physiological processes that interact to maintain homeostasis. Regulation of BP is focused on the autonomic nervous system, which controls vascular tone and cardiac output through sympathetic and parasympathetic pathways. Activation of the sympathetic nervous system can lead to vasoconstriction, increasing peripheral resistance and consequently BP. Conversely, the parasympathetic nervous system causes vasodilation and decreased heart rate. Additionally, RAAS is also responsible for long-term BP homeostasis by regulating blood volume and vascular resistance. Dysregulation of these mechanisms may lead to hypertension, which appears as vascular structural alterations, noted with endothelial dysfunction and arterial remodeling, thereby worsening cardiovascular risk factors of hypertensive heart disease (Cameron et al., 2016). The other essential component of regulation of BP is the natriuretic peptide (NP) system, a counter-regulatory mechanism to the RAAS. The NP family, comprising atrial natriuretic peptide (ANP), brain natriuretic peptide (BNP), and C-type natriuretic peptide (CNP), plays a central role in causing diuresis and vasodilation and reducing BP. These peptides exert their action on specific receptors, eliciting effects that inhibit premature renin secretion and increase sodium excretion.

These have been shown to preclude the development of hypertension and resultant target organ damage, including heart failure and renal damage. Investigation of the actions of natriuretic peptides also yields significant information about the mechanisms of hypertension pathogenesis and of possible therapeutic strategies for the control of hypertensive states (Forte et al., 2019). In addition to neurohormonal regulation, behavioral aspects significantly contribute to BP homeostasis. Dietary intake, exercise, and coping with stress are all central to the prevention of hypertension-related vascular dysfunction. Emerging evidence supports that nutritional patterns rich in fruit, vegetables, and whole grains, and low in sodium intake, can have marked lowering effects on BP. Physical activity helps not only in weight control but also enhances endothelial function and reduces arterial stiffness, maintaining vascular health. Additionally, stress-reducing practices such as mindfulness and relaxation exercises can reverse the physiological mechanisms underpinning BP elevation. In combination, these lifestyle treatments, along with pharmacologic interventions such as ACE inhibitors and calcium channel blockers, that directly attack vascular remodeling, are crucial to the management of hypertension and the prevention of hypertensive heart disease (Cameron et al., 2016) (Figure 7.10).

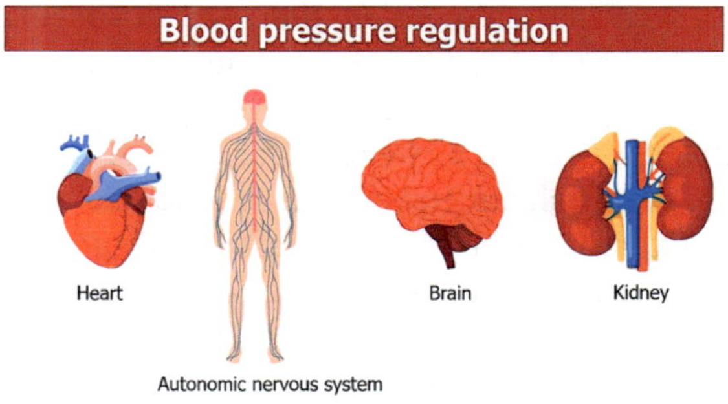

Figure 7.10. Blood pressure regulation.

Source: https://i.ytimg.com/vi/6n2aKipt4U0/maxresdefault.jpg?sqp=-oaymwEmCIAKENAF8quKqQMa8AEB-AH-CYAC0AWKAgwIABABGH8gFSgTMA8=&rs=AOn4CLAYYUu1Ys-PHH9EWUrJzSKDw9_uqQ.

7.3.2. Impact on the Cardiovascular System

Hypertension significantly impacts the cardiovascular system, exhibiting numerous undesirable features that can lead to long-term complications. Hypertension leads to increased vascular resistance, which increases the heart load and results in left ventricular hypertrophy. These changes can alter myocardial function over time, making the heart prone to failure and arrhythmias. Of particular interest, hypertension is not only a significant risk factor for cardiovascular disease but also exacerbates pre-existing cardiovascular disease. The interaction between elevated blood pressure and cardiovascular mortality makes active control interventions in high-risk groups essential to counteract these effects and prevent progression to hypertensive heart disease. Systemic alteration in lifestyle, along with drug therapy when indicated, is essential in the management of hypertension and in maintaining cardiovascular status. The effects of hypertensive disorders of pregnancy (HDP) also depict the interaction between hypertension and cardiovascular outcomes. Women suffering from gestational hypertension or preeclampsia have extreme changes in their cardiovascular systems that even persist many years after pregnancy. Studies reveal that women suffering from HDP are at a higher risk for cardiovascular diseases such as heart failure and ischemic heart disease twenty years after giving birth. This increase in risk is attributed to underlying cardiovascular risk factors and the direct action of HDP on maternal physiology. Of special concern is the severity and timing of such hypertensive complications, which are cardinal determinants of long-term cardiovascular health since early-onset and recurrent preeclampsia strongly predict adverse outcomes, including cardiovascular-related mortality, as stipulated in research evidence (Lailler et al., 2024). Additionally, harmful heart remodeling may be a part of the circulatory alterations in HDP, leading to heart failure with preserved ejection fraction. During and after pregnancy, patients with HDP are often noted to have impaired myocardial function and suboptimal biventricular performance. These alterations not only represent acute cardiovascular stresses but also suggest susceptibility to further metabolic and hemodynamic insults. Given growing awareness of cardiovascular risk among women with a history of HDP, early cardiovascular assessment is recommended. The question of standardization of protocols, however, remains problematic because of insufficient evidence. There is a necessity thus to acknowledge and address long-term cardiovascular implications of hypertensive pregnancy disorders to improve outcomes across women's lifespan (Ghossein-Doha et al., 2024).

7.3.3. Consequences of Chronic Hypertension

Chronic hypertension, also referred to as long-term high blood pressure, has profound implications that extend far beyond cardiovascular effects. The most direct single consequence is the heightened cardiac workload, in which the heart must pump against elevated arterial pressure. This may lead to left ventricular hypertrophy (LVH), a condition that entails an increase in left ventricular heart mass. LVH is a severe prognosticator of heart failure and arrhythmia and significantly raises morbidity and mortality risk in affected individuals. Moreover, the cardiac structural changes are further accentuated by functional impairments that may jeopardize cardiac output and lead to symptoms such as dyspnea and fatigue. As hypertension continues to place additional stress on the heart, the chances of developing hypertensive heart disease increase, thereby establishing a vicious cycle of deteriorating cardiac function. In addition to cardiac concerns, chronic hypertension also poses significant danger to the renal system. The kidneys have a sophisticated network of vessels to purify blood and maintain fluid balance, and prolonged high blood pressure has the consequence of injuring these intricate structures. The filtering units of the kidneys, the glomeruli, may over time undergo alterations leading to CKD. This is particularly troublesome because CKD can worsen hypertension, a two-headed monster: each worsens the other. As blood flow through the kidneys is diminished due to damage to the vessels, proteinuria occurs as an indicator of renal injury and a signal that proteins are passing into the urine. This is not only reflective of decreasing renal function but also a marker of cardiovascular risk, complicating further the care of patients with chronic hypertension and its consequences. Also, systemic effects of chronic hypertension are observed to involve multiple organ systems by exhibiting multiple complications outside the heart and kidneys. For instance, the risk of stroke is significantly increased due to the deleterious effects of high blood pressure on cerebral vasculature. Chronic stress can lead to the development of small vessel disease, leading to cerebrovascular accidents that may result in disabling cognitive deficits or death. In addition, injury to the retinal vessels may lead to hypertensive retinopathy, which can lead to irreversible blindness if untreated. This multifaceted effect of chronic hypertension highlights the vital importance of early diagnosis and efficient control measures. Through the active management of hypertension, medical practitioners can reduce the wide range of health impairments linked with this silent but deadly disease, finally enhancing the overall patient outcome in populations prone to hypertensive heart disease and related conditions (Figure 7.11).

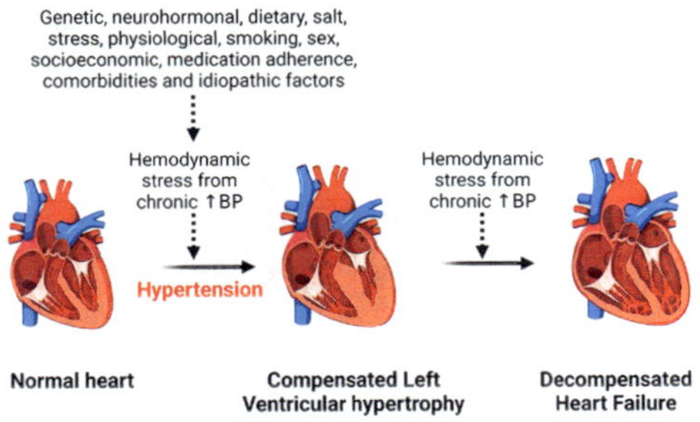

Figure 7.11. Effect of chronic hemodynamic stress on the heart. Chronic hypertension resulting from various stimuli leads to left ventricular hypertrophy as a compensation for the hemodynamic stress and metabolic demand on the heart. However, heart failure results when the heart can no longer withstand the persistent hemodynamic stress.

Source: https://www.frontiersin.org/files/Articles/1205475/fcvm-10-1205475-HTML-r1/image_m/fcvm-10-1205475-g001.jpg.

7.4. Symptoms and Diagnosis

Expression of symptoms in patients with hypertensive and hypertensive heart disease is often multifarious and heterogeneous, hence proving to be more complicated for diagnosis. Patients may present with non-specific symptoms like dyspnea, asthenia, palpitations, and edema that are similar to other illnesses. Development of such symptoms necessitates a high degree of clinical investigation to reach an appropriate diagnosis. The challenge lies in distinguishing between actual hypertensive heart disease and other potential diagnoses, such as pulmonary disease or coronary artery disease. Therefore, techniques such as echocardiography, natriuretic peptide levels, and functional testing prove priceless in addressing such diagnostic challenges. In addition, comprehension of the patient's history, such as demographics and related risk factors, plays a vital role in developing a proper diagnosis and individualized appropriate treatment interventions, thereby ensuring that management is consistent with the targeted pathophysiological mechanisms affecting the patient's individual presentation. Diagnosis of heart failure with preserved ejection fraction (HFpEF) still poses a complex challenge because of symptom heterogeneity as well as the absence of absolute non-invasive tests. Subsequent investigations have made it clear the value of specific diagnostic algorithms like H2FPEF and HFA-PEFF that utilize a battery of clinical markers in identifying HFpEF risk in symptomatic patients. In hypertension-related heart failure, subclassifying such presentations from other analogous conditions has therapeutic implications. An investigation in patients with HFpEF in the presence of hypertension revealed considerable disparities in myocardial strain and other CMR parameters concerning patients with uncomplicated hypertensive heart disease. Particularly, quantification of late gadolinium enhancement and extracellular volume fraction can reveal critical information about myocardial remodeling, thus illustrating the utility of advanced imaging modalities in fine-tuning the diagnostic approach to HFpEF and hypertensive heart disease (Rasalam et al., 2025). Providing additional impetus to the requirement of reliable diagnostic tools, research has shown that CMR-derived parameters are potentially capable of yielding valuable information about left and right ventricular dynamics required for assessment of the characteristic presentation of HFpEF-HTN.

The population under study showed marked reduction in longitudinal, circumferential, and radial strain values compared to the other groups and, therefore, exhibited compromised myocardial function characteristic of this syndrome. Higher N-terminal pro-brain natriuretic peptide levels were similarly correlated with increased functional class in such patients, highlighting the multifactorial pathophysiology of heart failure in hypertension (Li et al., 2024). Further, application of CMR parameters to assess myocardial strain and tissue properties not only enhances diagnostic sensitivity but also assists in clinical decision-making in managing hypertensive heart disease. The findings emphasize the need for focused diagnostic strategies that consider the profiles of individual patients, eventually resulting in more subtle treatment and improved health outcomes.

7.4.1. Common Symptoms of Hypertension

Hypertension, or the silent killer, typically does not have signs or minimal symptoms, hence the need for early diagnosis, prevention, and treatment. Hypertensive individuals may present with nonspecific symptoms such as headache, dizziness, or feeling of head pressure. The nonspecific nature typically hinders diagnosis as patients do not attribute them to hypertension. The insidious nature of hypertension can result in extensive organ damage before symptom detection is possible, particularly in instances of hypertensive heart disease. Risk subjects must be screened for blood pressure frequently to identify hypertension even in the absence of apparent symptoms, thereby facilitating intervention and management strategies that arrest extensive cardiovascular events (Babu et al., 2025). Hypertension sometimes precipitates more serious health issues reflecting its onset. Such health issues in the form of breathlessness on effort or pain in the chest may ensue, which can be premonitory signs of incipient heart issues in the form of hypertensive heart disease. Organ damage-type symptoms like blurred vision or a bleeding nose can ensue in more advanced situations, which are signs of end-organ damage due to prolonged high blood pressure. Recognition of these signs is crucial for supporting patient education, as they may be the impetus for medical assessment and treatment.

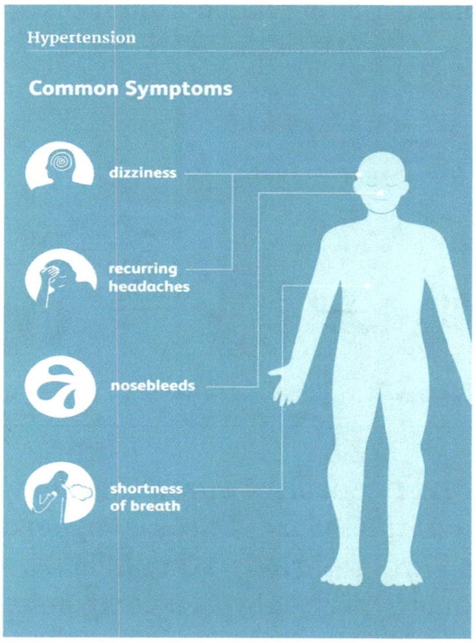

Figure 7.12. Symptoms of hypertension.

Source: https://www.verywellhealth.com/thmb/Y-cqfIBAn4pu7-X9aynK4BuNaU8=/750x0/filters:no_upscale():max_bytes(150000):strip_icc():format(webp)/hypertension-symptoms-5afedc4da9d4f90036e90344.png.

Moreover, an awareness that hypertension can also exacerbate pre-existing disease states, such as diabetes, adds importance to symptom recognition among at-risk populations. Intervention at the point of occurrence of such signs will significantly reduce the risk of progressing to more severe health complications (Babu et al., 2025). Hypertension is also capable of causing psychological symptoms due to its association with ongoing stress and tension. Some of the frequent symptoms manifested by patients resulting from the physiological stresses exerted on the body include mood changes, fatigue, or restlessness. The interplay between the psychological and physical determinants of health explains the necessity of an integrated approach in managing hypertension. Both physical symptom and mental health screening on a routine basis can make overall treatment outcomes better. Additionally, identification of pervasive symptoms of hypertension enhances not only patient education but also enhances active management of their illness. While primary focus may be on cardiovascular risks, recognition and treatment of the whole spectrum of symptoms may enable quality of life improvement and reduced disease burden (Torma et al., 2024) (Figure 7.12).

7.4.2. Diagnostic Procedures

Diagnosis methods for hypertension and hypertensive heart disease are critical in the initiation of early intervention and individualized patient management plans. Measuring blood pressure accurately is the foundation of hypertension diagnosis, and most often it is performed with sphygmomanometers. Nevertheless, the introduction of ambulatory blood pressure monitoring (ABPM) has dramatically changed the diagnosis of hypertension, as it allows the blood pressure to be evaluated under different conditions of daily life. ABPM is more comprehensive and is helpful in the diagnosis of white-coat syndrome or masked hypertension, which can significantly affect management. Furthermore, emphasis on accurate diagnosis has led to a recent guideline to reduce the target blood pressure. This shift points to the importance of precise and relentless blood pressure measures in the avoidance of hypertensive heart disease risk as expressed in current literature exploring novel strategies in maximizing cardiovascular outcomes (Wang, 2025). Beyond blood pressure measurement, various diagnostic procedures quantify target organ damage and cardiovascular risk from hypertension. Electrocardiogram (ECG) is also employed regularly to identify arrhythmias and evidence of left ventricular hypertrophy, an irreversible consequence of longstanding hypertension. Echocardiography is also crucial in imaging structural changes of the heart because of hypertensive heart disease and has proven helpful in identifying diastolic dysfunction and other myocardial derangements. Besides, advanced imaging techniques, including cardiac MRI and CT angiography, can provide detailed information regarding vascular changes and coronary artery disease. Systematic evaluation of such diagnostic modalities is central in that they not only direct therapy choice but are also integral to current risk stratification and patient management frameworks. The evolving character of hypertension diagnosis reflects a growing recognition of the imperative to conduct a careful evaluation within diverse cohorts of patients (Agarwal et al., 2024). Emerging guidelines are indicative of a broader understanding of hypertension as a multifactorial syndrome and thus the necessity to include cutting-edge diagnostic strategies in routine practice. New diagnostic categories, such as isolated diastolic hypertension, reflect the continuous progress in the notion of blood pressure-associated health hazard. The systematic review underscored the cardiovascular implications of different diagnostic criteria and illustrated how different guidelines yield various outcomes in the stratification of risk in patients. These findings reinforce the necessity of adherence to amended guidelines for accurate diagnosis to prevent the progression of hypertensive heart disease. Clinicians are encouraged to implement these findings to introduce preventive diagnostic strategies, emphasizing early diagnosis and treatment of hypertension in varying population segments. By strict adherence to diagnostic progress and evolving guidelines, healthcare workers can best curb the morbidity of hypertensive heart disease (Wang, 2025) (Figure 7.13).

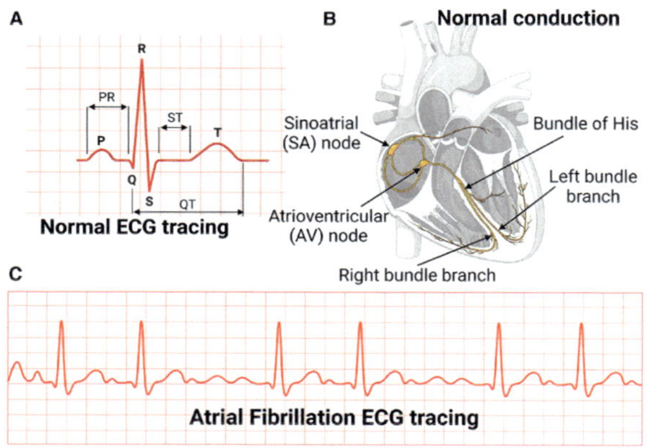

Figure 7.13. Electrocardiography and conduction system of the heart. (A) Normal Electrocardiography (ECG). (B) Conduction system of the heart. (C) Atrial Fibrillation ECG tracing.

Source: https://www.frontiersin.org/files/Articles/1205475/fcvm-10-1205475-HTML-r1/image_m/fcvm-10-1205475-g003.jpg.

7.4.3. Importance of Regular Monitoring

Regular blood pressure checks are a fundamental component of hypertension management and prevention of HHD. Hypertension remains asymptomatic, and hence regular monitoring to check for it early on and treat it is essential. Existing guidelines recommend a lower target systolic blood pressure value, between 120–129 mmHg, and this emphasizes the need for regular monitoring to achieve this. This early activation can significantly lower the threat of hypertension complications, including heart failure, stroke, and other cardiovascular events. Thus, a regular monitoring routine helps not only in assessing the success of treatment but also in enhancing the awareness of patients regarding their health status, ultimately resulting in better compliance with lifestyle modification and pharmacologic intervention (Wang, 2025). Along with this, the introduction of technology, such as wearable technology and telehealth systems, has made blood pressure monitoring an ongoing and easy procedure. AI-based monitoring systems guarantee real-time data analysis, notifying healthcare professionals to worrisome trends that can require immediate intervention. Since hypertension is a chronic ailment, being able to regularly check blood pressure levels from the comfort of one's home not only relieves the burden on medical facilities but also enables patients to take an active role in managing their condition. The technology not only facilitates early intervention but also enhances communication between patients and healthcare professionals, hence optimizing management protocols and outcomes (Igwama et al., 2024).

The value of routine monitoring, therefore, lies not in mere measurement but in synthesizing patient participation with professional knowledge. The value of routine monitoring also lies in the creation of individualized treatment plans that change over time based on unique patient information. Through regular monitoring of blood pressure measurements, clinical professionals can make informed judgments about the efficacy of prescribed treatments, make appropriate changes, and detect potential side effects. This evidence-based practice is also helpful in the identification of resistant hypertension, a situation that typically requires complex management. Patients who are motivated in their monitoring are most likely to understand their condition and appreciate the importance of adhering to treatment regimens. Consequently, constant monitoring is a cornerstone not just for on-site clinical evaluation but also for sustained interventions to forestall the dangers of hypertension, thus protecting against the development of hypertensive heart disease (Wang, 2025). In short, adoption of standardized monitoring practices is essential to achieving better patient outcomes in the management of hypertension (Figure 7.14).

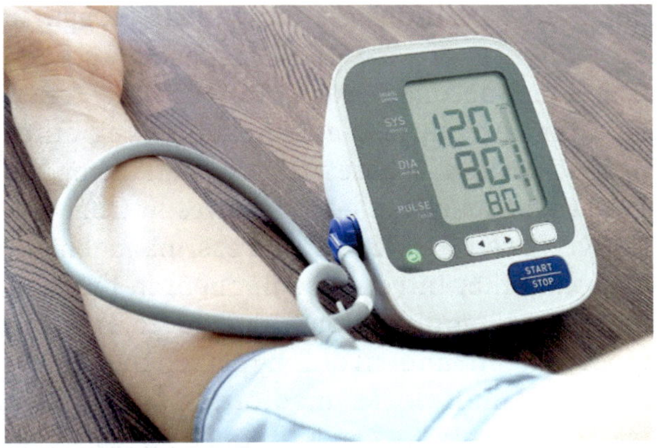

Figure 7.14. Regular monitoring of blood pressure.

Source: https://encrypted-tbn0.gstatic.com/images?q=tbn:ANd9GcQTW43K9Owp2MCBn38yQXLfUdgTF4J5bPRzEg&s.

7.5. Treatment Options

Treatment of hypertension includes a variety of drugs to lower blood pressure to avoid cardiovascular disease, as well as the development of hypertensive heart disease. Pharmacologic therapy remains the cornerstone of treatment, and numerous antihypertensive drugs are now available. The options are diuretics, ACE inhibitors, angiotensin II receptor blockers, beta-blockers, and calcium channel blockers that each target a different pathway involved in blood pressure regulation. Individual patient considerations can also guide the selection of a particular antihypertensive regimen, since some drugs are more beneficial or less toxic in terms of side effects about the individual profile of a patient. Thus, individualized management of drugs is essential in an attempt to maximize compliance and overall treatment success, as well as to prevent complications from chronic hypertension. In addition to pharmacologic treatment, lifestyle modification is a key component of the treatment of general hypertension. Dietary modification (e.g., use of the DASH diet), exercise, weight loss, and smoking abstinence can significantly enhance the control of blood pressure. Non-drug interventions not only lower blood pressure itself but also promote general cardiovascular health and hence possibly reduce the impact of hypertensive heart disease. Education and home-based self-management practices, including self-monitoring of blood pressure at home, can empower patients and facilitate compliance with medical therapy. A holistic strategy integrating pharmacotherapy with lifestyle modification is most critical to optimize treatment outcomes and prevent complications of uncontrolled hypertension. Novel concepts in personalized medicine have revolutionized the management of hypertension, now advocating more individualized care plans based on genetic, environmental, and lifestyle determinants.

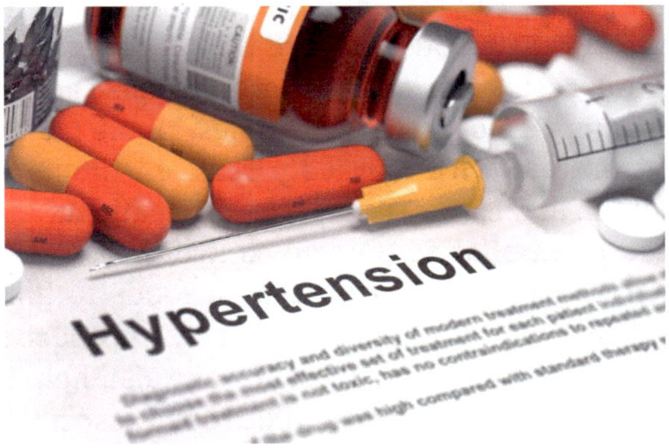

Figure 7.15. Hypertension treatment.

Source: https://static.s4be.cochrane.org/app/uploads/2016/01/Hypertension.jpg.

Study emphasizes the need for an individualized treatment protocol instead of a one-size-fits-all approach, particularly in light of the multiformity of hypertension and its varied expressions. For some of the risk factors in every patient, doctors can optimize therapeutic effects and minimize the risk of side effects, thereby promoting optimal compliance and outcomes. Additionally, systems biology and high-throughput technologies have facilitated personalized medicine through comprehensive assessments of patient-specific information that guide treatment decisions. This drift towards an individual approach reflects a broader movement in modern healthcare, one centered on the importance of tailored solutions to combat long-term illnesses like hypertension and their associated complications, including the development of hypertensive heart disease (Borghi et al., 2017; Khan et al., 2017) (Figure 7.15).

7.5.1. Lifestyle Modifications

Management of hypertension, particularly in the context of hypertensive heart disease, is a multidisciplinary approach with lifestyle modification forming a pivotal element in prevention as well as therapy. Use of a heart-healthy diet, e.g., the DASH diet, has been effective in lowering blood pressure and subsequently cardiovascular risk. The diet emphasizes more consumption of fruits, vegetables, whole grains, and protein with markedly reduced intake of sodium. In this regard, hypertensive patients also need to emphasize portion control and reduce their consumption of processed foods to limit total sodium intake. These dietary approaches not only lower blood pressure but also help in avoiding hypertensive complications associated with chronic hypertension, thereby highlighting the elementary role of such changes in managing total cardiovascular health (Baoum et al., 2024). Apart from dietary modification, regular exercise is also instrumental in combating hypertension and its resultant complications. At least 150 minutes of cardiovascular exercises such as walking, cycling, and swimming every week has been shown to enhance cardiovascular function greatly. Studies have established that exercise maintains blood pressure at a normal level, aids in weight maintenance, and reduces the risk of developing left ventricular hypertrophy, a common consequence of long-standing hypertension. Furthermore, incorporating strength training activities on more than two days a week improves health and metabolic conditions. As individuals recognize the benefits of sustained physical activity, compliance becomes crucial, as it not only treats hypertension but also aids in combating other lifestyle-related diseases, thereby enhancing the positive feedback cycle that can result from this change (Urs et al., 2022). Stress management is also another intrinsic component in the field of lifestyle modifications needed to manage hypertension and avoid hypertensive heart disease. Mindfulness meditation, yoga, and breathing exercises can all reduce stress levels to a considerable extent. Furthermore, these reduced stress levels can lead to lower blood pressure. Long-term stress has been reported to cause elevated heart rates and constriction of blood vessels, thus exacerbating hypertension. As individuals integrate these routines into their daily lives, they can observe better physical and emotional well-being, facilitating easier management of their condition. Notably, quitting smoking is also critical as tobacco use is a confirmed risk factor for hypertension and cardiovascular disease. By altering these lifestyle determinants, a person can create an effective strategy to combat hypertension and general cardiovascular health, as attested to by the sheer volume of evidence on behalf of these non-pharmacological interventions (Baoum et al., 2024).

7.5.2. Pharmacological Interventions

The management of hypertension has undergone a revolutionary change in the last two decades with the continuous advancement of pharmacologic interventions. Medications form the core for controlling blood pressure and retarding the growth of hypertensive cardiac disease, which can lead to serious cardiovascular pathology. Some of the most commonly employed groups of antihypertensive medications are diuretics, ACE inhibitors, angiotensin II receptor blockers (ARBs), calcium channel blockers, and beta-blockers. All drugs act through distinct mechanisms to promote vasodilation, reduce volume, or inhibit adverse cardiac remodeling. Recommendations from various organizations emphasize the importance of individualized treatment based on factors specific to the patient, including comorbidities, severity of hypertension, and overall cardiovascular risk, an all-inclusive approach to hypertensive therapy that balances maximum therapeutic effectiveness with minimum side effects (Williams et al., 2018). In the real world, GDMT models have been created that optimize pharmacological therapy for hypertension to help achieve this goal. These models benefit from extensive evidence from clinical trials, expert consensus, and systematic reviews to generate the treatment strategies that will yield better patient outcomes. The ACC/AHA guidelines, for instance, develop recommendations founded upon thorough evaluation of new scientific evidence, providing a good platform for clinical decision (Whelton et al., 2017). Through categorizing the strength of recommendations and the quality of evidence, the guidelines enable healthcare practitioners to select appropriate therapies, balancing possible benefits against harm. Notably, the recommendations are dynamic, shifting with the creation of new evidence and therefore accurately reflecting the dynamic process of hypertension control and the necessity for health professionals to remain current with the latest research. Not less important is the emphasis on compliance of the patient with medication regimens prescribed, and this has a significant bearing on the success of hypertension control. A multitude of causes, such as complicated dosing regimens, side effects, and insufficient patient education about the value of consistent treatment may disrupt adherence. Direct communication between healthcare professionals and patients may improve understanding and compliance with prescribed medicines. Pharmacists and other healthcare providers can play a valuable role in this educational aspect with access to medication use counseling, potential side effects, and long-term benefits of ideal blood pressure control. Therefore, interprofessional collaboration in pharmacologic management not only enhances patient understanding but also enables more enhanced health outcomes in hypertension management and prevention of hypertensive heart disease (Figure 7.16).

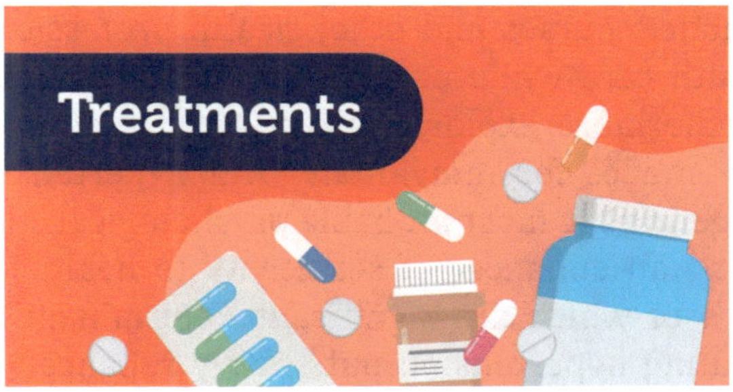

Figure 7.16. Hypertension medications and treatment options.

Source: https://cdn.myhealthteams.com/graphic/6617e63b02ac649572960fe8/woriginal/myPCOSteam_YourGuideToPCOS_Treatments-369095b1004c797c91c6a73612d98736.webp?1712842298.

7.5.3. Alternative Therapies

Within the context of treating hypertension, complementary treatments are in the limelight as adjuncts to standard pharmacological therapy. Their inclusion as part of the overall plan can optimize patient outcomes and improve the quality of life. For instance, non-pharmacologic interventions such as dietary modifications, regular exercise, and stress management techniques are often emphasized in clinical practice guidelines. The 2023 and 2024 European Society of Hypertension (ESH) and European Society of Cardiology (ESC) guidelines have ranked such lifestyle changes as primary drivers to control blood pressure and prevent HHD. In the process of clinicians grappling with these new alternatives, early identification and intervention take the front seat, in line with the guidelines' stringent blood pressure objectives calling for multidimensional interventions by the patient (Wang, 2025). Among the range of alternative therapies, music therapy has proven to be a significant intervention worth a shot. This non-invasive approach has the potential to diminish anxiety and decrease blood pressure in hypertensive individuals. It is indicated in research that listening to music can distract from stressors and induce relaxation, which can potentially play a vital role in the management of hypertension. According to studies evaluated in recent literatures, it has been established that music therapy is a powerful adjunct treatment that physicians can prescribe to their patients (Perawat et al., 2024). By incorporating music therapy into everyday practice, nurses and other health professionals can empower patients to become their agents of health care while providing them with helpful tools with which to lower blood pressure levels. Furthermore, exploring alternative treatments like mindfulness and meditation can offer significant advantages for individuals with hypertension. Mental well-being practices provide a means of targeting the most probable psychological causes for increased blood pressure. Mindfulness, beyond being an enhancer of sensitivity to health and one's body, is also a relaxant and stress reducer, both of which are significant determinants of reducing blood pressure. The evolving nature of treating hypertension puts heavy reliance on a comprehensive treatment approach that includes such alternative therapies. While healthcare professionals become more aware of HHD's intricate nature and risk factors, implementation of the same therapies as part of total care plans is crucial for achieving maximum patient outcomes and preventing hypertensive heart disease progression (Wang, 2025) (Figure 7.17).

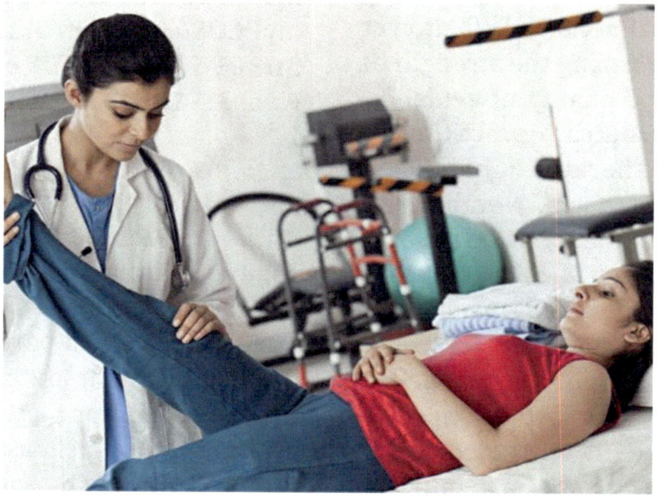

Figure 7.17. Alternative therapies help to treat hypertension.

Source: https://images.hindustantimes.com/rf/image_size_640x362/HT/p1/2013/04/16/Incoming/Pictures/1045324_Wallpaper2.jpg.

SUMMARY

Analysis of hypertension and its resulting complications, that is, HHD, signifies the significance of proper management and intervention strategies. As is revealed through the intricate relationship between LVH and clinical outcomes, identification of the underlying mechanism contributing to HHD is crucial for clinicians. The identification of the left ventricular mass-to-strain ratio (LV-MSR) as an early predictive indicator for altered cardiac geometry and prognosis is a welcome new advance in the follow-up of patients with hypertension. By its superior predictive ability to traditional measures, LV-MSR may potentially enable clinical practitioners to more effectively stratify risk, personalize treatment protocols, and thereby maximize patient outcomes, an integral component in the comprehensive treatment of hypertensive heart disease (Hwang et al., 2025). Moreover, cardiovascular health has an interlinked correlation with heart rate (HR) control in hypertensive patients. Research shows that lowering heart rate has a significant effect on the majority of cardiovascular outcomes in addition to controlling blood pressure. For example, a systematic review confirmed that therapies with HR reduction reduced coronary heart disease and heart failure rates while simultaneously reducing cardiovascular and all-cause deaths. However, clinicians must be careful with regard to their associated risks, such as increased discontinuations due to side effects, particularly in specific populations. Thus, determination of an optimal HR target for hypertensives—ideally in the 65–70 beats per minute range—is of utmost significance to balance therapeutic efficacy and safety (Sanidas et al., 2025). In brief, the interactive dynamics of hypertension, LVH, and HR demonstrate the complexity involved in the management of hypertensive heart disease. Congruent risk determination and individually adjusted therapeutic regimens should be directed towards harnessing innovative biomarkers such as LV-MSR along with traditional risk factors. In addition, incorporating HR management into the treatment process is crucial to combatting the morbidity and mortality associated with this prevalent condition. The shift to an individualized process in hypertension management can potentially lead to enhancements in clinical outcomes and quality of life of hypertensive heart disease patients, an aspect calling for further research and study in this significant field of cardiovascular health.

In investigating the association between HHD and hypertension, it is essential to note the most prominent points that reflect their association. Hypertension is a significant risk factor for most cardiovascular disorders, including hypertensive heart disease, which includes left ventricular hypertrophy and heart failure. The transition from high blood pressure to heart disease is frequently subtle and requires constant checks and early treatment to prevent complications. One of the key aspects of this interaction is the quantitation of how chronic elevation of blood pressure leads to structural and functional changes in the heart, contributing to increased morbidity and mortality. The impact of hypertension is heterogeneous within the population, so prevention must be targeted and consider the risk factors for the person and the availability of healthcare. The consequences of hypertensive disorders of pregnancy only serve to illustrate the serious consequences of hypertension in a specific group. Pregnant women with chronic hypertension have higher risks, including the development of severe maternal morbidity (SMM). Evidence indicates that preeclampsia in over 31% of pregnant chronic hypertension patients compared to merely 4.7% without chronic hypertension, and it reveals there is a direct association between chronic hypertension and complications of pregnancy. SMM risk was found to be five times higher for chronic hypertension with superimposed preeclampsia, and therefore, the necessity to follow cautious management and preventive measures in this group. Concurrently, the findings indicate the importance of detection and control of hypertension in reproductive health because it would also have a significant effect on maternal and fetal outcomes and therefore demand a wider health policy. The interaction of hypertensive heart disease with right ventricular function also needs to be noted, specifically about HFpEF. Such a condition, which is often compounded by advanced age and comorbidities, poses special challenges in managing the patient. Evidence shows that HFpEF patients tend to have pulmonary hypertension and right ventricular hypertrophy, making their clinical picture more complicated. Specifically, a new model of HFpEF presented data that metabolic stress combined with hypertensive challenge could lead to an adverse prognosis, characterized by vascular inflammation and simultaneous post- and precapillary pulmonary hypertension (CpcPH). These findings highlight the multifaceted nature of hypertensive heart disease and draw attention to the need for novel treatment strategies aimed at beneficial patient prognosis and quality of life. Knowledge of these pathophysiologic correlations is valuable for guiding future research and treatment strategies in hypertensive heart disease.

A CLOSER LOOK

COMPLICATIONS OF HYPERTENSIVE HEART DISEASE (HHD)

HHD is a significant public health condition since it potentially leads to disastrous cardiovascular morbidity. Recurrent or persistent hypertension imposes an unfair load on heart structure and function and is often followed by LVH or myocardial thickening. This alteration may lead to impaired cardiac pumping, congestive heart failure, arrhythmia, and predisposition to myocardial infarction. Further, with the progression of the condition, the frequency of sudden cardiac events rises significantly, affecting mortality among the infected. The interaction between cardiovascular-related complications and hypertension renders observation and management essential to curtail the economic cause of hypertensive heart disease among the patient population, more so with its astronomical estimate of accounting for around 8 million annual deaths (Siska et al., 2024). In addition to affecting cardiac function, hypertensive heart disease is also associated with systemic complications that further extend its impact throughout general health. For instance, hypertensive patients who have poorly controlled blood pressure are typically at high risk of developing kidney disease, stroke, and other cardiovascular diseases such as coronary artery disease. This is a complicated relationship in which a comprehensive approach to treatment and education of the patient, particularly in the context of lifestyle modification and adherence to drug therapy, is essential. Evidence shows that few patients have adequate knowledge regarding hypertension, complications of which further increase the risk of adverse health outcomes (Wake et al., 2024).

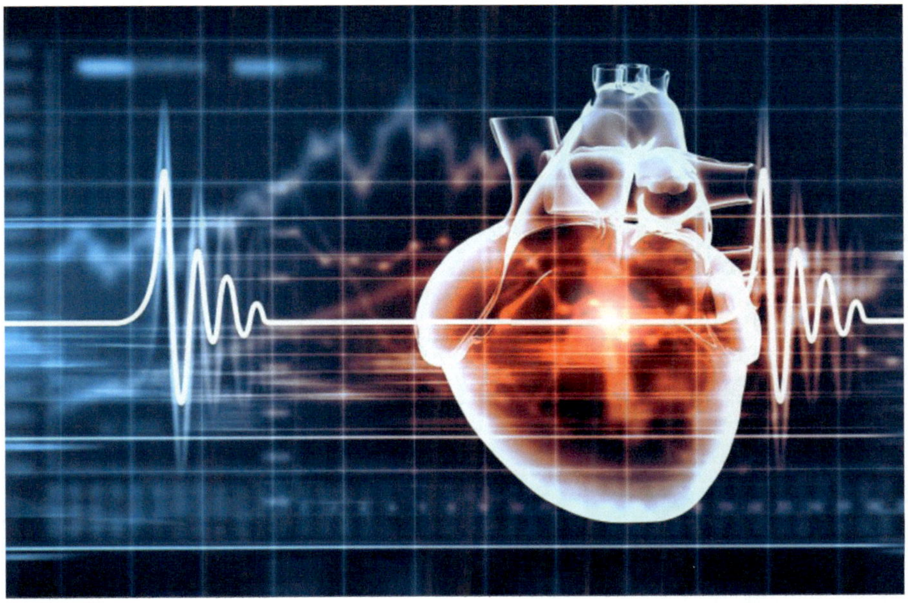

Figure 7.18. Complications of Hypertensive Heart Disease (HHD).

Source: https://www.drjimcollins.com/wp-content/uploads/2018/05/Myocardial-Infarction-770x500.jpg.

Enhancing patient understanding of the effect of hypertension can produce active disease management, ultimately leading to improved prognosis and reduced incidence of secondary complications. Furthermore, control of complications of hypertensive heart disease requires a multidimensional approach involving prevention strategies in high-risk populations. Large-scale public health interventions encouraging publicity of the hazards of hypertension along with its complications are necessary. Educational interventions for risk factors, such as diet, physical activity, and the avoidance of smoking, can provide patients with the knowledge necessary to make informed choices that minimize their risk of developing hypertensive heart disease. Daily health screening and early intervention approaches also can identify hypertension before it leads to irreparable complications. Through the reinforcement of a culture of healthcare that focuses on preventive care and patient engagement, the healthcare system is able to combat the hypertensive heart disease challenges effectively, thus finally putting an end to its colossal strain on the populace and society at large (Siska et al., 2024; Wake et al., 2024) (Figure 7.18).

References

1. Agarwal, A., Mostafa, M. A., Ahmad, M. I., & Soliman, E. Z. (2024). Isolated diastolic hypertension and cardiovascular outcomes across different diagnostic guidelines: a systematic review and meta-analysis. *The Egyptian Heart Journal, 76*(1). https://doi.org/10.1186/s43044-024-00556-5Ahuja, N., Pathania, M., Mohan, L., Mittal, S., Bhardwaj, P., & Dhar, M. (2025). The effect of Yoga Nidra intervention on blood pressure and heart rate variability among hypertensive adults: A single-arm intervention trial. *Cureus, 17.* https://www.semanticscholar.org/paper/aa86886aaf496dec718f1a2ea86d6896041cfdaf (accessed on 29th May 2025).
2. Arendshorst, W. J., Vendrov, A. E., Kumar, N., Ganesh, S., & Madamanchi, N. (2024). Oxidative stress in kidney injury and hypertension. *Antioxidants, 13.* https://www.semanticscholar.org/paper/8fd8312d7bf165d53e0d0f75504e2d63d8b6ebf6 (accessed on 29th May 2025).
3. Aryan, L., Eghbali, M., Medzikovic, L., Umar, S., et al. (2020). *Pregnancy-Associated Cardiac Dysfunction and the Regulatory Role of microRNAs.* https://core.ac.uk/download/323076335.pdf (accessed on 29th May 2025).
4. Babu, A., Uthaiah, C. A., Wasnik, P., Verma, N. R., Vijay-Kumar, M., & Abraham, J. (2025). Leveraging circulating DNase I activity to detect silent coronary artery disease among hypertensive diabetes individuals. *American Journal of Physiology. Heart and Circulatory Physiology*. https://www.semanticscholar.org/paper/44204dceeef58bd50e126b194a1d090b9bf380d6 (accessed on 29th May 2025).
5. Baoum, S. O., Anbarserri, F. M., Alhassan, S. E., Al Hani, H. F., Almutairi, F. N., Sulayman, M. L., Alfadhli, J. L., et al. (2024). Evaluating the impact of lifestyle modifications on hypertensive heart disease. *International Journal of Community Medicine and Public Health*. https://www.semanticscholar.org/paper/01e9ae17b80e151575be78c31d8f634f86cad52b (accessed on 29th May 2025).
6. Baumgartner, H., De Backer, J., Babu-Narayan, S. V., Budts, W., Chessa, M., Diller, G. P., Lung, B., et al. (2020). 2020 ESC guidelines for the management of adult congenital heart disease. *European Heart Journal, 42*, 563–645. https://doi.org/10.1093/eurheartj/ehaa554 (accessed on 29th May 2025).
7. Borghi, C., Grassi, G., Agabiti, R. E., Savoia, C., et al. (2017). *Personalized Medicine—A Modern Approach for the Diagnosis and Management of Hypertension.* https://core.ac.uk/download/96884785.pdf (accessed on 29th May 2025).
8. Cameron, A. C., Dobbin, S. J. H., Jones, R. J., Lang, N. N., et al. (2018). *Toxicity of Cancer Therapy: What the Cardiologist Needs to Know About Angiogenesis Inhibitors.* https://core.ac.uk/download/161514882.pdf (accessed on 29th May 2025).
9. Cameron, A. C., Lang, N. N., & Touyz, R. M. (2016). *Drug Treatment of Hypertension: Focus on Vascular Health.* https://core.ac.uk/download/46559725.pdf (accessed on 29th May 2025).
10. Chrysohoou, C., Skoumas, J., Georgiopoulos, G., Liontou, C., Vogiatzi, G., Tsioufis, K., Lerakis, S., et al. (2017). Exercise capacity and hemodynamic response among 12,327 individuals with cardio-metabolic risk factors undergoing treadmill exercise. *European Journal of Preventive Cardiology, 24*, 1627–1636. https://doi.org/10.1177/2047487317726069 (accessed on 29th May 2025).

11. Del Pinto, R., Giua, C., Keber, E., Grippa, E., Tilotta, M., & Ferri, C. (2023). Impact of 2021 ESC guidelines for cardiovascular disease prevention on hypertensive patients risk: Secondary analysis of Save Your Heart study. *High Blood Pressure & Cardiovascular Prevention, 30*, 167–173. https://www.semanticscholar.org/paper/741ed75d7e7577aa1f3bd7281cb8a8ff4702d143 (accessed on 29th May 2025).

12. Dodds, L., Feaster, D., Kiefe, C., Gunderson, E. P., Bello, N., Rundek, T., Paidas, M., et al. (2025). Abstract P1139: Lower pre-pregnancy cardiovascular health is associated with higher odds of hypertensive disorders of pregnancy: Coronary Artery Risk Development in Young Adults Study (CARDIA). *Circulation*. https://www.semanticscholar.org/paper/40f7ef4811f79061cf0c45afe4a9af420212ae8f (accessed on 29th May 2025).

13. Forte, M., Marchitti, S., Rubattu, S., Volpe, M., et al. (2019). Molecular implications of natriuretic peptides in the protection from hypertension and target organ damage development. *International Journal of Molecular Science*. https://core.ac.uk/download/195776786.pdf (accessed on 29th May 2025).

14. Ghossein-Doha, C., Thilaganathan, B., Vaught, A., Briller, J. E., & Roos-Hesselink, J. (2024). Hypertensive pregnancy disorder, an under-recognized women specific risk factor for heart failure? *European Journal of Heart Failure, 27*, 459–472. https://www.semanticscholar.org/paper/550f1a7b2052988429c20ab6f2a76ba90cee634e (accessed on 29th May 2025).

15. Groenewegen, A., Rutten, F. H., Mosterd, A., & Hoes, A. W. (2020). Epidemiology of heart failure. *European Journal of Heart Failure, 22*, 1342–1356. https://doi.org/10.1002/ejhf.1858 (accessed on 29th May 2025).

16. Gunderson, E. P., Greenberg, M., Najem, M., Sun, B., Alexeeff, S., Alexander, J., Nguyen-Huynh, M., et al. (2025). Severe maternal morbidity associated with chronic hypertension, preeclampsia, and gestational hypertension. *JAMA Network Open, 8*. https://www.semanticscholar.org/paper/73e6b8508245b6969bac9c23ea95ae521d0a5cbb (accessed on 29th May 2025).

17. Guzik, T. J., Mohiddin, S., Dimarco, A., Patel, V., Savvatis, K., Marelli-Berg, F. M., Madhur, M. S., et al. (2020). COVID-19 and the cardiovascular system: Implications for risk assessment, diagnosis, and treatment options. *Cardiovascular Research, 116*, 1666–1687. https://doi.org/10.1093/cvr/cvaa106 (accessed on 29th May 2025).

18. Hwang, I., Kim, H. M., Park, J., Choi, H. M., Yoon, Y. E., & Cho, G. (2025). Left ventricular mass-to-strain ratio to predict treatment response and prognosis in hypertensive heart disease. https://www.semanticscholar.org/paper/2299de72a7a7ab828c93e82132fd8942804724d3 (accessed on 29th May 2025).

19. Igwama, G. T., Nwankwo, E. I., Emeihe, E. V., & Ajegbile, M. D. (2024). AI-enhanced remote monitoring for chronic disease management in rural areas. *International Journal of Applied Research in Social Sciences*. https://www.semanticscholar.org/paper/7c8c0da47ca5672d5ace1aee8a4293453c9d13d3 (accessed on 29th May 2025).

20. Khan, F. H., & Khan, K. K. (2017). *Pulmonary Hypertensive Crisis and its Efficient Management: A Case Report and Literature Review*. https://core.ac.uk/download/132194203.pdf (accessed on 29th May 2025).

21. Lailler, G., Grave, C., Gabet, A., Joly, P., Regnault, N., Deneux-Tharaux, C., Tstsaris, V., et al. (2024). Early mortality, cardiovascular, and renal diseases in women's lives following hypertensive disorders of pregnancy: The prospective nationwide study CONCEPTION. *Journal of the*

American Heart Association: Cardiovascular and Cerebrovascular Disease, 13. https://www.semanticscholar.org/paper/fb6978456166a252e1b211a63c7fa039925aa660 (accessed on 29th May 2025).

22. Laukkanen, J., & Kunutsor, S. (2021). Fitness and reduced risk of hypertension—Approaching causality. *Journal of Human Hypertension, 35*, 943–945. https://www.semanticscholar.org/paper/232d65a3750b93c0b91f6440fe360b1747de535d (accessed on 29th May 2025).

23. Lees, C., Stampalija, T., Baschat, A., da Silva, C. F., Ferrazzi, E., Figueras, F., Hecher, K., et al. (2020). ISUOG practice guidelines: Diagnosis and management of small-for-gestational-age fetus and fetal growth restriction. *Ultrasound in Obstetrics and Gynecology, 56*, 298–312. https://doi.org/10.1002/uog.22134 (accessed on 29th May 2025).

24. Li, R., Lei, F., Liu, F., Cao, L., Cao, X., Niu, M., & Guo, S. (2024). The transition from hypertension to hypertensive heart disease and heart failure with preserved ejection fraction: A retrospective cross-sectional study of myocardial magnetic resonance strain and tissue characteristics. *Quantitative Imaging in Medicine and Surgery, 14*, 7684–7696. https://www.semanticscholar.org/paper/dc1e823d1294a2f7384881aa614e68e62b46743f (accessed on 29th May 2025).

25. Maron, B. A. (2015). Emerging hemodynamic signatures of the right heart (Third International Right Heart Failure Summit, part 2). *Pulmonary Circulation*. https://core.ac.uk/download/28952964.pdf (accessed on 29th May 2025).

26. Masenga, S., & Kirabo, A. (2023). Hypertensive heart disease: Risk factors, complications and mechanisms. *Frontiers in Cardiovascular Medicine, 10*. https://www.semanticscholar.org/paper/8374bf34b8f39febae09961a531f6dcccbfba9c4 (accessed on 29th May 2025).

27. Matin, M., Ali, I. A., & Haq, M. (2024). Hospital outcome of hypertensive non-ST elevation myocardial infarction patients in diabetic and non-diabetic groups. *Bangladesh Heart Journal*. https://www.semanticscholar.org/paper/78d64735848d2ea652b8aa67aa2a85e0f704be36 (accessed on 29th May 2025).

28. Mondol, A. S. M. R., Zaman, T., Anwar, M., Miah, M. H., Adiluzzaman, M. A. F. A., Banu, A., Jahan, S., et al. (2023). Prevalence of microalbuminuria and its association with left ventricular hypertrophy (LVH), ischemic heart disease (IHD), retinopathy, and stroke in hypertension. *Journal of Rangpur Medical College*. https://www.semanticscholar.org/paper/17d49893ddf90aa5a7f74bb9136eda4ebd06d07d (accessed on 29th May 2025).

29. Nastasa, A. (2023). Epidemiology of chronic kidney disease and comorbid illness in hospitalized geriatric patients. *Revista Medico-Chirurgicala*. https://www.semanticscholar.org/paper/d9b4c615cc2ccdfbd598498051bc802989b56368 (accessed on 29th May 2025).

30. Perawat, L., Runesi, O., & Sukihananto. (2024). Effectiveness of music therapy as an intervention in patients with hypertension: A literature review. *Lentera Perawat*. https://www.semanticscholar.org/paper/bd3151160c81bc6a1d9b33db7a3c1b19da4e769b (accessed on 29th May 2025).

31. Rasalam, R., Sindone, A. P., Deed, G., Audehm, R., & Atherton, J. J. (2025). State of precision medicine for heart failure with preserved ejection fraction in a new therapeutic age. *ESC Heart Failure*. https://www.semanticscholar.org/paper/b1f0f3c2c3e665b8dcc21ce1daa996681bad7fac (accessed on 29th May 2025).

32. Sanidas, E., Böhm, M., Oikonomopoulou, I., Dinopoulou, P., Papadopoulos, D., Michalopoulou, H., Tsioufis, K., et al. (2025). Heart rate-lowering drugs and outcomes in hypertension and/or

cardiovascular disease: A meta-analysis. *European Heart Journal*. https://www.semanticscholar.org/paper/a236123c5a2e6d62303d2f03a1b30d04a0b4ff8a (accessed on 29th May 2025).

33. Sharma, D., Goel, N., Lehl, S., Walia, D., Puri, S., Shukla, K., & Mishra, S. (2022). Prevalence and predictors of medication nonadherence among hypertensive patients. *International Journal of Noncommunicable Diseases, 7*, 71–75. https://www.semanticscholar.org/paper/9ab5ce1c5b709c7761fa1d96466f4bfd9c3974f3 (accessed on 29th May 2025).

34. Siegel, R. L., Miller, K. D., & Jemal, A. (2019). Cancer statistics, 2019. *CA: A Cancer Journal for Clinicians, 69*, 7–34. https://doi.org/10.3322/caac.21551 (accessed on 29th May 2025).

35. Siska, F., & Oktavia, T. (2024). Predictive analysis of hypertensive heart disease using a machine learning approach. *2024 International Conference on ICT for Smart Society (ICISS)*. https://www.semanticscholar.org/paper/72dd57d9833a0ce2ec4b3bf74a854b890b004df2 (accessed on 29th May 2025).

36. Su, H., Yang, M., Wan, C., Yi, L. X., Tang, F., Zhu, H. Y., Yi, F., et al. (2020). Renal histopathological analysis of 26 postmortem findings of patients with COVID-19 in China. *Kidney International, 98*, 219–227. https://doi.org/10.1016/j.kint.2020.04.003 (accessed on 29th May 2025).

37. Torma, D., Rinta-Harri, M., Ruotsalainen, A. K., & Yla-Herttuala, S. (2024). Gradual hypertensive response in aortic alterations and myocardial inflammatory activation in progressing HFpEF in mice. *European Heart Journal*. https://www.semanticscholar.org/paper/d128f4cfc7ba37d75936660601a8cc7112890d7d (accessed on 29th May 2025).

38. Urs, G., Bag, K., & Anand, L. (2022). Managing hypertension: An audit of local practice in a tertiary care hospital. *RGUHS Journal of Medical Sciences*. https://www.semanticscholar.org/paper/2d58ce69ddd22595f9051ceba360ebca77c66f70 (accessed on 29th May 2025).

39. Visseren, F. L. J., Mach, F., Smulders, Y. M., Carballo, D., Koskinas, K. C., Bäck, M., Bénétos, A., et al. (2021). 2021 ESC guidelines on cardiovascular disease prevention in clinical practice. *European Heart Journal, 42*, 3227–3337. https://doi.org/10.1093/eurheartj/ehab484 (accessed on 29th May 2025).

40. Wake, A. D., & Gebreyohannes, L. T. (2024). Hypertension complications: Common complications, awareness and associated factors in hypertensive patients in Ethiopia: Multicenter cross-sectional study. *Journal of Cardiology & Current Research*. https://www.semanticscholar.org/paper/7dbc6e5cec51d7ab4121cbe184e4095915d74039 (accessed on 29th May 2025).

41. Wändell, P., Crump, C., Li, X., Saleh, S. N., Carlsson, A., Sundquist, J., & Sundquist, K. (2024). Hypertension in pregnancy among immigrant and Swedish women: A cohort study of all pregnant women in Sweden. *Journal of the American Heart Association: Cardiovascular and Cerebrovascular Disease, 13*. https://www.semanticscholar.org/paper/b9a6cc1aad0e209bd16d66dac6d971f755258739 (accessed on 29th May 2025).

42. Wang, B. (2025). Diagnosis and management of hypertensive heart disease: Incorporating 2023 European Society of Hypertension and 2024 European Society of Cardiology guideline updates. *Journal of Cardiovascular Development and Disease, 12*. https://www.semanticscholar.org/paper/f95dc02c3a186b733c7b0a483428a1bc3ab2ed73 (accessed on 29th May 2025).

43. Weng, J., Ji, L., Jia, W., Lu, J., Zhou, Z., Zou, D., Zhu, D., et al. (2016). Standards of care for type 2 diabetes in China. *Diabetes/Metabolism Research and Reviews, 32*, 442–458. https://doi.org/10.1002/dmrr.2827 (accessed on 29th May 2025).

44. Whelton, P. K., Carey, R. M., Aronow, W. S., Casey, D. E., Collins, K. J., Himmelfarb, C. D., DePalma, S. M., et al. (2017). 2017 ACC/AHA/AAPA/ABC/ACPM/AGS/APhA/ASH/ASPC/NMA/PCNA guideline for the prevention, detection, evaluation, and management of high blood pressure in adults: A report of the American College of Cardiology/American Heart Association Task Force on Clinical Practice Guidelines. *Hypertension, 71*. https://doi.org/10.1161/hyp.0000000000000065.

45. Wijayanti, Y. T., Sasarari, Z. A., Sumiyati, S., Prasetyowati, P., & Rusli, R. (2024). Motivation can improve medication adherence in hypertension patients. *Jurnal Edukasi Ilmiah Kesehatan*. https://www.semanticscholar.org/paper/d78390273800d107a477cc56b1ecca2c96b5db97 (accessed on 29th May 2025).

46. Williams, B., Mancia, G., Spiering, W., Agabiti, R. E., Azizi, M., Burnier, M., Clement, D. L., et al. (2018). 2018 ESC/ESH guidelines for the management of arterial hypertension. *European Heart Journal, 39*, 3021–3104. https://doi.org/10.1093/eurheartj/ehy339.

47. Xu, Z., Shi, J., Deng, D., Zhang, W. S., Liu, X., & Lin, J. H. (2019). Initial-onset symptoms of preeclampsia and their relation to pregnancy outcomes. *Journal of Obstetrics and Gynecology, 40*, 947–952. https://www.semanticscholar.org/paper/e35b42d624f7e89c35b00f2ee6737abe9486ccd1 (accessed on 29th May 2025).

48. Yang, H. O., Wang, A., Hu, H., & Li, Y. (2025). Nursing future horizon: Simultaneous continual nursing model and homemade dialogue tool for controlling cardiac function and blood pressure in hypertensive heart diseases. *Patient Preference and Adherence, 19*, 661–672. https://www.semanticscholar.org/paper/b9e32d4854539eced37bea6e697877159479e882 (accessed on 29th May 2025).

49. Zhao, J., Wang, M. H., Li, N., Luo, Q., Yao, L., Cai, X., Yue, N., et al. (2023). Development and validation of a novel model for predicting coronary heart disease in snoring hypertensive patients with hyperhomocysteinemia. *International Heart Journal*. https://www.semanticscholar.org/paper/330908ee9965d0bc43aee0ccd194a5bcfeb0a926 (accessed on 29th May 2025).

50. Zimmermann, L., Mueller, R., Gnatzy-Feik, L., Berghausen, E., Zierden, M., Vantler, M., Baldus, S., et al. (2024). Pathobiological characterization of pulmonary hypertension associated with heart failure with preserved ejection fraction. *European Heart Journal*. https://www.semanticscholar.org/paper/cb2092ab44e246f7856a854ab08dcb745d6eb2c2 (accessed on 29th May 2025).

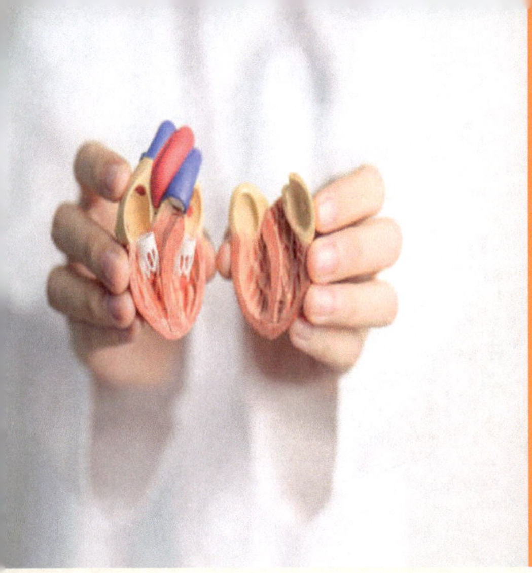

Chapter 8

VALVULAR HEART DISEASES

Contents

Introduction

The valvular heart disease diagnosis should involve a holistic understanding of structural and functional abnormalities that can take place in cardiac valves. Such diseases are full of anomalies such as stenosis, regurgitation, and congenital malformations, with the capacity to inflict very disruptive effects on cardiac function. Such conditions as the double-chambered right ventricle (DCRV) should be noted in defining the complexity of such disorders, where the right ventricle is divided into two chambers because of the anomalous band of muscle. DCRV is traditionally diagnosed most in the childhood stage, but in others, it can even manifest in adulthood, making diagnosis more challenging due to potential nonspecific symptoms that may be diagnosed late (Hesarur, 2018). Clinicians are advised to be vigilant when examining cardiac symptoms, particularly in vulnerable groups where these might otherwise be overlooked, and to place a lot of emphasis on proper clinical assessment for early diagnosis. The pathophysiology of valvular heart disease is more or less associated with the hemodynamic changes that arise due to valvular abnormalities. For instance, in conditions such as aortic stenosis or mitral regurgitation, resulting pressure overload or volume overload can induce maladaptive remodeling of the heart, with resulting development of heart failure if left untreated. These include biomarkers like B-type natriuretic peptide (BNP) and N-terminal fragment of BNP (NT-proBNP), which also prove to be helpful in the diagnostic evaluation of these conditions. These peptides have been correlated with the severity of cardiac insufficiency by being found at higher levels. They also provide essential information regarding prognosis and treatment of valvular disease patients, allowing clinicians to intervene appropriately (Christ et al., 2008).

Thus, comprehension of the complicated interaction of systemic expression and valvular illness is paramount to achieving maximal patient outcome. Lastly, early diagnosis and best treatment of valvular heart disease are essential in reducing morbidity and improving quality of life in patients. Surgical treatments, including valve replacement and repair, are often successful both in the restoration of normal function and in relief of symptoms but are subject to careful selection of patients based on clinical presentation and hemodynamic evaluation.

The heterogeneity of clinical presentation among populations underscores the need for a better technique of diagnosis and treatment. Ongoing research into long-term outcomes following surgical and medical therapy will continue to define the current gold standard for treating these challenging diseases. Through forging interdisciplinary cooperation between surgeons, cardiologists, and general practitioners, ideal management for patients with valvular heart disease can be optimized, culminating in enhanced prognostic features and improved quality of life (Figure 8.1).

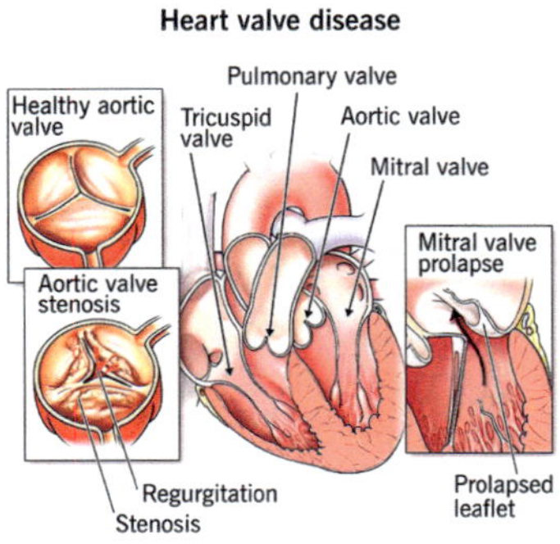

Figure 8.1. Heart valve disease includes issues like leaky or stretchy flaps that keep your valves from opening and closing correctly.

Source: https://my.clevelandclinic.org/-/scassets/images/org/health/articles/17639-valve-disease.

Definition of Valvular Heart Diseases (VHD)

VHD encompasses a broad spectrum of disorders that affect the valves of the heart, responsible for providing regular circulation of blood between the chambers of the heart. The conditions predominantly result from structural abnormalities or functional injury to one or more of the four heart valves, which include the mitral, aortic, tricuspid, and pulmonary. Failure of these valves may result in significant hemodynamic consequences, which can ultimately induce heart failure or other cardiovascular diseases. Valvular heart diseases in clinical practice can be categorized generally into two categories: stenosis, under which the valve fails to open completely, hindering blood circulation, and regurgitation, under which the valve fails to close properly, and blood leaks in a backward direction. Knowledge of the intricate dynamics of these conditions is crucial for effective diagnosis, treatment, and maximizing patient outcomes in cardiovascular medicine practice. The historical context of valvular heart diseases suggests a transformation of the understanding and classification of the diseases. Early classification of cardiac disease was straightforward, with the complexity of valvular pathology being treated as secondary.

Medical imaging and surgical technologies have transformed the management of VHD into a feasible possibility, to the extent of enhancing the complexity of understanding how these diseases affect patients. Terms like rheumatic heart disease suggest the impact of infectious pathology on the valves, while diseases like degenerative valve disease emphasize the role of age and degenerative processes in valve material. In addition, recent insight into genetic susceptibility to certain types of VHD adds another level of sophistication to the definition of these illnesses. These advancements necessitate ongoing research and discussion within the medical community about best practice treatment and intervention in VHD patients (Rubis, 2023). As valvular heart diseases advance both in terms of technology and knowledge, accurate definitions and classifications remain a central part of effective clinical practice. Understanding that VHD can be due to a broad array of etiologies, such as congenital malformations, inflammatory causes, or degenerative processes, allows clinicians to tailor management according to the patient-specific needs. Moreover, the implications of VHD extend far beyond mere anatomic descriptions; they significantly impact patients' quality of life, morbidity, and mortality. Then, an integrated strategy with regular follow-up and assessment of valve functioning is essential to achieve improved clinical results. Recognition of current research findings and medical practices, along with the integration of new diagnostic devices, can further enhance our understanding of VHD and support improved treatment patterns in affected patients (Maisch et al., 2020) (Figure 8.2).

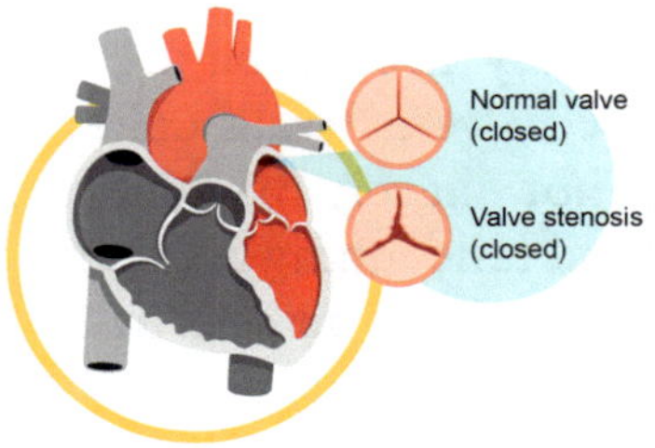

Figure 8.2. Valvular heart disease (VHD).

Source: https://www.pantai.com.my/images/pantaihospitalmalaysialibraries/specialties/cardiology/valvular_heart_disease_infobanner_1.png?sfvrsn=b60ed829_7.

8.1. Anatomy of the Heart Valves

The heart valves are vital structures of the circulatory system responsible for unidirectional blood flow and preventing regurgitation. Each valve—comprising the mitral, tricuspid, aortic, and pulmonic valves—is specifically designed anatomically to allow it to carry out its specific function. The mitral valve, in particular, is constructed of two leaflets and exists between the left atrium and left ventricle. Its complex geometry allows it to endure varied conditions of pressure during the cardiac cycle. Disequilibrium in structure or function in any of the valves can lead to valvular heart disease, which can lead to serious morbidity. These illnesses stress the importance of understanding valve anatomy as a foundation of effective diagnosis and treatment protocols designed to limit the impact of valvular disease and improve the patient's outcomes (Berry et al., 2017). Also, every valve shares a close relationship with the surrounding cardiac structures and the hemodynamics imposed on them. The aortic valve, located at the juncture of the left ventricle and the aorta, regulates systemic blood flow. Thus, the aortic valve must withstand pressure conditions accommodating hemodynamic changes occurring between systole and diastole. Similar crucial functions about pulmonary circulation are possessed by the pulmonic valve as well. Collectively, these valves are not merely passive tubes; their movement and functioning are a direct function of physical forces associated with the heart. This nuance is further compounded in stenosis or regurgitation, which in themselves may precipitate further cardiovascular pathology. Biomechanics of heart valves thus may inform prevention of valvular heart disease (Höglund et al., 2007). New developments in computational modeling of the mechanics of heart valves have shed light on their biomechanical performance under healthy and disease conditions.

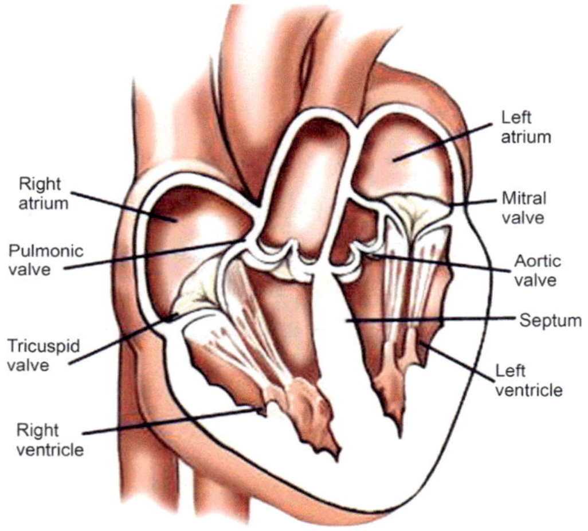

Figure 8.3. The anatomy of your heart includes four chambers.

Source: https://my.clevelandclinic.org/-/scassets/images/org/health/articles/heart-blood-vessels-valves-insideheart2.ashx.

These models have enabled improved hypotheses to be formulated regarding the possible causes and effects of valve-related conditions, especially for the mitral valve, which is the most under-researched valve despite its impact on clinical outcomes. Modern imaging technologies have also provided insights into the dynamic interactions among the valves and adjacent structures, which once again emphasize the importance of integrative anatomical studies. Such data are invaluable to the design of new therapies that might potentially move diagnostic and therapeutic interventions for valvular heart disease patients forward. By a deep understanding of valve anatomy and heart function, health professionals can more effectively treat the clinical complications produced by these critical cardiac structures' disease (Berry et al., 2017) (Figure 8.3).

8.1.1. Types of Heart Valves: Aortic, Mitral, Pulmonary, and Tricuspid

The heart consists of four main valves: the aortic, mitral, pulmonary, and tricuspid valves, all of which play essential roles in regulating blood flow in the cardiovascular system. The aortic valve, positioned between the left ventricle and the aorta, ensures that oxygenated blood cannot flow back into the body. Functional valvular impairment can lead to aortic regurgitation or stenosis, both of which are causes of severe morbidity due to alteration of the dynamics of blood flow. Similarly, the mitral valve between the left atrium and left ventricle must be present to prevent backflow during ventricular contraction. Conditions such as mitral stenosis predominantly occur due to rheumatic heart disease, which points towards the susceptibility of valves to grossly impact global heart function diseases (Dhanalakshmi et al., 2014). The pulmonary valve, situated between the pulmonary artery and the right ventricle, plays the role of channeling deoxygenated blood to the lungs to be oxygenated. Pulmonary valve failure, which is less common than aortic or mitral valve failure, will similarly lead to serious consequences such as pulmonary stenosis or regurgitation, impacting the right heart and pulmonary circulation in and of itself. The tricuspid valve between the right atrium and proper ventricle functions to prevent backflow with ventricular contraction, as well as its counterparts. Tricuspid valve pathology, though often overlooked, plays a crucial part in determining right ventricular output and the overall cardiac efficiency. To effectively manage valvular heart disease, it is essential to identify the individual function and dysfunction of every valve (N/A, 2019). Enhanced echocardiographic techniques are often needed to comprehensively assess the valves and ascertain their particular structure and function. Transthoracic echocardiography is one of the first-line non-invasive techniques for the evaluation of heart valve morphology and functional dynamics. With various modes of imaging, physicians can detect changes that reflect stenosis, regurgitation, and other valvular heart disease-related conditions. For example, valvular abnormalities like rheumatic heart disease have the mitral valve as their preferred target, underscoring the importance of specific echocardiographic assessment to determine the degree of compromise of the valve (Dhanalakshmi et al., 2014). Moreover, an understanding of the function of several valves under various conditions highlights the multifaceted nature of valvular disease, which again demands the best possible comprehension of each valve's unique nature and the effect of their disease on cardiac well-being (N/A, 2019) (Figure 8.4).

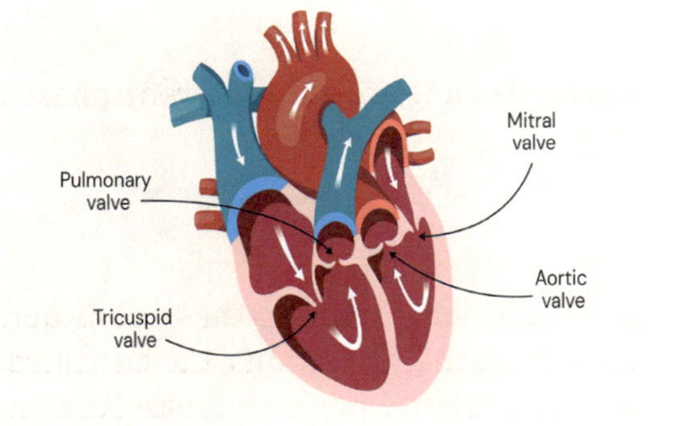

Figure 8.4. The heart has four valves; pulmonary valve, mitral valve, tricuspid valve, and aortic valve.

Source: https://guysandstthomasspecialistcare.co.uk/wp-content/uploads/2024/02/267_RBH_Illustrations_Heart-Valves_v1.jpg.

8.1.2. Function of Each Valve in the Cardiac Cycle

Throughout the cardiac cycle, the four valves of the heart—the tricuspid, pulmonary, mitral, and aortic valves—allow essential functions in blood flow direction and hemodynamic stability. The tricuspid and mitral valves are the atrioventricular (AV) valves, which would enable one-way blood flow from the atria to the ventricles. These two valves open during diastole to allow blood to fill the ventricles. Conversely, when ventricles are contracting during systole, mitral and tricuspid valves close to prevent flow back, and hence blood is permitted to exit from the heart through the pulmonary and aortic valves. This coordinated opening and closing is critical for effective pumping and forms the foundation to learn about valvular heart diseases, where in any dysfunction or structural loss of such valves can significantly inhibit the cardiac cycle and overall circulatory efficiency. Pulmonary and aortic valves are part of the group of semilunar valves and are responsible for regulating blood flow from the ventricles to the pulmonary artery and aorta, respectively. During ventricular systole, the pulmonary valve opens to allow deoxygenated blood from the right ventricle to pass into the lungs for oxygenation. The aortic valve also opens for oxygenated blood to be pumped into systemic circulation from the left ventricle simultaneously. The moment the contraction of the ventricles ceases, the valves close to prevent backflow of the blood to the ventricles. This illustrates the importance of these valves in guaranteeing the forward flow of blood and the fact that oxygenated blood will be delivered to vital organs. Abnormalities in these valves caused by stenosis or regurgitation can lead to severe cardiac diseases, and that is why clinical significance in this instance of valvular heart diseases is so crucial. The synchronized action of all four valves is essential to a healthy cardiovascular system, and any malfunction can radically alter the cardiac cycle dynamics. As an instance, valvular heart diseases can result in mitral valve prolapse or aortic stenosis, and, if not treated, can lead to heart failure in the long term. Such diseases often manifest with specific clinical features, such as shortness of breath, fatigue, and palpitations. For appropriately diagnosing these conditions, medical practitioners need to adhere to updated clinical guidelines and literature to evaluate the patients correctly. Adhering to these guidelines, yet crucially considering each patient's context, is necessary to deliver maximum patient care and devise appropriate treatment in cases of valvular heart diseases (Whelton et al., 2017; Baumgartner et al., 2020) (Figure 8.5).

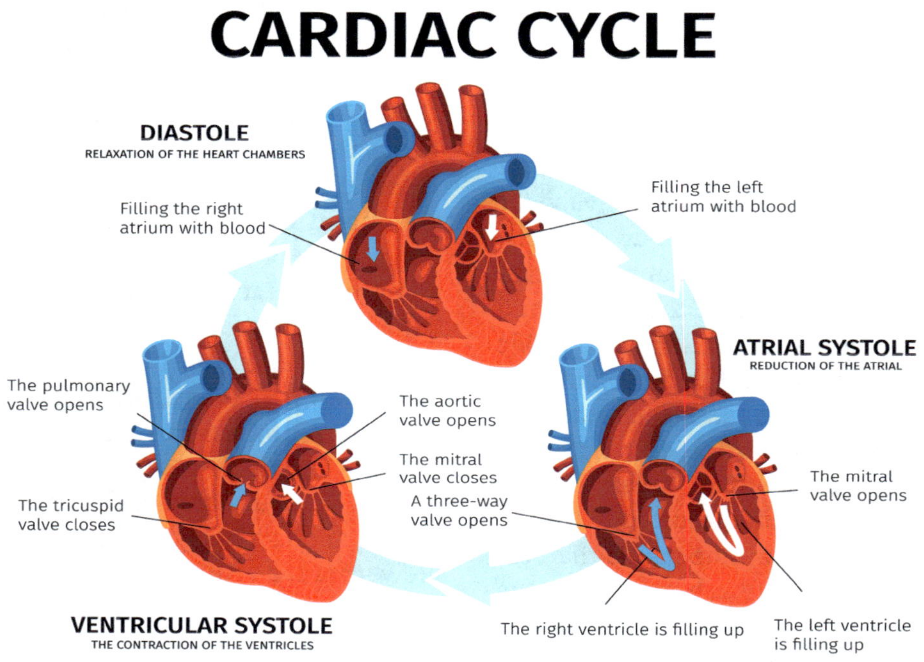

Figure 8.5. Cardiac cycle.

Source: https://artemiscardiac.com/blog/66dfd57c14c16Large-what-are-the-different-phases-of-the-cardiac-cycle.jpg.

8.1.3. Common Anatomical Abnormalities

The prevalence of usual anatomical malformations of the cardiovascular system also has a considerable impact on the development of valvular heart diseases. Among these malformations, the classification of congenital heart defects like aortic stenosis and mitral valve prolapse plays a pivotal role. Aortic stenosis, in veterinary medicine, is generally defined as the most common congenital cardiac defect in certain breeds of dogs, which sets up a working familiarity with the condition in human and veterinary medicine. Fixed sub-valvular lesions or distorted valvular structure may lead to progressive obstruction of blood flow, hence increased cardiac workload with the possibility of causing heart failure. The implications of the abnormalities underscore the importance of early detection and diagnosis, which is by the universal objectives of current cardiology. Additionally, the anatomical variations of cardiac anatomy can manifest in numerous ways, which disrupt standard treatment protocols. Valvular abnormalities are not only represented as congenital defects, but also as acquired states based upon other associated comorbidities. For instance, exercise intolerance and syncope, which occur in patients with the condition, are clear indicators of the necessity for further investigation (Chintala et al., 2005). As a non-invasive diagnostic technique, echocardiography plays a vital role in assessing valvular malformations, allowing clinicians to measure hemodynamic severity and improve patient outcomes. Step by step, understanding the interrelation between anatomy and function is crucial to direct therapeutic intervention that can minimize the danger of these common anatomical abnormalities in the context of valvular heart diseases. Foremost, the multifactorial pathogenesis of valvular heart diseases, commonly based on anatomical abnormalities, calls for an extended scope for treatment efficacy evaluation. Studies with striking examples, like a 19-month-old patient with Kawasaki Disease who had developed giant coronary artery aneurysms, illustrate the range and severity of usual anatomical defects that occur even after birth (Chintala et al., 2005). Complications based on such anatomical abnormalities make it difficult to predict prognosis and management. As we delve further into the topic, it is clear that the definition of such abnormalities will enhance our understanding of their pathological roles in the heart and demand advancement in therapeutic approaches. More studies will be of most tremendous significance in establishing precise guidelines for diagnosis and management and, ultimately, enhancing patient care in human and veterinary cardiology.

8.2. Types of Valvular Heart Diseases (VHD)

VHD can be divided into several principal types with various etiologies and clinical relevance. The most common are aortic stenosis (AS), mitral regurgitation (MR), and tricuspid regurgitation (TR), each with distinct diagnostic and management issues. Aortic stenosis, i.e., aortic valve narrowing, typically presents as age-related calcific degeneration or rheumatic fever. Clinically, patients can present with exertional dyspnea, angina, and syncope, and, therefore, end up affecting their quality of life immensely. Mitral regurgitation, however, is referred to as retrograde left ventricular to left atrial blood flow in systole secondary to degenerative valvular disease or ischemic causes. Clinicians should pay attention to these differences to guide relevant therapeutic interventions and enhance patient outcomes. A further form of valvular cardiac disease that is worth noting includes mitral stenosis, which is mainly caused by rheumatic heart disease. This condition involves the mitral valve narrowing, thereby causing blood to flow from the left atrium to the left ventricle in a way that is obstructed. The elevated pressure of the left atrium can cause atrial fibrillation, pulmonary hypertension, and heart failure in the long run. Notably, the presentation is insidious, with symptoms of fatigue, palpitations, and right heart failure. Mitral stenosis may be treated with a range of medical therapy to percutaneous balloon mitral valvuloplasty or surgery based on the severity of stenosis and the general clinical status of patients. The prognostic implications of untreated mitral stenosis can be disastrous, and hence these types of patients need to be monitored carefully, and intervention must be done in a timely fashion when required. Tricuspid regurgitation is another significant valvular heart disease that most often develops secondary to other cardiac disease. Unlike the valvular disease discussed above, TR is most frequently associated with right-sided heart failure and is caused by etiologies such as idiopathic dilation, rheumatic heart disease, or pulmonary hypertension. The pathophysiology is venous blood flow retrograde into the right atrium during ventricular contraction, producing signs and symptoms of peripheral edema, ascites, and jugular venous pressure elevation. The treatment approaches for tricuspid regurgitation are usually directed toward treating the underlying cause, with surgery in the case of severe right heart failure. The prevalence of severe valvular heart disease, including tricuspid regurgitation, has been extensively examined, and its adverse impact on survival and quality of life is well proven, particularly in high-risk patients (Samaras et al., 2021; Waleed, 2020) (Figure 8.6).

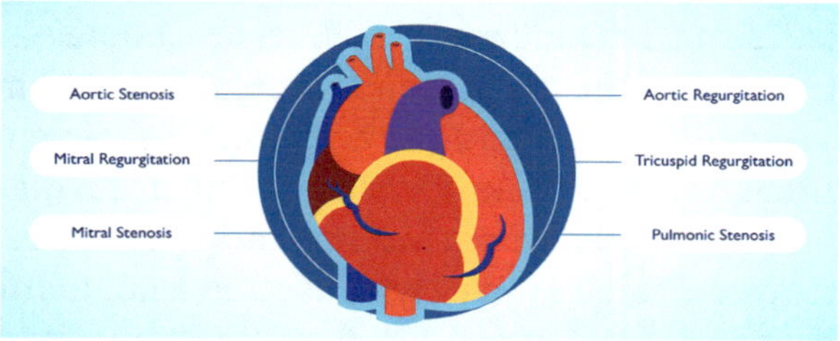

Figure 8.6. Types of valvular heart diseases (VHD).

Source: https://images.ctfassets.net/eexbcii1ci83/53qAjVhBTD9grPJ58WR9aD/4f90929ccfefc691ae2e26fea1f22711/Types_of_Valvular_Heart_Disease.jpg.

8.2.1. Stenosis: Definition and Causes

Stenosis, an emergent condition best explained in valvular heart disease, is a pathological thickening of heart valves, obstructing the flow of blood and causing several cardiovascular morbidities. It predominantly affects the aortic and mitral valves, although calcific aortic stenosis most frequently affects the elderly. In this context, the mechanical obstruction in the cardiac cycle can cause the resultant augmented load on the heart, in the long run, resulting in myocardial hypertrophy and consequent heart failure if left unchecked. Understanding the mechanics of stenosis is fundamental to determining viable treatment pathways, particularly because the condition is typically asymptomatic in its initial stages and is often diagnosed incidentally during routine echocardiographic evaluation. The etiology of stenosis is multifactorial, with both congenital and acquired etiologies.

Congenital malformations, such as a bicuspid aortic valve at birth, make the patient susceptible to early-onset aortic stenosis. Acquired etiologies, such as rheumatic fever and degeneration of valves with aging, also contribute. In particular, rheumatic heart disease resulting from untreated streptococcal infections causes inflammatory changes in the heart valves, which in turn causes stenosis. Of interest is calcific degeneration, which is influenced by hypertension, dyslipidemia, and alterations in calcium metabolism with advancing age. Awareness of such predisposing causes is essential in making specific therapeutic strategies to prevent or slow stenotic heart disease, as exemplified in primary valvular pathology discussions (Small et al., 2024). Furthermore, the impact of stenosis on patient outcomes can significantly vary based on demographic factors like age and gender. Studies indicate that women may present with some characteristics of valvular cardiac disease, particularly mitral stenosis, at an advanced age and with increased symptoms compared to men, which will influence treatment modalities and prognostic results. Specifically, studies have found women to be less concordant with evidence-based treatments for diseases like mitral stenosis and primary mitral regurgitation, a care disparity (Mascherbauer et al., 2024). Such an appreciation of sex-specific differences in disease and treatment presentation highlights the imperative need for individualized strategies in valvular heart disease management, particularly in terms of stenotic lesions. Addressing these disparities easily is vital for improving overall patient care and ensuring equitable access to interventions (Figure 8.7).

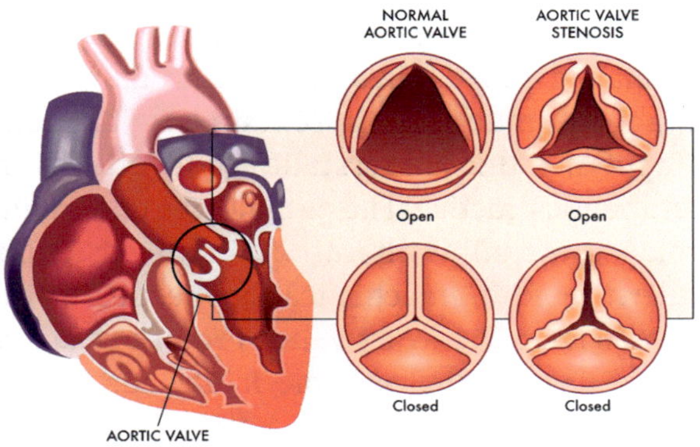

Figure 8.7. Aortic stenosis.

Source: https://drraghu.com/wp-content/uploads/2022/04/Aortic-stenosis.jpg.

8.2.2. Regurgitation: Definition and Causes

Regurgitation of valvular heart disease is a term employed to describe the backflow of blood due to improper closure of heart valves. It may occur in any heart valve, i.e., the aortic, mitral, and tricuspid valves, and causes severe hemodynamic consequences. Etiology of regurgitation typically encompasses intrinsic causes, ie, structural valve leaflet abnormalities, and extrinsic causes, ie, left ventricular dilation affecting valve function. Nonfunctioning valves result in volume load for the heart and induce symptoms such as dyspnea and exercise intolerance. Understanding the pathophysiologic mechanisms of regurgitation is required to devise proper management and improve patient outcomes in patients with valvular heart diseases. TR is usually observed in patients with severe left-sided VHD. Increased right heart pressure due to volume overload might result in dilation of the tricuspid valve annulus and thus deterioration of the regurgitant flow. As described in recent literature, the prevalence of TR should be assessed attentively as it has significant implications on the overall clinical outcome since its treatment. The interdependence of TR with left-sided VHD emphasizes the integration of cardiac structure and function, underlining the importance of detailed evaluations in the affected patients. Worsening symptoms in the affected patients can accompany TR, ultimately necessitating interventions ranging from medical management to surgical valve repair or replacement (Dreyfus et al., 2024). In addition, the nature of TR can be determined by its etiology. Atrial secondary TR is most commonly found in conjunction with right atrial enlargement due to a variety of reasons, including atrial fibrillation and pulmonary hypertension. Ventricular secondary TR is typically found in conjunction with left-sided heart illness, which includes reduced left ventricular ejection fraction and ischemic heart disease (Muraru et al., 2024). This is significant as it enables the use of specific therapy strategies tailored to the patient's profile and disease etiology. The appreciation and understanding of these differences improve diagnostic accuracy and therapeutic interventions in the treatment of regurgitation due to valvular heart disease. Lastly, a close knowledge of the etiology and nature of regurgitation allows clinicians to manage the complexity of valvular heart disease and provide the optimal possible care to these patients (Figure 8.8).

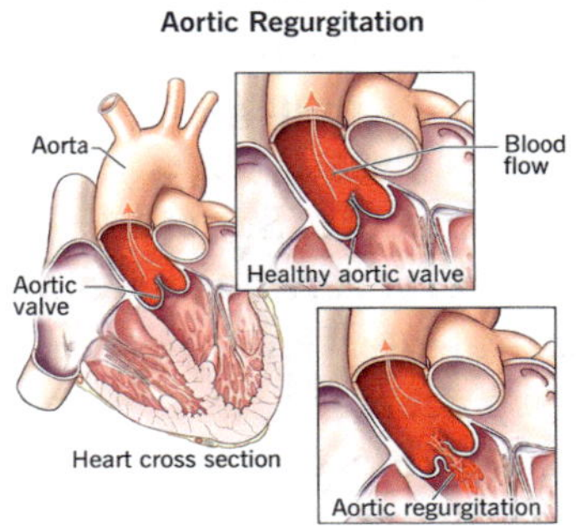

Figure 8.8. Aortic regurgitation.

Source: https://my.clevelandclinic.org/-/scassets/images/org/health/articles/aortic-regurgitation.

8.2.3. Prolapse: Definition and Causes

Prolapse within valvular heart disease is the pathologic displacement of a heart valve out of its usual position within the cardiac cycle. The condition most frequently involves the mitral and tricuspid valves and occurs as a result of elongation of the leaflets or injury to supporting structures, such as the chordae tendineae. The cause of the prolapse can be quite dissimilar, with genetic factors, degenerative changes, or functional heart diseases playing a key role. In the majority, mitral valve prolapse is idiopathic with a familial predisposition. Those with connective tissue disorders such as Marfan syndrome are more at risk, indicating that congenital or genetic factors also have a significant role to play in its development. Knowledge of the mechanisms of prolapse is critical, as it can lead to complications such as regurgitation and, if left untreated, heart failure. The effects of prolapse on cardiac function cannot be overstated since it has the potential to develop into severe valvular diseases. Mitral valve prolapse, for instance, can result in mitral regurgitation, where non-closure of the valve results in backflow of blood into the left atrium. The presentation may range from asymptomatic to those manifesting with signs and symptoms of heart failure, including palpitations, fatigue, and shortness of breath, which can undoubtedly affect the patient's quality of life. As evidenced in the literature, severe valvular heart diseases require surgical intervention in the form of valve repair or replacement, thus emphasizing the importance of early detection and monitoring through echocardiography. Of relevance, ongoing research still helps clarify molecular mechanisms underlying these changes, as evidenced by ongoing studies examining the cellular organization of heart valves and molecular pathways involved in primary valvular disease, including prolapse (Small et al., 2024). The multifactorial etiology of prolapse also recognizes a deficit in holistic patient management approaches. While advances in medical imaging and the understanding of valvular disease have increased diagnostic capability, much work remains to be done in applying this understanding to effectively therapeutic practice. The pathologies underlying prolapse, including alterations in the structural integrity and biomechanical properties of the tissue within the heart valve, require research toward discovering possible molecular targets for therapy (Agarwal et al., 2024). Moreover, enhancing clinical registries for tracking patients with valvular heart diseases can provide valuable data on the epidemiology of conditions like prolapse, which will prove helpful for public health surveillance as well as better management strategies. Finally, addressing the causes and effects of prolapse is also essential not only to optimize individual patient outcomes but also to minimize the public health burden of valvular heart diseases (Figure 8.9).

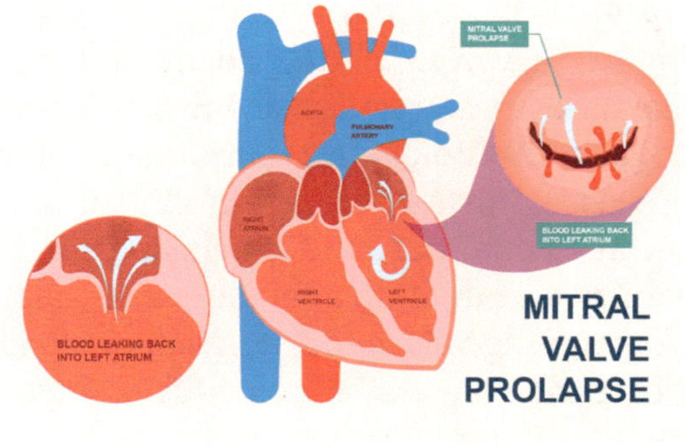

Figure 8.9. Mitral valve prolapse.

Source: https://www.okheart.com/wp-content/uploads/2024/10/hri-2021-06-01.jpg.

8.3. Risk Factors and Epidemiology

VHD encompasses a range of conditions that affect the functioning of the heart valve. It is crucial to research their epidemiology as a precursor to identifying risk factors and maximizing outcomes. Recent studies have highlighted the aging population as a strong determinant of VHD prevalence. Findings in a multicenter registry study conducted in rural Italy indicated that close to 75% of individuals aged above 65 years had one or more valvular defects and that the prevalence rose dramatically in individuals 75 years and older. This shifting population emphasizes the requirement for focused public health measures, particularly as the population becomes older. Additionally, the prevalence of left-sided valvular heart diseases, including aortic stenosis and mitral regurgitation, points towards the fact that degenerative changes in old age play a significant role in the etiology of these conditions, and thus preventive measures in the elderly population are necessary (Amico et al., 2024). Apart from age, various factors predispose patients to valvular heart disease. There is a strong correlation between pre-existing heart disease and the prevalence of VHD. For instance, findings from studies indicate that congenital heart disease and degenerative heart disease are related to VHD, wherein high proportions of infected patients have these conditions. Furthermore, healthcare-related risk factors such as hospitalization, invasive cardiac procedures, and intravenous drug use have emerged as major elements in the epidemiology of infective endocarditis, which is a complication of valvular heart disease. These associations necessitate an integrated approach to patient care and surveillance, particularly among vulnerable groups where preventive interventions can be best executed (Arslan et al., 2024). The pathophysiology of valvular heart disease necessitates an ongoing assessment of its epidemiology and risk factors to improve clinical outcomes. Research indicates that age and comorbidities are major determinants, necessitating enhanced vigilance and early intervention among groups with these risk factors. By forging cooperative strategies among healthcare practitioners, researchers, and local government health agencies, VHD awareness can be enhanced to enable early detection and targeted prevention interventions for different populations. The co-action of individual risk factors such as lifestyle and biological susceptibility, and population epidemiologic trends demonstrates the imperative role of community-based prevention and education initiatives to combat this rising public health concern (Amico et al., 2024; Arslan et al., 2024) (Figure 8.10).

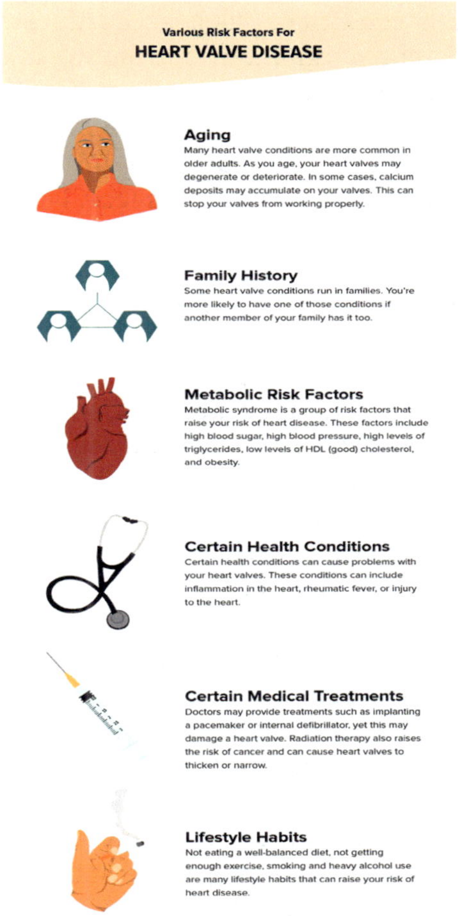

Figure 8.10. Risk factors for heart valve disease.

Source: https://post.healthline.com/wp-content/uploads/2022/04/heart-valve-disease-1296x3601-body.20220426220931496-1-scaled.jpg.

8.3.1. Age and Gender-Related Prevalence

The epidemiology of VHD is most marked by age and gender, with significant implications for patient management and the distribution of healthcare resources. In populations with increasing age, the incidence of VHD significantly increases, particularly among older people. Studies indicate that approximately 65.9% of individuals aged 65 years and above exhibit some form of valvular disease, with other common conditions such as aortic stenosis and mitral regurgitation contributing to a very high percentage of the instances. The pattern of increased prevalence of disease with age underscores the importance of continued screening and monitoring, especially in older patients who often have more than one comorbid condition to cloud diagnosis and management strategies. Prompt identification of these conditions has the potential to enhance patient outcomes significantly, and hence demographic variation awareness is essential to cardiovascular medicine clinicians (Hieda et al., 2023). Gender variance also illuminates the case of the prevalence of VHD since evidence shows that the prevalence of valvular heart diseases is higher in women than in men. Women were noted to have an incidence of valvular disease that is approximately 1.3–2.5 times greater than their male counterparts. The disparity is explained by biological, hormonal, and lifestyle factors that have different effects on the cardiovascular status in women and men. Also, with increasing life expectancy, women will survive longer and thus be more susceptible to age-related cardiac diseases like VHD. Understanding these disparities is crucial; healthcare professionals must tailor prevention practices and treatments not only according to demographics but also to gender-specific risk profiles. This differential strategy is required for improving access to care and developing better health outcomes among men and women (Mehrabinejad et al., 2022). The implications of understanding age- and gender-specific patterns of prevalence extend beyond the treatment of individual patients and involve broader public health matters.

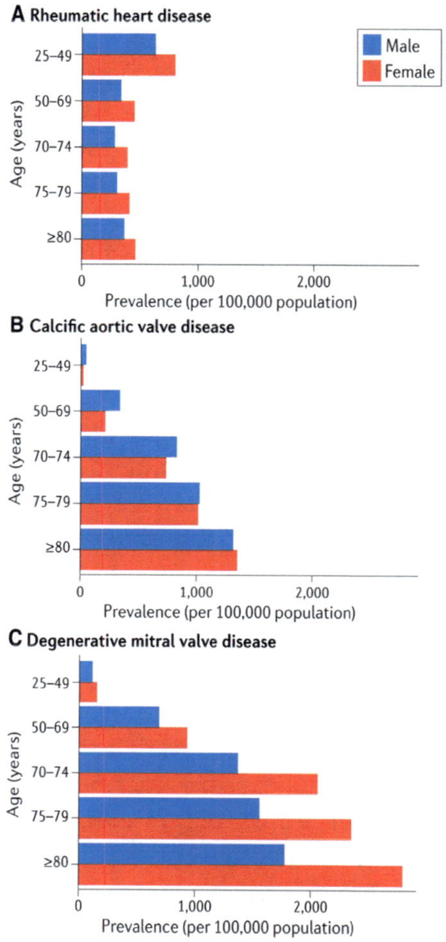

Figure 8.11. Age- and sex-specific global prevalence for (A) rheumatic heart disease, (B) calcific aortic stenosis, and (C) degenerative mitral valve disease.

Source: https://www.ahajournals.org/cms/10.1161/CIRCRESAHA.121.319914/asset/e829daba-3819-45c3-8e57-238af4c3b544/assets/graphic/circresaha.121.319914.fig02.jpg.

With the increased burden of non-rheumatic valvular heart diseases (NRVHDs), especially amongst the elderly, the healthcare systems need to be altered in response to these new demands. The evaluation of healthcare quality indicators and accessibility reveals disparities that correlate with age and gender, calling for an active management of VHD. For instance, a remarkable chart based on global health statistics demonstrates an acceptable quality of care index (QCI) for NRVHDs regardless of gender. Yet, prudence is still needed for low sociodemographic index (SDI) regions. Through the correction of these disparities, an equitable system can be formulated that effectively targets the at-risk populations most susceptible to valvular heart diseases (Mehrabinejad et al., 2022; Hieda et al., 2023) (Figure 8.11).

8.3.2. Genetic Predispositions and Family History

Knowledge of genetic predispositions about family history is essential in understanding valvular heart diseases, given that both elements have a significant contribution to disease susceptibility. A family history of heart disease may indicate a genetic factor that affects one's risk of developing the condition. Genetic predispositions may be the result of various gene mutations that are inherited from one generation to the next, thereby increasing the likelihood that offspring will also develop these cardiovascular complications. For instance, specific gene variants for disease conditions such as inherited cardiomyopathy or arrhythmogenic right ventricular dysplasia can increase the susceptibility to developing valvular complications. As science moves forward, it is essential to discover these genetic links in designing preventative measures and tailored therapy for patients with a significant family history of heart disease. The nature of genetic susceptibilities extends beyond solely heritable disease because environment and lifestyle come into the picture, along with family history. Therefore, it is essential to quantify both genetic and environmental variables while assessing an individual's risk for valvular heart disease. Notably, categorizing patients based on familial background gives a clearer picture of potential predispositions. In addition, studies have shown that some gene variations may offer higher chances of associated cardiovascular issues that are, in turn, manifested in the heart valves. As an example, it has been shown that there exists a relationship between gene effects and the susceptibility to developing rheumatic heart disease among those predisposed through family connections. Thus, understanding such dynamics not only sheds light on disease pathology but also encourages evidence-based clinical practice for intervention and management. Novel evidence suggests the role of specific genes and hereditary connections in the etiology of valvular heart diseases, further lending support to enhanced research into genetic markers. Findings from studies on recurrent cardiac ailments suggest that a significant percentage of patients with a hereditary history carry pathogenic or putatively pathogenic genetic mutations that influence disease behavior. These findings call for the use of genetic screening in subjects with family histories to facilitate early detection and intervention strategies specifically tailored to forestall threats to valvular heart disease. Furthermore, the finding of genetic differences through modern technologies, such as whole exome sequencing, supports the integration of genetic counseling into clinical practice. Detection of genetic components may one day transform the area of cardiovascular medicine, with potential for improved outcomes with tailored healthcare interventions (Collini et al., 2024; Hassan et al., 2025).

8.3.3. Lifestyle Factors: Diet, Exercise, and Smoking

Lifestyle factors such as diet, physical activity, and smoking are significant determinants in the development and management of VHD. Individuals who adopt a poor diet, involving high saturated fats, sodium, and processed foods, are at greater risk of developing cardiovascular disease, including VHD. Research has indicated that dietary habits play a significant role in influencing phenotypic age acceleration, which is directly correlated with the occurrence of most heart diseases. Also, the inclusion of dietary modifications, like the DASH diet, can reduce hypertension and overall cardiac health, thus reducing the risk of valvular malfunction. In doing so, a healthy diet is not merely essential for overall well-being but also a determining component in avoiding VHD-related complications, revealing the strong interconnections between lifestyle and cardiac health in affected patients (Liu et al., 2025). Physical exercise is another basic lifestyle factor that has a significant influence on the occurrence and management of VHD. Cardiovascular fitness is promoted, stress is reduced, and normal weight is maintained through exercise, which in turn decreases the risk factors of heart disease. For instance, studies found that subjects who engaged in strenuous exercise had reduced hazard ratios for VHD occurrence compared to their sedentary counterparts. Regular use of aerobic and resistance training can assist in controlling blood pressure and cholesterol levels, thereby ensuring a healthy cardiovascular system. Therefore, the program of regular exercise is not only necessary for the prevention of valvular dysfunction but also for maximizing the well-being of patients with underlying cardiac disease (Wei et al., 2024). Smoking, an established risk factor for most cardiovascular disorders, carries grave implications for patients with or at risk of valvular heart diseases. Tobacco smoking adversely affects endothelial function and promotes arterial stiffness, aggravating the risk of aortic stenosis or regurgitation. Evidence indicates that both current smokers and former smokers possess elevated hazard ratios for new onset VHD compared to never smokers, supporting the value of smoking cessation intervention. This life modification is also validated through the intersections of socioeconomic problems, wherein lower socioeconomic populations are more likely to have higher smoking prevalence, associated with increased prevalence of VHD and poorer health. Therefore, regulation of smoking as a modifiable risk factor is central to primary and secondary prevention in the management of valvular heart diseases (Liu et al., 2025) (Figure 8.12).

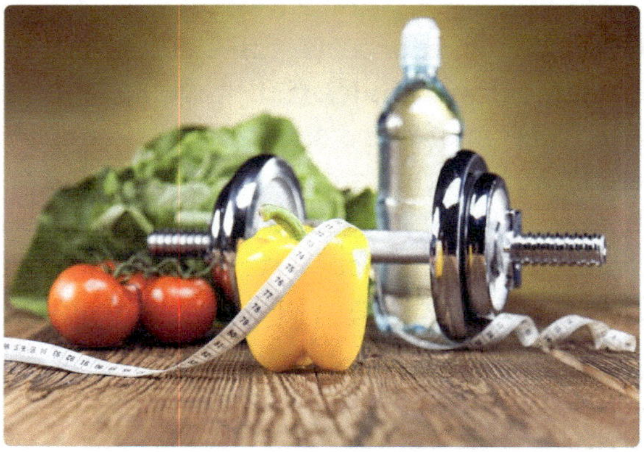

Figure 8.12. Lifestyle factors of valvular heart disease.

Source: https://d2jx2rerrg6sh3.cloudfront.net/image-handler/picture/2019/9/shutterstock_160379219.jpg.

8.4. Symptoms and Diagnosis

VHD often has a prodromal type of symptoms that are subtle and imprecise, so early diagnosis is challenging. Fatigue, dyspnea, palpitation, and chest pain are some symptoms, compromising normal function and raising the suspicion of other cardiac abnormalities. Particularly in conditions of mitral regurgitation or aortic stenosis, these symptoms worsen over some time, pointing to a background pathology requiring investigation. Early identification of the symptoms is essential, as they are usually the earliest signs of valvular malfunction. Moreover, the complex presentation of symptoms is further compounded by the patient's comorbid conditions, which can mask or simulate the symptoms of valvular heart diseases, a factor that underscores the importance of clinical acumen in diagnosis (Kovalev, 2025). Diagnosis of valvular heart diseases is based mainly on extensive clinical assessment complemented by imaging studies, which in most cases is tiered in structure. History and physical examination are front and center in the initial case, where auscultation can reveal pathological cardiac sounds such as murmurs that indicate valve dysfunction. On raising suspicion, non-invasive imaging techniques such as echocardiography play pivotal roles in the evaluation of valvular function and integrity. Echocardiography especially allows physicians to visualize the morphology and hemodynamics of heart valves and facilitate distinguishing among different types of valve diseases. These findings, however, may not necessarily be straightforward and require skill on the part of physicians to equate clinical symptoms with findings obtained through echocardiography, because long-term conditions are involved (Kovalev, 2025). As the incidence of valvular heart diseases, particularly aortic stenosis, becomes more prevalent, urgent and accurate diagnostic measures are a necessity in providing optimal patient outcomes. Aortic stenosis, the most frequent valvular disease in industrialized nations, has its diagnosis inevitably delayed due to the elusive nature of the disease. Intervention is necessary, since patients then lose significant survival time after symptom appearance, with identification of diagnostic problems paramount. A variety of diagnostic techniques, including cardiac catheterization and stress testing, alongside echocardiography, can provide additional information regarding the extent of disease and guide treatment. Detection and treatment are emphasized in the 2021 European guidelines as early and essential, with recognition of the pitfalls of misdiagnosis and resultant adverse prognostic impact on patients with aortic stenosis.

8.4.1. Common Symptoms Associated with Valvular Heart Diseases (VHD)

VHD can typically be identified by a constellation of symptoms that reflect the hemodynamic derangements that cause valve dysfunction. Exertional dyspnea, or shortness of breath with effort, is the characteristic symptom with which the patient comes to the doctor. This is caused by increased pulmonary pressures from reduced cardiac output or volume overload and represents the heart's failure to pump blood effectively. In addition to dyspnea, patients may also report palpitations or an abnormal rhythm, typically resulting from atrial fibrillation, which is apt to arise as a consequence of left atrial enlargement. These symptoms help emphasize the necessity for early diagnosis and treatment because valvular disease, if not treated, will progress to lead to heart failure and other severe complications and thus tremendously impact patients' quality of life and overall prognosis. Another pronounced symptom of valvular heart disease is pain in the chest, which could be in the form of atypical or anginal pain. This symptom could be associated with impaired myocardial perfusion, especially where there has been involvement of the aortic or mitral valve. More specifically, aortic stenosis, the most common valvular heart disease, by recent estimates, is distinguished by this symptom, along with fatigue and syncope. Chest pain necessitates an appropriate clinical evaluation to differentiate between valvular and other potential causes, such as coronary artery disease. Accurate identification and timely intervention on the basis of updated clinical guidelines are essential to avoid valvular heart disease-associated morbidity, underlining the importance of recognizing and interpreting these significant symptoms in clinical practice (Rana, 2022). Patients of severe valvular heart disease may also manifest signs of systemic involvement, such as ascites and peripheral edema. These findings occur when there is right heart compromise leading to fluid accumulation due to elevated venous pressures. Fatigue is also a frequent complaint in all forms of valvular dysfunction and typically arises from reduced cardiac output and secondary exercise intolerance. Identification of these common presentations is crucial for clinical professionals, as they are the most critical signs that justify referral for further diagnostic testing and therapeutic management. Proper treatment modalities must be employed to treat these signs, i.e., pharmacological management and surgery where necessary, thus improving patient outcome and overall quality of life (Bembey et al., 2024) (Figure 8.13).

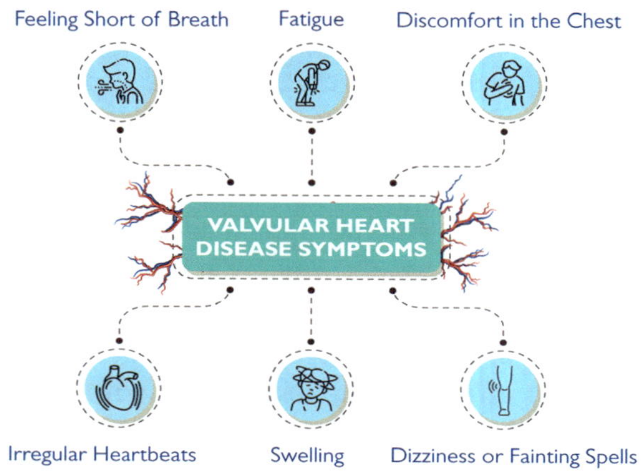

Figure 8.13. Valvular heart disease (VHD) symptoms.

Source: https://images.ctfassets.net/eexbcii1ci83/5UTlIgjCjDD5YQVPufOIyJ/fef6f15392c406ebdae51472bda1ead6/Valvular_Heart_Disease_Symptoms.jpg.

8.4.2. Diagnostic Tests: Echocardiogram, MRI, and X-Rays

The diagnostic domain of valvular heart diseases is supported by different imaging modalities, one of the most important being echocardiography. It is a non-invasive procedure that utilizes ultrasound to generate in-real-time images of the structure and function of the hearts, thereby enabling clinicians to evaluate valve morphology, motion, and hemodynamic importance. Echocardiograms enable clinicians to detect abnormalities like stenosis or regurgitation, critical for diagnosing conditions like aortic stenosis or mitral valve prolapse. Furthermore, advances in Doppler echocardiography provide insight into hemodynamics and gradients through valves. Such accurate evaluations are crucial because the early detection of valvular pathology significantly influences patient treatment and therapeutic approach and could even improve long-term outcomes in patients with valvular heart conditions like those of Höglund et al. (2007) or analogous congenital defects, as demonstrated in the literature. As an adjunct to echocardiography, magnetic resonance imaging (MRI) is a powerful tool in the assessment of valvular heart diseases, particularly for cases with complexity or where the outcome of echocardiography is not definitive. Cardiac MRI is noninvasive and offers better visualization of cardiac anatomy, including valve structure and the surrounding tissues. It is superior to quantify blood flow and myocardial strains, which are useful in detecting valve dysfunction complications. Of significant interest is the role MRI plays in the evaluation of patients with bicuspid aortic valve so that associated aortic dilation and other morphological changes can be extensively appraised, as the case is with Al-Razik et al. (2022). Such extensiveness lends a more comprehensive understanding of the disease, allowing specialized treatment plans to be formulated. Ultimately, MRI is a valuable component in the non-invasive diagnostic process, complementing echocardiography and enhancing the accuracy in the diagnosis of valvular heart disease. X-rays are still used as an auxiliary, not a conclusive, imaging tool in the clinical evaluation of valvular heart disease. Chest radiographs can provide information on the size, shape, and related pulmonary disease of the heart, however X-rays cannot image the heart valves. When the patient has severe valvular disease, X-rays may show cardiomegaly or pulmonary congestion, implying pressure overload or heart failure. X-ray findings mentioned above can aid clinicians in evaluating the extent of cardiac involvement and planning for further diagnostic procedures. Though less specific than echocardiography or MRI, their accessibility and simplicity render X-rays an indispensable component of initial evaluation in suspected valvular heart disease. Through comprehensive integration with newer imaging modalities, clinicians can form an integrated profile that dictates effective management for affected individuals (Figure 8.14).

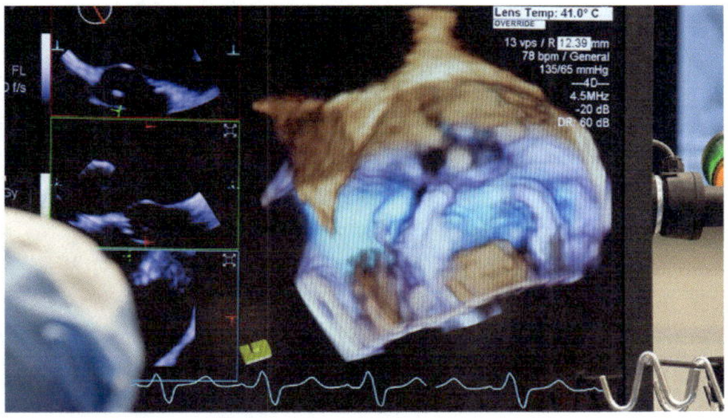

Figure 8.14. Diagnosing mitral valve disease.

Source: https://nyulangone.org/files/mitral-valve-imaging.jpg.

8.4.3. Importance of Early Detection and Monitoring

The significance of early detection and monitoring in valvular heart diseases cannot be overstressed since it is directly proportional to patients' outcomes and quality of life. Early detection enables appropriate interventions, which can significantly reduce morbidity and mortality. Through technology advancements, equipment such as wearable devices and smartphone apps is increasingly being utilized to monitor patients from remote sites. The potential of these technologies to identify people at risk of cardiovascular diseases implies proactive management opportunities, cutting down on diagnosis delays, and enhancing patient treatment in the long term. Research indicates that there is higher awareness and availability of monitoring technology that encourages better health outcomes among patients, particularly those with chronic conditions such as pulmonary arterial hypertension (PAH) (Delgado-SanMartin et al., 2025). Other than technology, traditional diagnostic methods are still essential in the initial detection of valvular heart diseases. Cardiac auscultation, an old but tried practice, is still a significant tool for clinicians. By listening to and analyzing heart sounds and recognizing atypical patterns, doctors can gather important information regarding the cardiac condition of a patient. The phonocardiogram (PCG), a tool that captures and displays heart sound signals, is helpful in the detection of some cardiac abnormalities, including valvular disease. Technological progress in automated systems such as Automatic Computerized Auscultation (ACA) enhances the accuracy and effectiveness of such old-fashioned methods, providing physicians with instantaneous diagnostic information. Such progress indicates the importance of integrating conventional diagnostic techniques with modern technology to facilitate a comprehensive monitoring system for high-risk populations (Singh et al., 2024). Installation of a multi-faceted approach to early diagnosis and ongoing surveillance of valvular heart disease is paramount. This combination of innovative technology and established practice not only aids in the detection of possible abnormalities but also helps in the continuous monitoring of disease progression. Continuous monitoring aids practitioners in dynamically adjusting treatment strategies, enhancing patient care. With progressing clinical expertise on these diseases, the implementation of combined approaches for detection and monitoring continues to be a priority. Ultimately, the merging of new monitoring technology with existing knowledge results in an enhanced understanding of valvular heart disease and the way to improve patient outcomes and a healthier healthcare system devoted to cardiovascular well-being.

8.5. Treatment Options

Effective treatment interventions for valvular heart illnesses are crucial in providing improved patient outcomes as well as minimizing the complications of such normally disabling diseases. Treatment is usually dependent on the targeted valve, the seriousness of the disease, and the overall general well-being of the patients. For minor illnesses, treatment can be performed using drugs alone, for instance, diuretics, beta-blockers, or anticoagulants, to control symptoms and prevent complications. Nonetheless, intervention is needed in advanced stages when surgical interventions, including valve replacement or correction, are required. Decisions are intricate and entail profound considerations on the risk and benefit of each form of treatment, with the necessity of ensuring an individualized treatment for the patient emphasized. Surgical interventions can significantly improve the quality of life for valvular heart disease patients. Referring to the aortic and mitral valves, valve repair or complete valve replacement can be done. Valve repair is the first choice if feasible, as it is minimally associated with morbidity and is also anatomically sparing. If repair is not possible, valve replacement with prosthetic valves may then be employed using either mechanical or biological valves. Every treatment modality carries unique benefits and complications, such as durability and the need for anticoagulation therapy, necessitating significant patient education and postoperative care. Increased awareness and technological advancement also contribute to improving survival and functional outcomes in patients who receive these interventions. Emerging computational modeling technologies have opened up new avenues to tailor treatment alternatives for mitral valve disease in particular. These models enable improved understanding of the complex biomechanics around the mitral valve and its coupling with blood dynamics and ventricular mechanics. Increased sophistication in modeling strategies has the potential to yield more effective preventative and therapeutic interventions, including personalized surgical planning and innovative interventions. Recent efforts have highlighted the growing enthusiasm in the area, indicating the necessity of ongoing exploration and application of advanced computational methodologies to advance therapeutic interventions. Balancing these new technologies against established medical modalities will be essential to optimizing total management of valvular heart disease and addressing patients' individualized needs (Berry et al., 2017; Kitsiou et al., 2013) (Figure 8.15).

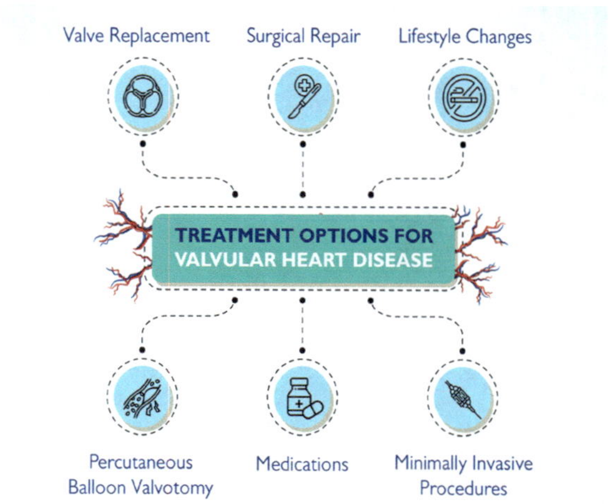

Figure 8.15. Treatment options for valvular heart disease (VHD).

Source: https://images.ctfassets.net/eexbcii1ci83/HMZwSyhODvNZWoiatHwzu/5503ce031d8de794b1ba63f19134b982/Treatment_Options_for_Valvular_Heart_Disease.jpg.

8.5.1. Medical Management: Medications and Lifestyle Changes

Medical therapy of valvular cardiac diseases is a complex intervention involving both pharmacologic treatment and lifestyle modifications. Drugs play a crucial role in symptom palliation and disease prevention. For instance, patients typically benefit from the use of anticoagulants in managing the risk of thromboembolic events, particularly in patients with atrial fibrillation secondary to valve disease. Furthermore, comorbid illness medication such as hypertension and hyperlipidemia with a variety of antihypertensive agents and statins is essential. Not only do these drugs enhance quality of life, but they are also central to lowering morbidity and mortality rates among infected patients. Utilization of drugs that have been individually profiled is a further plus to the central treatment method in treating the complexities of valvular heart disease. Besides pharmacotherapy, lifestyle change is crucial for valvular heart disease patients. Better food choices, exercise, and cessation of smoking can have dramatic impacts on the cardiovascular system. Weight control is specifically relevant; obesity may exacerbate heart disease and complicate its management medically. As quoted, the best intervention options are caloric restriction and increased physical activity, which can reduce obesity and thus lower the load on the heart as a whole (Bai et al., 2010). Further, promoting adherence to a heart-friendly diet, i.e., the Mediterranean diet, can improve metabolic parameters and promote best outcomes. By encouraging lifestyle modifications, health professionals can empower patients to become engaged with their health, thereby enhancing their control over their disease. The interaction between lifestyle modifications and pharmacotherapy is particularly observed in comorbid patients, such as those with Type II diabetes mellitus (T2DM), who are also prone to heart failure due to valvular heart diseases. Studies demonstrate that such patients are characterized by elevated inflammatory markers and depression, which make their clinical picture more complicated (Greenberg et al., 2019). Therefore, medical treatment must address the physical aspects of valvular heart disease as well as the psychological and metabolic dimensions of comorbidities. This comprehensive strategy is crucial in maximizing treatment regimens and providing patients with proper intensive care tailored to their individual needs. With this unification of drugs and lifestyle therapy, valvular heart diseases can be well managed, eventually enhancing patient outcomes and quality of life (Figure 8.16).

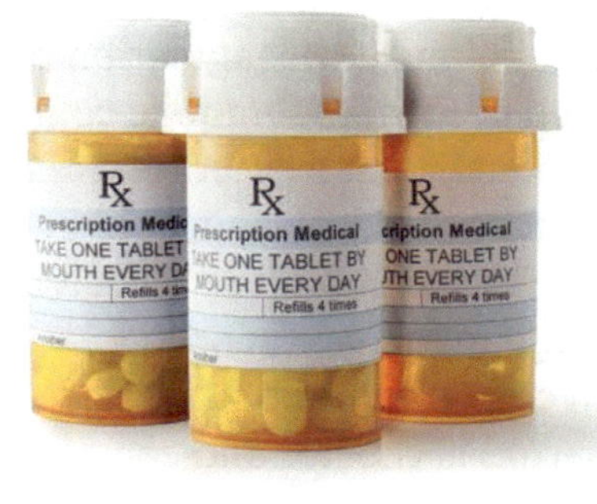

Figure 8.16. Medication for heart valve disease.

Source: https://www.heart-valve-surgery.com/Images/medication-treat-heart-valve-disease.jpg.

8.5.2. Surgical Interventions: Valve Repair and Replacement

Surgical interventions for valvular heart disease are overwhelmingly made up of valve repair and replacement techniques, which are required for the return to normal cardiac function. These are most important for the mitral and aortic valves, in which impairment has the potential to result in significant morbidity and mortality. Valves are usually repaired when possible because it usually preserves the patient's native tissue and permits normal hemodynamics. For instance, advances in technology and surgery have significantly improved the performance of mitral valve repairs. An understanding of mitral valve biomechanics has enabled the development of more sophisticated surgical methods and highlighted the importance of applying computational models and imaging modalities to surgical planning and execution (Berry et al., 2017). Such technologies enhance the accuracy of repair and assist in more tailored treatment for patients with valvular disease. Where valve repair is not feasible, valve replacement has to be done to ensure adequate blood supply and prevent complications. Operations have traditionally involved mechanical or biological bioprosthetic valves, which have both advantages and disadvantages. Mechanical valves, while durable, must be treated with lifelong anticoagulation to decrease the likelihood of thromboembolic complications. Biological valves, constructed of animal tissue, provide a more natural solution but are less durable. Advances in surgical procedures, such as minimally invasive techniques, have also altered valve replacement surgeries so that the recovery period is shorter and complications are fewer. With valvular heart disorders becoming increasingly common in elderly patient groups, as reflected by the increasing number of interventions, cardiovascular surgeons find it imperative to adapt these new techniques and make use of novel technologies in an attempt to optimize patient outcomes (Hudorović et al., 2008). Additionally, the development of catheter-based therapies, which provide less invasive substitutes for conventional surgical surgery, is also altering the nature of interventions. These transcatheter techniques, including transcatheter aortic valve replacement (TAVR) and mitral valve repair, are similarly being adopted in clinical practice. These techniques are particularly beneficial for high-risk individuals who cannot tolerate open-heart surgery. This transition to less invasive techniques necessitates an interaction among cardiovascular surgeons and interventional cardiologists to offer comprehensive care for patients with valvular heart disease. The faster evolution of surgical techniques emphasizes the importance of ongoing education and research on the subject. While surgeons adjust to new techniques, integration of technology and their ability will be key to maximizing treatment for valvular heart disease victims and, in the long term, improving patient survival rates and quality of life (Hudorović et al., 2008) (Figure 8.17).

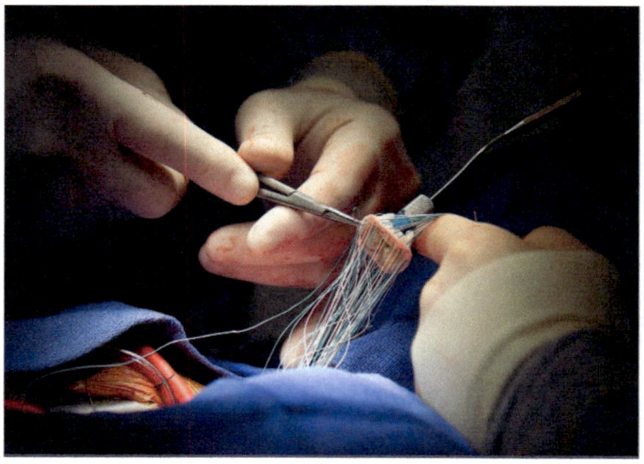

Figure 8.17. Heart valve replacements.

Source: https://onewelbeck.com/media/ihaj5uzv/image1435.jpg.

8.5.3. Emerging Therapies: Transcatheter Interventions

The evolution of transcatheter therapy of valvular heart disease has revolutionized the landscape of cardiovascular treatment. In the past, patients with advanced mitral and tricuspid regurgitation were often relegated to surgery, which was of higher risk, especially in the elderly and those with comorbidities. New technology, such as the MitraClip® system, has provided a minimally invasive solution for these high-risk patients. Regulatory bodies have approved this technology and is also being utilized on a large scale in patients with functional mitral regurgitation, demonstrating a paradigm shift in the treatment strategy. Advances in the technology of transcatheter valves are not limited to the mitral valve; there are rising exploratory procedures for tricuspid valve repair and replacement, which indicate a rose-tinted future for patients having complex valvular heart disease (Benito-González et al., 2017). With the progress of cardiovascular medicine, transcatheter aortic valve implantation (TAVI) has established itself as an anchor therapy for aortic valve disease, particularly severe aortic stenosis. With the increasing population of the elderly and increasing burden of heart failure, not only does TAVI symptomatically relieve but also significantly improves quality of life and survival. Studies indicate that TAVI is particularly effective in patients at high risk of traditional surgical techniques, for instance, those with multiple comorbidities. Moreover, TAVI has been employed in uncommon conditions, namely, in individuals with aortic regurgitation and poor ventricular function, to effectively reduce the burden of the left ventricle (Loforte et al., 2021). The relentless growth of the indications for TAVIs and their application across different settings of clinical practice demonstrates their importance in modern cardiac treatment. The prospect of transcatheter treatment is promising as ongoing research keeps addressing unsatisfied clinical needs. More sophisticated devices and techniques are being explored to optimize outcomes in patients with functional mitral regurgitation and other valvular conditions. Besides, percutaneous mitral valve repair is now becoming a viable option for patients not only to enhance prognosis but also quality of life, most particularly as a bridge to left ventricular assist device or heart transplantation. New technologies, including transcatheter technology, are being increasingly used to treat patients with chronic heart failure. These advancements are a significant step towards less-invasive, but effective, therapies for the management of valvular heart disease and herald a new era for cardiovascular intervention (Benito-González et al., 2017; Loforte et al., 2021).

SUMMARY

Overall, valvular heart diseases are a significant public health problem, particularly among the elderly. This age group exhibits high rates of various cardiovascular conditions, including hypertension and congestive heart failure as common complaints. Research findings, for example, at Muhimbili National Hospital, have indicated that the vast majority of elderly patients present with cardiac diseases, and this highlights the need to diagnose and treat early to minimize associated morbidity and disability. Because cardiovascular diseases are typically underdiagnosed upon hospital admissions for non-cardiac causes, systemic screening recommendations must be implemented to ensure complete patient care and improved clinical outcomes in older adults (Kisenge et al., 2011). Furthermore, the severity of valvular heart diseases, particularly involving the mitral valve, underscores the need for further research and innovative treatment approaches. Emerging advances in computational modeling have opened up new avenues for understanding the mitral valve biomechanics, critical to establishing effective treatment and prevention programs. With the help of sophisticated modeling involving fluid-structure interactions, researchers can model and predict valve behavior more effectively, leading to enhanced diagnostic precision. These advancements are essential in addressing the complex issues presented by valvular diseases, thereby generating optimism for improved management and patient care in the future (Berry et al., 2017). Finally, the integration of clinical practice and research into valvular heart diseases supports the imperative of a multi-faceted approach towards this shared issue. There is a necessity for greater interaction among clinicians, scientists, and technologists to drive the understanding, diagnosis, and treatment of these multi-factorial diseases. Increased research into valvular heart disease and rigorous screening practices will allow the healthcare industry to counteract the mounting morbidity burden resulting from these disorders and strive towards reducing cardiovascular-related mortality rates. The future efforts must be focused not only on educating healthcare providers regarding the nuances of valvular disease but also on eliciting patient education and engagement to foster an active approach to heart health (Kisenge et al., 2011; Berry et al., 2017).

The management and perception of VHD have significantly evolved, including the use of clinical guidelines and new therapies that enhance patient outcomes. Among the most contentious issues is the diagnostic approach, headed by echocardiography, which remains the cornerstone of VHD assessment. The non-invasive imaging modality provides invaluable information regarding valvular structure and function, permitting the detection of stenosis and regurgitation. Also, it allows for real-time monitoring of disease progression, which is required for early treatment. Recent guidelines have also pointed out individualized treatment regimens, which are tailored to the specific characteristics of each patient's valvular disease and hence enable more effective management regimens. Another important area highlighted in the discussion of valvular heart diseases is the coordination of anticoagulation therapy, particularly among patients with a likelihood of developing atrial fibrillation (AF) due to VHD. The availability of non-vitamin K antagonist oral anticoagulants (NOACs) has transformed the methodology of anticoagulation with certain advantages over traditional vitamin K antagonists (VKAs) as they have predictable pharmacokinetics and require less monitoring. As noted by the European Heart Rhythm Association, this has involved a concerted attempt to deal with issues of practical clinical scenarios regarding the use of NOAC, so both patients and doctors can feel at ease with options for anticoagulation treatment in AF in terms of VHD (Steffel et al., 2018). This trend in more accessible anticoagulation therapy indicates the emphasis on patient safety and treatment compliance. Finally, controversy about the surgical treatment of VHD underscores the value of a multidisciplinary approach to the management of patients. Valve repair and replacement have both reduced morbidity and mortality significantly in their results when done in a timely fashion. Selection of patients for surgery cannot be overvalued since comorbid status, age, and lifestyle all contribute significantly to clinical outcomes. In addition, post-operative management and long-term follow-up are essential elements in maintaining long-term benefits from surgical interventions. As recommendations change and new evidence arises, healthcare practitioners are urged to stay abreast of updated research to provide improved decision-making for VHD patients (Vahanian et al., 2021). This integrated approach ultimately seeks to improve the quality of life of VHD patients.

A CLOSER LOOK

COMPLICATIONS AND PROGNOSIS

Complications of valvular heart diseases, particularly AS, are severe and have the potential to impact the patient's prognosis markedlyAS is characterized by a very long asymptomatic course, which, without the presence of symptoms, may evolve into serious complications at the onset of symptoms. The evolution from symptom-free to symptomatic status involves a sudden worsening of the patients' prognosis in general. Severe complications of AS include heart failure, arrhythmias, and sudden cardiac death, which indicate that early treatment is necessary. With an increased population age, AS, along with its complications, increases, and therefore, more information regarding disease progression and management is required. Such a scenario indicates the necessity of monitoring patients regularly in order to balance risks related to the disease and make the right decisions regarding surgical interventions, previously represented by aortic valve replacement as the gold standard of treatment (Smirnova et al., 2021). Recent years have witnessed advancements in minimal invasive interventions, e.g., TAVI, which have completely changed the practice of AS treatment. TAVI is particularly beneficial in high-risk or elderly patients who are intolerant to conventional surgical methods due to comorbidities.

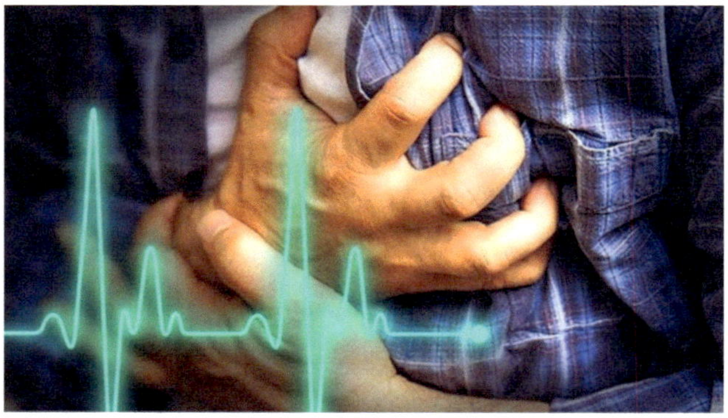

Figure 8.18. Complications of valvular heart diseases.

Source: https://www.hindustantimes.com/ht-img/img/2023/11/28/550x309/salt_1660564880632_1701156895106.jpg.

This advance emphasizes the clinical significance of creating therapies that reduce complications and improve prognostic outcomes. Studies indicate that TAVI use has been correlated with fewer postoperative complications than conventional surgical methods. However, understanding of TAVI selection criteria and possible complications remains relevant in an attempt to optimize patient outcomes. Furthermore, a multidisciplinary approach to evaluate and treat patients with AS should be employed to determine that the advantages of TAVI over surgical replacement are maximized, especially with heterogeneous risk profiles among patients (Smirnova et al., 2021). Valvular heart diseases, particularly within the context of autoimmune rheumatic diseases, introduce a complex interplay of systemic manifestations and cardiac issues. Such diseases are likely to manifest through a variety of cardiac presentations like valvular malfunction and heart failure, thus necessitating the use of adequate diagnostic methods like echocardiography. Utilizing newer image acquisition technologies, doctors can precisely diagnose cardiac function as well as disease progression. Echocardiography is enormously valuable for assessing valvular heart disease-associated complications that are significant for the development of appropriate treatment options. It aids practitioners in determining the effectiveness of current treatments, with special emphasis on parameters such as valvular function and pulmonary artery pressures. Because of this intricacy, proper knowledge of symptoms, treatment options, and prognostic factors is essential in successfully managing patients with valvular heart diseases (Figure 8.18).

References

1. Elsaka, O., Noureldean, M. A., M, A. G., M, T. G., H, A. a. A., & Hisham, D. (2022). PATHOPHYSIOLOGY, INVESTIGATIONS, AND TREATMENT OF PATIENTS WITH BICUSPID AORTIC VALVE. *Zenodo (CERN European Organization for Nuclear Research)*. https://doi.org/10.5281/zenodo.7636740Agarwal, A., Tromp, J., Almahmeed, W., Angermann, C. E., Chandramouli, C., Cho, H., Choi, D., et al. (2024). Toward a universal definition of etiologies in heart failure: Categorizing causes and advancing registry science. *Circulation: Heart Failure, 17*, e011095. https://www.semanticscholar.org/paper/9c9690980f038852f4fe00302ac72caa3487f3e8 (accessed on 29th May 2025).

2. Allan, V. (2018). *Exploiting Electronic Health Records for Research on Atrial Fibrillation: Risk Factors, Subtypes, and Outcomes*. https://core.ac.uk/download/158170726.pdf (accessed on 29th May 2025).

3. Amico, M. A., Busi, G., Vannini, M., Bruscoli, F., Marchionni, N., Boccanelli, A., & Carrabba, N. (2024). PREVASC: Prospective registry of epidemiology of valve disease in asymptomatic Italian subjects. *European Journal of Preventive Cardiology*. https://www.semanticscholar.org/paper/20f61ef140a7c2387088b102886cfc60aa25ffe8 (accessed on 29th May 2025).

4. Arslan, M., Kaleli, İ., & Kutlu, M. (2024). Prospective clinical follow-up results of infective endocarditis. *Infectious Diseases & Clinical Microbiology*, *6*, 133–140. https://www.semanticscholar.org/paper/b60ee13b7ce4ead65b702083972b693646b08cf7 (accessed on 29th May 2025).

5. Bai, B., & Wang, Y. (2010). *The Use of Lorcaserin in the Management of Obesity: A Critical Appraisal*. https://core.ac.uk/download/pdf/8515525.pdf (accessed on 29th May 2025).

6. Barman, L., Dhankhar, K., Goyal, N., & Das, A. (2024). Low-dose fractionated spinal anesthesia for elective caesarean section in a patient with large atrial septal defect, severe pulmonary hypertension and preeclampsia: A case report. *Journal of Clinical and Diagnostic Research*. https://www.semanticscholar.org/paper/aadde900597244886b371437aa299a57f458dd03 (accessed on 29th May 2025).

7. Baumgartner, H., De Backer, J., Babu-Narayan, S. V., Budts, W., Chessa, M., Diller, G. P., Lung, B., et al. (2020). 2020 ESC guidelines for the management of adult congenital heart disease. *European Heart Journal, 42*, 563–645. https://doi.org/10.1093/eurheartj/ehaa554 (accessed on 29th May 2025).

8. Bembey, R., & Babu, R. (2024). Cardiomyopathy in a nutshell: From etiopathogenesis and diagnosis to treatment. *International Journal of Research in Medical Sciences*. https://www.semanticscholar.org/paper/7adb9c160f553ae1b0bc5aad0fb8db079c109bb8 (accessed on 29th May 2025).

9. Benito-González, T., Cardona, J. G., Estévez-Loureiro, R., Fernández-Vázquez, R., et al. (2017). *Percutaneous Treatment of Mitral and Tricuspid Regurgitation in Heart Failure*. https://core.ac.uk/download/322430893.pdf (accessed on 29th May 2025).

10. Berry, C., Danton, M., Feng, L., Gao, F., et al. (2017). *Modeling Mitral Valvular Dynamics – Current Trend and Future Directions*. https://core.ac.uk/download/74230677.pdf (accessed on 29th May 2025).

11. Chintala, K., Forbes, T. J., & Reddy, S. V. (2005). *Cardiovascular Involvement in Kawasaki Disease*. https://core.ac.uk/download/46602916.pdf (accessed on 29th May 2025).

12. Christ, M., & Mueller, C. (2008). Use of natriuretic peptide assay in dyspnea. *Deutsches Arzteblatt International, 105*(6), 95–100. https://www.semanticscholar.org/paper/dba1f30d85f297802ad1798af9fc74bdfbc3edae (accessed on 29th May 2025).

13. Collini, V., Faletra, F., Zucco, J., Mio, C., Carraro, M., Gava, A. M., De Biasio, M., et al. (2024). Whole exome sequencing in patients with recurrent pericarditis. *European Heart Journal*. https://www.semanticscholar.org/paper/9b22462cdf90cde65af2b73c720db7225974e598 (accessed on 29th May 2025).

14. Delgado-SanMartin, J. A., Errington, N., Schuetz, N., Johnson, A., Kim, D. S., Gupta, V., Hershman, S., et al. (2025). *Remote Monitoring of Physical Activity Captured by the MyHeart Counts App Identifies Pulmonary Arterial Hypertension*. https://www.semanticscholar.org/paper/06ada0995dad5b160896c4792e92f014d750a5f9 (accessed on 29th May 2025).

15. Dhanalakshmi, C., Manjunath, C. N., Ravindranath, K. S., Srinivas, S., et al. (2014). Incidence and patterns of valvular heart disease in a tertiary care high-volume cardiac center: A single center experience. *Indian Heart J*. https://core.ac.uk/download/pdf/82755521.pdf (accessed on 29th May 2025).

16. Dreyfus, J., Komar, M., Attias, D., De Bonis, M., Ruschitzka, F., Popescu, B., Laroche, C., et al. (2024). Tricuspid regurgitation: Frequency, clinical presentation, management and outcome among patients with severe left-sided valvular heart disease in Europe. Insights from the ESC-EORP Valvular Heart Disease II survey. *European Journal of Heart Failure, 26*. https://www.semanticscholar.org/paper/ee49d83c52e3d16d0dd36c17bceab3ddb72dfeae (accessed on 29th May 2025).

17. Greenberg, B. H., Lunde, O., Maisel, A., Mills, R., et al. (2019). *Depressive Symptoms in Asymptomatic Stage B Heart Failure with Type II Diabetic Mellitus*. https://core.ac.uk/download/323066773.pdf (accessed on 29th May 2025).

18. Hassan, H., Rahman, T., Bacon, A., Knott, C., Allen, I., Huntley, C., Loong, L., et al. (2025). Long-term outcomes of bilateral salpingo-oophorectomy in women with personal history of breast cancer. *BMJ Oncology, 4*. https://www.semanticscholar.org/paper/32a640077d0a04c69a4d70429372548d97984e64 (accessed on 29th May 2025).

19. Hesarur, V. (2018). Clinical and hemodynamic characteristics of double chambered right ventricle in adult patients. *Journal of Medical Science and Clinical Research, 6*. https://www.semanticscholar.org/paper/de8a220034d67d5d43aa59b30b739c9931ac065a (accessed on 29th May 2025).

20. Hieda, M., Rikumaru, K., Yamamoto, Y., Futami, S., Yamashita, K., Maruyama, T., & Hara, H. (2023). Abstract 16869: Prevalence of valvular heart disease in the elderly as observed in a large-scale echocardiographic database. *Circulation*. https://www.semanticscholar.org/paper/5227aac326dd114c198690ac07c0381f127731d4 (accessed on 29th May 2025).

21. Höglund, K. (2007). *Systolic Ejection Murmurs and the Left Ventricular Outflow Tract in Boxer Dogs*. https://core.ac.uk/download/11695170.pdf (accessed on 29th May 2025).

22. Hudorović, N. (2008). *Aortic Valve Surgery: What is the Future?* https://core.ac.uk/download/pdf/82413667.pdf (accessed on 29th May 2025).

23. Kisenge, P. R. (2011). Pattern of cardiovascular diseases among elderly patients admitted in medical wards at Muhimbili National Hospital Dar es Salaam, Tanzania. https://core.ac.uk/download/pdf/16666639.pdf (accessed on 29th May 2025).

24. Kitsiou, A., Caforio, A. L. P., Porta-Sanchez, A., Vahanian, A., Iung, B., Carrera, C., Szymanski, C., et al. (2013). *ESC Core Curriculum for the General Cardiologist (2013).* https://core.ac.uk/download/55756305.pdf (accessed on 29th May 2025).

25. Kovalev, D. S. (2025). Clinical picture, diagnosis and treatment of mitral valvular disease. *Spravočnik Vrača Obŝej Praktiki (Journal of Family Medicine).* https://www.semanticscholar.org/paper/eca925389b37c6e897eaf4d9ac341be1d3226a4c (accessed on 29th May 2025).

26. Liu, X., Luo, D., Hu, Z., Tian, H., Jiang, H., & Chen, J. (2025). The association between biological aging markers and valvular heart diseases. *Zhejiang Da Xue Xue Bao. Yi Xue Ban = Journal of Zhejiang University. Medical Sciences.* https://www.semanticscholar.org/paper/efb560227be540b922495e91e7e46e3adeb22817 (accessed on 29th May 2025).

27. Loforte, A., Pacini, D., & Saia, F. (2021). *Innovative Transcatheter Procedures for the Treatment of Heart Failure.* https://core.ac.uk/download/573436016.pdf (accessed on 29th May 2025).

28. Machado, A. C. V. (2018). *A Retrospective Review of Aortic Stenosis in 274 Dogs in Scotland: Clinical Presentation and Diagnosis.* https://core.ac.uk/download/154344390.pdf (accessed on 29th May 2025).

29. Maisch, B., & Bauersachs, J. (2020). Cardiomyopathies—Past, present, future. *Herz, 45,* 209–211. https://www.semanticscholar.org/paper/c4c708905a829737d6661e31c33edd2e8b1e9846 (accessed on 29th May 2025).

30. Makavos, G., Varoudi, M., Papangelopoulou, K., Kapniari, E., Plotas, P., Ikonomidis, I., & Papadavid, E. (2020). Echocardiography in autoimmune rheumatic diseases for diagnosis and prognosis of cardiovascular complications. *Medicina, 56.* https://www.semanticscholar.org/paper/d18a4db0a890a51a11c0834378914d2cd5f2e59c (accessed on 29th May 2025).

31. Marek, J., Chocholová, B., Rob, D., Paleček, T., Masek, M., Dostálová, G., & Linhart, A. (2023). Three-dimensional left ventricular strain analysis in Fabry disease: Correlation with heart failure severity, myocardial scar and impact on long-term prognosis. *European Heart Journal – Cardiovascular Imaging.* https://www.semanticscholar.org/paper/a32e61ae3782a77a36c504366582899ab92481c8 (accessed on 29th May 2025).

32. Margonato, D., Ingallina, G., Belli, M., Tavernese, A., Ricchetti, G., Ancona, F., Stella, S., et al. (2024). Tricuspid regurgitation in the context of severe concomitant left-sided valvular heart disease: Patients characteristics and long-term clinical and interventional outcomes. *European Heart Journal.* https://www.semanticscholar.org/paper/f2604cde4dd7ba0b530d584849d38a653af78d92 (accessed on 29th May 2025).

33. Mascherbauer, J., Kammerlander, A., Nitsche, C., Bax, J., Delgado, V., Evangelista, A., Laroche, C., et al. (2024). Sex-related differences in severe native valvular heart disease: The ESC-EORP Valvular Heart Disease II survey. *European Heart Journal, 45,* 3818–3833. https://www.semanticscholar.org/paper/808f5aeeac83d496b89b0a68ad9c8de7ae119ca2 (accessed on 29th May 2025).

34. Mehrabinejad, M., Ahmadi, N., Mohammadi, E., Shabani, M., Sherafati, A., Aryannejad, A., Rezaei, N., et al. (2022). Global and regional burden and quality of care of non-rheumatic valvular heart diseases: A systematic analysis of Global Burden of Disease 1990–2017. *International*

Journal for Quality in Health Care, Journal of the International Society for Quality in Health Care. https://www.semanticscholar.org/paper/79073185538f2d966509961eec505ff1715f9ea5 (accessed on 29th May 2025).

35. Mihaljević, J., Mihaljević, D., Drenjančević, I., & Sitaš, Z. (2024). The role of miRNAs in the regulation of oxidative stress and microvascular reactivity in chronic kidney disease. *Proceeding of the Shevchenko Scientific Society. Medical Sciences.* https://www.semanticscholar.org/paper/feabccd712157dabf0a4a6e632fd1f83fd8e1067 (accessed on 29th May 2025).

36. Muraru, D., Badano, L., Hahn, R., Lang, R. M., Delgado, V., Wunderlich, N. C., Donal, E., et al. (2024). Atrial secondary tricuspid regurgitation: Pathophysiology, definition, diagnosis, and treatment. *European Heart Journal, 45*, 895–911. https://www.semanticscholar.org/paper/a51066914f8251a7374f1a3ef8bb360474f1da68 (accessed on 29th May 2025).

37. N/A. (2019). *Echocardiography in Adults.* https://core.ac.uk/download/286334724.pdf (accessed on 29th May 2025).

38. Rana, M. (2022). Aortic valve stenosis: Diagnostic approaches and recommendations of the 2021 ESC/EACTS guidelines for the management of valvular heart disease – A review of the literature. *Cardiology and Cardiovascular Medicine, 6*, 315–324. https://www.semanticscholar.org/paper/00ba414fd8e8ad82bbe3c0c8d6a6b09a15465f8b (accessed on 29th May 2025).

39. Rubis, P. (2023). Low-normal systolic function and hypertrophic cardiomyopathy. *Heart, 109*, 732–733. https://www.semanticscholar.org/paper/ae316efa65be56e93c71322f9b7157730ed35ec7 (accessed on 29th May 2025).

40. Samaras, A., Vrana, E., Kartas, A., Moysidis, D., Papazoglou, A., Doundoulakis, I., Fotos, G., et al. (2021). Prognostic implications of valvular heart disease in patients with non-valvular atrial fibrillation. *BMC Cardiovascular Disorders, 21.* https://www.semanticscholar.org/paper/3889390d850048760b5b5a43cb1595801a6ce68c (accessed on 29th May 2025).

41. Schwartz, J. D. (2005). *The Prevalence of Comorbid Chronic Disease in Virginia's Adult Patient Population During the Years 2001 and 2004.* https://core.ac.uk/download/51292489.pdf (accessed on 29th May 2025).

42. Singh, H., & Agarwal, V. (2024). *Heart Condition Monitoring Using Phonocardiogram and Murmurs Analysis by CNN.* 2024 2nd International Conference on Advancements and Key Challenges in Green Energy and Computing (AKGEC). https://www.semanticscholar.org/paper/8bd20dca405130ab359bda7105ddbde1a9db1a7b (accessed on 29th May 2025).

43. Small, A. M., Yutzey, K., Binstadt, B., Key, K. V., Bouatia-Naji, N., Milan, D., Aikawa, E., et al. (2024). Unraveling the mechanisms of valvular heart disease to identify medical therapy targets: A scientific statement from the American Heart Association. *Circulation.* https://www.semanticscholar.org/paper/74cd2fab51605579b4c17bf2e2bf225e0e2d38a3 (accessed on 29th May 2025).

44. Smirnova, E., Terekhina, A., Filonenko, S. P., & Muranchik, E. N. (2021). Calcific aortic valve stenosis: Potentials and complications of surgical treatment. *I.P. Pavlov Russian Medical Biological Herald.* https://www.semanticscholar.org/paper/9026ee2ab2a29931374874cecf1a5f25c8ec1f31 (accessed on 29th May 2025).

45. Steffel, J., Verhamme, P., Potpara, T., Albaladejo, P., Antz, M., Desteghe, L., Hæusler, K. G., et al. (2018). The 2018 European Heart Rhythm Association practical guide on the use of non-vitamin K antagonist oral anticoagulants in patients with atrial fibrillation. *European Heart*

Journal, 39, 1330–1393. https://doi.org/10.1093/eurheartj/ehy136 (accessed on 29th May 2025).

46. Vahanian, A., Beyersdorf, F., Praz, F., Milojevic, M., Baldus, S., Bauersachs, J., Capodanno, D., et al. (2021). 2021 ESC/EACTS guidelines for the management of valvular heart disease. *European Heart Journal, 43*, 561–632. https://doi.org/10.1093/eurheartj/ehab395 (accessed on 29th May 2025).
47. Waleed, M. (2020). Prevalence of different types of valvular heart disease and other cardiac pathologies of the heart in high-risk patients with suspicion of heart failure: A retrospective cohort study. *Clinical Cardiology and Cardiovascular Interventions, 3*, 1–7. https://www.semanticscholar.org/paper/c4164bbf494351b24f779c006929a2350423bb26 (accessed on 29th May 2025).
48. Wei, Y., Sun, D., Jaiswal, S., He, Y., Liu, X., & Wang, J. (2024). Association of lifestyle with valvular heart disease progression and life expectancy among elderly people from different socioeconomic backgrounds. *BMC Medicine, 22*. https://www.semanticscholar.org/paper/be94ed08cee97bfda8fc5788eb865680479b9045 (accessed on 29th May 2025).
49. Whelton, P. K., Carey, R. M., Aronow, W. S., Casey, D. E., Collins, K. J., Dennison, H. C., DePalma, S. M., et al. (2017). 2017 ACC/AHA/AAPA/ABC/ACPM/AGS/APhA/ASH/ASPC/NMA/PCNA guideline for the prevention, detection, evaluation, and management of high blood pressure in adults: A report of the American College of Cardiology/American Heart Association Task Force on Clinical Practice Guidelines. *Hypertension, 71*. https://doi.org/10.1161/hyp.0000000000000065 (accessed on 29th May 2025).

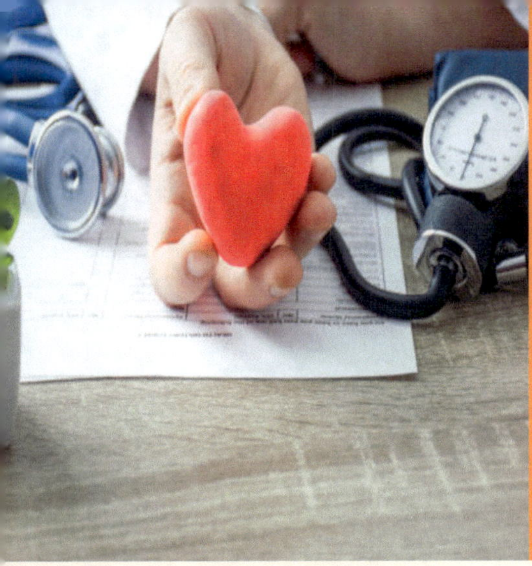

Chapter 9

CONGENITAL HEART DISEASES

Contents

Introduction

Congenital heart diseases (CHDs) should be studied because they have a direct impact on children's health and affect an estimated 1 in 100 live births. The illnesses encompass a broad group of structural heart anomalies that range from simple defects to complicated malformations and, in some cases, necessitate immediate intervention. Understanding the pathophysiology of cardiac abnormalities is crucial in the development of the best treatment plans and minimizing morbidity and mortality rates. With advances in diagnostic imaging and genetic investigation, doctors are now able to diagnose and treat CHDs at an earlier stage in life, which ultimately results in higher survival and better quality of life for the individual. With awareness about the conditions on the rise, it is now more evident that there is a requirement for comprehensive care, including medical, surgical, and psychosocial intervention. These multidisciplinary approaches ensure the patient receives total care as may be required for their specific needs. In management and treatment, congenital heart diseases present unique challenges varying wildly with the type and extent of the defect. Those individuals afflicted by these diseases can require anything from regular checkups to complex surgical procedures like heart transplantation, especially in cases involving non-repairable defects or declining heart function. For instance, cardiac transplantation in children is now a life-saving intervention in infants and children with end-stage heart failure due to diseases such as cardiomyopathy or complex congenital malformations. Management after transplant is essential, with long-term follow-up for the diagnosis of complications such as arrhythmias that even in the symptom-free state may arise, necessitating regular follow-up through the use of Holter ECG monitoring and other studies (Doğan et al., 2024).

The ongoing research into emerging treatment strategies aims to reduce risks from complications and enhance the quality of life for CHD patients. Additionally, it is essential to clarify the role of genetic causes in congenital heart disease etiology. Genomic studies have indicated that there are patients with CHDs who can be traced back to specific genetic mutations or syndromic presentations, providing an improved understanding of the etiology and heterogeneity of particular phenotypes. This provides for better screening and early diagnosis, which subsequently results in early interventions. Also, awareness of anomalous coronary artery origins, such as anomalous origin of the right coronary artery, underscores the intimate association between anatomical heart disease and sudden death risk, particularly among otherwise healthy young individuals (Solangi et al., 2024). Hence, interprofessional collaboration among cardiologists, geneticists, and pediatricians is required to optimize care pathways for congenital heart disease patients so that interventions become effective and tailored to specific patient requirements (Figure 9.1).

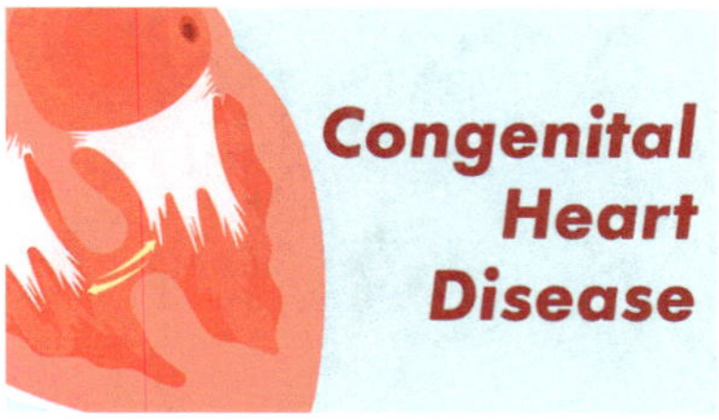

Figure 9.1. Congenital heart diseases (CHDs).

Source: https://ausmed-images.s3.ap-southeast-2.amazonaws.com/ausmed.com/ausmed-articles/20180418_cover_2.jpg.

Definition of Congenital Heart Diseases (CHDs)

CHDs are a group of structural and functional cardiac abnormalities apparent at birth. They can affect the chambers of the heart, the valves, and the vessels, and lead to abnormal blood circulation and impaired cardiac function. The CDC estimates that CHD complicates approximately 1 in 100 live births, rendering the condition one of the most prevalent congenital malformations. CHD types are usually graded based on complexity and the severity of the abnormalities present, e.g., atrial septal defect, ventricular septal defect, or complex defects like transposition of the great arteries. These differences in presentation and etiology account for the necessity of early diagnosis and treatment to improve outcomes and reduce the effects of the condition on the family and healthcare system. The pathogenesis of CHD is multifactorial, with both genetic and environmental etiologic factors. Genetic elements, such as chromosomal abnormalities and syndromes, play a significant role in the pathogenesis of CHD. Environmental elements, such as maternal status and exposure to teratogens, also play important roles in the equation. Recent literature has demonstrated a robust correlation of air pollution with an increased incidence of CHD, pointing towards the necessity for further research in environmental modifiable risk factors. Furthermore, studies have indicated that exposure to harsh heat during pregnancy holds high promise for increasing CHD risk in children, with research citing odds ratios describing an alarming correlation (Krishnakumar et al., 2024). As our knowledge of such intricate interactions evolves, it can have implications for targeted prevention and better clinical outcomes in high-risk groups. With improved survival rates among patients with CHD, it is essential to study not only the short-term medical management but also the long-term effects of such congenital abnormalities. Surgical management has been revolutionary in terms of better outcomes, yet new evidence suggests that sex differences in surgical mortality and neurodevelopmental outcome are conceivable (Crain et al., 2025). The treatment of CHD is complex outside the operating room since most patients have to contend with concomitant issues of health, development, and quality of life for a whole lifetime. Increased insight into the potential neurodevelopmental disabilities, particularly in vulnerable populations, could influence health care policies and determine patient care protocols. Thus, an interdisciplinary understanding of CHD, its heterogeneous presentation, and late intervention effects remains fundamental to optimizing patient treatment and improving overall quality of life in subjects with these complex cardiovascular anomalies (Figure 9.2).

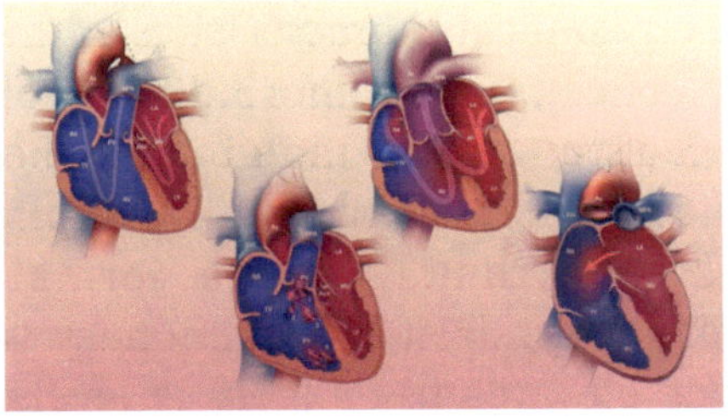

Figure 9.2. Understanding Congenital Heart Disease.

Source: https://stgaccinwbsdevlrs01.blob.core.windows.net/newcorporatewbsite/blogs/october2023/detail-main-Congenital-Heart-Disease.jpeg?w=3840&q=75.

9.1. Types of Congenital Heart Diseases (CHDs)

Several types of CHD can significantly affect the cardiovascular system of a patient and, therefore, manifest with a variety of clinical presentations and management challenges. Some of the most common are atrial septal defects (ASDs), ventricular septal defects (VSDs), and patent ductus arteriosus (PDA). In ASDs, the dividing wall between the two upper chambers of the heart fails to close during development, producing an abnormal connection between the atria. This is typically overlooked on the initial occurrence, though it can contribute to over-circulation of the lungs and ultimately heart failure. VSDs, where there is an opening between the lower chambers of the heart, also result in oxygen and deoxygenated blood mixing, leading to pulmonary artery pressure. PDAs, a residue of the ductus arteriosus postnatally, may also cause heart complications and necessitate early diagnosis and treatment to prevent adverse consequences, as indicated by findings from studies reporting rates of such disorders among infants (Golalipour et al., 2011). In addition to these more prevalent defects, CHDs comprise various other forms of complicated malformations that need meticulous medical assessment and management. Diagnoses such as tetralogy of Fallot, a four-component defect involving a VSD and pulmonary stenosis, present unique challenges due to how they impact the flow and oxygenation of blood. Moreover, the critical congenital heart defects (CCHDs) that often require urgent surgical interventions shortly after birth highlight the requirement for early diagnosis. Current research has highlighted the importance of improved mechanisms for screening, since early detection has been found to affect survival rates and long-term health results significantly. Advances in neonatal care and procedures have made a critical contribution to making prognostic results better, creating a model for the management of complicated CHD cases (Golinowska et al., 2012). The epidemiology of congenital heart disease exhibits striking variations among populations due to factors in genetics, environmental exposure, and maternal health. A longitudinal study in A Gorgan, Northern Iran, presented an 8.6 per 1,000 live births prevalence rate, suggesting a lower prevalence compared to other parts and particularly to Europe and the Middle East (Golalipour et al., 2011). This disparity points to the necessity to treat the different influences on the prevalence of CHDs, including genetic susceptibilities observed in involved families and the potential impact of socio-environmental factors. Also, the identification of congenital heart diseases as significant public health challenges highlights which policies aimed at prevention, early detection, and general management strategies need to be framed, incorporating health services that uniquely address the complexity of CHD patterns across different populations.

9.1.1. Atrial Septal Defect (ASD)

ASD is a severe form of congenital heart defect involving an atrial septal defect that establishes an abnormal pathway between the heart's chambers. It results in a left-to-right shunt, whereby oxygenated blood from the left atrium shunts to the right atrium with a high risk for secondary clinical complications. While ASDs could be asymptomatic for years, their undiagnosed state could lead to progressive alterations such as enlargement of the right atrium and right ventricle, pulmonary hypertension, and eventual heart failure in the long run. Early detection is therefore essential since prolonged exposure to these hemodynamic alterations can profoundly affect a patient's long-term prognosis. Familiarity with the pathology of the disease and its clinical presentation is a necessary consideration for directing management and treatment strategies, facilitating improved patient care in both pediatric and adult populations (Crișan et al., 2024). The current approach to ASD diagnosis relies heavily on advanced imaging modalities, where transthoracic and transesophageal echocardiography are significant players. These modalities form the core of identifying the presence and severity of the defect, evaluating right heart measurements, and defining blood flow patterns. Cardiac magnetic resonance imaging (CMR) also turns out to be a valuable modality, particularly for comprehensive evaluation before surgical interventions. Despite imaging advancements, ASD diagnosis can turn out to be challenging, especially in adults, where the presentation is attributed to other diseases, such that it can be delayed to diagnose and treat. Incorrect interpretation of clinical presentations can mimic other cardiovascular diseases, thus making it a rough ride to a correct diagnosis. It emphasizes that there must be a high index of suspicion of ASD in patients with manifestations of unexplained exertional dyspnea or right ventricular dysfunction (Cherkasova et al., 2024). The management of ASD has advanced significantly, and surgical correction is now available to repair the defect and restore normal hemodynamics. Percutaneous closure techniques have become popular due to their minimally invasive nature, which is characterized by quicker recovery and shorter hospital stays as opposed to traditional open-heart surgery. However, the suitability of such a procedure is dependent on various factors, including the size and anatomical characteristics of the defect and any concomitant comorbidities. Following the procedure, careful monitoring should be performed to detect potential complications such as arrhythmia or the formation of Eisenmenger syndrome, if pulmonary vascular resistance elevates to dangerous levels. Long-term follow-up is crucial because ASD patients can tolerate long-term complications that need multidisciplinary teams of caregivers to manage their care throughout different stages of life, striking a balance between quality of life and lifespan (Crișan et al., 2024) (Figure 9.3).

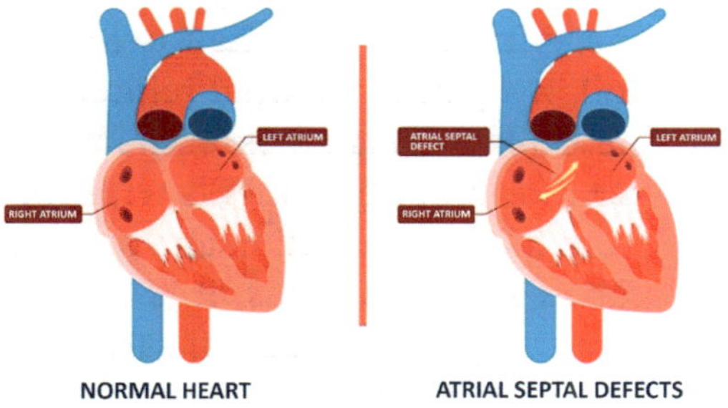

Figure 9.3. Atrial septal defect (ASD).

Source: https://punecardiologist.com/images/atrial-septal-defectsd.webp.

9.1.2. Ventricular Septal Defect (VSD)

The anatomy of congenital cardiac abnormalities lists VSD as a frequent malformation, representing a high percentage of diagnosed illnesses. With an imperfection in the septum that separates the ventricles of the heart, VSDs can result in left-to-right shunt, creating increased pulmonary flow of blood and potentially overloading the pulmonary vasculature. Early diagnosis is crucial since spontaneous defects can result in heart failure, pulmonary hypertension, and delayed development in children. The gravity of VSDs necessitates a collaborative treatment approach, not just for acute clinical needs but also for lasting health outcomes. Effective management strategies involve inter-professional collaboration between pediatric cardiologists, surgeons, and nursing professionals, each of whom plays an indispensable role towards optimal patient healing and quality of life (Calderón Rodríguez et al., 2025). The latter few years have witnessed appreciable advancement in diagnostic and interventional methods that have transformed the management of VSDs, particularly with the advent of transesophageal echocardiography (TEE) in minimal invasiveness therapy. TEE facilitates improved definition of , defect morphology, and inter-structural spatial relations, and enhances procedural planning accuracy. One study highlighted that during the period from June 2019 to June 2022, TEE-guided VSD closure using fully biodegradable occluders was 100% successful, indicating that careful preoperative evaluation can lead to successful outcomes. Most patients in the group had no residual shunt following surgery, which underlines the effectiveness of this procedure. These innovations not only improve surgical results but also reduce trauma associated with traditional approaches, thus being by the emerging standards of pediatric cardiac care (Zhang et al., 2024). Additionally, implications of VSD care extend beyond the operating room, targeting postoperative care and family instruction. Routine practice of prolonged follow-up is essential in monitoring recovery and diagnosing complications, such as residual shunts or arrhythmias. Family education plays a critical role in providing awareness and treatment protocol compliance. Interventions like emotional care for caregivers and outreach programs can address gaps in accessibility of health care, especially among families in rural settings where limited specialized services are available. Interventions applied in countries like Peru highlight the function of specialized care units and protocols in enhancing recovery and quality of life among VSD patients. By addressing comprehensive care, including family involvement and targeted follow-up, the course of congenital heart disease treatment, particularly for VSD, can be significantly altered (Calderón Rodríguez et al., 2025) (Figure 9.4).

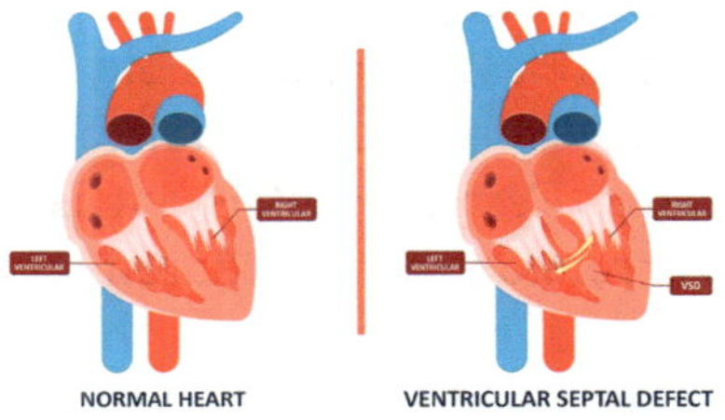

Figure 9.4. Ventricular septal defect (VSD).

Source: https://punecardiologist.com/images/Ventricular-Septal-Defect.webp.

9.1.3. Tetralogy of Fallot (ToF)

Among the various types of congenital heart disease, ToF is one of the most clinically significant due to its unique combination of structural defects. Ventricular septal defect, pulmonary stenosis, right ventricular hypertrophy, and overriding aorta are the fundamental findings of ToF. These defects collectively impair normal blood flow, resulting in cyanosis due to reduced systemic circulation oxygen saturation. Although the definitive etiology of ToF is still largely idiopathic, it is found to be related to genetic predisposition and fetal exposures during intrauterine life, thereby highlighting the significance of maternal well-being in fetal life. As the understanding of these determinants progresses, early intervention measures become increasingly vital to the management of this condition and in striving for improved outcomes for affected neonates. Diagnosis of Tetralogy of Fallot is typically made through echocardiography, the mainstay for cardiac morphology and function imaging. The presentation can vary, but the signs tend to be cyanosis, feeding intolerance, and, in others, cyanotic spells of great depth. Prompt recognition and therapy are critical because untreated ToF can cause severe complications such as heart failure or sudden cardiac death. In the age of the dynamic clinical scenario, improvements in imaging technology during the recent past have rendered diagnosis more precise and earlier, allowing clinicians to modify interventions based on disease severity and patient needs. Thus, understanding and management of ToF complexities are essential to enable streamlined treatment protocols in the pediatric population. Treatment for Tetralogy of Fallot is primarily surgical correction of the anatomical defects, with complete repair being the definitive operation performed in early infancy or childhood, which corrects the ventricular septal defect and solves the right ventricular outflow obstruction. While general success rates for this operation, it leaves some patients with residual morbidity, such as pulmonary regurgitation or right ventricular dysfunction, which need ongoing follow-up and potential reintervention later in life. Follow-up is an essential part over the long term, as repaired patients with ToF will require more medical attention and monitoring for associated sequelae. Thus, it is imperative that an interdisciplinary group of cardiologists, surgeons, and pediatricians is important to maximize the quality of life in such patients with this congenital cardiac malformation, ultimately enabling them to lead rewarding, fulfilling lives throughout elderly age (Figure 9.5).

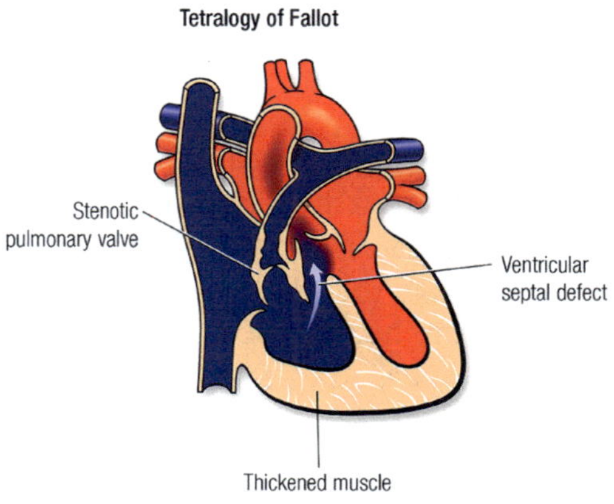

Figure 9.5. Tetralogy of fallot (ToF).

Source: https://www.heart.org/-/media/Images/Health-Topics/Congenital-Heart-Defects/50_1683_51_ToF.jpg?sc_lang=en.

9.2. Causes and Risk Factors

CHDs are congenital cardiac malformations, and their various causes and risk factors should be understood to diagnose and prevent them accordingly. Certain chromosomal anomalies, such as trisomy 21 (Down syndrome) and trisomy 18, and maternal genetic predisposition, have been proven to be powerful causes of CHDs. Maternal pathological conditions like diabetes and obesity can also enhance the risk of congenital anomalies. After these genetic factors, specific prenatal environmental exposures—teratogenic medications, alcohol consumption, and tobacco use—have been linked with increased incidence of CHDs. In this manner, the combination of ecological insult and genetic susceptibility significantly contributes to the risk profile for congenital heart malformations. Mother's health and behavior contribute beyond traditional risk, with nuanced interplay between biochemical pathways and congenital heart disease. Metabolomics research has elucidated potential biomarkers in mothers' urine that can serve as markers of CHD risk, particularly for the second and third trimesters. The discovery of molecules such as 4-hydroxybenzeneacetic acid and uric acid not only gives us a better insight into how metabolic disturbances might be linked to CHDs, but also indicates why monitoring maternal health as a whole across pregnancy is critical. These findings bring into focus the importance of early screening and intervention processes that target environmental as well as genetic risk factors, potentially altering the trajectory for high-risk pregnancies and facilitating neonatal health outcomes in the case of congenital heart diseases (Xie et al., 2019). For some populations, establishing risk factors at the individual level is necessary to treat congenital heart diseases. Surgical outcomes of pediatric CHD patients often highlight the complexity of the case. For instance, varying etiologies of extubation failure, such as airway stenosis, diaphragmatic dysfunction, and pulmonary infection, necessitate tailored treatment approaches according to the unique challenge of each patient. A recent investigation had shown that individualized treatment protocols greatly enhanced extubation success rates, demonstrating the value of individualized interventions based on the specific needs that each group of congenital heart defect presents (Wu et al., 2022). By recognizing and resolving these patient-specific risk factors, clinicians can enhance postoperative recovery and overall patient health, eventually improving quality of life for patients afflicted with these life-altering conditions (Figure 9.6).

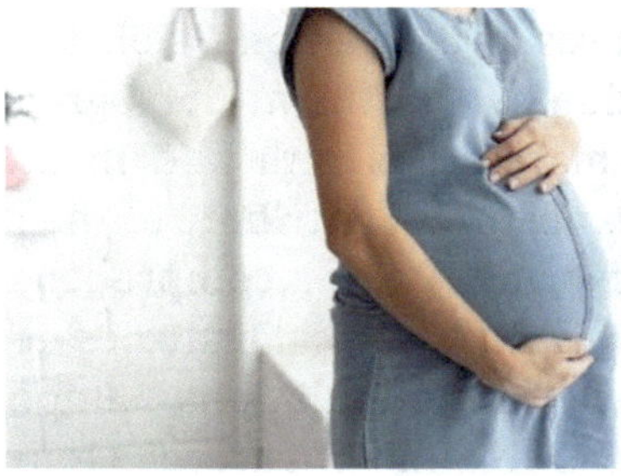

Figure 9.6. Causes of congenital heart disease (CHD).

Source: https://punecardiologist.com/images/Pregnant-Women.webp.

9.2.1. Genetic Factors and Family History

In the case of CHD, it is essential to identify the family history and the genetic factors because the etiology and heritability of the conditions are affected by genetic variation. The ability to quantify the genetic basis of CHD has been given to medical practitioners through genomic research. For instance, targeted genetic testing is now more frequent, particularly in young populations in whom high diagnostic yield often corresponds to specific genetic variation. One particular study of note identified that a large percentage of patients with congenital heart defects have positive genetic findings, particularly in those with extracardiac lesions associated with a strong family history. This underscores the importance of early genetic diagnosis as part of clinical assessment to individualize treatment routes efficiently and to make families aware of important information regarding the likelihood of recurrence of CHD in subsequent generations (Morrish et al., 2025). Family history is usually an important factor in evaluating patients with congenital heart disease. Studies have indicated that individuals with a family history of CHD have higher probabilities of developing similar congenital conditions. Genetic testing according to family history is also likely to raise diagnostic rates significantly, as in patients with genetic predispositions who may also present with phenotypic features of CHD among their family members. Additionally, pertinent demographic data, including maternal health and in utero environmental exposures, contribute to the risk profile of the offspring. Thus, a comprehensive understanding of family medical histories helps clinicians identify risk populations, supports informed decision-making regarding genetic counseling, and facilitates the implementation of proactive measures to preclude expected adverse effects on the family (Onorato et al., 2024). In consideration of these genetic and familial factors, it is clear that developing a comprehensive evaluation framework is crucial to manage congenital heart diseases better. The addition of genetic counseling to clinical practice can help facilitate communication regarding the implications of genetic results and the potential effects on family structure. As medical research has been advancing, patients and families have shown greater interest in genetic testing in large percentages, prioritizing its importance to prepare for a future pregnancy. It's particularly seen in patients with adult congenital heart disease, who unconsciously link their condition with their offspring's potential state of health. Therefore, encouraging improved understanding of genetic factors and family history will not only enhance patient care but also strengthen family support structures by familiarizing them with the essential knowledge needed to overcome the challenges of congenital heart diseases (Onorato et al., 2024).

9.2.2. Environmental Influences During Pregnancy

Prenatal environmental conditions have far-reaching implications for fetal growth, especially in the case of CHD. Other studies have shown that maternal health and lifestyle patterns have a significant influence on fetal success. For instance, research exploring the correlations between maternal 25-hydroxyvitamin D (25(OH)D) levels and CHD suggests a complex relationship;. At the same time, some observational data have demonstrated that increased vitamin D status may be connected with lower risk of CHD, the lack of robust evidence in support of a causative relationship challenges the size of vitamin Ds protective effect (Walker et al., 2025). Further, confounding variables such as maternal age, smoking, and body mass index must be controlled for because they can individually impact the levels of 25(OH)D and CHD incidences separately, making it challenging for us to study this intricate relationship. Apart from nutritional factors, exposure to environmental endocrine disruptors (EEDs) during perinatal development has emerged as a significant area of concern regarding CHD. A meta-analysis of numerous studies demonstrates an absolute connection between prenatal exposure to toxic chemicals—such as polycyclic aromatic hydrocarbons and pesticides—and heightened risks for CHD in children. Specifically, elevated odds ratios emphasize the relationships between these poisonous chemicals and specific congenital heart malformations, such as tetralogy of Fallot and septal defects, demonstrating a concerning trend (Pan et al., 2024). These findings underscore the importance of education for pregnant women regarding potential environmental risks, promoting public health efforts to reduce exposure to EEDs and improving maternal outcomes. An understanding of these environmental influences on pregnancy reinforces the necessity of integrating preventive approaches in maternal healthcare practice. Nutritional status, exposure to toxins, and overall maternal well-being interact in ways that necessitate an interdisciplinary approach to prenatal care. Encouraging healthy dietary practices, supplementation of required nutrients, and policy intervention to minimize environmental pollutants are primary steps towards the prevention of CHD risk. With further advancements in research, the identification of modifiable risk factors assumes greater importance, offering hope for the prevention of congenital heart diseases and healthier pregnancies overall. Coordinated effort from healthcare workers, policymakers, and families is required to address the multicausal etiology of congenital heart disease and enhance the health of future generations (Figure 9.7).

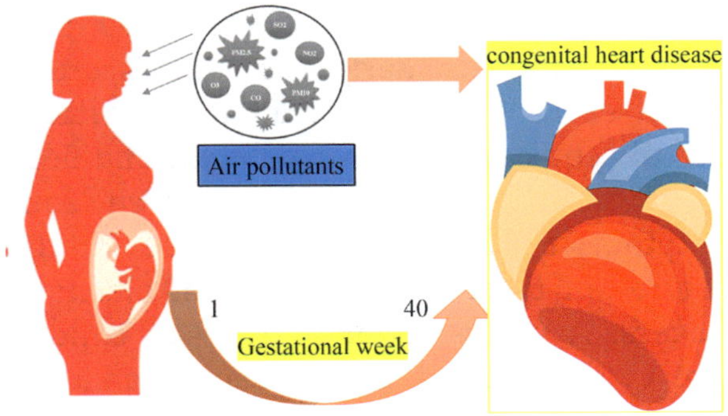

Figure 9.7. Associations between weekly air pollution exposure and congenital heart disease (CHD).

Source: https://ars.els-cdn.com/content/image/1-s2.0-S0048969720373526-ga1_lrg.jpg.

9.2.3. Maternal Health Conditions

The interplay of maternal health status and CHD underscores the significance of preconceptional care and prenatal diagnosis. Various maternal conditions, from chronic diseases such as diabetes, hypertension, and obesity, have been implicated in the etiology of CHD in the child. Research shows that maternal diabetes, for instance, has a two- to three-fold risk of fetal heart anomalies. Besides, maternal illness can have epigenetic impacts on fetal development through mechanisms that are not genetic but also contingent upon maternal states of metabolism and the environment. This demands an integrative policy for maternal care that entails ongoing monitoring, risk stratification, and management plan implementation during pregnancy to mitigate potential risks associated with CHD to enhance fetal outcomes in vulnerable populations, emphasized in recent literature (Wilde et al., 2022). Apart from metabolic disorders, the participation of placental well-being in the outcome of congenital heart disease is a novel area of interest. The placenta plays a significant role in fetal growth, and placental dysfunction may cause growth and health impairment of the fetus. Specifically, studies indicate that pregnancies complicated with CHD may be associated with abnormal placental morphology that disrupts normal development. The role of placental health is particularly relevant since, in addition to that of a conduit for oxygen and nutrients, it also answers to the distinct needs of the growing fetus. Placental dysfunction often follows that of maternal health conditions, thereby creating a feedback loop that enhances the risk of fetal heart defects. Better understanding of placental function has the potential to provide new insights into the multifactorial determinants behind unfavorable results seen in CHD, ultimately informing clinical practice based on maternal health (Andescavage et al., 2021).

Furthermore, maternal mental health throughout pregnancy is also increasingly recognized as an essential component of maternal health that can influence fetal heart formation. Anxiety, depression, and chronic stress are associated with poor pregnancy outcomes, which may potentiate risk factors for congenital heart disease. Stress responses at the physiological level may affect not only maternal health but also fetal physiology through changes in placental function and hormone regulation. Adequate maternal care that includes mental health support may prevent or reduce the severity of congenital heart malformations in the neonate. Mental health being treated as an element of prenatal care becomes important in framing an integrated strategy for improving maternal and infant outcomes. By the detection and treatment of physical as well as mental elements, healthcare providers are in a better position to manage the complexities associated with maternal health disorders and how they affect congenital heart diseases (Wilde et al., 2022) (Figure 9.8).

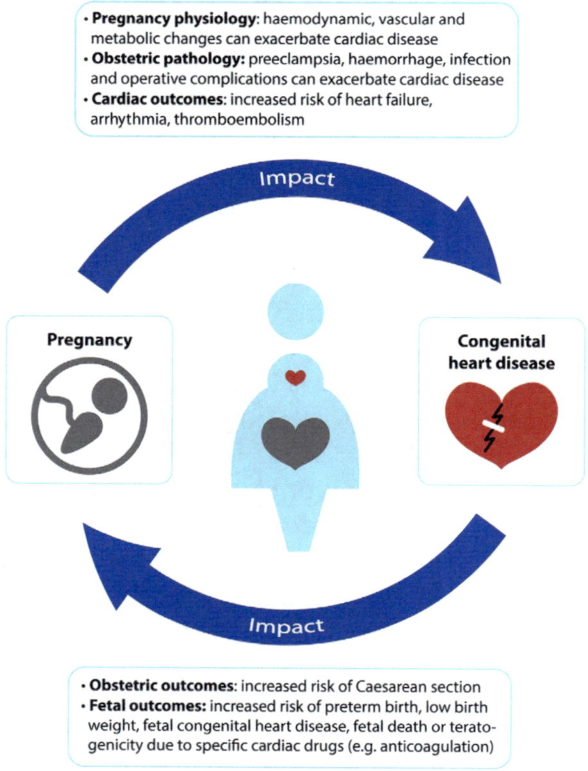

Figure 9.8. The interplay between maternal congenital heart disease and pregnancy.

Source: https://www.researchgate.net/publication/347468483/figure/fig1/AS:971916106006530@1608734265564/The-interplay-between-maternal-congenital-heart-disease-and-pregnancy.ppm.

9.3. Symptoms and Diagnosis

The CHD diagnosis is most often complicated and needs to be approached in a multidimensional manner, as the presenting symptoms in infants and children differ. One of the most common first-line approaches to diagnosis is by clinical evaluation of cyanosis, respiratory distress, and indications of poor feeding. These signs are either subtle or easily overlooked at birth and can lead to severe complications if they are not correctly identified. Pulse oximetry screening, in particular, has gained prominence as a valuable diagnostic tool in the first 24–48 hours of life. It detects CCHDs by measuring the degree of oxygen saturation of blood and, hence, hypoxemia despite the absence of overt clinical symptoms. Early detection is crucial as untreated conditions lead to devastating clinical sequelae like cardiac failure and death (Sonawane et al., 2022). In children, some symptoms change with time as the children mature, and these typically guide the diagnostic process. A cross-sectional study of children with cyanotic CHDs, for instance, highlighted cyanotic spells as the significant presenting symptom in emergency presentations, revealing a clear need for immediate assessment and intervention. Presenting symptoms typically present as fever, respiratory distress, and other manifestations that are systemic and tend to mask the underlying cardiac condition. The most common diagnosis among the involved children was tetralogy of Fallot, then tricuspid atresia and pulmonary atresia. This heterogeneity, aside from making clinical presentation challenging, also demands a high level of suspicion by clinicians to facilitate timely intervention that can significantly improve patient outcomes (Ilyas et al., 2021). The application of advanced imaging techniques, such as echocardiography, is important in diagnosing the condition after the suspicion of CHD. Echocardiography is a minimally invasive and very informative test that provides accurate anatomical and functional data about the heart. This imaging test can determine the existence of structural abnormalities such as septal defects or valvular abnormalities, and also determine the extent to which the heart is functioning. Early diagnosis and adequate management, including medical stabilization and surgery, are paramount in the prognosis of children with congenital heart disease. Thus, continued education of healthcare professionals on the scope of symptoms, rapid referral mechanisms to advanced imaging, and multidisciplinary follow-up care are instrumental in addressing the issues resulting from congenital heart disease (Sonawane et al., 2022).

9.3.1. Common Symptoms in Infants and Children

The clinical presentation of CHDs in infants and children can be very heterogeneous, and timely diagnosis is crucial for effective management. One of the most common presentations is cyanosis, in which one will notice a bluish hue to the skin and lips, indicating inadequate oxygenation of blood. It is especially prevalent in conditions such as ASD, where the abnormalities in circulation can lead to decreased oxygenation in systemic circulation. In one such reported case, a seven-year-old child came with cyanosis along with breathlessness, and timely action was taken to avoid further complications. The detection of such symptoms at an early level ensures that physicians can undertake necessary diagnostic measures and therapeutic processes, e.g., surgery or medication, to correct underlying issues and achieve healthier outcomes for affected children (Hakim et al., 2024). Furthermore, these symptoms of shortness of breath with feeding or only with light exercise are particularly sinister in children. Pediatric patients with left-to-right shunt lesions like ASD or ventricular septal defect also commonly present with shortness of breath and thus suffer from poor weight gain and chronic fatigue. While evaluating cardiac status, a complete clinical examination supported by imaging techniques such as chest X-rays may reveal underlying pathology not necessarily apparent. A study of congenital heart disease highlighted the importance of clinical examination, contrasting clinical presentations of cardiac enlargement with imaging results. This emphasizes the importance of an integrated strategy in identifying symptomatic children, giving those with CHDs early treatment to avoid increasing risk to their health (Tinh et al., 2024). Other significant symptoms to consider are palpitations or irregular heart rhythms in children, which most often indicate arrhythmias associated with some of the congenital heart defects. Such abnormalities are caused by structural heart defects that disrupt normal electrical conduction pathways, resulting in feelings of a rapid or irregular heartbeat. Palpitations in children may also involve reporting episodes of dizziness or syncope that a doctor must immediately evaluate. It is essential to understand the interaction between these symptoms and the congenital heart diseases in the formulation of treatment plans that address each patient's requirements. As in the case of the girl above with ASD, timely diagnosis and correct management procedures are crucial to improving the quality of life and minimizing long-term complications with regard to presentations of congenital heart disease in children (Hakim et al., 2024) (Figure 9.9).

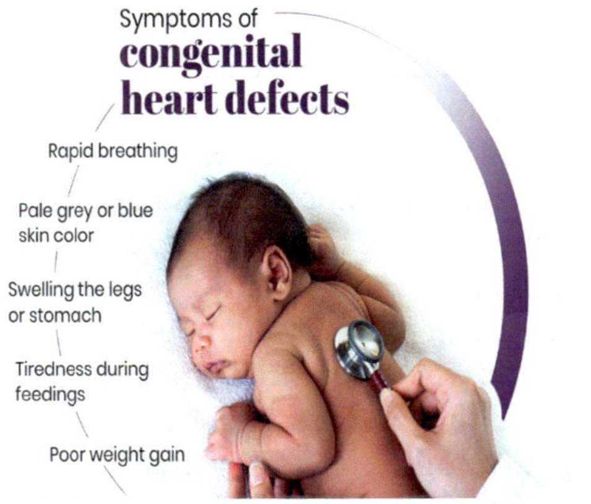

Figure 9.9. Symptoms of congenital heart defects (CHDs).

Source: https://kdahweb-static.kokilabenhospital.com/kdah-2019/tips/1644583788.jpg.

9.3.2. Diagnostic Imaging Techniques

The diagnostic imaging discipline plays a critical role in the diagnosis and treatment of CHDs. Of all the methodologies available, echocardiography has in the past been extolled as the first-line imaging tool, especially for children. The method is free from invasiveness as it utilizes ultrasound waves to generate real-time images of the heart, whereby clinicians can monitor cardiac structures and their function. Significant heart defects such as ASD and VSD can be accurately diagnosed using echocardiographic assessments. During a comparison of echocardiography with MDCTA, both imaging procedures demonstrated superior correlation in imaging structural defects, while echocardiography was particularly useful in the visualization of intracardiac defects (Ahamd et al., 2025). Thus, integration of these imaging modalities enhances our ability to diagnose congenital heart disease accurately and effectively. As technology becomes more advanced, MDCTA has been an effective complement to echocardiography in the assessment of congenital heart disease. MDCTA can produce high-quality images that allow for detailed visualization of the heart and vasculature. MDCTA is particularly helpful in assessing complex cardiac disease and extracardiac abnormalities that are not optimally visualized on echocardiography. Evidence showed that while MDCTA was better for the diagnosis of anatomical abnormalities (Ahamd et al., 2025), echocardiography remained the predominant diagnostic modality for the assessment of definitive intracardiac anomalies. The application of MDCTA enhances the sensitivity of diagnosis and allows for preoperative planning, with complete information about the patient's individual cardiac anatomy and guiding therapeutic interventions. MDCTA is applied to image the heart. Cardiac magnetic resonance imaging (MRI) is another important diagnostic imaging modality in the evaluation of congenital heart disease. MRI offers high spatial resolution in addition to the ability to evaluate both cardiac shape and function without the ionizing radiation of CT scans. The imaging process is particularly advantageous for those patients requiring frequent examinations over a long period, minimizing total radiation exposure. Cardiac MRI is superior in the evaluation of myocardial viability and hemodynamic function, thereby yielding information about the impact of congenital anomalies on overall cardiac performance. A pictorial chapter highlights the advantage of cardiac CT in illustrating the complexity of various congenital heart diseases, showing the spectrum of anomalies encountered in clinical practice. Combined, these new modalities significantly enhance the clinician's diagnostic, treatment, and individualized treatment plan design capability for patients with congenital heart disease (Figure 9.10).

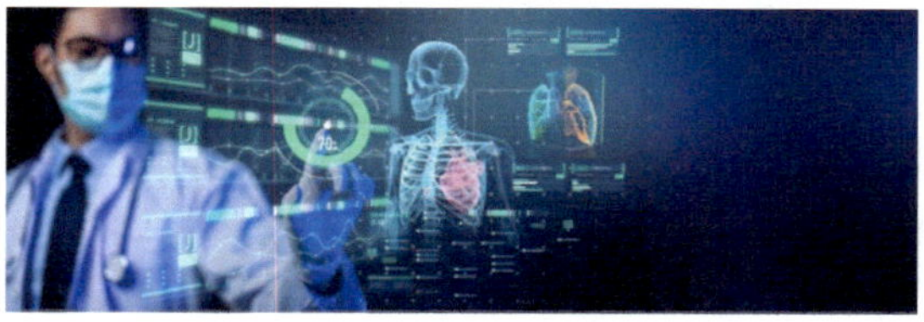

Figure 9.10. Diagnosis of congenital heart disease (CHD).

Source: https://punecardiologist.com/images/Diagnosis-of-Congenital-Heart-Disease.webp.

9.3.3. Role of Echocardiography (ECG) in Diagnosis

Echocardiography offers a basis for diagnosis of CHDs in the form of a non-invasive, real-time cardiac anatomy and hemodynamic performance imaging. This method enables clinicians to visualize both fetal and postnatal cardiac defects well, a consideration in the context that CHDs are the most common congenital condition in infants and account for the most infant mortality of congenital malformations. The ability of echocardiography to define cardiac anatomy enables early diagnosis and intervention strategies, ultimately improving patient outcomes. As shown in studies, echocardiography not only evaluates heart anatomy and physiology but also serves to monitor during the child's growth, thus demonstrating its vital position in ongoing clinical management of pediatric patients with suspected or established CHDs (Megahed et al., 2023). The use of echocardiography is particularly crucial in prenatal care, where it becomes essential for the diagnosis of congenital cardiac abnormalities of the developing fetus. Fetal echocardiography, performed between the second trimester, allows clinicians to see anatomical malformations, as well as critical insight into postnatal management strategies. Despite its advantages, echocardiography may be hindered by technical challenges, including maternal habitus and fetal position. To combat these issues, fetal cardiac MRI is used routinely as an adjunct imaging modality, enhancing report accuracy by providing additional information on cardiac and extra-cardiac structures (Megahed et al., 2023). This combination of modalities highlights the role of echocardiography as the backbone for comprehensive fetal cardiac assessment, optimizing prenatal diagnosis of congenital anomalies. Apart from prenatal diagnosis, echocardiography has roles to play beyond this because, even in infancy, it remains a valuable tool in both the assessment and follow-up of congenital heart disease. Under clinical conditions, echocardiography lies at the core of the diagnostic evaluation of murmurs or other cardiovascular presentations. For instance, a study in Dongguan, China, concluded that comprehensive prevalence of CHD was ascertained through systematic screening, corroborating the indispensable nature of echocardiographers' role in the detection and classification of such defects at an early stage. Echocardiography proved especially valuable in diagnosing prevalent forms of CHD, such as ventricular septal defects and atrial septal defects, and thus influencing the treatment plan and follow-up (Kang et al., 2023). As a result, echocardiography contributes significantly to the clinical management and long-term outcome of diagnosed patients with congenital heart disease, indicating its central position in the health care system.

9.4. Treatment Options

The management of CHDs is a multi-faceted approach with both surgical and non-surgical options. Surgical procedures are often at the center stage, especially for complex heart defects with significant impairment of cardiac function or oxygenation. Atrioseptal defect repair or Fontan procedures, for instance, aim to restore normal physiologic function and improve quality of life. These therapeutic surgeries must be appropriately timed, as early intervention can be more successful, but risks involved in surgery must also be carefully weighed against each child's specific condition. Also, planning before and after surgery must be incorporated as a combination to minimize complications and improve recovery, showing the complexity involved in effectively treating this cohort (Pribadi et al., 2023). Barring surgical intervention, the role of pharmacologic therapy in the management of CHD cannot be underestimated. Diuretics, ACE inhibitors, and beta-blockers are a few of the drugs that are employed to alleviate symptoms of heart failure and reduce the workload on the heart. This form of therapy is especially significant in the preoperative phase, stabilizing patients and preparing them for surgery. Long-term follow-up treatment also entails modification of medication therapy, as the patient's response to the therapy might be modified with time. Comprehensive management of congenital heart disease includes a combination of surgical and medical strategies to optimize patient outcomes and offer effective care throughout the life cycle (Pribadi et al., 2023). The study of alternative treatments, such as xenotransplantation, has become a reality in addressing the growing shortage of children in need of heart transplants. Since there is always a lack of donor organs, particularly children's organs, scientists are increasingly considering genetically engineered animal organs, such as pigs, as the best candidates for transplantation. Clinical trials have been initiated under the FDA's expanded access program, emphasizing the urgency to find alternatives for vulnerable neonates and infants who otherwise stand no hope of survival. This new approach introduces ethical and medical issues to consider, including informed consent and transmission risks of zoonotic diseases. With ongoing advancements in research in this area, hopes are for widening horizons for the treatment of congenital heart disease as well as improving survival rates for this vulnerable population (Figure 9.11).

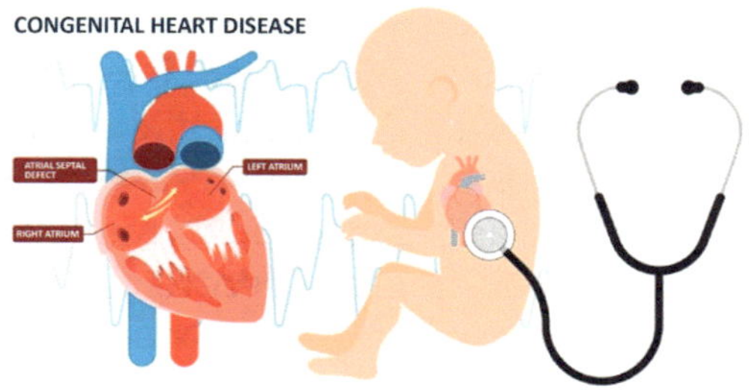

Figure 9.11. Congenital heart disease (CHG) treatment.

Source: https://punecardiologist.com/images/Congential-Heart-Disease.webp.

9.4.1. Medical Management and Medications

Effective medical management of CHD calls for a multi-dimensional approach that includes both pharmacologic treatment and comprehensive care programs. Pharmacologic therapy plays a central role in the management of symptomatic expression of CHD, particularly in ensuring optimal cardiac function and hemostatic balance. The medications prescribed include diuretics like Furosemide, which are crucial to manage fluid overloads, and ACE inhibitors like Captopril, which are employed to reduce afterload and increase cardiac output. These medications are also frequently used in combination to optimize patient outcomes, particularly in children in whom the potential for adverse effects might be higher. It is essential to monitor the side effects and efficacy of these treatments closely because CHD in children is found to have a unique therapeutic pattern compared to adults, so it is prudent to have a broader and more cautious treatment regimen. The combination of clinical evaluation and appropriate medication management is the key to the facilitation of not only the immediate health of CHD patients but also the long-term outcome. There has been an observational study aimed at determining patterns of antihypertensive medication usage in 92 children with CHD, which revealed Furosemide usage in 44.9% of the study participants, attributing its predominance in therapeutic regimens (Ali et al., 2024). Furthermore, research showed dosing and adherence to therapy as prescribed to be of high importance, with 98.9% effectiveness ratings. This suggests that while prescribing would be well-informed, problems of compliance remain barriers to be overcome. The complexities involved with CHD necessitate a synergistic effort on the part of medical providers, including pediatric cardiologists, pharmacists, and caregivers, to give a multifaceted form of care that remains responsive to evolving needs. Despite the availability of enhanced medical management, patient education and follow-up are still necessary variables for the optimization of health outcomes in children with congenital cardiac disease. Continued interaction with patients and guardians facilitates understanding of treatment regimens, drug compliance, and the need to identify side effects. Regardless of how current research calls for the potentiality of the inaccuracy of AI-designed learning materials in the medical field, appropriate utilization and assessment of tools can improve the learning experience for both healthcare professionals and patients (Temsah et al., 2024). Ultimately, building a culture of cooperation, wherein contributions from various fields can converge, will persist to maximize medication management in CHD, such that therapeutic strategies are maximally effective and attuned to the unique challenges presented by this heterogeneous collection of disorders.

9.4.2. Surgical Interventions

Surgery is a cornerstone in the management of CHD, repairing anatomical abnormalities that may essentially impair cardiac function. Operations range from subtle interventions like balloon atrial septostomy to extremely complicated procedures such as total correction of defects like tetralogy of Fallot or great vessel transposition. The timing of such operations is of significance; in some instances, early intervention in life, at an age in infancy or early childhood, may significantly enhance long-term function and quality of life. With advancing technology in surgical intervention and care after operation, cardiologists and child surgeons are increasingly capable of managing the unique challenges posed by CHDs. However, the intricacy that accompanies such patients demands an integral care process with the multiparametric management of potential complications following surgery, such as arrhythmias and heart failure, which are essential to the long-term success of such procedures. Lifesaving though such surgical procedures are, they carry risks that demand extensive preoperative investigation and postoperative monitoring. The most serious among these issues is the risk for surgical site infections (SSIs) that contribute negatively to recovery time and overall health status. A systematic review of the impact of targeted nursing interventions on surgical site infection rates among children having surgery for CHD found significant reductions in infection rates and improved wound healing for those patients receiving exceptional care. Observation group recorded a high SSI rate of 1.7% against 11.6% in the control group, emphasizing the importance of postoperative all-round management. These findings illustrate how tailored nursing treatments can act as an important essential adjunctive modality to surgery and positively influence patient recovery trajectories, emphasizing the interconnectedness of surgical and nursing interventions in maximizing patient outcomes for CHD (He et al., 2024). Apart from addressing short-term surgical risks, long-term follow-up care remains a fundamental component of managing congenital heart disease following intervention. Patients will often require regular surveillance for potential complications, including heart failure and the need for further surgical intervention in adulthood. Moreover, advances in technology such as cardiovascular imaging and biomarker analysis have provided clinicians with tools for assessing heart function comprehensively, guiding subsequent management modalities. These new procedures not only enhance the precision of existing surgical methods but also contribute to the development of personalized medicine approaches, culminating in enhanced life expectancy and life quality for subjects with congenital heart disease. As knowledge concerning CHDs increases, the unification of surgical and postoperative treatment methodologies and ongoing investigation of new therapies will be pivotal in advancing care (Netala et al., 2024) (Figure 9.12).

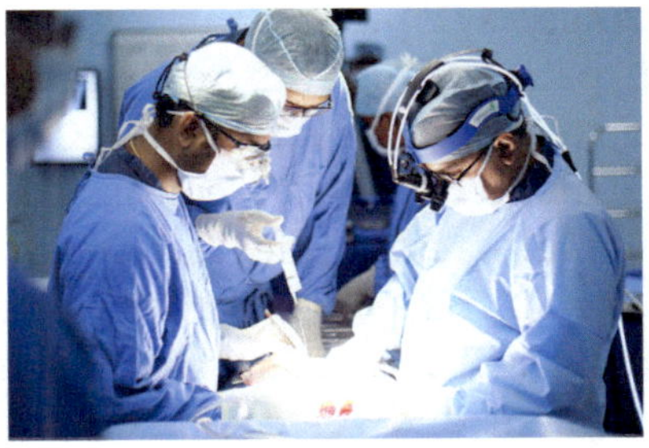

Figure 9.12. Surgical management of coronary artery disease.

Source: https://www.bcmch.org/asset/uploads/common/93228970861bc4cffa63d0.jpg.

9.4.3. Long-Term Care and Follow-Up

The treatment of CHDs far surpasses the initial treatment, requiring an active long-term care and follow-up plan specific to each patient's needs. Most patients with CHD, as they enter adulthood, will need ongoing surveillance because of possible complications that could occur due to their conditions. This long-term care is imperative since it can have a great deal of influence on morbidity and mortality rates in this group of individuals. Routine follow-up clinic visits allow assessment of cardiac function, detection of arrhythmias, and recognition of heart failure manifestations, which are prevalent among subjects with complex anatomic heart defects. Furthermore, the process of building a relationship between patients and multidisciplinary treatment teams comprised of cardiologists, primary care providers, and psychiatrists/psychologists may enhance treatment compliance and general health outcomes. Long-term follow-up thus becomes a cornerstone in the management of CHD, giving comprehensive care throughout the whole life of an individual. Transition to adult care in the evaluation of long-term results for patients with congenital heart disease is plagued with unique challenges. According to recent evidence, a significant proportion of ACHD patients present severe symptoms that result in emergency department visits. For instance, symptoms and signs such as dyspnea, palpitation, and heart failure have been reported to be prevalent in these patients, justifying the necessity for continued medical attention. Multifactorial heart defects also put patients at risk of developing complications and readmission, which indicates the necessity for early treatment and referral pathways. There should also be periodic psychological and social assessments incorporated into long-term follow-up protocols because emotional health can significantly influence treatment adherence and overall quality of life. It's therefore essential to have a comprehensive plan for long-term care among ACHD patients to mitigate risks and ensure good health outcomes throughout life. The requirement for sound long-term care and follow-up is well warranted based on literature highlighting the complexity of caring for congenital heart disease. Evidence suggests that meticulous assessment and individualized management plans have a good ability to enhance patients' outcomes in the long term. For example, longitudinal studies demonstrate that the majority of CHD patients undergoing systematic follow-up can adjust more easily to their health condition, resulting in fewer instances of serious complications and hospitalization. Moreover, emerging treatments and advances in healthcare provision are continually emerging, necessitating ongoing education and the integration of novel therapies into long-term treatment plans. These advancements require close integration of healthcare professionals of multiple specialties, such that patients are given holistic care. Lastly, the importance of long-term follow-up in the case of congenital heart diseases is that it can enhance patients' survival and quality of life, thereby reiterating the importance of close medical care and monitoring throughout their lives (Figure 9.13).

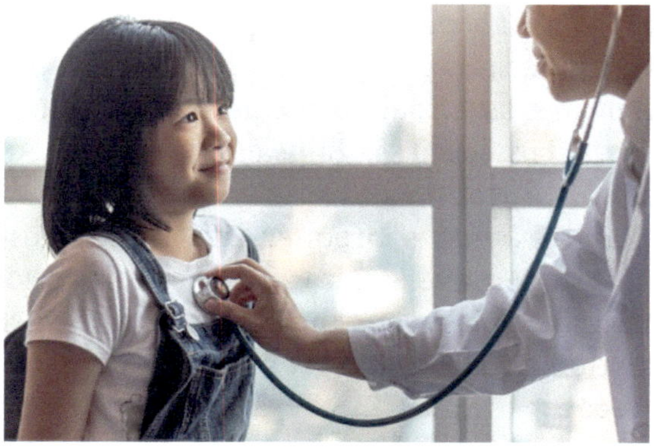

Figure 9.13. Treatment of Congenital Heart Disease.

Source: https://punecardiologist.com/images/Treatment-of-Congenital-Heart-Disease.webp.

SUMMARY

Overall, the intricacies of CHDs mandate patient management by a multidisciplinary team with early diagnosis, timely intervention, and ongoing management. The emergence of pulmonary arterial hypertension (PAH) in PAH patients with CHD adds another dimension of intricate challenges, significantly influencing their prognosis and quality of life. Current studies have highlighted the importance of early diagnosis and intervention strategies, such as congenital portosystemic shunt closure, in mitigating the severity of PAH and improving clinical outcomes. Understanding the correlation between clinical presentation, e.g., portal vein hypoplasia and hepatic dysfunction, and PAH advancement is central to optimizing treatment modalities and patient management protocols (Matsuoka et al., 2024). Secondly, the growing body of evidence points towards the necessity of standardized guidelines that address the management of PAH in CHD. While advances in medicine continue to increase the survival of patients with such conditions, there is a compelling need to develop integrative algorithms that consider the personalized nature and prognostic factors observed in PAH-CHD. These frameworks will encourage not only more specialized interventions by healthcare practitioners but also enhance the quality of care for an increasingly expanding population. By integrating advanced treatment modalities and diagnostic technology into practice, practitioners can facilitate better patient outcomes and more efficient management paradigms (Vasilyeva et al., 2024). Lastly, to confront the difficulties presented by congenital heart diseases, multidisciplinary teams must ally with cardiologists, surgeons, and allied healthcare workers. As new findings on PAH pathophysiology and clinical presentation in patients with CHD are released through ongoing research, it is now imperative that these be translated into feasible interventions. Increased awareness and knowledge among healthcare providers will ensure that patients with congenital heart diseases receive timely, optimal care suited to their respective conditions. Such a multi-level plan will not merely decrease the effects of congenital heart diseases as well as their complications but also provide long-term optimal well-being and health to the affected (Vasilyeva et al., 2024).

The complexity of CHDs is multi-dimensional, and they encompass not only the inherent physiological and anatomical challenges, but also the potential for resulting health complications. Of note is how conditions that are present before a CHD can lead to abnormal presentations of patients, particularly in the young. For instance, a case under discussion demonstrates the significance of taking unexplained back pain into account within the patient's cardiology history, and here indicates the association of congenital aortic stenosis and subsequent infective endocarditis. The interaction of these diagnoses emphasizes the necessity for differential diagnoses in clinical evaluation, as the symptoms can be caused by unforeseen cardiac malformations suffered by the patient (Ali et al., 2024). Furthermore, the role of other factors, such as genetic predispositions, must not be underestimated when the issue of CHD is being considered. The presence of markers like HLA B27 is a well-known indication of potential inflammatory diseases, but its relationship with infectious processes must be interpreted very carefully. For patients with congenital heart anomalies, the occurrence of infection may dominate the clinical setting very significantly. The case presentation underscores how an initial diagnosis would be easily predisposed towards musculoskeletal etiology when, in reality, the etiology was infective in origin due to the underlying cardiac pathology. Hence, detailed investigations, including imaging and microbiological swabs, are critical to create an ideal management plan (Ali et al., 2024). Lastly, management of congenitally diseased patients, especially those with arrhythmias, also poses some difficulties. Atrial tachycardias often present as recurrent complications in patients with specific anatomical alterations due to surgical interventions or due to congenital anomalies. Effective treatment, such as radiofrequency catheter ablation, can be complicated by abnormal venous anatomy, requiring a high-level understanding of these variations to ensure effective treatment. A case exemplifying a complex anatomic arrangement indicates how specialized techniques and multidisciplinary practice are essential for optimal patient outcomes. With increasingly advanced procedural methods, the integration of diverse medical specialties remains necessary to address the complex demands of this unusual patient population in depth.

A CLOSER LOOK

IMPACT ON QUALITY OF LIFE

CHDs significantly affect the quality of life (QoL) of the patients involved in various ways, including physical, psychological, and social conditions. Research has indicated that adults with CHD report lower QoL compared to their healthy counterparts, primarily due to the ongoing medical complications and psychosocial problems associated with the condition. For instance, depression and anxiety are common among this population, which plays a significant factor in their overall satisfaction and performance daily. Moreover, many may have difficulty with restrictions in physical functioning, which may affect their ability to engage in social and leisure activities. The cumulative effect of the above issues reiterates the supreme significance of comprehensive healthcare approaches addressing both the medical and emotional aspects of life in patients with CHD (Mahmod et al., 2024). Besides, the effect of CHD on quality of life extends beyond physical health and plays a distinct role in the attainment of developmental milestones, particularly in pediatric populations. Children with CHD can be plagued by developmental delays and psychosocial complications that impact their motor function and social interactions. For instance, it is described how children with Down syndrome will experience exacerbation of these challenges when combined with CHD, particularly in the early childhood period. Measurement of QoL in these subjects shows that while significant effects on motor function are present at younger ages, these discrepancies become progressively less pronounced with advancing age, suggesting the potential for benefit from early intervention to augment benefit to long-term development. Yet the possibility of early impairment highlights the difficulties involved in successful management of CHD and emphasizes the importance of holistic approaches to care (Alhaddad et al., 2023).

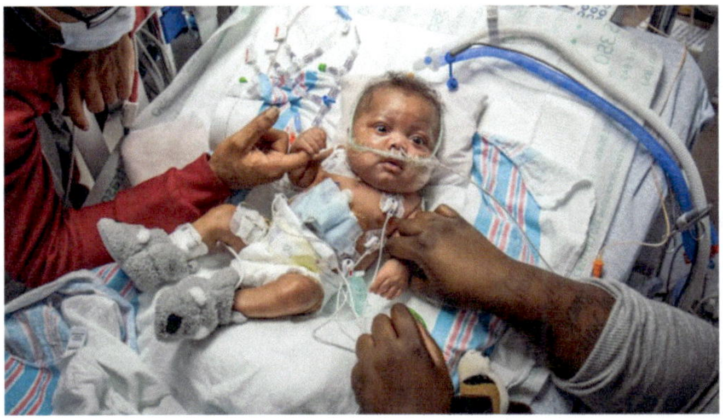

Figure 9.14. Quality of Life in Patients with Congenital Heart Disease.

Source: https://assets.clevelandclinic.org/transform/LargeFeatureImage/35aff0ba-b96e-4f53-a873-df35705d8089/CCC-2251608_07-12-21_069_LDJ-jpg.

At different life stages, the relationship between their medical condition and quality of life remains prevalent. Adulthood also presents another batch of problems associated with it since most young adults face more job worries, relationship problems, and general independent living, all of which are affected by their cardiac condition. This transition phase is also critical since it usually sets their adaptability capacity and long-term mental health status. Proper support mechanisms and resources become essential in maintaining resilience and improving QoL in this period. Thus, managing the multifaceted impact of CHD on quality of life not only involves medical care but demands the establishment of psychological support and education interventions that strive to optimize coping skills, ultimately leading to better life results for the affected individuals in their pursuit of a purposeful life (Mahmod AMA et al., 2024) (Figure 9.14).

References

1. Kochovska, S., Luckett, T., Agar, M., & Phillips, J. L. (2017). Impacts on employment, finances, and lifestyle for working age people facing an expected premature death: A systematic review. *Palliative & Supportive Care, 16*(3), 347–364. https://doi.org/10.1017/s1478951517000979Ahamd, B., Ashraf, R., Naseem, C., Ullah, K., Ali, S., & Raza, M. (2025). Correlation of multidetector computed tomography and transthoracic echocardiography in the diagnosis of congenital cyanotic heart diseases. *Kashf Journal of Multidisciplinary Research*. https://www.semanticscholar.org/paper/6db9f9c10e40161f26cef9aeee2dd9b5f263a3de (accessed on 29th May 2025).
2. Alhaddad, F., Alkhushi, N., Alharbi, A. M., Al Talib, S. A., Sultan, S. M., & Bahawi, Y. O. (2023). Quality of life among Down syndrome patients with and without congenital heart disease at King Abdulaziz University Hospital, Jeddah, Saudi Arabia. *Cureus, 15*. https://www.semanticscholar.org/paper/ba8277c2b5328f1112e893a1ef6f0e5fa088716a (accessed on 29th May 2025).
3. Ali, R. H. E., Warrell, C., & Manson, J. (2024). P16: Concurrent sacroiliitis and infective endocarditis in a young male with congenital aortic stenosis: A diagnostic challenge and learning points. *Rheumatology Advances in Practice, 8*. https://www.semanticscholar.org/paper/cb19696b75a815a13dd3429da9549bf40468196b (accessed on 29th May 2025).
4. Ali, S., Sobhan, A., & Pathak, A. (2024). Evaluating the efficacy and safety of antihypertensive drugs in the treatment of congenital heart disease in pediatric patients: A comprehensive study. *Journal of Medical and Health Studies*. https://www.semanticscholar.org/paper/ca6322b73fdfa99116f479c023fdea37bf68e0a6 (accessed on 29th May 2025).
5. Alkahtani, H., Haq, I., Ghadi, Y., Innab, N., Alajmi, M., & Nurbapa, M. (2024). Precision diagnosis: An automated method for detecting congenital heart diseases in children from phonocardiogram signals employing deep neural network. *IEEE Access, 12*, 76053–76064. https://www.semanticscholar.org/paper/3c1e2165909562860ea36f0216ec80d07f82a0b1 (accessed on 29th May 2025).
6. Andescavage, N., & Limperopoulos, C. (2021). Placental abnormalities in congenital heart disease. *Translational Pediatrics, 10*, 2148–2156. https://doi.org/10.21037/tp-20-347 (accessed on 29th May 2025).
7. Baráth, S., Nagy, O., & Ujfalusi, A. (2019). *The Role of microRNAs in Congenital Heart Disease*. https://core.ac.uk/download/220110021.pdf (accessed on 29th May 2025).
8. Barradas, P. A., Krishnathasan, K., Constantine, A., & Dimopoulos, K. (2024). Cardiopulmonary exercise testing in adult congenital heart patients: A new data-focused approach to predict mortality. *European Heart Journal*. https://www.semanticscholar.org/paper/fbb5aa2ea5a3d36bfc9e5d3be47438022646ac24 (accessed on 29th May 2025).
9. Bobier, C., Cleveland, D., Cleveland, J. D., Hurst, J., et al. (2024). *Pediatric Cardiac Xenotransplantation and Expanded Access: Ethical Considerations*. https://core.ac.uk/download/639364754.pdf (accessed on 29th May 2025).
10. Calderón, R. A. D., Arredondo, M. E., & Reinoso, H. M. G. (2025). Comprehensive nursing care for pediatric patients with congenital heart diseases: A focus on ventricular septal defect.

SCT Proceedings in Interdisciplinary Insights and Innovations. https://www.semanticscholar.org/paper/d1d1f7ca93afd22c6aeb8749eebbb451dc9d7faf (accessed on 29th May 2025).

11. Cherkasova, O., & Krykhtina, M. (2024). *Congenital Heart Defects and Eisenmenger's Syndrome in Adults – Diagnostic Difficulties (Clinical Case).* Reports of Vinnytsia National Medical University. https://www.semanticscholar.org/paper/f33f37842c835daeadf88069c66183bc1d65f1a0 (accessed on 29th May 2025).

12. Crain, A. K., Lim, Z. N., Sarfatis, C. J., Arias, M., Holder, T., Moreira, A. G., Corno, A. F., et al. (2025). Meta-analysis on sex differences in mortality and neurodevelopment in congenital heart defects. *Scientific Reports, 15.* https://www.semanticscholar.org/paper/86d582010b755172c658bf27b8c14fd39bbffc68 (accessed on 29th May 2025).

13. Crea, F. (2021). The central role of amygdala in stress-related cardiac diseases and an update on long-COVID. *European Heart Journal, 42*(19), 1813–1817. https://www.semanticscholar.org/paper/32241aefa763d34669da313f103697eb8d1d544f (accessed on 29th May 2025).

14. Crişan, S., Băghină, R. M., Luca, S. A., Pătru, O., Lazăr, M., Văcărescu, C., Rus, M., et al. (2024). From ECG to imaging: Challenges in the diagnosis of adult congenital heart diseases. *Journal of Clinical Medicine, 13.* https://www.semanticscholar.org/paper/bf13fe1ce4fd24d8fb16f91604368853a69d85b4 (accessed on 29th May 2025).

15. Doğan, E., Ergin, F., Beyter, M., Kaşıkçı, G. K., Ön, Ş. Ş., Ay, O., Levent, R., et al. (2024). Arrhythmias in children undergoing orthotopic heart transplantation. *Frontiers in Cardiovascular Medicine, 10.* https://www.semanticscholar.org/paper/2a7891a73130aa1b75e4f0b571bf46e6ccd1537c (accessed on 29th May 2025).

16. Dziewczapolski, G. (2020). Cure CMD, a patient-centered organization: Pivotal role to help move emerging therapeutics into clinical practice for the congenital muscular dystrophies. *12, 2020.* https://www.semanticscholar.org/paper/1666a371e905c0488c2854ba237f94cdc7f3128f (accessed on 29th May 2025).

17. Elmustfa, A. A. M., & Koko, S. H. M. (2024). Adult congenital heart diseases: Systematic review/meta-analysis. *Annals of Medicine and Surgery, 86*, 1606–1612. https://www.semanticscholar.org/paper/7729a8a4ef262f949115db78ed72cde0e9941fe7 (accessed on 29th May 2025).

18. Golalipour, M. J., Mirfazeli, A., Nikyarspi-Sup, B., Qourbani, M., et al. (2011). *Prevalence and Pattern of Congenital Heart Disease Among Neonates in Gorgan, Northern Iran (2007–2008).* https://core.ac.uk/download/52204847.pdf (accessed on 29th May 2025).

19. Golinowska, S., & Sowa, A. (2012). *Health Status, Functional Limitations and Disability: Changes in Poland.* https://core.ac.uk/download/30436254.pdf (accessed on 29th May 2025).

20. Hakim, A. N. A., Adnaya, A. A. N. M., Prasetyo, A. B., Pikir, R. R., Diarsvitri, W., Suhadi, A. R., & Dita, A. (2024). Atrial septal defect. *Surabaya Biomedical Journal.* https://www.semanticscholar.org/paper/fc9fe33c2d85f30cb8bdb46e5a26a5972d809dfe (accessed on 29th May 2025).

21. He, P., & Hai, Y. (2024). The efficacy of nursing interventions in preventing surgical site infections in patients undergoing surgery for congenital heart disease. *International Wound Journal, 21.* https://www.semanticscholar.org/paper/5614d23597a2c3f27d133e6419ac1d96cf447271 (accessed on 29th May 2025).

22. Ilyas, S., Rehman, Y., Hussain, I., Khan, A., Ahmed, T., & Akbar, A. (2021). Emergency department presentation and outcome of children with cyanotic congenital heart diseases. *Cureus, 13.*

https://www.semanticscholar.org/paper/c9a7822a8fb98747435a7169fd51919d48e5f12d (accessed on 29th May 2025).

23. Kang, G., Xiao, J., Wang, J., & Zhang, H. (2023). Prevalence and pattern of congenital heart diseases in school children in Dongguan, China. *World Journal for Pediatric and Congenital Heart Surgery, 14*, 442–445. https://www.semanticscholar.org/paper/d64af552762565a4c59b1a56113227bec18f1127 (accessed on 29th May 2025).

24. Kitsiou, A., Caforio, A. L. P., Porta-Sanchez, A., Vahanian, A., Iung, B., Carrera, C., Szymanski, C., et al. (2013). *ESC Core Curriculum for the General Cardiologist (2013).* https://core.ac.uk/download/55756305.pdf (accessed on 29th May 2025).

25. Krishnakumar, M., Hari, A., Gutjahr, G., Bendapudi, P., Ahamed, H., Prabhakaran, P., Kumar, R. K., et al. (2024). Impact of exposure to extreme heat events during pregnancy on the incidence of congenital heart disease in offspring: A meta-analysis. *BMJ Pediatrics Open, 8.* https://www.semanticscholar.org/paper/a7b37c6bea76882597a6378f44f2be0eb42bc783 (accessed on 29th May 2025).

26. Matsuoka, R., Nagata, H., Kobayashi, M., Uike, K., Nagatomo, Y., Terashi, E., Hirata, Y., et al. (2024). Abstract 4139896: Prognosis of pulmonary arterial hypertension after treatment for congenital portosystemic shunt in children. *Circulation*. https://www.semanticscholar.org/paper/0ea1fa0fbd1ee01ac1a4395bfacc54cdcbb35616 (accessed on 29th May 2025).

27. Megahed, S. R., Ibrahim, A., & Hassan, H. (2023). Role of fetal cardiac MRI in assessment of congenital heart diseases in comparison to fetal echocardiography. *QJM: An International Journal of Medicine*. https://www.semanticscholar.org/paper/7dd50f877ca40b963548259b421667b0686ad3b1 (accessed on 29th May 2025).

28. Morrish, A. M., O'Malley, B. R., Hilton, D. C. K., Webb, A. E., Bennetts, B., Sholler, G. F., Smith, J., et al. (2025). Outcomes and experiences of genetic testing in children with congenital heart disease. *Journal of Medical Genetics*. https://www.semanticscholar.org/paper/0dddecbf7589960458fc53a4f75c55aa14269f72 (accessed on 29th May 2025).

29. Netala, V. R., Teertam, S., Li, H., & Zhang, Z. (2024). A comprehensive review of cardiovascular disease management: Cardiac biomarkers, imaging modalities, pharmacotherapy, surgical interventions, and herbal remedies. *Cells, 13*. https://www.semanticscholar.org/paper/308135f5cf36d96b4e2d99c8fad92729ba89260d (accessed on 29th May 2025).

30. Onorato, A., Vannatta, K., Texter, K., Spayde, K., Gosselin, R., Chaudhari, B., Kistler, I., et al. (2024). Abstract 4141963: Patient perspectives of genetic testing in adult congenital heart disease. *Circulation*. https://www.semanticscholar.org/paper/b662469c33c8d64ec6ef973622f5c3ec61fe15d2 (accessed on 29th May 2025).

31. Pan, K., Xu, J., Wang, C., Mao, Z., Xu, Y., Zhang, H., & Yu, J. (2024). Association between maternal exposure to environmental endocrine disruptors and the risk of congenital heart diseases in offspring: A systematic review and meta-analysis. *Environmental Research Letters, 19*. https://www.semanticscholar.org/paper/3554ae8d32799b6a2efc6bfc9c895b2a0a683149 (accessed on 29th May 2025).

32. Piazza, I., Memaj, I., Della, B. L., Preti, C., Bassareo, P., Cosentini, R., & Ferrero, P. (2024). Emergency care of adult patients with congenital heart disease: Are we prepared? Data from a tertiary center and long-term follow-up. *Emergency Care Journal*. https://www.

semanticscholar.org/paper/5d02553c5dd1822d1aaf280c1ba0aded114c43db (accessed on 29th May 2025).

33. Pidaparti, M., Geddes, G. C., & Durbin, M. D. (2024). Clinical genetic and genomic testing in congenital heart disease and cardiomyopathy. *Journal of Clinical Medicine, 13*. https://www.semanticscholar.org/paper/03ca6253deab7294a91620b24644a8e294b68f9c (accessed on 29th May 2025).

34. Pribadi, A. (2023). *Women with a History of Congenital Anomaly: Preparation for Next Pregnancy*. https://core.ac.uk/download/570905628.pdf (accessed on 29th May 2025).

35. Ruddarraju, P., Ayapaneni, D. R., & Moorthy, N. L. N. (2024). Exploring the uncommon: A pictorial journey through rare congenital heart diseases via cardiac CT imaging. *International Journal of Advanced Research*. https://www.semanticscholar.org/paper/3e0455252b640baee9e6d56555d4cb36e45ecc3b (accessed on 29th May 2025).

36. Siregar, F., Hartopo, A. B., & Mubarika, S. (2024). Recent progress in the roles of microRNAs in pulmonary arterial hypertension associated with congenital heart disease. *Narra J., 4*. https://www.semanticscholar.org/paper/86538d85e06f68ba285c58924111b2d798a4bf68 (accessed on 29th May 2025).

37. Solangi, A. A., & Khan, N. K. (2024). Case report: A case of an anomalous right coronary artery arising from the left coronary cusp. *The Journal of Cardiovascular Diseases*. https://www.semanticscholar.org/paper/5c29b3c4017d4fbabbcc1ea2839fd845da0333f9 (accessed on 29th May 2025).

38. Sonawane, R., Shah, R., Sonawane, S., & Gaikwad, R. (2022). Screening of newborn by pulse oximetry at birth for the critical congenital heart disease. *MVP Journal of Medical Sciences*. https://www.semanticscholar.org/paper/cefe579eb4992d4d4b9e0e99bf907261c3fbfcf5 (accessed on 29th May 2025).

39. Temsah, M., Alhuzaimi, A. N., Almansour, M., Aljamaan, F., Alhasan, K., Batarfi, M. A., Altamimi, I., et al. (2024). Art or artifact: Evaluating the accuracy, appeal, and educational value of AI-generated imagery in DALL·E 3 for illustrating congenital heart diseases. *Journal of Medical Systems, 48*, 1–13. https://www.semanticscholar.org/paper/17feee9b2888193ab6ff7948b8500d96ff37baf7 (accessed on 29th May 2025).

40. Terzic, A., & Waldman, S. A. (2019). *Health Care Evolves from Reactive to Proactive*. https://core.ac.uk/download/213444739.pdf (accessed on 29th May 2025).

41. Thakur, Y., Meshram, R., & Taksande, A. (2024). Navigating pediatric cor pulmonale: A comprehensive review of diagnosis and management. *Cureus, 16*. https://www.semanticscholar.org/paper/0c55d708784169569baf14219459599de5d6815e (accessed on 29th May 2025).

42. Thunström, S., Wide, U., Landin-Wilhelmsen, K., Berntorp, K., Bryman, I., Krantz, E., Wahlberg, J., et al. (2024). Psychiatric disorders and comorbidity in women with Turner syndrome: A retrospective national cohort study. *Translational Psychiatry, 14*. https://www.semanticscholar.org/paper/fb93e85895dbd9c50f7957e86fcf9ae503ea4438 (accessed on 29th May 2025).

43. Tinh, T. D. H., Phan, T. T., & Nguyen, T. P. C. (2024). The role of combining clinical skills and chest X-ray in detecting pediatric congenital heart diseases. *Journal of Medicine and Pharmacy*. https://www.semanticscholar.org/paper/6a72d79433adebbe00f5a8f748237c6c5be8863f (accessed on 29th May 2025).

44. Turan, O. E., Yılancıoğlu, R. Y., Inevi, U., & Özcan, E. E. (2023). Pre-procedural imaging and atrial tachycardia ablation in a patient with complex congenital heart disease. *Pacing and Clinical Electrophysiology*, *46*, 510–514. https://www.semanticscholar.org/paper/47b60402d33a1c4a8258fc70a648c389e537c680 (accessed on 29th May 2025).

45. Vasilyeva, L. I., Kalashnykova, O. S., Smolianova, O., & Shashko, O. V. (2024). Pulmonary arterial hypertension associated with congenital heart disease: Rationale for management algorithm based on a literature review. *Art of Medicine*. https://www.semanticscholar.org/paper/08e4fc69546b38437198840cb158ced014ac1807 (accessed on 29th May 2025).

46. Walker, K., Specht, I., Hjortdal, V., Christesen, H. T., Heitmann, B. L., Santorelli, G., West, J., et al. (2025). Circulating 25-hydroxyvitamin D levels during pregnancy and risk of congenital heart diseases: Multivariable and Mendelian randomization analyses using 3 birth cohorts. *Journal of the American Heart Association*. https://www.semanticscholar.org/paper/a6c7826711b19d9edf64e08b434a2f13e9cfebb2 (accessed on 29th May 2025).

47. Wang, G., Deng, H., Peng, P., Zheng, H., Tian, B., & Zhu, C. (2024). Compound heterozygosity for Southeast Asian hereditary persistence of fetal hemoglobin and β^0-thalassemia results in thalassemia intermedia: Pedigree analysis and genetic research in a family from South China. A case report. *Medicine*, *103*. https://www.semanticscholar.org/paper/ce1fd3b295dde3d9ce30e632b6695aec36c32288 (accessed on 29th May 2025).

48. Wilde, A. A. M., Semsarian, C., Márquez, M. F., Sepehri, S. A., Ackerman, M. J., Ashley, E. A., Sternick, E. B., et al. (2022). European Heart Rhythm Association (EHRA)/Heart Rhythm Society (HRS)/Asia Pacific Heart Rhythm Society (APHRS)/Latin American Heart Rhythm Society (LAHRS) expert consensus statement on the state of genetic testing for cardiac diseases. *Heart Rhythm*, *19*, e1–e60. https://doi.org/10.1016/j.hrthm.2022.03.1225 (accessed on 29th May 2025).

49. Wu, X., Chen, J., Iroegbu, C., Liu, J., Wu, M., Xie, X., Xiang, K., et al. (2022). Individualized analysis and treatment of difficult weaning from ventilation following open cardiac surgery in young children with congenital heart disease. *Frontiers in Cardiovascular Medicine*, *9*. https://www.semanticscholar.org/paper/c664bcc29a81e89f4dada53a0cabc83c33cb4b01 (accessed on 29th May 2025).

50. Xie, D., Luo, Y., Xiong, X., Lou, M., Liu, Z., Wang, A., Xiong, L., et al. (2019). Study on the potential biomarkers of maternal urine metabolomics for fetus with congenital heart diseases based on modified gas chromatograph–mass spectrometer. *BioMed Research International*, *2019*. https://www.semanticscholar.org/paper/4f56e036e7b5d43bafd13ba3152b5f29585a3b1e (accessed on 29th May 2025).

51. Yaseen, M., Hasan, G., & Bakhsh, Z. L. (2023). Experiences of adults with congenital heart disease: An interpretative phenomenological analysis. *Pakistan Journal of Humanities and Social Sciences*. https://www.semanticscholar.org/paper/78c052523c6fc9b52f468b7af8628cd8cad31e4f (accessed on 29th May 2025).

52. Zhang, Q., Zhou, J., Zhu, S., Liu, H., Mao, Y., Tang, Y., Mo, X., et al. (2024). Safety, effectiveness, and complications of the first-in-human minimally invasive transthoracic ventricular septal defect closure using a bioabsorbable occluder: A cohort study with 12-month follow-up. *Cardiovascular Diagnosis and Therapy*, *14*, 630–641. https://www.semanticscholar.org/paper/b570c9fce5ee7b95eef7ac1ed00386db06b4dad0 (accessed on 29th May 2025).

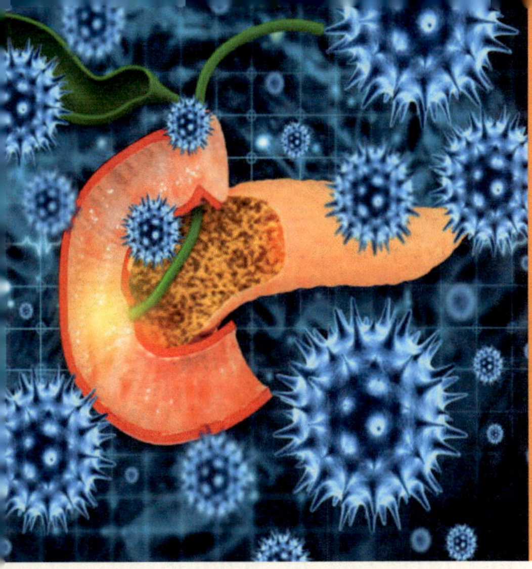

Chapter 10

INFLAMMATORY HEART DISEASES

Contents

Introduction

Inflammatory heart disease has been an emerging topic of research in recent years, reflecting the intricate relationship between inflammation and cardiovascular disease. These diseases, which are an inflammation of the cardiac muscle or the covering membranes, may exist in the forms of myocarditis or pericarditis. The etiologies would range from infection, including viral infection, to autoimmune responses, rendering diagnosis and treatment of these diseases particularly challenging. With researchers putting their best efforts into unraveling these complexities, there is a great need to adopt an interdisciplinary approach, combining information from cardiology, immunology, and infectious disease. This multidisciplinary perspective is hardly less crucial for the understanding of the pathophysiology of inflammatory heart disease than for planning effective therapeutic intervention strategies to modulate morbidity and mortality in these diseases. In addition to clinical contexts, there are also some factors in society involved in managing inflammatory heart illnesses. The health information of the patient that is reported to healthcare professionals can give a clue regarding treatment and outcomes. Remote patient monitoring, for instance, can offer continuous monitoring of the status of the patients beyond a usual healthcare situation, and this can enhance compliance on the part of the patients as well as clinical management. Studies have established that some patient groups, such as patients with heart failure, are greatly helped by remote monitoring systems, and the need for healthcare innovation has been highlighted (Wartenberg et al., 2025). While the developments provide prospective avenues for improvement in patient care, they also highlight the necessity of further studies to evaluate the effectiveness of the intervention across different groups of patients with inflammatory heart disease. In addition, emerging evidence about interventions and procedural outcomes in interventional cardiology testifies to an emerging discipline that increasingly incorporates the therapy of inflammatory heart disease.

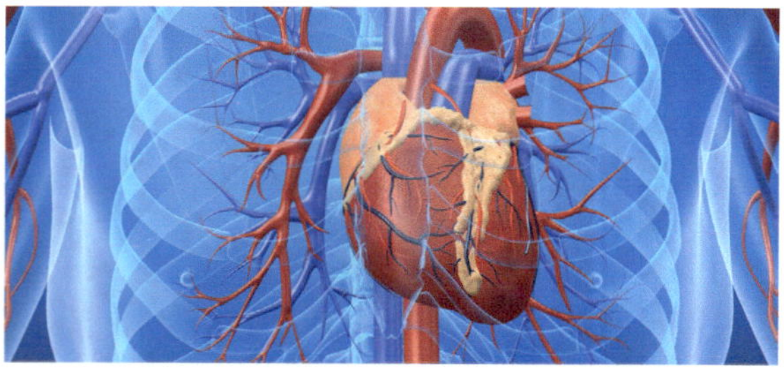

Figure 10.1. Inflammatory heart diseases (IHD).

Source: https://medizinonline.com/wp-content/uploads/2015/08/herz_kreislauf_2.jpg.

The most recent annual report on the activity of the Interventional Cardiology Association includes an emerging recognition of the need to address congenital heart diseases and inflammatory pathologies (Tejerizo et al., 2024). Such blending of therapy with novel procedures allows for enhanced patient treatment using sophisticated means by which ischemic episodes associated with inflammation may be lessened. Thus, it can be seen that knowledge of etiology, treatment options, and clinical courses of inflammatory heart diseases is necessary to treat patients effectively. A multidisciplinary approach, coupled with technological progress and routine practices, will eventually offer improved outcomes for patients afflicted by such complex heart diseases (Figure 10.1).

Definition of Inflammatory Heart Diseases

Inflammatory heart conditions include an array of disorders with myocardial, pericardial, or adjacent structure inflammation. These conditions primarily include myocarditis, pericarditis, and endocarditis. Myocarditis, for example, is usually brought about by viral infections, autoimmune disorders, or exposure to certain environmental toxins. The inflammation can severely alter cardiac function, leading to clinical manifestations such as chest discomfort, dyspnea, and in the worst-case scenario, sudden cardiac death. In contrast to other forms of heart disease, inflammatory heart diseases usually require individually adapted clinical examinations to understand their etiology and properly guide therapeutic strategies. As such, clinical definitions and classifications of the diseases have evolved, by advancements in medical technology and knowledge, as detailed in recent reviews of the challenges of myocarditis and related disorders diagnosis (Hracs et al., 2024). The clinical presentation and course of inflammatory heart diseases can vary significantly based on the etiology and extent of inflammation. While some patients thus have slow-moving manifestations that resolve spontaneously, others go on to develop ultimate heart failure or slow-moving complications necessitating prolonged treatment. In addition, the inflammatory process may lead to true cardiac structural abnormalities like scarring or fibrosis, further complicating the clinical picture. The importance of accurate diagnosis cannot be overemphasized, as incorrect diagnosis can lead to inappropriate treatment and undesirable outcomes. Recent studies emphasized the need for precise definitions that specify the different stages and intensities of such conditions, such as in models suggested for inflammatory bowel disease (Hracs et al., 2024). Such precision becomes critical to advancing patient care and clinical practice guidelines. Treatment of the inflammatory heart conditions is usually a multidisciplinary procedure determined by the specific disease and degree of inflammation. The therapeutic management can be made up of anti-inflammatory medications, immunosuppressants, or supportive therapy procedures meant to control the symptoms and prevent complications. Guidelines given by health authorities place special emphasis on the assessment of each patient's unique presentation to ensure maximum outcomes.

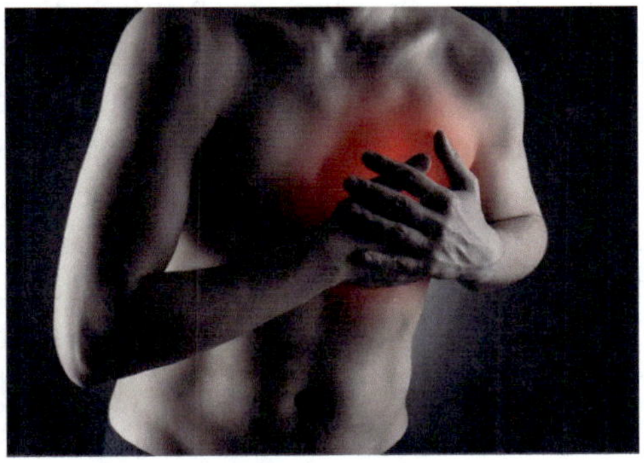

Figure 10.2. Inflammatory heart conditions.

Source: https://chblob.icloudhospital.com/thumbnails/2-5eb41d33-b959-4211-8866-117077169331.webp.

As highlighted in systematic reviews, the enormous shortfall in uniform clinical guidelines on the diagnosis and management of these complex disorders, particularly in myocarditis (Blagova et al., 2021), persists. The dynamic nature of these recommendations translates to a growing recognition of the complexities in the treatment of inflammatory heart diseases, ultimately to a balance between the treatment of acute inflammation and preserving long-term cardiac health (Figure 10.2).

10.1. Types of Inflammatory Heart Diseases

Chronic inflammatory heart diseases are a heterogeneous group of diseases with certain specific pathological processes and clinical manifestations. The most prominent among these is myocarditis, which is an inflammatory condition of the heart muscle and can be caused by viral infections, autoimmune response, or toxins. Clinical presentation of myocarditis is highly varied and often mimics symptoms of acute coronary syndrome, such as chest pain, shortness of breath, and palpitations. Moreover, the intensity of inflammation can lead to myocardial failure, potentially resulting in heart failure. Recent studies emphasize the significance of early diagnosis and etiological differentiation of myocarditis since treatment methods may be heterogeneous based on etiology. Cervical identification is essential as early treatment can prevent complications, enhancing patient prognosis and quality of life. Pericarditis, another severe type of inflammatory heart disease, is characterized by inflammation of the pericardial sac that covers the heart. It may be caused by infection, autoimmune diseases, or secondary to systemic disease such as cancer or renal failure. Severe, pleuritic chest pain that tends to be worse with inspiration or recumbency and improves with sitting up and leaning forward is the characteristic symptom of pericarditis. In most cases, pericardial effusion—fluid within the pericardial sac—may complicate the clinical picture with the potential for cardiac tamponade if left untreated. Diagnosis relies on clinical examination, imaging, and sometimes laboratory investigation to identify the etiology. Successful management may include non-steroidal anti-inflammatory drugs (NSAIDs) or corticosteroids to suppress symptoms, illustrating the importance of understanding the nuances of this inflammatory disease in maximizing therapeutic effects. Lastly, valvular heart disease also has an inflammatory cause, particularly in rheumatic heart disease and infective endocarditis. Infective endocarditis, characterized by microbial infection of the heart valves, leads to the formation of vegetations that can cause abnormalities in normal hemodynamics and trigger systemic embolic events. It has manifestations ranging from fever and malaise to more sinister presentations such as heart failure and heart murmurs. Rheumatic heart disease arises as a sequela of rheumatic fever, typically as a result of untreated streptococcal infection. Severe and chronic inflammation of rheumatic valvulitis may cause irreversible damage to heart valves, with surgical intervention needed in severe instances. Being aware of these types, particularly those associated with specific mechanisms of inflammation and their resultant effects, is central to the optimal management of inflammatory heart diseases, thereby enabling improved clinical outcomes and preventive measures (Figure 10.3).

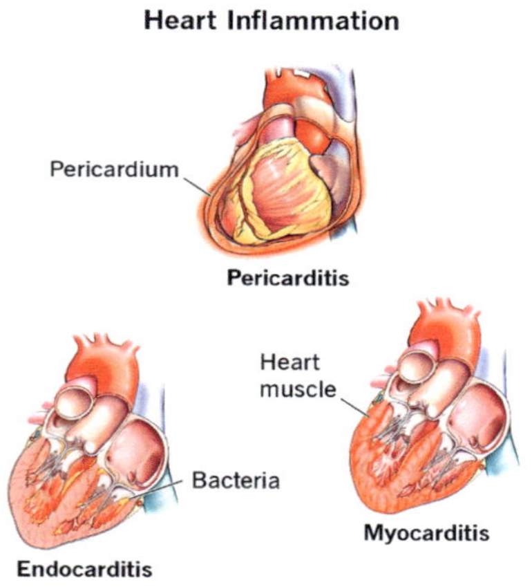

Figure 10.3. Three types of heart inflammation.

Source: https://my.clevelandclinic.org/-/scassets/images/org/health/articles/23052-heart-inflammation.

10.1.1. Myocarditis

Myocarditis, an inflammatory cardiac muscle process, is caused by a vast spectrum of etiologic causes, including viral infections, autoimmune disorders, and toxic exposures. Myocarditis pathophysiology involves an interaction of multifactorial infectious and host immune mechanisms leading to both acute and chronic myocardial tissue injury. Of significance, immediate removal of a viral pathogen may temper severe complications. At the same time, suboptimal immune resolution may allow for the establishment of chronic inflammatory processes to ensue, resulting in exacerbating myocardial dysfunction. The severe complications of the condition highlight the pivotal role of swift diagnosis and therapy, as the clinical presentation is often masked by other cardiology illnesses, rendering timely and effective treatment burdensome (Gil et al., 2017). By understanding these fundamental mechanisms, clinicians are better able to tackle the treatment and management of myocarditis within the broader context of inflammatory heart disease. The presentation of myocarditis is highly variable, making it difficult to diagnose. Symptoms range from mild fatigability and chest pain to more subtle findings like heart failure and arrhythmias. Due to its heterogeneity, diagnosis of myocarditis requires critical evaluation that transcends the typical clinical presentation and imaging techniques. Histological, immunohistochemical, and molecular studies play an essential role in establishing the diagnosis, indicating the mechanisms of inflammation and cell injury of the myocardium. Its multicentric character often results in underdiagnosis, particularly when overlapping with symptomatology of other cardiovascular diseases, hence the necessity for extensive diagnostic methods (Gil et al., 2017). Increasing awareness of the diverse clinical presentations of myocarditis can ultimately translate into improved patient outcomes and more advanced treatment modalities. Of the various forms of myocarditis, giant cell myocarditis is one of the more aggressive types that requires urgent treatment and management strategies. It is characterized by the presence of multinucleated giant cells within the myocardium and can occur variably from an acute to a sub-acute presentation, thereby complicating diagnosis and management. Although early detection and care are now possible because to advancements in circulatory support and imaging diagnostics, ideally effective regimens are still not well characterized. Improved results for impacted individuals necessitate tailored therapy, which includes immunosuppressive management augmented by supportive care. This highlights the importance of ongoing research and clinical innovation, as advocated by novel forms of treatment challenging the complex interaction of immune response with cardiac damage in giant cell myocarditis. It is therefore imperative to understand such minute features for improving the prognosis and management protocol of patients affected with this lethal condition (Figure 10.4).

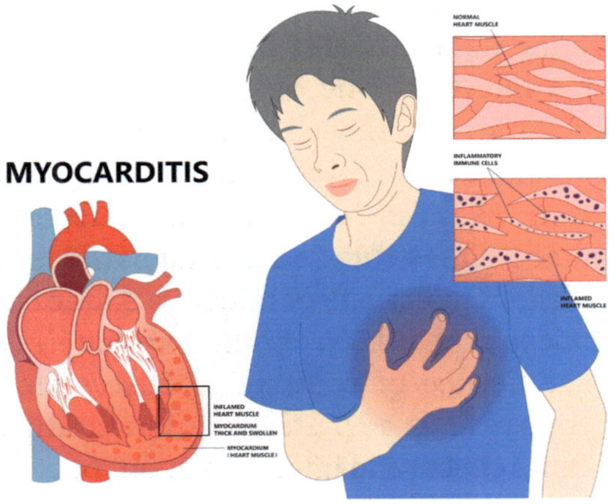

Figure 10.4. Myocarditis.

Source: https://chblob.icloudhospital.com/thumbnails/5-74df4616-d024-41bc-b556-f68f31320dcc.webp.

10.1.2. Pericarditis

The pericarditis is inflammation of the pericardium and is a significant clinical condition in the broader context of inflammatory heart disease. Pericarditis may be due to various etiologies involving infections, autoimmune processes, and post-inflammatory changes. Viral infections, particularly those caused by respiratory diseases, are the most common causative factor. Bacterial infections, including tuberculous pericarditis, are also delineated in their significance, more so in certain geographical regions. The characteristic features of pericarditis are paroxysmal stabbing pain in the chest and dyspnea, commonly exacerbated by deep inspiration or cough. Diagnosis is often a synergy of clinical assessment, imaging, and investigation, which may reveal typical electrocardiographic features or pericardial effusion on echocardiography. Early diagnosis is crucial for maximum management, especially with the danger of complications if left untreated. Treatment of pericarditis also largely depends on the etiology and severity of the disease. As an initial approach, treatment is focused on anti-inflammatory drugs like NSAIDs and corticosteroids to ease symptoms and reduce inflammation. If the disease is relentless or there are complications like effusion, then pericardiocentesis would be necessary to minimize cardiac pressure and improve hemodynamics. Pericardiectomy is an alternative for chronic or fibrotic conditions. Current literature indicates an integrated approach to pericarditis management is necessary, with novel biomarkers like interleukin-10 potentially enhancing diagnostic yields in more difficult cases. As such, a thorough understanding of the disease's pathophysiology and treatment is essential to optimize patient outcomes. As a new area of interest, the interaction between pericarditis and other inflammatory diseases, such as multisystem inflammatory syndrome in children (MIS-C), warrants further investigation. For instance, cardiac manifestation of MIS-C often presents with manifestations similar to those of pericarditis, including myocarditis and pericardial effusion. This overlap emphasizes the importance of diligent clinical evaluations, e.g., through the use of high-technology imaging modalities such as cardiac magnetic resonance imaging, which demonstrates essential information regarding myocardial damage and pericardial disease. While cardiovascular manifestations of MIS-C, i.e., coronary artery lesions and pericarditis, are representative of the disease complexity, prognosis in children with these findings appears good, particularly if appropriately treated. Awareness of these associations guides practitioners in developing an integrated strategy for both pericarditis diagnosis and treatment in response to the evolving dynamics of inflammatory cardiovascular diseases (Maggio et al., 2024; Ahmad et al., 2025) (Figure 10.5).

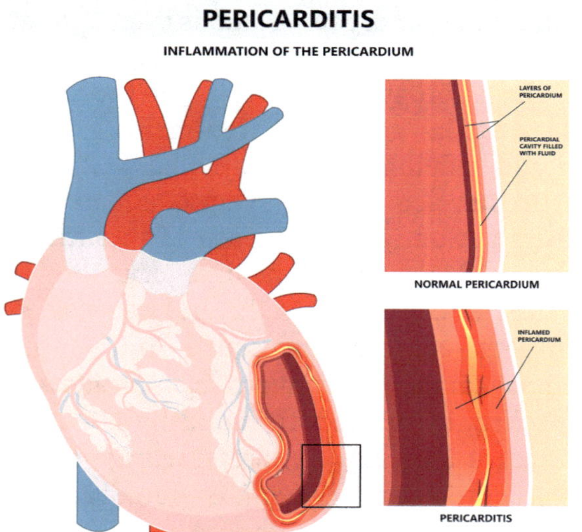

Figure 10.5. Pericarditis.

Source: https://chblob.icloudhospital.com/thumbnails/4-ea67c189-9aa0-4d1b-a776-2aaa74eb0657.webp.

10.1.3. Endocarditis

Endocarditis, as an inflammatory heart disease, is a significant clinical challenge since it can potentially lead to severe complications and high mortality. Endocarditis results from infection of the endocardial surfaces of the heart, typically the heart valves. Pathogenesis of endocarditis involves invasion of these surfaces by microorganisms that will result in vegetative growth, resulting in disruption of the normal heart function. It is essential to note that the microbiologic spectrum of infective endocarditis pathogens has evolved over the last decades, necessitating up-to-date awareness and knowledge from clinicians. The study revealed a recent finding where most cases are accounted for by gram-positive bacteria, Staphylococcus spp., and Enterococcus spp., documenting the importance of positive microbiologic blood cultures in diagnosis and the direction of appropriate antimicrobial therapy (Koltunova et al., 2024). Risk factors for the development of endocarditis include a wide range that most often overlap with preexisting health conditions that compromise the immune system. Patients with preexisting heart defects, artificial valves, or a history of endocarditis are at greater risk. Intravenous drug use, nosocomial infections, and poor dental health are also risk factors for this infection. One of the alarming trends observed in recent clinical reports is the development of antibiotic-resistant organisms, including oxacillin-resistant and vancomycin-resistant isolates cultured among patients with complicated infections of infective endocarditis (Koltunova et al., 2024). This finding underscores the significance of continuous observation of microbial resistance patterns to suit treatments to optimal effects and improve patient outcomes. Endocarditis clinical presentation may range from mild to severe, with several organ systems being involved secondary to embolic phenomena disseminated in the body. Valvular insufficiency, heart failure, and systemic embolization with possible infarction of organs distant from the initial clinical presentation are some of the complications that could occur. The distinction between acute and subacute endocarditis is particularly crucial, since acute endocarditis can cause rapid clinical deterioration. Recent findings have also indicated the association of endocarditis with MIS-C, particularly following COVID-19 infections, with implications for an active interaction between infectious and inflammatory mechanisms affecting cardiovascular health. Hence, insight into a detailed understanding of the complex interactions that underpin the initiation and establishment of endocarditis is critical to the development of effective prevention and management strategies in a multicomponent population base (Figure 10.6).

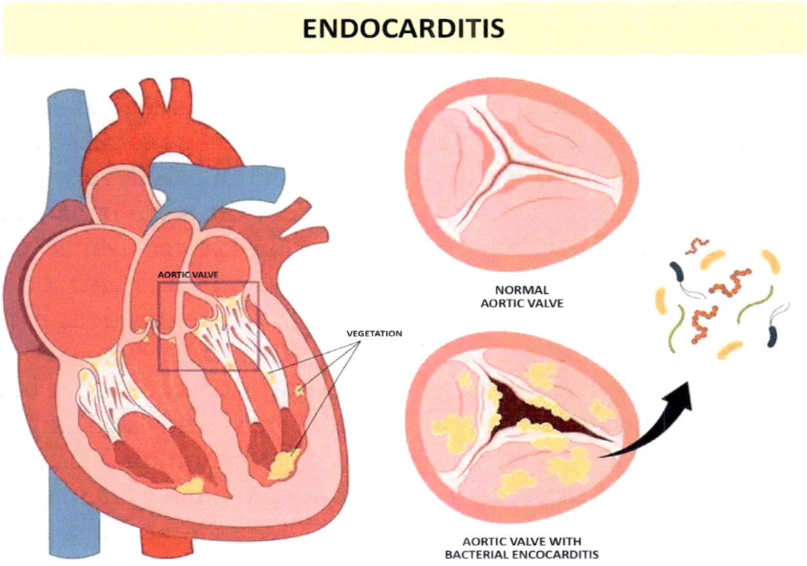

Figure 10.6. Endocarditis.

Source: https://chblob.icloudhospital.com/thumbnails/6-d3143553-86dc-4dfa-99ee-8be8f525fd35.webp.

10.2. Causes and Risk Factors

The multifactorial etiology of inflammatory heart diseases highlights the importance of familiarizing oneself with the varied causes and risk factors underlying their causation. One of the predominant among these is anemia, which has emerged as a robust independent risk factor for adverse cardiovascular outcomes. The World Health Organization reports that approximately 24.8% of the global population is susceptible to the onset of anemia, one of the most prominent among its causes being iron deficiency. Notably, anemia has been reported to be responsible for the exacerbation of coronary heart disease, complications of acute myocardial infarction, and increased risk of heart failure progression. Accordingly, anemia treatment and iron deficiency correction are central to cardiovascular risk attenuation in such groups (Bondareva et al., 2018). The relationship between anemia and inflammatory heart disease not only reflects the complexity of cardiovascular health but also the urgent need for holistic treatment approaches. The second major risk factor for inflammatory heart diseases is sleep disturbances, especially insomnia. Difficulty sleeping or staying asleep can lead to numerous physical and emotional ailments, including exacerbating cardiovascular issues. Environmental reasons, primarily nocturnal traffic noise, are primary reasons for sleep disturbance. Recent epidemiologic evidence indicates that environmental noise can be responsible for disturbed vascular function and increased stress hormones, established risk markers for cardiovascular disease. Alarmingly, ecological noise is reported by the European Environment Agency to be responsible for a high proportion of cases of ischemic heart disease and triggers premature mortality on an annual basis. Hence, adequate management of sleep disorders and environmental triggers is essential in reducing inflammatory heart disease risk and enhancing global cardiovascular well-being (Daiber et al., 2021). In addition, chronic diseases and inflammatory processes are underlying causes of inflammatory heart disease. Chronic renal failure, infections, and neoplasms are capable of contributing significantly to the etiopathogenesis of cardiovascular diseases. In pre-existing cardiac patients, the development of chronic inflammatory conditions may contribute to the risk, continuously creating a vicious circle of worsening health status. At least 58% of anemia in cardiac patients is attributed to chronic conditions, which indicates how various factors of health become interdependent. Prevention of other cardiovascular disorders requires ensuring proper evaluation and treatment of chronic conditions. Such an integrative approach acknowledges the intricate interaction between cardiovascular disease and inflammatory processes with varied emphasis on the significance of preventive strategies in combating these threats (Bondareva et al., 2018).

10.2.1. Infectious Agents

The pathogenesis of the inflammatory heart diseases occurs through the action of infectious agents in multiple ways, with new evidence also indicating their role in triggering and amplifying autoimmune responses. Particularly, specific viral and bacterial pathogens were discovered to trigger immune responses that harm the cardiac tissue. Infectious agents and autoimmunity interact in a complex manner whereby pathogens can provoke responses via mechanisms such as molecular mimicry and bystander activation. This means that the immune response, in its attempt to destroy the causative agent of infection, may inadvertently target the heart tissue, leading to inflammation and even heart disease. Thus, understanding the mechanisms of infection leading to these immune responses is essential towards developing interventions that will aid against the impact of infectious agents on cardiovascular health (Deidda et al., 2011). Oxidative stress is also a primary mechanism through which infectious pathogens participate in inflammatory heart diseases. Specific infectious pathogens have been shown to play a role in stimulating signaling cascades increasing the production of reactive oxygen species (ROS), ultimately leading to cellular damage and inflammation. Chlamydia pneumoniae is one such bacterium that has been identified as a primary etiologic agent of vascular oxidative stress, paving the way for atherosclerosis, an inflammatory arteriopathy. This oxidative setting not just induces endothelial dysfunction but also induces foam cell formation, which is key in the pathogenesis of atherosclerotic plaques. Furthermore, the association with Porphyromonas gingivalis highlights the intricate relationship between oral and cardiovascular risk, hence consolidating the idea that infection control may be beneficial in the prevention of inflammatory heart disease (Pietro et al., 2017). The relationship between infectious disease and inflammatory cardiovascular illnesses transcends the immediate mechanisms of tissue damage to suggest broader epidemiologic consequences. Awareness of the infectious pattern offers better insight into individual risk factors of heart disease, including genetic susceptibility and environmental factors. As advances proceed in clarifying the interrelation between specific infections and myocardial inflammation, the potential for directed preventive intervention becomes increasingly plausible. Efforts will be made towards vaccination tactics and appropriate management of established infectious risks, as treating these underlying issues can help decrease the occurrence of inflammatory heart diseases as a whole. Therefore, at the point where infectious pathogens and heart wellness intersect, there is a need for a coordinated public health approach to advocate for awareness and intervention (Deidda et al., 2011; Pietro et al., 2017) (Figure 10.7).

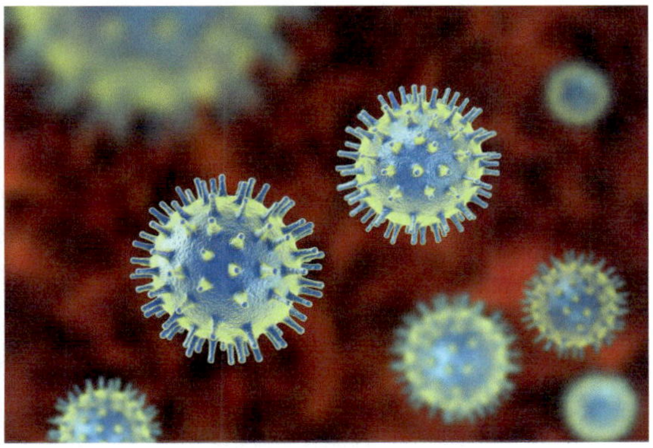

Figure 10.7. Infectious agents.

Source: https://images.nationalgeographic.org/image/upload/t_edhub_resource_key_image/v1638891947/EducationHub/photos/virus.jpg.

10.2.2. Autoimmune Disorders

The overlap between inflammatory heart disease and autoimmune disorders is a rich area of research, since the two diseases have reciprocal effects upon one another through complex mechanisms. Autoimmune diseases, in which the immune systems of the body launch an inappropriate attack on the body's tissues, can create chronic inflammation and tissue damage that are the dominant factors in inflammatory heart disease pathogenesis. Disease conditions such as rheumatoid arthritis (RA) and lupus are classically known to be associated with cardiovascular complications. Research indicates that systemic inflammation caused by autoimmune diseases can increase atherogenesis and thus increase cardiovascular disease risk, including myocardial infarction and heart failure. Such association suggests that it might be essential to manage autoimmune diseases adequately, not only to preserve joint and tissue integrity but also to suppress associated cardiovascular risks. Therefore, knowledge of these relationships can have a crucial influence on patient monitoring and the treatment approach. The contribution of inflammation in autoimmune diseases also comes into play regarding its role in cardiac disease. Long-standing inflammation, characteristic of most autoimmune diseases, is involved in changing the normal physiology of endothelial cells, which line the blood vessels. Interference with this endothelial layer can cause increased vascular permeability, with a cascade of inflammatory events causing heart disease. For example, in patients with systemic lupus erythematosus (SLE), inflammation can be a factor in pericarditis and myocarditis, where the heart muscle itself is involved. In addition, it has been reported that the presence of some autoantibodies can contribute to cardiac risk by the induction of fibrosis and coronary artery disease. It is essential for healthcare practitioners to recognize these correlations, as they highlight the need for regular cardiovascular assessments among these patients, enabling the initiation of proper intervention and management to prevent adverse heart outcomes. Emerging studies also investigate the potential mechanistic pathways between gut microbiota, autoimmune disorders, and inflammatory heart disease. The intestinal microbiome plays a significant role in systemic inflammation, modulating immune responses, and the development of autoimmune disease. Dysbiosis, or an imbalance of the intestinal microbial community, is linked with autoimmune diseases, which further contributes to the inflammation processes involved in cardiovascular health. Recent research suggests that gut bacteria-produced metabolites can enhance gut barrier function, thereby modulating inflammatory responses and possibly reducing cardiovascular risk from autoimmune conditions. Dietary or probiotic regulation of intestinal health may therefore emerge as a new therapeutic strategy. As our understanding of these complicated relationships deepens, the emphasis in treating autoimmune patients is the requirement for interdisciplinarity in treating patients for both the treatment of systemic inflammation and cardiovascular care to have better overall patient outcomes (Figure 10.8) ultimately.

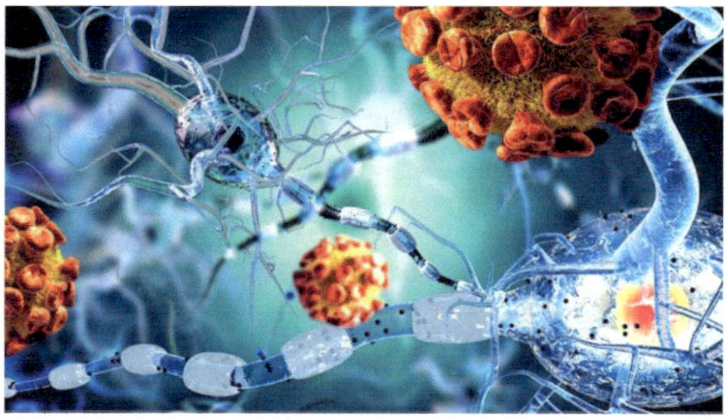

Figure 10.8. Autoimmune disorders.

Source: https://www.uchealth.com/content/dam/uchealth/images/media-room/articles/the-inside-story-on-autoimmune-disorders.jpg/jcr:content/renditions/cq5dam.web.767.431.jpg.

10.2.3. Environmental Factors

Environmental factors are the keystone in the pathogenesis of inflammatory heart diseases, particularly through their action on systemic inflammation. A case in point is the influence of gut microbiota composition on cardiovascular disease. Altered gut microbiota composition or dysbiosis has been implicated in numerous cardiovascular disease phenotypes, such as valvular heart disease (VHD). Gut dysbiosis has also been found to lead to a chronic inflammatory state with inflammatory cell infiltration of heart valves, followed by structural remodeling such as calcification and fibrosis. Therapeutic interventions in modifying the microbiotic environment, such as dietary modification and consumption of probiotics, hold potential in mitigating these detrimental inflammatory conditions and improving cardiac health and revealing an integrative system that bridges environmental factors with prognosis for heart disease (Nayak et al., 2024). Apart from microbiota influence, other environmental factors contribute to inflammatory heart diseases, such as air pollution and diet. Epidemiological evidence reveals that air pollution exposure triggers systemic inflammation, leading to increased cardiovascular morbidity and mortality. Delicate particulate matter and other air pollutants can induce oxidative stress and endothelial dysfunction, promote atherogenesis, and enhance inflammatory processes. This relationship highlights the need for public health measures to reduce air pollution levels and protect cardiovascular well-being. Furthermore, dietary habits, particularly those involving a high saturated fat and low antioxidant content, can also contribute to inflammation as well as the subsequent risk of heart disease. Awareness of such interaction between these environmental determinants is crucial in developing effective prevention strategies through changes in lifestyles that can reduce the occurrence of inflammatory heart diseases (Stolzer et al., 2019). The interaction between environmental exposures and genetic susceptibility also hints at the complexity of inflammatory heart diseases. For instance, various genetic profiles can alter individuals' responses to exposures such as certain dietary patterns or in the presence of specific microbial communities. In murine models, including gene-deficient murine models related to inflammatory bowel disease, both environmental influences and genetic predisposition have been reported to work in concert to determine the character and severity of the inflammatory response. This suggests that therapy has to be addressed to counteract both genetic tendencies and environmental influences, thereby allowing more selective therapeutic intervention. Lastly, understanding of how ecological exposures interact with genetic backgrounds is essential to foster research and clinical practice progress for relief of inflammatory heart diseases and better patient care (Nayak et al., 2024).

10.3. Symptoms and Diagnosis

The categorization of inflammatory cardiac disease is primarily based on the recognition and interpretation of a heterogeneous group of signs that occur in symptomatic patients. Often, they have chest pain, dyspnea, fatigue, palpitations, and sometimes fever, which make the clinical presentation difficult and may lead to misdiagnosis of more prevalent conditions such as coronary artery disease. For instance, MIS-C presents with clinical manifestations that mimic Kawasaki disease, with cardiovascular complications including myocarditis and arrhythmia, necessitating thorough clinical assessment using ECG and echocardiography at presentation and follow-up (Maggio et al., 2024). The similarity of clinical manifestations requires the employment of comprehensive diagnostic methods by health practitioners to differentiate among various inflammatory heart diseases effectively. Diagnostic modalities of inflammatory heart disease include a combination of imaging tests and laboratory studies aimed at identifying underlying pathophysiological processes. Cardiac magnetic resonance imaging (MRI) has emerged as a key tool, revealing vital information on myocardial damage and inflammatory activity. In MIS-C case studies, for instance, cardiac MRI identified significant pathological findings like pericardial effusion and myocardial edema that guided treatment. Nevertheless, the low cohorts of patients imaged with cardiac MRI highlight clinicians' challenges in clinical practice for everyday diagnostics (Maggio et al., 2024). Consequently, application of echocardiography and imaging with metabolism, such as positron emission tomography (PET), is typically undertaken as a necessary step to gain more diagnostic certainty, particularly in complex cases where cardiac involvement is suspected but cannot be excluded with certainty. Moreover, the integration of sophisticated diagnostic techniques is critical in handling the nuances of specific inflammatory cardiac illnesses. In systemic amyloidosis, tissue biopsy remains the gold standard for specific diagnoses, though invasive and technically demanding, and can lead to delays in obtaining critical information. New non-invasive methods, such as the application of F-18-Flutemetanol PET scans, provide promising avenues through being both sensitive and specific for the imaging of amyloid deposition in cardiac tissue. Such advances lay the groundwork for the necessity of further investigation and utilization of new diagnostic modalities to enable earlier detection and intervention and consequently improve patient outcomes in the area of inflammatory heart diseases (Figure 10.9).

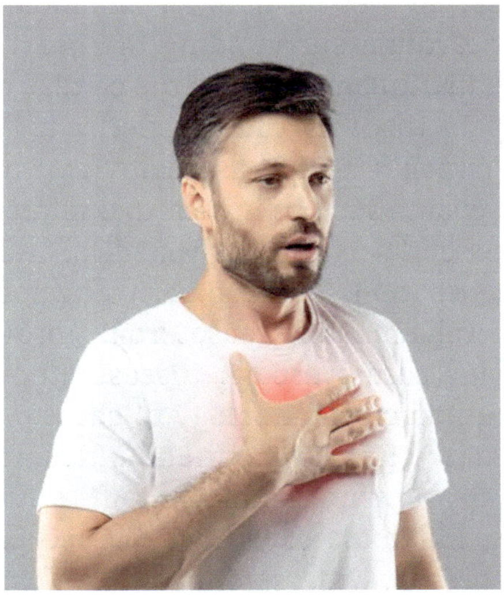

Figure 10.9. Dyspnea.

Source: https://chblob.icloudhospital.com/thumbnails/3-fe6972f6-9eb1-409b-b127-04713f0e3b8a.webp.

10.3.1. Common Symptoms

Inflammatory heart diseases are a collection of conditions of the heart tissue and structures related to it with inflammation. Among the most common patient complaints is fatigue. This is a result of the body trying to resist inflammation and leads to a general decrease in energy. The patients also typically report a general tiredness that is not improved by rest. Besides, the fatigue can also affect the quality of life of the patients and render them incapable of performing everyday tasks or maintaining social relationships. Moreover, the mental pressure that chronic fatigue is liable to impose tends to exacerbate the situation and result in frustration and isolation. The detection and treatment of fatigue in inflammatory heart disease patients are also imperative in keeping their overall health and well-being intact. Chest pain is another frequent symptom that is suggestive of potential inflammatory heart disorders. Patients may have varying degrees of pain, ranging from a stabbing or stinging quality to a dull ache, which is often exacerbated by exercise. It may be caused by pericarditis, an inflammation of the pericardium surrounding the heart, or by myocarditis, inflammation of the cardiac muscle. Chest pain tends to cause significant distress in that patients tend to associate it with major cardiac events such as myocardial infarction. It is thus essential to have early medical evaluation in such situations because early diagnosis will separate inflammatory causes from more serious underlying cardiovascular disease. Knowledge of the multifactorial etiology of chest pain can significantly improve patient outcomes and guide appropriate management strategies. Besides, inflammatory heart disease patients usually present with respiratory manifestations, for instance, shortness of breath, particularly during exercise. Such a symptom may arise from the compromised ability of the heart to efficiently deliver blood due to inflammation, leading to pulmonary congestion. Since the heart lacks full functionality, the patient can notice reduced exercise tolerance and largely debilitated activity status. In a few cases, they shall experience forceful breathing or the feeling of chest heaviness when exerting themselves. These respiratory symptoms are imperative indicators of the inflammatory processes in progress and warrant extensive evaluation to develop suitable management programs. Given the multifactorial nature of inflammatory heart diseases, their identification and treatment will enhance care and enhance the health-related quality of life in patients, as it has been described on the significance of holistic management of conditions that have a wide range of manifestations like in individuals with General variable immunodeficiency (Lepekhina et al., 2024) and congenital heart disease (Benrabah et al., 2024) (Figure 10.10).

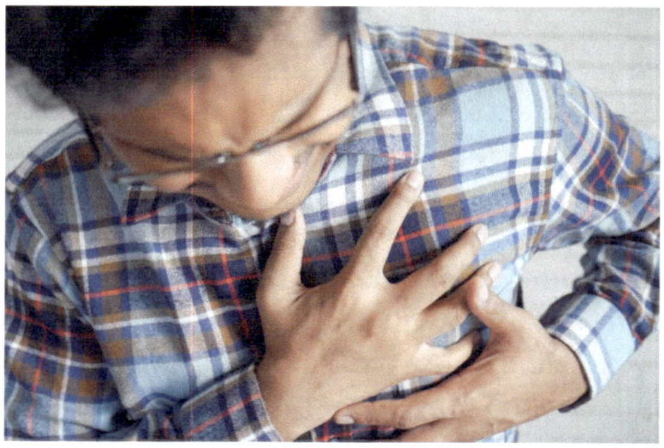

Figure 10.10. Symptoms of inflammatory heart diseases.

Source: https://mysiloam-api.siloamhospitals.com/storage-down/file-web-cms/17284397668683564.webp.

10.3.2. Diagnostic Tests

Diagnosis of inflammatory heart disease is greatly supported by the application of diagnostic tests, particularly those of specific pathophysiologic processes like myocarditis and heart failure. New imaging techniques like cardiac magnetic resonance (CMR) provide critical data about myocardial inflammation and functional deficits. For instance, in children with multisystem inflammatory syndrome (MISC) after COVID-19, they had some degree of left ventricular dysfunction as evident from CMR imaging. The fact that CMR can detect the presence of cardiac involvement makes clinicians capable of individualizing intervention, reflective of the necessity for a complete cardiac evaluation in exposed patients. Furthermore, biochemical tests for troponin, BNP, and inflammatory markers like C-reactive protein are supplementary to the understanding of the disease severity and prognosis, proving the use of an extensive diagnostic process in treating inflammatory heart disease (Alipour et al., 2024). The utility of biomarkers in the diagnosis of inflammatory heart diseases cannot be overstated. Biomarkers are handy markers of cardiovascular inflammation that make it easier to differentiate among various etiologies of heart disease. For instance, serum levels of some inflammatory markers, i.e., sCD40, sCD40L, and s4-1BB, have been measured and proven to be associated with severe heart failure and rejection of the allograft in heart transplant patients. Their presence at higher levels in severe heart failure patients suggests their use for prognostication and disease monitoring. Moreover, correlation analysis between these biomarkers and the remaining clinical parameters provides a better understanding of the inflammatory processes at play and assists in directing therapeutic interventions accordingly. Thus, incorporation of biomarker analysis into routine diagnostic investigations can improve patient outcomes by promoting personalized therapy based on the inflammatory status of the heart (Monteiro et al., 2024). As cardiology advances, the creation and use of novel diagnostic techniques are essential for treating inflammatory heart conditions. The progress of cardiac imaging technology and the discovery of biomarkers allow for improved diagnostic accuracy and insight into the pathophysiological mechanisms behind. In addition, the investigation into the performance of these tests continues to influence clinical practice, calling for updated guidelines and consensus recommendations. The combination of imaging studies, laboratory tests, and emerging biomarkers creates a common platform for the evaluation of patients with inflammatory heart diseases, thus resulting in improved management and outcomes. This not only reinforces the significance of continuous advances in diagnostic testing but emphasizes their role towards greater understanding and treatment efficiency in complex cardiovascular diseases (Alipour et al., 2024; Monteiro et al., 2024) (Figure 10.11).

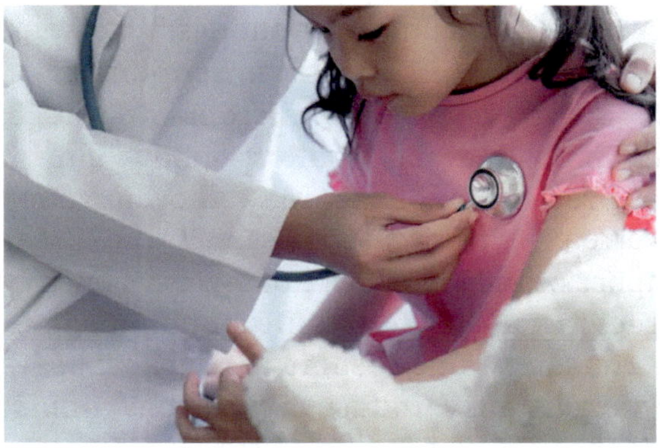

Figure 10.11. Diagnosis of inflammatory heart disease.

Source: https://chblob.icloudhospital.com/thumbnails/8-7f2e46d0-4019-4774-803e-ceb17b2482f5.webp.

10.3.3. Differential Diagnosis

Differential diagnosis is a valuable process in the diagnosis of inflammatory heart diseases with common clinical presentations and more than one etiology. Identification of the exact nature of the inflammation is based on a detailed analysis of a patient's history, physical examination, and results from applicable diagnostic studies. Myocarditis, an autoimmune-mediated myocardial inflammation, is one condition that necessitates an exhaustive differential diagnosis. Researchers have argued that the detection of immune cell subpopulations in the microenvironment of myocarditis can significantly enhance diagnostic accuracy. For instance, differential expression analysis has identified genes that are related to immune function and inflammation, which can enable clinicians to distinguish myocarditis from other cardiomyopathies or diseases of the heart that present with similar symptoms, such as heart failure or ischemic heart disease (Li et al., 2025). A broad differential diagnosis also includes the use of newer technologies, such as next-generation sequencing. This enables clinicians to identify potential infectious agents responsible for inflammatory heart conditions, with more targeted therapeutic interventions. With studies utilizing differential metatranscriptomics, one can attribute various microbial pathogens with inflammatory cardiomyopathy, showing that previously commensal pathogens may be involved in the disease process. These findings emphasize the importance of intensive microbial screening as part of differential diagnosis, particularly since some of the causative pathogens may induce a vigorous immune response in susceptible hosts. It is therefore essential to distinguish between infectious and autoimmune causes of heart inflammation to ensure appropriate interventions and improve patient outcomes (Huang et al., 2024). Moreover, differential diagnosis must be interdisciplinary to include both clinical findings and laboratory information. Identification of differential fibroblast and immune cell subpopulations within the myocarditis microenvironment—along with the presence of specific genetic variants—can uncover information about a patient's susceptibility to inflammatory heart disease development. It encourages an in-depth understanding of the disease mechanisms and enhances the ability to predict disease development or drug response. Therefore, inclusion of advanced diagnostics, including genomic profiling and imaging research, is most crucial in rationalizing the differential diagnosis. Such an extensive approach not only aids in the identification of the specific type of inflammatory heart disease but also assists in guiding targeted therapeutic strategies, thereby improving overall therapy of engaged patients (Li et al., 2025).

10.4. Treatment Options

Management of inflammatory heart diseases encompasses an array of therapeutic maneuvers to modulate inflammation, control symptoms, and ultimately improve patient outcomes. Pharmacologic therapy is significant in this respect, with corticosteroids and NSAIDs tending to be employed to block inflammatory processes. In addition, more targeted therapies such as disease-modifying antirheumatic drugs (DMARDs) are helpful by addressing underlying autoimmune mechanisms underlying conditions such as myocarditis. Furthermore, lifestyle modification, such as food modification, exercise, and smoking cessation, is also part and parcel of symptom control and reduction of exacerbations. This multi-factorial approach not only aims to reverse acute clinical features but also addresses precipitating risk factors for more complications, thereby maximizing the overall efficacy of treatment and maximizing patient quality of life in the long term. When inflammatory heart disease advances to severe complications, more advanced therapeutic methods may be necessary. Heart transplantation is a lifesaving procedure for patients who end up with end-stage heart failure, but it also has its challenges. The ischemia-reperfusion injury (IRI) that occurs during transplantation, along with the immune responses against the graft, significantly hinders achieving optimal results. New therapies to address these challenges are under development. For instance, the newly discovered delivery of plant-derived vesicle-like nanoparticles has the potential to modulate IRI while concurrently helping to modulate the immune system. The nanoparticles can be designed to home actively and deliver therapeutic drugs—such as rapamycin—to the heart graft selectively, thereby enhancing the therapeutic index and reducing the risk of post-transplant rejection complications. Such sophisticated studies illustrate the promising future of personalized treatment strategies in the management of inflammatory heart disease, particularly in complex clinical scenarios. Understanding the heart–brain axis is crucial to guide treatment in patients with inflammatory heart disease, particularly because inflammatory heart disease tends to occur in conjunction with neurological complications. Recent research highlights how both organ systems can be affected by inflammation at the same time, with one's dysfunction causing unfavorable events in the other. This interconnectedness provides a foundation for addressing inflammation through an integrative approach, leading to better clinical outcomes. Future research into the intricacies of this interaction could leverage our knowledge of the heart–brain axis to produce better upstream and downstream treatments, both for cardiovascular and neurological manifestations of inflammatory diseases. Additionally, knowledge gleaned from this relationship could give rise to novel prevention care strategies, ultimately increasing the arsenal of options for practitioners to choose from. Thus, it is hoped that patients will be encouraged to derive more benefits from a more integrated and holistic approach to the management of inflammatory heart disease (Figure 10.12).

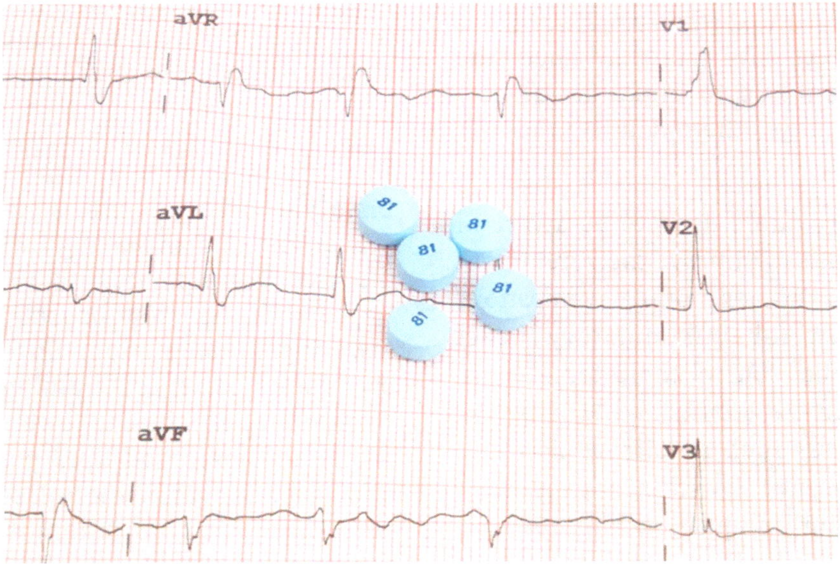

Figure 10.12. Treatment for inflammatory heart disorders (IHD).

Source: https://thumbnails.icloudhospital.com/tr:w-1024,f-webp,q-75/1-770e2000-9aee-4088-b898-04351fa8ee8c.webp.

10.4.1. Medications

Since many inflammatory heart diseases are caused by inflammation, medications are very important for their management. Many times, anti-inflammatory drugs like corticosteroids and NSAIDs are used to treat the inflammation that causes heart damage. Especially, corticosteroids can help control inflammation in the body, which supports better heart function and better outcomes for patients. Recent studies indicate that these drugs might make other treatments more effective by providing a better setting for healing. Even so, taking anti-inflammatory medications for a long time can cause unwanted effects, so patients should be overseen to weigh the advantages against the risks. As we learn more, finding the best set of drugs for each type of patient remains a primary concern. Besides the usual anti-inflammatory drugs, targeted therapies have now become a significant part of treating inflammatory heart diseases. Biologic agents which are tailored to block specific inflammatory pathways, are now widely used because they are precise and effective in relieving symptoms and improving life quality. They usually interfere with cytokines or their receptors, which reduces inflammation and stops heart disease from worsening. Recent studies suggest that using certain biologics may significantly reduce hospitalizations for acute episodes of inflammation. However, since these drugs are very expensive and may have side effects, people continue to argue about how easy it should be to get them and use them as part of treatment.

Healthcare providers need to be aware of recent developments to improve their treatment methods regularly. Another group of medications that is important for inflammatory heart diseases is those that control cholesterol levels. Proprotein convertase subtilisin/kexin type-9 (PCSK9) inhibitors, such as alirocumab and evolocumab, represent a significant advancement in the management of lipid levels, impacting cardiovascular health. Evidence shows that these drugs decrease low-density lipoprotein cholesterol and may also help by reducing inflammation. Inhibiting PCSK9 enables these therapies to enhance the function of hepatic LDL receptors, leading to reduced cholesterol levels and fewer inflammatory markers in the blood vessels. Because of this dual action, it could be helpful in managing inflammatory heart diseases, mainly in patients who also have dyslipidemia. As the understanding of these medications deepens, their role in comprehensive care strategies continues to evolve, contributing to improved outcomes for patients at risk of cardiovascular complications (Figure 10.13).

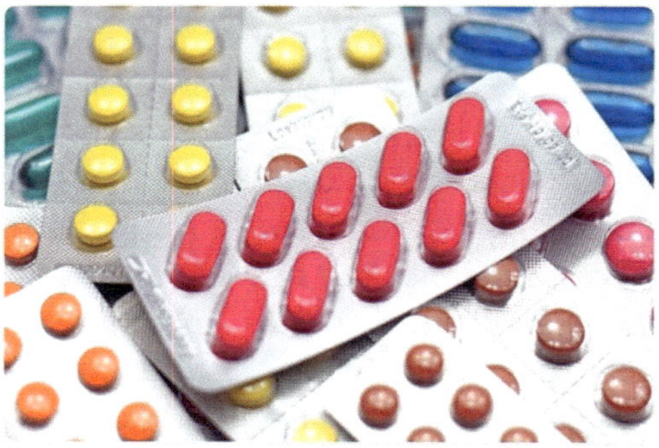

Figure 10.13. Nonsteroidal Anti-Inflammatory Drugs (NSAIDs).

Source: https://www.news-medical.net/image-handler/picture/2021/9/shutterstock_1034648131.jpg

10.4.2. Lifestyle Modifications

Lifestyle changes are significant in both preventing and managing inflammatory heart diseases. Doing physical activity regularly helps improve the heart by boosting blood flow and lowering inflammation. Engaging in aerobic exercises, resistance training, and flexibility workouts contributes to lower body mass index (BMI) and improved lipid profiles, which are critical for mitigating the risk of heart disease. In addition, eating a diet that includes lots of fruits, vegetables, whole grains, and lean proteins is known to reduce inflammation. Eating in this way can help lower cholesterol and improve heart health, which can lower the risk of heart problems. Evidence suggests that individuals who integrate these modifications into their daily routines not only experience better health outcomes but also exhibit a reduced risk of co-morbidities related to both cardiovascular conditions and chronic diseases, as affirmed by research suggesting a complex interplay between chronic inflammation and lifestyle choices (Abrignani et al., 2025). Also, stopping smoking and drinking less alcohol are important for controlling inflammatory heart diseases. Smoking tobacco is a known risk for heart disease because it causes more inflammation and problems with the endothelium. Not smoking reduces the risk of heart disease and its consequences, and it also makes the lungs work better and increases the body's ability to exercise. Also, drinking too much alcohol can result in high blood pressure and put someone at risk for heart rhythm disturbances. Drinking alcohol only in moderation can significantly decrease a person's risk of heart disease. Following these lifestyle changes can be supported by regular health check-ups, which are essential for checking your heart health and finding any early signs of disease. Such proactive measures are conducive to long-term health and well-being, aligning with current recommendations for heart disease prevention (Fahimi, 2024). Psychological health should not be ignored when talking about making lifestyle changes for inflammatory heart diseases. Long-term stress and anxiety can cause serious issues for the heart, such as raising inflammation and risk factors. Managing stress through mindfulness, yoga, or cognitive behavioral therapy can help reduce psychological stress and improve overall well-being. Also, having a strong network of friends or family can make it easier to support emotional health and choose better habits. Taking care of mental, emotional, and physical needs is necessary for people who have inflammatory heart diseases. By integrating all these dimensions, individuals can develop a more comprehensive plan for health management that not only addresses immediate concerns but also promotes sustainable, long-term lifestyle changes (Abrignani et al., 2025).

10.4.3. Surgical Interventions

Surgical intervention plays a critical role in the management of inflammatory heart diseases, particularly if medical interventions in the form of standard drugs cannot control symptoms or structural problems arise. Infections such as infective endocarditis, which entails inflammation and infection of the heart valves, may need to be operated on to repair or replace the valves. Such interventions are essential in the prevention of morbidity and mortality as a consequence of valve dysfunction, particularly for those with severe obstructions or regurgitations. With advancing surgical techniques, outcomes of these procedures have also improved, demonstrating the importance of early intervention in stabilizing patients with complicated inflammatory processes on cardiac structures. This highlights a critical aspect of the management of inflammatory heart disease extending beyond drug therapy, suggesting the value of a multi-disciplinary approach with surgical expertise to address the complications of progressing disease optimally. For inflammatory bowel disease after transplant, patients who have developed cardiac complications after solid organ transplant can also require surgery. The interaction between IBD and cardiac diseases can complicate the clinical presentation to the extent that a thorough evaluation is necessary to establish treatment modalities, including surgery when indicated. A case in point is that gastrointestinal symptoms secondary to IBD can be indistinguishable from symptoms due to the heart, complicating diagnosis and curative intervention strategies by extension. Surgical interventions could be called for should medical treatment fail or secondary complications like abscesses and strictures occur. As noted from studies comparing results in pediatric solid organ transplantation recipients, careful monitoring and prophylactic surgical intervention can lead to good clinical outcomes, illustrating the interconnectedness of inflammatory disease processes affecting multiple organ systems and the place of focused surgical treatment as indicated (Wenzel et al., 2024). Also, surgical procedures for inflammatory cardiac conditions must be managed with consideration of the patient's underlying immunological status, especially in chronic inflammatory illness that can have systemic implications. For instance, people with autoimmune diseases that cause myocarditis would need to be managed with anything from steroid medication to invasive surgery if their heart function drastically declines. The management and assessment of such patients are not easy; therefore, collaboration between cardiologists, rheumatologists, and cardiothoracic surgeons is vital to achieving maximum postoperative outcomes. Evidence shows that patients with persistent symptoms following medical management failure in the aspect of incomplete response experience benefits from re-establishing normal cardiac function with surgery (Plymoth et al., 2024). This underscores the value of personalized therapy in preoperative planning to achieve comprehensive care for patients with the double jeopardy of inflammation and impaired cardiac function (Figure 10.14).

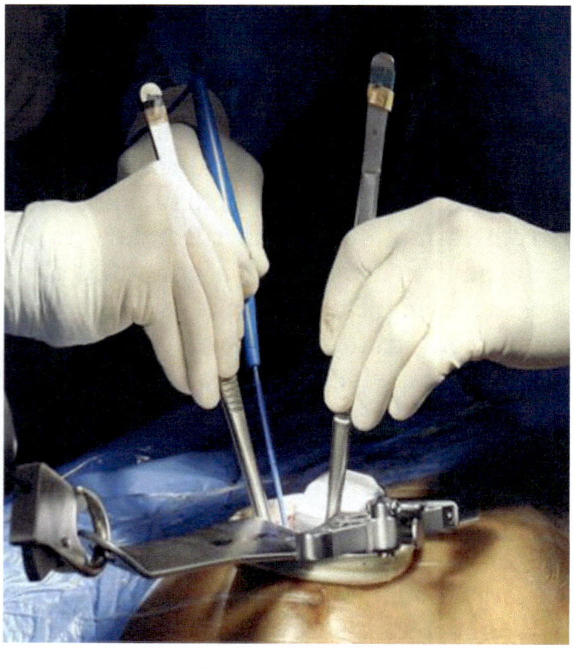

Figure 10.14. Inflammation and heart surgery.

Source: https://www.frontiersin.org/image/researchtopic/38563.

10.5. Prevention Strategies

Optimal prevention of IHD is central to the reduction of the worldwide burden of cardiovascular morbidity and mortality. A triad of strategy consists of lifestyle modification, early detection, and targeted pharmacologic treatment. Healthy lifestyle habits, such as physical activity, a well-balanced diet with anti-inflammatory agents, and smoking cessation, are central to the reduction of risk factors for IHD. Secondly, the utilization of extensive cardiovascular risk assessment can identify those at greater risk, where specific preventive measures can be put in place. Improved patient and public education regarding how lifestyle influences the heart is most important in encouraging healthy habits ahead of time, resulting in overall prevention. Recent developments towards understanding immunological processes that underlie IHD have enormous potential for fresh approaches to prevention. Immune cells such as monocytes and neutrophils have been brought to light in research on the etiopathogenesis of cardiovascular disease, highlighting the importance of inflammation targeting in prevention (Tercan, 2025). Investigation of processes behind clonal hematopoiesis and trained immunity continues to underscore the importance of individualized approaches in risk prediction and management. By integrating such new understanding into practice, clinicians can adjust and improve their preventive interventions, thereby reducing the prevalence and severity of inflammatory heart diseases. In addition to this, continued research into anti-inflammatory pharmacotherapies, such as colchicine, uncovers novel mechanisms by which inflammation can be treated, suggesting a multifaceted prevention program reaching beyond traditional cardiovascular risk factors. Lastly, the recognition of systemic inflammatory processes, such as those that play a role in heart failure, highlights the necessity of multimodal prevention involving both the physiological and immune aspects of IHD. The recent identification of PANoptosis as a novel target for therapy highlights how comprehending underlying mechanisms of pathophysiologic processes, such as PANoptosis, can lead to effective, evidence-based prevention (Jia et al., 2024). Health systems can enhance their preventative measures by focusing on cutting-edge treatments for the inflammatory factors that contribute to heart disease. The need to establish more interdisciplinary teamwork is no longer debatable as science continues to uncover the complex connections between inflammation and heart disease. This convergence can drive the development of both public health interventions and individual therapeutic therapies, hence providing a solid groundwork for inflammatory heart disease prevention.

10.5.1. Vaccination

Inflammatory heart diseases caused by viruses are mitigated by vaccination, which has become very important. With the arrival of COVID-19, people have seen that respiratory illnesses and heart problems are often linked. Studies indicate that the severe acute respiratory syndrome coronavirus 2 (SARS-CoV-2) infection may lead to long-term health issues, including inflammatory responses that can increase the risk of myocarditis and other heart-related conditions (Ren et al., 2024). So, getting vaccinated against COVID-19 helps prevent the primary infection and also reduces the chances of developing inflammatory heart problems after a COVID-19 infection. For people with pre-existing diseases such as hypertension or diabetes, vaccination is vital because these conditions increase their risk of contracting COVID-19. Complications resulting from the virus, such as hyperinflammatory syndrome and cardiac failure, can severely affect overall health outcomes (Kemerley et al., 2024). Such programs are necessary to reduce the risk of severe illness and heart problems in these people. Research has shown that vaccination may play a key role in preventing myocarditis and other heart problems, which could mean that vaccination helps reduce the burden of illness and death from heart diseases. Besides helping people with heart conditions, vaccination can be a part of strategies to lower the number of inflammatory heart diseases in the community. With the emergence of the MIS-C related to COVID-19, awareness and vaccination efforts can foster a proactive approach towards protecting younger demographics (Kemerley et al., 2024). Vaccination not only protects individuals, but also helps the community by allowing herd immunity and protecting those at greater risk. Thus, enhancing vaccination coverage is a strategic public health imperative that addresses both immediate infectious diseases and their potentially devastating long-term cardiovascular consequences, emphasizing the critical intersection of vaccination initiatives and strategies to combat inflammatory heart diseases (Figure 10.15).

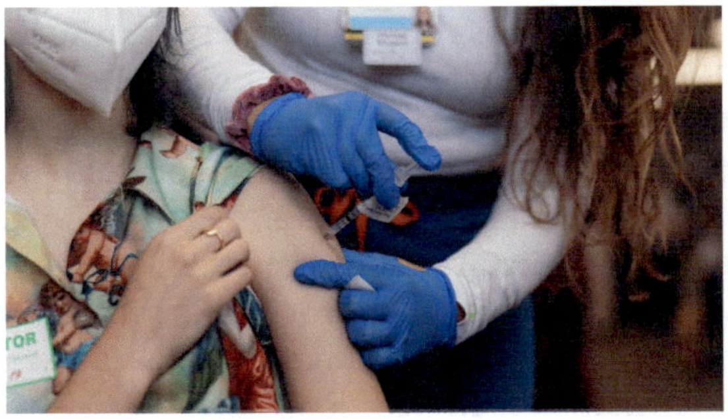

Figure 10.15. Vaccination.

Source: https://static01.nyt.com/images/2021/05/22/us/22virus-myocarditis-youth/22virus-myocarditis-youth-videoSixteenByNineJumbo1600.jpg.

10.5.2. Healthy Lifestyle Choices

A significant way to prevent inflammatory heart diseases is by choosing a healthy lifestyle. Regular exercise is necessary because it helps the heart and also reduces the body's overall inflammation, which is related to heart disease.

Eating a Mediterranean diet, which includes a lot of fruits, vegetables, whole grains, fish, and healthy fats, is linked to a reduced risk of heart disease. What we eat is very important for our weight and cholesterol, which affects our heart health significantly. The European Society of Cardiology has emphasized these aspects in its guidelines, advocating for lifestyle modifications to mitigate the risks associated with heart diseases (Visseren et al., 2021). In general, making healthy diet and exercise choices can lower inflammation and help keep the heart healthy which supports a complete strategy for disease prevention. As well as eating well and exercising, managing stress is an integral part of a healthy lifestyle. Long-term stress raises the amount of cortisol and other stress hormones, which can cause more inflammation and raise the risk of heart problems. Mindfulness, yoga, and other relaxation methods have been found to reduce stress and improve the health of the heart. In addition, having strong social bonds can give people emotional support, which helps them handle stress better. The European Society of Hypertension offers similar recommendations that align with the promotion of a lifestyle geared toward reducing risk factors associated with heart disease (Williams et al., 2018). Looking after mental health and strengthening against stress can help people improve their heart health as part of a complete inflammatory heart disease prevention plan. In addition, staying away from smoking and drinking too much alcohol is very important for your heart. Smoking directly causes inflammation in the heart and blood vessels, which leads to chronic illnesses and speeds up the wear and tear on arteries. At the same time, moderate drinking could help the heart, but drinking too much increases your risk of hypertension, cardiomyopathy, and additional serious health problems. Choosing not to smoke and watching your drinking can significantly lower inflammatory markers in the body. For this reason, incorporating these healthy choices into your daily habits can significantly benefit your heart. Health professionals, as indicated in the guidelines, should actively promote these lifestyle changes, recognizing that they are essential components in the fight against inflammatory heart diseases and are integral to cultivating long-term health (Visseren et al., 2021) (Figure 10.16).

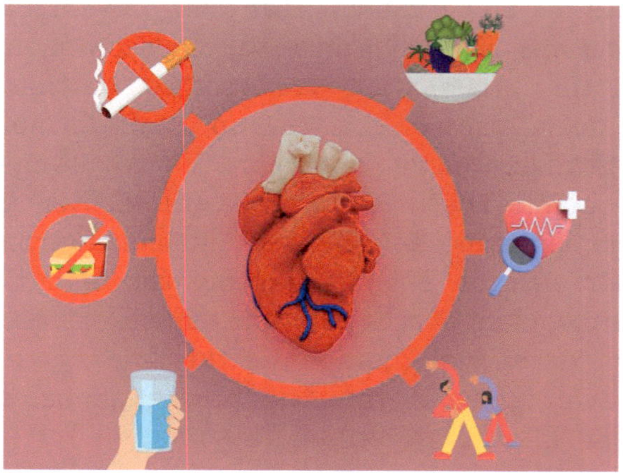

Figure 10.16. Healthy Lifestyle Choices.

Source: https://hsmc.com.au/wp-content/uploads/2024/02/Heart-health-4x3-1.jpg.

10.5.3. Regular Medical Check-Ups

Regular follow-up by a physician is a key component of preventive care, particularly in inflammatory cardiac disease. Such conditions, while characteristically accompanied by systemic inflammation, have the potential for serious cardiovascular complications if they remain undetected. Follow-up allows physicians to evaluate risk factors such as blood pressure, lipid levels, and markers of inflammation. In particular, measurement of lipoprotein(a) levels is increasingly recognized as a significant cardiovascular risk factor. Although the levels as mentioned above are not typically measured during regular check-ups, recommendations have proposed inclusion to stratify risk further (Baran et al., 2024). Therefore, regular check-ups not only facilitate early diagnosis but also empower patients with individualized guidelines that promote worldwide cardiovascular well-being. Incorporation of regular medical check-ups into healthcare is crucial for the prevention as well as the management of inflammatory heart diseases. These positions provide channels through which health workers can educate patients on lifestyle changes that can minimize risk, such as diet and exercise interventions. Literature shows that educational support significantly improves patient outcomes, especially among those grappling with chronic inflammatory diseases (Khatoon et al., 2024). By creating a culture of surveillance and well-being, patients can play more active roles in their health, adhering to necessary lifestyle modifications and medical interventions. Hence, these check-ups change from mere evaluation into detailed sessions capable of determining long-term health outcomes. Moreover, the role of healthcare practitioners extends beyond individual assessment; it's about integrating patient education into routine check-ups. As more is learned about inflammatory heart diseases and their underlying root cause risk factors, healthcare practitioners bear an additional responsibility of empowering patients through education. This approach can demystify clinical technical terminology and instill a sense of empowerment in patients when making health-related decisions. To be specific, informing patients of the necessity for measuring lipoprotein(a) and its effect on cardiovascular risk can assist in bridging the knowledge gap that is traditionally present in patient management (Baran et al., 2024). Through a focus on education alongside regular medical check-ups, healthcare systems can encourage educated patients who will be able to manage their health and reduce the prevalence of inflammatory heart diseases (Figure 10.17).

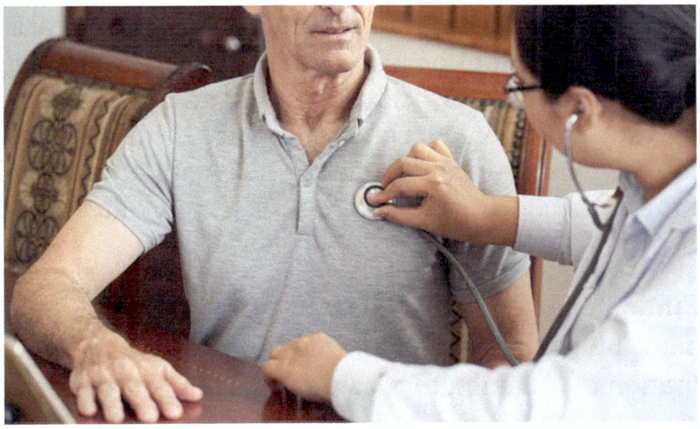

Figure 10.17. Regular medical check-ups.

Source: https://health-e.in/wp-content/uploads/2022/12/what-are-the-benefits-of-regular-heart-check-ups.webp.

SUMMARY

The pathophysiology of inflammatory heart disease illustrates a complex interplay of forces that have direct implications for patient outcomes. New reports identify the emerging adulthood of remote patient monitoring as a potential adjunctive treatment for these diseases. Systematic reviews do indicate some patient benefit, mainly in select populations like heart failure, but evidence overall is sparse for other diagnoses. The use of remote patient monitoring can help improve patient engagement and possibly lower healthcare expenditures but needs rigorous studies to evaluate its effectiveness across a broader range of inflammatory heart diseases (Wartenberg et al., 2025). Therefore, these findings highlight an important gap in clinical practice that requires remedies through strong clinical trials and long-term follow-up investigations. Moreover, the relationship between lifestyle habits and inflammatory heart diseases cannot be overstated. Existing studies establish that lifestyle habits and eating patterns trigger inflammatory reactions that exacerbate heart conditions. Of particular concern is the Western lifestyle, characterized by a diet high in fat and minimal exercise, which contributes to increased metabolic inflammation. This connection necessitates that treatment modalities adopt an integrated model, managing not just the inflammatory component but also promoting patients with better lifestyle practices. By understanding the overall mechanisms associating metabolic disease with inflammatory heart conditions, clinicians are able to design more effective, integral modes of treatment (Adolph et al., 2024). Briefly, further research into inflammatory heart diseases is needed, emphasizing the interaction between technological monitoring and traditional lifestyle modification. As the shape of healthcare in the future is molded, taking advantage of remote patient monitoring technologies and enhancing metabolic health will be integral to improving patient outcomes. The existing limited evidence suggests that while new approaches are promising, they must be underpinned by substantial research to demonstrate safety and effectiveness in various patient groups. The future lies in an interdisciplinarity to bridge these gaps, ultimately leading to improved practice and better health outcomes for inflammatory heart disease patients.

The contribution of inflammatory mechanisms to cardiac illnesses, and particularly coronary heart disease (CHD), cannot be overemphasized. One of the outstanding characteristics of such a correlation is the participation of inflammatory cytokines, which have been incriminated as playing pivotal roles in CHD pathogenesis. Research utilizing techniques such as Mendelian randomization (MR) has demonstrated the ability of specific cytokines to serve as upstream regulators of CHD risk, with robust correlation between increased levels and development of cardiovascular complications. For example, cytokines including eotaxin (CCL11) and C–C motif chemokine ligand 20 (CCL20) have been shown to increase risk significantly, thereby underlining the significance of continued research geared toward exploring therapeutic interventions including these inflammatory mediators, as evident from recent evidence in cardiovascular pathology (Kyryk, 2024). In addition to the direct effect of inflammatory cytokines, the emergence of advanced cellular and tissue technologies has revealed avenues for novel therapeutic approaches to inflammatory heart diseases. Stem cell therapy is a valuable avenue for myocardial regeneration in patients with cardiac pathologies. These are multipotent mesenchymal cells and tissue-specific progenitors, which are promising due to their low immunogenicity and ability to exert trophic, anti-inflammatory, and immunomodulatory properties. The best route of administration for such cells, and ongoing clinical trials, remain paramount to optimizing the safety and efficacy of cell therapy, which is increasingly regarded as a key component of modern regenerative medicine (Kyryk, 2024). The multifactorial condition of inflammatory heart disease demands an interdisciplinary solution that combats both the inflammatory processes and the potential for regenerative therapy. Additional research of the interaction between inflammatory mediators and the cardiovascular system is needed for novel prevention and treatment. Impressions from current research suggest that therapeutic intervention of pro-inflammatory cytokines can lower the incidence of CHD. Concurrently, the development of stem cell therapy as a possible therapeutic modality highlights the necessity of a two-way approach towards the alleviation of established inflammatory conditions, together with the facilitation of myocardial repair. In this regard, the therapeutic progress made can be a significant contributor towards diminishing the effect of cardiovascular morbidity and mortality resulting from inflammation-caused heart ailments (Lv et al., 2024).

A CLOSER LOOK

COMPLICATIONS OF INFLAMMATORY HEART DISEASES (IHD)

Complications from IHD in the form of myocarditis present stern clinical challenges and can lead to calamitous outcomes. The disease, which is inflammation of the heart muscle, can manifest in a spectrum of severity ranging from mild to fatal. The symptoms will vary from imperceptible manifestations such as chest pain or weakness to severe heart failure requiring immediate medical intervention. The heterogeneity in clinical presentation renders diagnosis challenging, and hence, health professionals must utilize a multi-modal approach with history, clinical evaluation, and advanced imaging techniques to identify the disease and its severity effectively. Further, even though supportive care is of utmost significance, the need for aggressive management in severe myocarditis once again underscores the potential complications of this inflammatory disease. Recognition of such complexities is vital to improving results for affected patients because varied underlying etiologies have a significant influence on management and results (Zafeiri et al., 2024). Another important concern of inflammatory heart disease complications is their association with systemic conditions, particularly under SARS-CoV-2 infection conditions. With the onset of COVID-19, the interaction between viral infections and myocarditis has come into focus because of the evidence of myocardial damage even in patients with no history of cardiovascular disease. Such a complication, including myocarditis and hyperinflammatory syndromes, is responsible for increased morbidity and mortality rates among patients, particularly those with comorbidities like hypertension and diabetes.

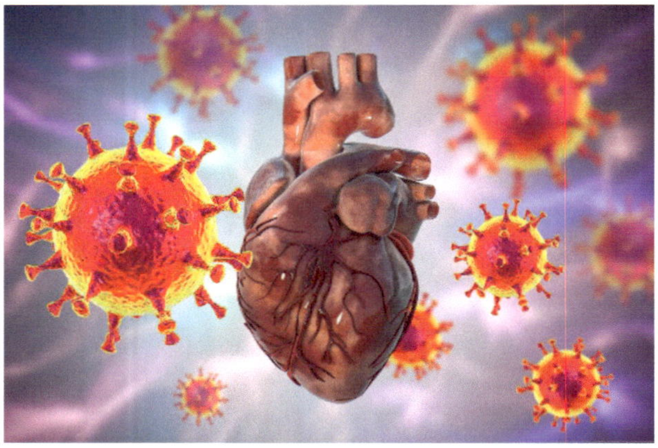

Figure 10.18. Complications of Inflammatory Heart Diseases (IHD).

Source: https://www.nih.gov/sites/default/files/news-events/research-matters/2024/20240402-heart-damage.jpg.

Besides, children have presented unique inflammatory responses, including multisystem inflammatory syndrome, that are increasingly linked to prior COVID-19 infection. Such linking highlights the importance of ongoing research to unravel the mechanisms by which viral pathogens trigger inflammatory heart disease. It further leads to severe cardiovascular complications (Kemerley et al., 2024). The late consequences of inflammatory heart disease are possibly the most concerning, in the sense that they can lead to chronic cardiovascular illness, including dilated cardiomyopathy and heart failure. The pathophysiologic mechanisms of such illness are commonly the consequence of persistent inflammation leading to remodeling of cardiac tissue structure and function. Chronic myocarditis can cause progressive deterioration in cardiac function, necessitating interventions ranging from pharmacologic therapy to surgical interventions like heart transplant in severe cases. Furthermore, chronic inflammation increases the likelihood of arrhythmias and thromboembolic consequences, which makes patient care and outcomes even more challenging. Continued research into the fundamental immunopathological mechanisms, supported by well-conducted clinical studies, is critical for the development of rationale therapeutics and the improvement in long-term prognosis of patients with inflammatory heart disease (Zafeiri et al., 2024) (Figure 10.18).

References

1. Abrignani, M. G., Lucà, F., Abrignani, V., Nucara, M., Grosseto, D., Lestuzzi, C., Mistrangelo, M., Passaretti, B., Rao, C. M., & Parrini, I. (2025). Risk factors and prevention of cancer and CVDs: a chicken and egg situation. *Journal of Clinical Medicine, 14*(9), 3083. https://doi.org/10.3390/jcm14093083Adolph, T., Meyer, M., Jukic, A., & Tilg, H. (2024). Heavy arch: From inflammatory bowel diseases to metabolic disorders. *Gut, 73*, 1376–1387. https://www.semanticscholar.org/paper/291b0f43a2f660a5140078683b50fe9e3eaa2adb (accessed on 29th May 2025).
2. Ahmad, F. A. J., Abdi, S. I. A., Verma, T., Barsinge, T., Banderas, E. W. M., Sampath, N., Fathima, A., et al. (2025). A comprehensive review of effusive-constrictive pericarditis, diagnosis, and management. *Cardiology in Review*. https://www.semanticscholar.org/paper/312a79eb4e1b0c40adeda58f02f4b6c2a04f16ca (accessed on 29th May 2025).
3. Alipour, A., Akhavein, F., Rahimpour, F., Naghibi, S. M. R., & Alizadeh, B. (2024). Imaging evaluation of clinical and subclinical myocarditis in multisystem inflammatory syndrome of children with COVID-19 using cardiac magnetic resonance: The results and prognosis. *Iranian Journal of Radiology*. https://www.semanticscholar.org/paper/065483a011e39ae9e486e849588a81c38bf87778 (accessed on 29th May 2025).
4. Ballesteros, T. F., Coserría, S. F., Jurado-Román, A., Cruz-González, I., Álvarez-Fuente, M., Amat-Santos, I., Betrián, B. P., et al. (2024). Spanish cardiac catheterization in congenital heart diseases registry: Third official report from the ACI-SEC and the GTH-SECPCC (2022). *REC: Interventional Cardiology (English Edition)*. https://www.semanticscholar.org/paper/bb19bf22d35d6a0f40e2f7a563c0353e21fa24bb (accessed on 29th May 2025).
5. Baran, J., Garbacz, K., Krawczuk, V. W. J., Maciąg, A., et al. (2024). *The Role of Lipoprotein a in Cardiac Risk Stratification and Evaluation of Hypolipemizing Treatment*. https://core.ac.uk/download/636385413.pdf (accessed on 29th May 2025).
6. Benrabah, O., Ait Mouheb, T., Dahmoune, R., Bellouti, S., Ait Mokhtar, L., Amine, Z., & Maoudj, A. (2024). Congenital heart diseases with neonatal onset: Prevalence and circumstances of diagnosis in the newborn. *International Journal of Science and Research Archive*. https://www.semanticscholar.org/paper/f44197683961659c5861147dcd7d65348b5305df (accessed on 29th May 2025).
7. Blagova, O., Moiseeva, O., & Paleev, F. (2021). Controversial and open issues of diagnosis and treatment of myocarditis (based on the discussion of Russian national recommendations). *Russian Journal of Cardiology*. https://www.semanticscholar.org/paper/fb33e0f4cce257feb30b97cd92d1f3631d505bd7 (accessed on 29th May 2025).
8. Bondareva, O. O., Dolnik, M. Yu., Ryazanova, O. V., Tyshchenko, T., et al. (2018). *Some Aspects of the Latent Iron Deficiency Diagnosis in the Patients with Cardiac Pathology*. https://core.ac.uk/download/304693522.pdf (accessed on 29th May 2025).
9. Calabrese, A., Ghisletti, A., Gori, M., Iorio, A., Giammarresi, A., Quarta, G., Cirelli, C., et al. (2024). AL-amyloidosis related advanced heart failure diagnosed through F-18-flutemetamol PET scan. *European Heart Journal Supplements*. https://www.semanticscholar.org/paper/85fa51198223982adffd4899b22fb57e4793af4a (accessed on 29th May 2025).

10. Chang, M. L., Mi, K. L., Cunningham, R. R., Catterall, W. A., Yared, M. A., Siegel, C. A., & Yen, R. W. (2025). The efficacy of traditional Chinese medicine for Crohn's disease treatment: A systematic review and meta-analysis. *Journal of Gastrointestinal and Liver Diseases: JGLD, 34*(1), 98–107. https://www.semanticscholar.org/paper/209068d2b54b1f149246b5d6188f6f133b65c54e (accessed on 29th May 2025).

11. Daiber, A., Hadad, O., Munzel, T., Röösli, M., et al. (2021). *Nachtlärminduzierte Schlafstörungen und Herz-Kreislauf-Risiko.* https://core.ac.uk/download/551516252.pdf (accessed on 29th May 2025).

12. Deidda, S., Delitala, G., Delogu, L. G., Manetti, R., et al. (2011). *Infectious Diseases and Autoimmunity.* https://core.ac.uk/download/11692556.pdf (accessed on 29th May 2025).

13. Di Pietro, M., Falasca, F., Filardo, S., Sessa, R., et al. (2017). *Infectious Agents in Atherosclerotic Cardiovascular Diseases Through Oxidative Stress.* https://core.ac.uk/download/153366001.pdf (accessed on 29th May 2025).

14. Dunn, S. P., Fallon, J. M., Kennedy, J. L. W., Parker, B., et al. (2020). *A Giant Mystery in Giant Cell Myocarditis: Navigating Diagnosis, Immunosuppression, and Mechanical Circulatory Support.* https://core.ac.uk/download/323063243.pdf (accessed on 29th May 2025).

15. Dutka, M., Zimmer, K., Ćwiertnia, M., Ilczak, T. P., & Bobiński, R. (2024). The role of PCSK9 in heart failure and other cardiovascular diseases—Mechanisms of action beyond its effect on LDL cholesterol. *Heart Failure Reviews, 29*, 917–937. https://www.semanticscholar.org/paper/8518e909634484a98d92ee71430378a1226c8451 (accessed on 29th May 2025).

16. Fahimi, B. (2024). Atrial fibrillation and lifestyle modification: Charting new courses for cardiovascular health. *Clinical Research and Clinical Trials.* https://www.semanticscholar.org/paper/6f7f6e6b2db31e658e5103bdba8b6720ba878f01 (accessed on 29th May 2025).

17. Fonseca De, A. E. V. F., Cassia Da, L. G. C. L. G., Alex Bezerra Da, S. M. A. B. S. M., Jefferson, V. J. V., Vanderson, S. V. S., Allyson, G. A. G., Guilherme Peixoto Tinoco Areas, G. P. T. A. (2024). Higher inflammatory cytokines in long-COVID with cardiovascular symptoms after acute severe COVID-19? A two-year, pre-vaccine, longitudinal, exploratory, nested cohort. *European Journal of Preventive Cardiology.* https://www.semanticscholar.org/paper/4c4185f5864e931e73c8f968aeaf2e6456b49f6b (accessed on 29th May 2025).

18. Ghosh, S., Whitley, C. S., Haribabu, B., & Jala, V. R. (2021). Regulation of intestinal barrier function by microbial metabolites. *Cellular and Molecular Gastroenterology and Hepatology, 11*, 1463–1482. https://doi.org/10.1016/j.jcmgh.2021.02.007 (accessed on 29th May 2025).

19. Gil, R. J., & Pawlak, A. (2017). *Infective Cardiomyopathy.* https://core.ac.uk/download/322428717.pdf (accessed on 29th May 2025).

20. Goto, S., Angchaisuksiri, P., Bassand, J., Camm, A., Dominguez, H., Illingworth, L., Gibbs, H., et al. (2019). Management and 1-year outcomes of patients with newly diagnosed atrial fibrillation and chronic kidney disease: Results from the prospective GARFIELD-AF registry. *Journal of the American Heart Association: Cardiovascular and Cerebrovascular Disease, 8.* https://www.semanticscholar.org/paper/d13e4a8bbada3267a4f5278f3859f0d14e2e3952 (accessed on 29th May 2025).

21. Hracs, L., Windsor, J., Gorospe, J., Buie, M., Quan, J., Caplan, L., Markovinović, A., et al. (2024). Machine learning classification of the epidemiologic stages of inflammatory bowel

disease across geography and time. *Gastroenterology*. https://www.semanticscholar.org/paper/b457a8e69c01854ce0eb4a73afea291fd8902e31 (accessed on 29th May 2025).

22. Huang, W., Yin, C., Lento, P. A., Adem, P. V., Dimitrova, N., & Fallon, J. T. (2024). Differential deep RNA sequencing for diagnostic detection of microbial infections in inflammatory cardiomyopathy. *Circulation: Genomic and Precision Medicine*. https://www.semanticscholar.org/paper/c50bad423816c865e3e44ac505bdd39de3e77d83 (accessed on 29th May 2025).

23. Jia, Y., Liu, Y., Zuo, Y., Zhang, J., Li, Y., Liu, X., & Lv, S. (2024). The potential therapeutic prospect of PANoptosis in heart failure. *Journal of Inflammation Research*, *17*, 9147–9168. https://www.semanticscholar.org/paper/479d998da0ba5342de3fdbe982f07e43768d524d (accessed on 29th May 2025).

24. Kemerley, A., Gupta, A., Thirunavukkarasu, M., Maloney, M., Burgwardt, S., & Maulik, N. (2024). COVID-19 associated cardiovascular disease—Risks, prevention and management: Heart at risk due to COVID-19. *Current Issues in Molecular Biology*, *46*, 1904–1920. https://www.semanticscholar.org/paper/70451ec9d42f33c36238ad5991d199687c1e4fc4 (accessed on 29th May 2025).

25. Khatoon, J., & Saha, J. K. (2024). *Nursing Care for Inflammatory Bowel Disease: Patient Support and Symptom Management – A Scoping Review*. https://core.ac.uk/download/638724139.pdf (accessed on 29th May 2025).

26. Kirchhof, P., Benussi, S., Kotecha, D., Ahlsson, A., Atar, D., Casadei, B., Castellá, M., et al. (2016). 2016 ESC guidelines for the management of atrial fibrillation developed in collaboration with EACTS. *European Heart Journal*, *37*, 2893–2962. https://doi.org/10.1093/eurheartj/ehw210 (accessed on 29th May 2025).

27. Koltunova, H., & Chyzh, K. (2024). Microbiological spectrum of infective endocarditis complicated by heart failure. *Pain, Anesthesia & Intensive Care*. https://www.semanticscholar.org/paper/faca823905accc998ecf19deb03b304353b00efb (accessed on 29th May 2025).

28. Kyryk, V. (2024). Stem cell therapy for cardiac regeneration: Key points. *Cell and Organ Transplantology*. https://www.semanticscholar.org/paper/6a1b536f3691ad0d162e4187a4a2e2ffd1507b5f (accessed on 29th May 2025).

29. La Vecchia, G., Del Buono, M. D., Bonaventura, A., Vecchié, A., Moroni, F., Cartella, I., Saponara, G., et al. (2024). Cardiac involvement in patients with multisystem inflammatory syndrome in adults. *Journal of the American Heart Association: Cardiovascular and Cerebrovascular Disease*, *13*. https://www.semanticscholar.org/paper/db8a1adc198ab6f265322e7f7fe16356f3c8c7c5 (accessed on 29th May 2025).

30. Lauinger, A. R., & Sepe, J. J. (2025). Vascularization, innervation, and inflammation: Pathways connecting the heart–brain axis and implications in a clinical setting. *Biomedicines*, *13*. https://www.semanticscholar.org/paper/aeb4c7afe6a3b797f066aa706d8c0b14d9c783d3 (accessed on 29th May 2025).

31. Lepekhina, E. S., Nadey, E. V., & Usacheva, E. V. (2024). A clinical case of a patient with common variable immune deficiency. *Clinical Review for General Practice*. https://www.semanticscholar.org/paper/3b368d98d60af471ff7d99ed48b7cc0fb1d66e29 (accessed on 29th May 2025).

32. Li, Y., He, S., Wu, J., Liu, S., Liu, R., Du, Y. P., Han, D., et al. (2025). Integrated transcriptomic and single-cell analysis reveals key immune-related genes and cellular crosstalk in the myocarditis

microenvironment. *European Journal of Inflammation*. https://www.semanticscholar.org/paper/1ccd61897a0d9c0975b6322d5514e8225184e8e7 (accessed on 29th May 2025).

33. Liu, S., & Gu, Y. (2024). INFLA score: A novel inflammatory marker for assessing cardiometabolic disease risk in obese individuals. *Diabetology & Metabolic Syndrome, 16*. https://www.semanticscholar.org/paper/ffb9ccc6e5a5663d0e9f6517157648b1758a7d2d (accessed on 29th May 2025).

34. Lu, X., Xu, Z., Shu, F., Wang, Y., Han, Y., Yang, X., Shi, P., et al. (2024). Reactive oxygen species responsive multifunctional fusion extracellular nanovesicles: Prospective treatments for acute heart transplant rejection. *Advanced Materials*. https://www.semanticscholar.org/paper/60001e201ce10462759b074b4cce601bf19d5a6f (accessed on 29th May 2025).

35. Lv, L., Guo, Y., Zheng, Z., & Li, B. (2024). Exploring causal correlations between inflammatory cytokines and coronary heart disease: A Mendelian randomization study. *Medicine, 103*. https://www.semanticscholar.org/paper/1ed75d4937b0be9626092423e25f4416f8e79f89 (accessed on 29th May 2025).

36. Maggio, M., Lembo, A., Finazzo, F., Alaimo, A., Benfratello, G. F., Corsello, G. (2024). Cardiovascular involvement in children with COVID-19 temporally related multisystem inflammatory syndrome (MIS-C): Can cardiac magnetic resonance arrive to the heart of the problem? *Italian Journal of Pediatrics, 50*. https://www.semanticscholar.org/paper/cfaf6ac194cba89ef3aa05e64f0abb1e08416a15 (accessed on 29th May 2025).

37. Monteiro, V., Torres, L., Carneiro, R., Cunha, C., Figueira, F., Matta, M., Silva, I., et al. (2024). Evaluation of serum levels of sCD40, sCD40L and s4-1BB in advanced heart failure and after heart transplant. *European Heart Journal*. https://www.semanticscholar.org/paper/eac705daac377bff431da636fb1d42a5b049ac15 (accessed on 29th May 2025).

38. Nayak, G., Dimitriadis, K. S., Pyrpyris, N., Manti, M., Kamperidis, N., Kamperidis, V., Ziakas, A., et al. (2024). Gut microbiome and its role in valvular heart disease: Not a "gutted" relationship. *Life, 14*. https://www.semanticscholar.org/paper/8abb80aa16dac035c4ffa3d869c8902be0a422a3 (accessed on 29th May 2025).

39. Nazrin, T., & Hassan, M. (2023). Infective endocarditis associated with multisystem inflammatory syndrome in children (MIS-C): Two case studies. *Pulse*. https://www.semanticscholar.org/paper/d1df817c62a9dec88acf774b67e3e48ecf54647e (accessed on 29th May 2025).

40. Plymoth, M., Lundquist, R., Nystedt, A., Sjöstedt, A., & Gustafsson, T. N. (2024). Targeting tularemia: Clinical, laboratory, and treatment outcomes from an 11-year retrospective observational cohort in northern Sweden. *Clinical Infectious Diseases: An Official Publication of the Infectious Diseases Society of America, 78*, 1222–1231. https://www.semanticscholar.org/paper/4c5aa9b2cb77bc960434a7d9fb7d8384b44b71f2 (accessed on 29th May 2025).

41. Ren, Z., & Li, G. (2024). A comprehensive review on the association and prevention of long-term COVID-induced heart failure: A review. *Medicine, 103*. https://www.semanticscholar.org/paper/79169cc760bfbd87c9357fd11a2350797b937179 (accessed on 29th May 2025).

42. Rinella, M. E., Neuschwander-Tetri, B. A., Siddiqui, M. S., Abdelmalek, M. F., Caldwell, S. H., Barb, D., Kleiner, D. E., et al. (2023). AASLD practice guidance on the clinical assessment and management of nonalcoholic fatty liver disease. *Hepatology, 77*, 1797–1835. https://doi.org/10.1097/hep.0000000000000323 (accessed on 29th May 2025).

43. Sandireddy, R., Sakthivel, S., Gupta, P., Behari, J., Tripathi, M., & Singh, B. (2024). Systemic impacts of metabolic dysfunction-associated steatotic liver disease (MASLD) and metabolic dysfunction-associated steatohepatitis (MASH) on heart, muscle, and kidney related diseases. *Frontiers in Cell and Developmental Biology, 12*. https://www.semanticscholar.org/paper/640458bb2418cc956da7f6df2d2a7d621bbede23 (accessed on 29th May 2025).

44. Stolzer, I., Kaden-Volynets, V., Ruder, B., Letizia, M., Bittel, M., Rausch, P., Basic, M., et al. (2019). Environmental microbial factors determine the pattern of inflammatory lesions in a murine model of Crohn's disease-like inflammation. *Inflammatory Bowel Diseases*. https://www.semanticscholar.org/paper/5490654aaf82e248ca64a21727f1f46b7e108ffc (accessed on 29th May 2025).

45. Tercan, H. (2025). *Regulation of the Innate Immune Phenotype in Atherosclerosis: Navigating the Inflammatory Landscape*. https://www.semanticscholar.org/paper/54b2c16f39d5af23fbc56a4b27f6bccabf399c9d (accessed on 29th May 2025).

46. Theodoropoulou, T., Apostolos, A., Ktenopoulos, N., Koliastasis, L., Tsalamandris, S., Mourouzis, I., Pantos, C., et al. (2025). Impact of chronic inflammatory diseases on clinical outcomes in patients undergoing aortic valve replacement: A systematic review and meta-analysis. *Angiology*. https://www.semanticscholar.org/paper/6840e033b0ce5e58355e2dc88b3c7cca9df3abda (accessed on 29th May 2025).

47. Visseren, F. L. J., Mach, F., Smulders, Y. M., Carballo, D., Koskinas, K. C., Bäck, M., Bénétos, A., et al. (2021). 2021 ESC guidelines on cardiovascular disease prevention in clinical practice. *European Heart Journal, 42*, 3227–3337. https://doi.org/10.1093/eurheartj/ehab484 (accessed on 29th May 2025).

48. Wartenberg, C., Elden, H., Frerichs, M., Jivegård, L. L., Magnusson, K., Mourtzinis, G., Nyström, O., et al. (2025). Clinical benefits and risks of remote patient monitoring: An overview and assessment of methodological rigor of systematic reviews for selected patient groups. *BMC Health Services Research, 25*. https://www.semanticscholar.org/paper/fef7b4712606ee7633b949b29eb4f84c0d1f9839 (accessed on 29th May 2025).

49. Wenzel, A. A., Saul, S., Kodiak, T., Whitehead, B., Strople, J., Brown, J., & Cohran, V. (2024). Posttransplant inflammatory bowel disease after successful solid organ transplantation: Not out of the woods yet. *Journal of Pediatric Gastroenterology and Nutrition*. https://www.semanticscholar.org/paper/71d639fb5b1f490a48bb7ee0e661bc261d0fc648 (accessed on 29th May 2025).

50. Williams, B., Mancia, G., Spiering, W., Agabiti, R. E., Azizi, M., Burnier, M., Clement, D. L., et al. (2018). 2018 ESC/ESH guidelines for the management of arterial hypertension. *European Heart Journal, 39*, 3021–3104. https://doi.org/10.1093/eurheartj/ehy339 (accessed on 29th May 2025).

51. Williams, S. A., Murthy, A., DeLisle, R. K., Hyde, C., Malarstig, A., Ostroff, R., Weiss, S. J., et al. (2017). Improving assessment of drug safety through proteomics. *Circulation, 137*, 999–1010. https://www.semanticscholar.org/paper/5abd584d011cc5b9183f6640a2850b02f2620588 (accessed on 29th May 2025).

52. Zafeiri, M., Knott, K., & Lampejo, T. (2024). Acute myocarditis: An overview of pathogenesis, diagnosis and management. *Panminerva Medica*. https://www.semanticscholar.org/paper/99506d6909d5a816e3bad9acd1c178aacfded47d (accessed on 29th May 2025).

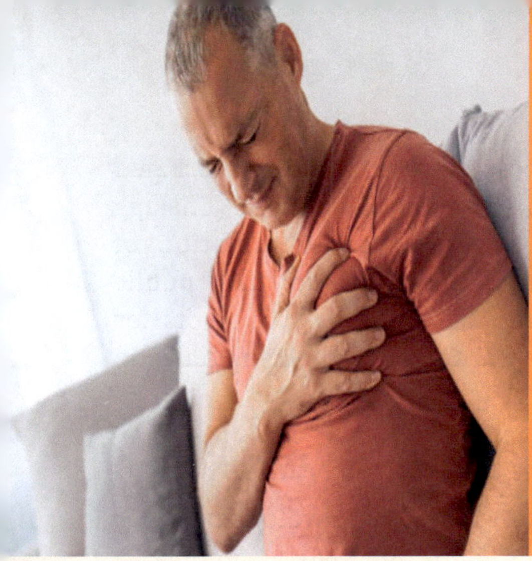

Chapter 11
CARDIOMYOPATHIES

Contents

Introduction

Cardiomyopathies are a diverse group of heart muscle diseases with structural and functional alterations that impair the heart's ability to pump. Cardiomyopathies are caused by a variety of etiologic substrates, including genetic mutations, metabolic disorders, or systemic illness, and manifest with many different clinical syndromes. It is paramount to understand how complex cardiomyopathies are to justify appropriate therapeutic regimens and improve outcomes in patients. Recognition of the diverse causes, such as those of herpesviruses, for infant deaths outside hospitals, as evidenced in recent studies, creates an avenue for widespread research into how infectious pathogens may be the cause of such cardiac ailments (Chalapa et al., 2024). The multifactorial etiology of cardiomyopathies justifies the demand for multidisciplinary practice and research. The cardiomyopathies are also subdivided into various subtypes, such as hypertrophic, dilated, and restrictive cardiomyopathy, each with differential pathophysiologic mechanisms and clinical importance. For instance, transthyretin amyloidosis (ATTR) has become an important condition characterized by protein misfolding deposition, causing cardiac impairment and typically associated with neuropathic manifestations. The identification of specific genetic mutations that define ATTR highlights the importance of genetic screening in understanding cardiomyopathy phenotypes (Stinson et al., 2023). The standard diagnosis of cardiomyopathies must evolve to incorporate genetic testing and advanced imaging techniques that can provide information regarding disease progression and inform the treatment plan.

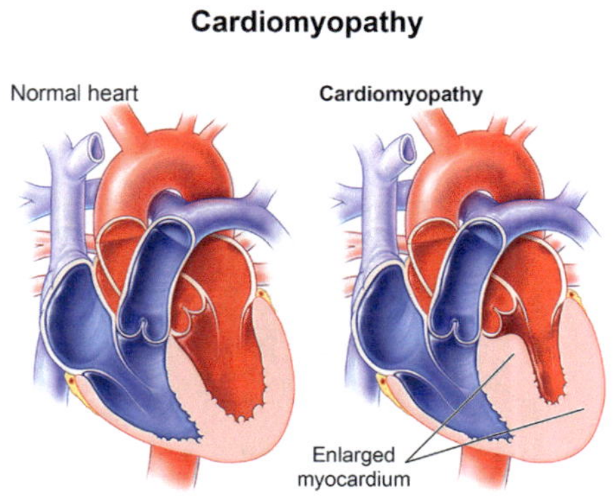

Figure 11.1. A heart with cardiomyopathy gets larger and weaker and can end up in heart failure.

Source: https://my.clevelandclinic.org/-/scassets/images/org/health/articles/16841-cardiomyopathy-illustration.

Cardiomyopathies research and clinical practice must address not just the biological and genetic origins of such disorders but also the public health aspects. Effective cardiomyopathy management is closely linked with early diagnosis and individualized treatment regimens, which can enhance patient quality of life considerably. As has been observed from the most recent evidence validating the role of viral infections in infant mortality, increased research on the infectious and environmental determinants possibly feeding into exacerbated heart conditions is highly warranted (Chalapa et al., 2024). An in-depth examination of such associations may generate new public health intervention and strategy concepts for minimizing the burden of cardiomyopathies in at-risk groups (Figure 11.1).

Definition of Cardiomyopathies

A detailed understanding of cardiomyopathies requires a clear definition that encompasses various heart diseases characterized by structural and functional changes in the myocardium. They are at risk to develop severe complications like heart failure, and arrhythmias, having a last effect on the patients' quality of life and their elevated risk of death. Cardiomyopathies are typically classified into several types, including dilated, hypertrophic, restrictive, and arrhythmogenic right ventricular cardiomyopathy (ARVC). Each type possesses distinct pathophysiological mechanisms, etiologies, and prognoses, which complicate their diagnosis and treatment all the more.

Defining such classifications enables clinicians to develop specific interventions and optimize patient outcomes with precise management procedures adapted to the type of cardiomyopathy. Of all the cardiomyopathies, diabetic cardiomyopathy (DbCM) is especially significant due to its increasing prevalence in diabetic patients. Initially explained as ventricular dysfunction independent of coronary artery disease or hypertension, the complexity of DbCM has created ongoing research to investigate in detail its definition. Recent literature shows that diastolic dysfunction, with associated alterations in myocardial metabolism, characterizes this disorder. The interaction of glucose metabolism and cardiac function offers critical information regarding how diabetes is altering mechanisms of heart disease. Moreover, heterogeneity of DbCM understanding justifies the need for intensive clinical assessment, where patient reactions can be significantly different, thus making individualized therapy a requirement for treating diabetic patients (Heather et al., 2024). Dilated cardiomyopathy (DCM) has a unique position in cardiomyopathy types as a primary etiology of heart failure worldwide. The intricate interaction between environmental factors and genetic background renders the clinical presentation of DCM a complicated one, with phenotypes in the affected individuals possibly being extremely heterogeneous. Advanced genetic testing has illuminated genotype-phenotype correlations, with prognostication tailor-made for each individual. Better risk stratification models involving genetic and clinical factors enhance the clinician's ability to predict outcomes, for instance, hospitalization for heart failure or fatal ventricular arrhythmias (LTVA) (Sammani et al., 2021). These innovations underscore the merit of the application of detailed assessment tools, including cardiac imaging technologies, to optimize patient care and develop targeted treatment protocols that include consideration of specific genetic hazards. Continuous improvement of DCM's definition thus reflects continued research and practical use in cardiomyopathies (Figure 11.2).

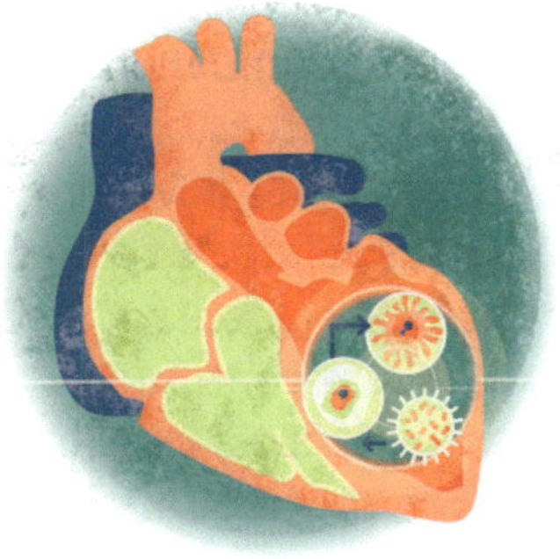

Figure 11.2. Cardiomyopathy.

Source: https://assets.medpagetoday.net/media/images/97xxx/97961.png?width=0.8.

11.1. Types of Cardiomyopathies

The classification of cardiomyopathies primarily includes various categories, including dilated cardiomyopathy (DCM), hypertrophic cardiomyopathy (HCM), and restrictive cardiomyopathy. Dilated cardiomyopathy is characterized by ventricular dilation and systolic dysfunction, which most commonly leads to heart failure. In DCM, genetic disorders are the most contributing factor, and mutations in several genes account for its pathophysiology. Studies applying next-generation sequencing techniques have described numerous genetic mutations associated with DCM, including plakophilin-2 and myosin-binding protein C-3, illustrating the heterogeneous genetic etiology of the disorder (Lombardo et al., 2020). Identification of the causative mutations can facilitate the establishment of personalized treatment strategies, ultimately optimizing patient outcomes. Hypertrophic cardiomyopathy, on the other hand, is an abnormally thickened heart muscle, most often the left ventricle. HCM can be genetic, typically with mutations in genes encoding sarcomeric proteins. It can range from asymptomatic to dramatic presentation, like arrhythmia and sudden death. Athletes are particularly at risk, occult inherited cardiomyopathies being prevalent among them (Lombardo et al., 2020). The challenge in anticipating those who are at risk has underpinned the proposal of predictive medicine, which couples traditional diagnostic equipment with genetic analysis. By knowing the causative genetic abnormalities, medical practitioners can predict the risk of sudden cardiac arrests more precisely, so that preventive management can be maximized on an individual basis, especially in high-risk groups such as competitive athletes. Restrictive cardiomyopathy is less common but worthy of mention owing to its unique pathology. This type is characterized by hardening of the heart muscle, which renders it incapable of filling usually at diastole, leading to symptoms of heart failure. Unlike DCM and HCM, restrictive cardiomyopathy is more likely to arise as a result of systemic diseases such as amyloidosis or hemochromatosis. The diverse etiologies underscore the requirement of a multi-factorial diagnostic approach, which can include genetic testing where appropriate. As research continues to advance in demarcating cardiomyopathies' genetic origin, novel information on restrictive cardiomyopathy could become imminent. For example, upcoming achievements in genetic screening can potentially make it possible to treat and diagnose earlier, ultimately maximizing treatment outcomes and patient benefits (Amr et al., 2014) (Figure 11.3).

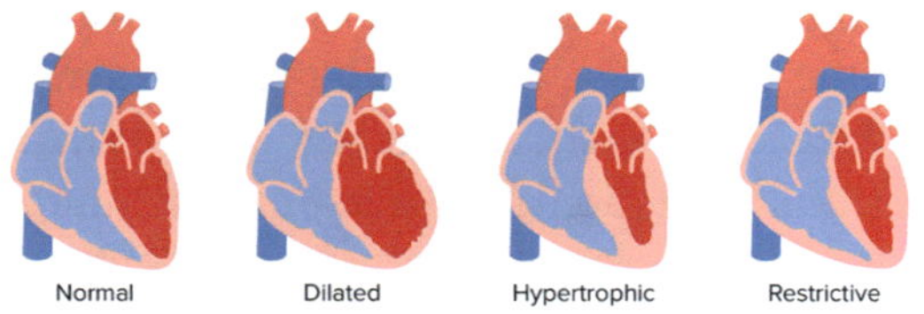

Figure 11.3. Morphological classification of cardiomyopathies.

Source: https://cdn.lecturio.com/assets/Overview-of-cardiomyopathies-01-1536x556.png.

11.1.1. Dilated Cardiomyopathy (DCM)

DCM is the most prevalent type of cardiomyopathy and is essentially typified by left ventricular dilation and systolic dysfunction. It often leads to a significant diminishment of the heart's pumping function, which can be quantified as heart failure and arrhythmias. Clinically, DCM can present heterogeneously, with certain patients being asymptomatic while others are highly symptomatic and result in sudden cardiac death. Following recent publications, DCM patients may have cardiovascular mortality rates of as much as 40% at 10 years, a reflection of the severity and heterogeneity of this disease (Arenja et al., 2019). Recognition of the varied clinical presentations of DCM is critical in ensuring early intervention and management. Dilated cardiomyopathy's pathophysiologic mechanisms are complex and multifactorial. Genetic factors play a significant role, with familial DCM illustrating the hereditary component of some presentations of DCM. Gene mutations affecting cardiac muscle function can disrupt the normal structure and function of the heart. Additionally, there are also various non-genetic reasons, such as viral infections, alcoholism, and metabolic disorders, involved in the pathogenesis of DCM (Arenja et al., 2019). The interplay between these environmental and genetic reasons is responsible for the heterogeneous presentation and prognosis in patients, for which diagnosis and management are particularly challenging. Given the heterogeneity of DCM expression, a proper understanding of these mechanisms is critical for clinicians seeking to tailor effective care. From a therapeutic standpoint, management of dilated cardiomyopathy is as diversified as its expression. No surefire cures are available, but various modalities of treatment can be used to alter manifestations and improve quality of life. Conventional approaches typically consist of the use of heart failure medications such as angiotensin-converting enzyme (ACE) inhibitors, beta-blockers, and diuretics. In extreme cases, individuals can be eligible for novel therapies such heart transplants or implanted cardioverter-defibrillators. Notably, disease-modifying therapy studies have been promising, particularly in cases related to genetic mutation or particular etiologies (Arenja et al., 2019). Even as healthcare workers continue to endeavor to enhance patient outcomes, continued research into these treatment modalities will be at the forefront, alongside individually chosen management based on patient and disease course (Figure 11.4).

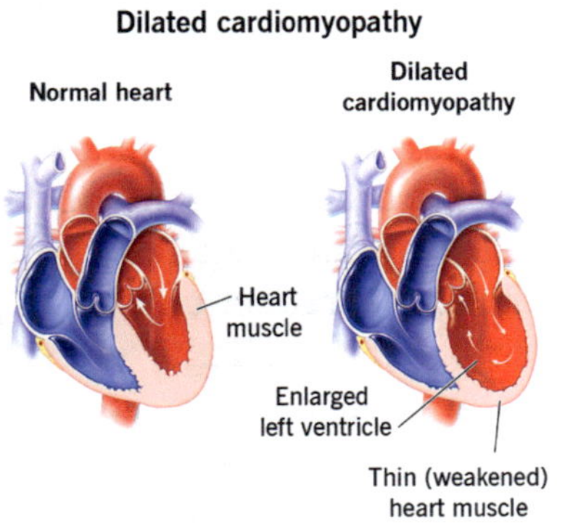

Figure 11.4. Dilated cardiomyopathy (DCM).

Source: https://my.clevelandclinic.org/-/scassets/images/org/health/articles/16932-dilated-cardiomyopathy.

11.1.2. Hypertrophic Cardiomyopathy (HCM)

HCM is the most frequent presentation of primary cardiomyopathy, referring to the abnormal thickening of the myocardium, particularly in the left ventricle. HCM is typically asymptomatic, hence challenging to diagnose and treat early. The symptoms, if any, include exertional dyspnea, nonspecific chest pain, and syncope that together impair the patient's quality of life. Sudden cardiac death (SCD) is primarily a significant concern, particularly among young athletes, and heightened awareness and screening are thus mandatory.

The pathophysiologic substrate of HCM is typically genetic with sarcomeric protein mutations, emphasizing the use of genetic counseling and testing in involved families. With advances in the area of predictive medicine, it calls a need to have genetic testing included, which could potentially allow for earlier diagnosis and preventive strategies in at-risk individuals (Lombardo et al., 2020). Clinical diagnosis of HCM demands a multidisciplinary approach, with accurate patient history, physical examination, and sophisticated imaging techniques. Electrocardiogram (ECG) typically reveals characteristic changes, while echocardiography plays a vital role in visualizing ventricular hypertrophy and functional impairment. In more recent times, the advent of next-generation sequencing (NGS) technology has enabled us to screen for specific genetic mutations predisposing to HCM. The molecular data make precision medicine more realistic, where treatment can be individualized based on the patient's genetic makeup. Also, early identification of relatives by genetic testing can lead to preventive measures being undertaken, ultimately to reduce morbidity and mortality as a consequence of HCM.

Due to the intricate interaction between genetics and clinical presentation, HCM demonstrates the merit of a multidisciplinary strategy to its management (Lombardo et al., 2020). Treatment of hypertrophic cardiomyopathy is predominantly symptomatic and stage-based, with the primary goal of alleviating symptoms and preventing ill outcomes. Initial treatment is typically by change of lifestyle and medical therapy, such as beta-blockade and calcium channel blockade, to reduce myocardial oxygen demand. In the more complex forms, septal myectomy or alcohol septal ablation may be indicated to relieve left ventricular outflow obstruction. Application of implantable cardioverter-defibrillators (ICDs) in high-risk patients for SCD also remains a critical factor, as these devices reduce the risk of sudden cardiac events. Continued advances in genetic research and individualized treatment protocols offer encouraging avenues for improved prognosis, justifying aggressive treatment of HCM. Physicians need to remain vigilant for high-risk patients and encourage patient education regarding the significance of this disease (Babu et al., 2024) (Figure 11.5).

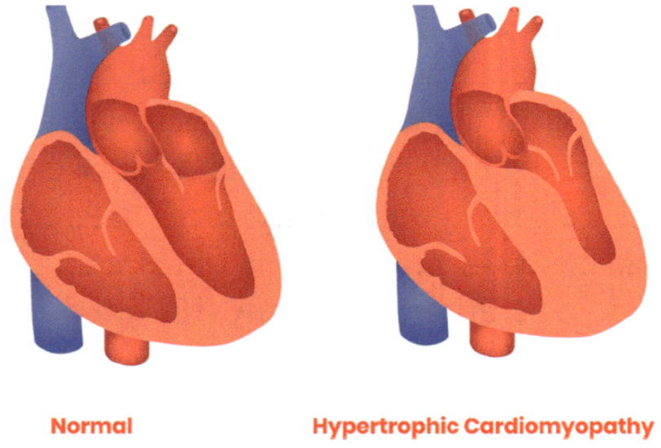

Figure 11.5. Hypertrophic cardiomyopathy (HCD).

Source: https://www.thekeyholeheartclinic.com/wp-content/uploads/2021/04/HOCM.jpg.

11.1.3. Restrictive Cardiomyopathy (RCM)

RCM is also reported to be one of the less common forms of cardiomyopathy, representing as few as 2%–5% of all occurrences. It possesses a stiff and inelastic myocardium, which restricts the ability of the heart to fill with blood during diastole. This impaired filling will often lead to symptoms of heart failure, such as exertional shortness of breath, fatigue, and fluid overload. In contrast to dilated cardiomyopathy, where the chambers of the heart are enlarged, in RCM, the size can be normal; however, the function of the heart considerably worsens. Diagnosis is generally by a complete assessment encompassing echocardiography, which will detect diastolic dysfunction, and other imaging modalities. As clinicians have noted, early identification of RCM is part of controlling its course and related complications (Babu et al., 2024). The pathogenesis of restrictive cardiomyopathy is typically associated with systemic diseases and hence distinct from other cardiomyopathies. The etiology is predominantly infiltrative disorders such as amyloidosis and fibrosis, but also non-infiltrative disorders like radiation therapy effects. These conditions cause stiffening of the myocardium and consequently produce partial diastolic relaxation and increased intracardiac pressures. What is significant is that RCM may also occur due to genetic etiologies, but these are less frequent compared to dilated or hypertrophic cardiomyopathy. RCM treatment typically involves management of the underlying disease, causing a reduction of symptoms of heart failure. Pharmacologic intervention to control blood pressure and achieve optimal hemodynamics is a key to reducing morbidity for the disease (Babu et al., 2024). Though uncommon, restrictive cardiomyopathy is a challenging disease for clinicians and patients alike due to the complexity of the disease and the need for treatment. Prognosis in diagnosed patients with RCM is highly variable based on etiology and the rapidity of management of the treatable causes. Generally, patients may wind up requiring vigorous therapy, including heart transplantation, especially as the disease progresses and conventional measures are not beneficial. Along with that, genetic testing and family screening are particularly valuable in cases of hereditary conditions. With increasing knowledge regarding restrictive cardiomyopathy, more studies are needed to enlighten on more effective diagnostic and management methods to improve patient outcomes (Ciarambino et al., 2021) (Figure 11.6).

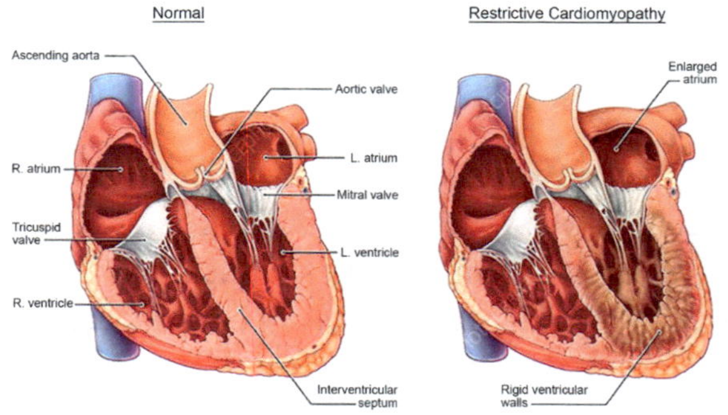

Figure 11.6. Restrictive cardiomyopathy (RCM).

Source: https://cdnintech.com/media/chapter/1188806/1730301094-529054099/media/F4.png.

11.2. Causes and Risk Factors

It is essential to understand the etiology and risk factors for cardiomyopathies so that they can be diagnosed at an early stage, and this group of heart diseases can be well managed. Cardiomyopathies are genetic and acquired, and each makes a different contribution to the disease course. The to disease is made by genetic causes, primarily through mutations in genes governing cardiac structure and function, which render individuals susceptible to conditions such as hypertrophic cardiomyopathy and arrhythmogenic right ventricular cardiomyopathy. In addition to its genetic causes, cardiomyopathies may also be induced or exacerbated by environmental factors, such as exposure to infection and toxins, thus also emphasizing the disease's multifactorial etiology. Investigation into its etiologic determinants not only allows for targeted prevention strategies but also unmasks the complex dynamics involved in the onset of various types of cardiomyopathies. Another significant topic to address is demographic factors like sex, age, and ethnicity on developing cardiomyopathy. Research indicates that men tend to develop certain cardiomyopathies more than women, perhaps due to hormonal influences.

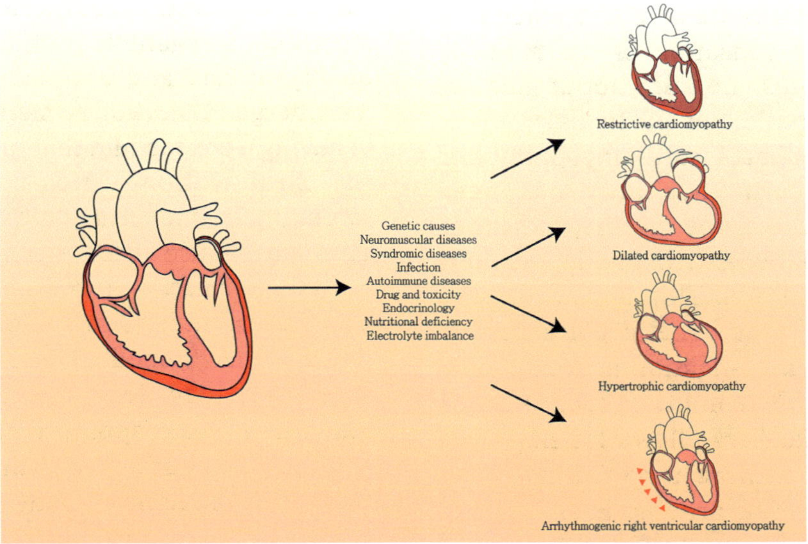

Figure 11.7. Risk factors of the four major types of cardiomyopathy.

Source: https://www.researchgate.net/publication/332492008/figure/fig1/AS:11431281213082202@1702939312044/Risk-factors-of-the-four-major-types-of-cardiomyopathy.tif.

This difference is particularly observed in ischemic cardiomyopathy, which tends to develop due to coronary heart disease, which is more prevalent in the elderly and men. Also, ethnic variation identifies other risk factors in that some groups experience elevated rates of cardiomyopathies that are linked to genetic susceptibilities. This intersection between population and risk for cardiomyopathy highlights the importance of tailored approaches in clinical practice and public health initiatives to effectively address the varying presentations of risk among groups. Also, lifestyle, as well as comorbidities, is responsible for a significant part in the development of cardiomyopathies. Diseases such as diabetes, obesity, and hypertension are equally known to be contributing causes since they place the heart under undue strain over the years. Additionally, self-determinant behaviors like physical inactivity, smoking, and diet also exacerbate these diseases, weaken cardiac function. According to the latest evidence, approximately 40% of cardiac arrests are sudden and have no apparent reason, typically backtracking to underlying hereditary cardiomyopathies and arrhythmias that predispose patients to life-threatening events (Bai et al., 2024). On this note, detection of the complex interaction between risk factors is critical in designing effective prevention interventions and measures to contain the burden of cardiomyopathies among vulnerable populations (Figure 11.7).

11.2.1. Genetic Predispositions

Genetic predispositions are of most tremendous significance to the causation of the majority of cardiomyopathies, notably about familial incidence. Participation of particular genetic mutations within dilated cardiomyopathy and arrhythmogenic cardiomyopathy has been identified as a cause of the disease, indicating increased risk in patients with family members who have the condition. This familial history indicates a significant genetic contribution, leading to further investigation into the genes that contribute to the condition. Identification of these genetic markers allows for improved risk estimation and more targeted screening strategies in high-risk groups. Early genetic testing can result in successful anticipatory management strategies and inform clinical management, as is frequently necessary because of the often variable clinical course of such conditions among affected persons and their relatives. The need for efficient screening procedures is appreciated, considering the importance of early cardiomyopathy detection in individuals with a genetic predisposition. Utilization of newer technology, such as echocardiographic deformation imaging and cardiac magnetic resonance imaging, holds the potential to reveal subclinical disease expression numerous years before clinical manifestation. Asselbergs et al. (2021) bring to prominence the point that non-invasive discovery of biomarkers has much potential for improved diagnostic yield and patient outcome. However, it remains essential to optimize and integrate these diagnostic methods in everyday clinical practice to offer patients timely evaluation of the complexities of genetic penetrance and expressivity. With further investigation in this field, concordance between genetic information and high-tech imaging modalities promises to reduce cardiomyopathy-related morbidity and mortality. Furthermore, personalized medicine is emerging as an essential approach in the treatment of individuals with genetic predispositions to cardiomyopathies. Tailoring screening and treatment protocols by individualized genetic profiles will enhance the quality of care and optimize health outcomes. Asselbergs et al. (2021) mention the necessity of having a consortium that targets personalized risk stratification, which may lead to viable screening frequencies and treatment regimens. Through the use of long-term electronic health record information in conjunction with genetic and clinical information, clinicians can identify those at heightened risk of heart failure and sudden cardiac death more accurately. This multi-disciplinary approach not only encourages early therapy but also coordinates patient care with their specific genetic settings, offering a customized pathway for treating these potentially deadly disorders.

11.2.2. Environmental Influences

Environmental determinants have a significant role to play in the etiopathogenesis of cardiomyopathies, determining cardiovascular disease and health incidence. Of the many environmental toxins, polychlorinated biphenyls (PCBs) have been implicated due to their relative environmental persistence and adverse biological effects. The bioaccumulation in wildlife and along polluted habitats, such as the upper Hudson River, has introduced harmful changes to the cardiovascular systems of affected animals. Notably, embryonic exposure to PCBs in avian models has shown significant cardiomyopathies, including teratogenic heart wall formations and arrhythmias. This justifies the need to study the interference of environmental contaminants with cardiac structure and function and has significant implications beyond cardiovascular disease because comparable modes of exposure to these chemicals also happen in specific occupational and environmental exposures (Carro et al., 2012). Moreover, the familial basis of cardiomyopathies highlights the synergism between environmental exposures and genetic factors. Research has indicated that individuals with a genetic predisposition to heart failure are at a considerably higher risk of hospitalization and mortality, particularly in sibling carriers of the disease. Heritability of heart failure, while representative of genetic susceptibility, further suggests that there may be a role of common environmental influences that could be responsible for disease progression and outcomes between families. This interactive effect of environment and genetics points to the complexity of cardiomyopathies, which calls for a more in-depth exploration of how lifestyle, environmental pollutants, and even socioeconomic status can interact synergistically to advance heritable risk (Lindgren et al., 2020). In this regard, awareness of environmental factors is critical for identifying individuals at high risk and creating prevention interventions. Preventing cardiomyopathies needs to be multifaceted in its approach and be aware of the multicausal causes of the diseases. Reducing exposure to environmental contaminants such as PCBs is paramount in protecting vulnerable groups, particularly at sensitive stages of development. Public health interventions at the community level, including the restriction of contaminant discharge into the environment and stringent regulation of chemical production and disposal, can prevent harm from toxic exposures. Further, promoting awareness of the contribution of environmental factors to cardiovascular disease can gain broader engagement in prevention from the general population. By including genetics and environmental toxicity assessments within cardiovascular health care plans, physicians are better able to respond to the complexity of cardiomyopathies, facilitating enhanced early detection and therapeutic intervention in diverse populations (Carro et al., 2012) (Figure 11.8).

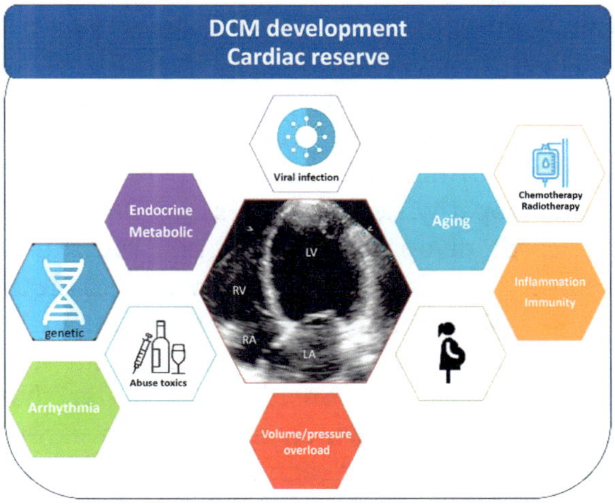

Figure 11.8. Schematic representation of the interplay of environmental and genetic factors participating in the development of dilated cardiomyopathy (DCM).

Source: https://www.mdpi.com/jcm/jcm-09-01702/article_deploy/html/images/jcm-09-01702-g001.png.

11.2.3. Comorbid Conditions

The presence of comorbid conditions significantly complicates the clinical management and prognosis of cardiomyopathies. Commonly observed comorbidities include hypertension, diabetes, and chronic kidney disease, which are often interconnected and exacerbate heart failure symptoms. For instance, hypertension, a prevalent condition among cardiomyopathy patients, can lead to maladaptive cardiac remodeling and worsen the overall heart function. In addition to this, diabetes also has an association with insulin resistance and metabolic derangement, impacting heart muscle function. Because these comorbidities frequently co-occur, their interaction should be quantified as a crucial aspect of developing personalized therapy. As heart failure with preserved ejection fraction (HFpEF) comes into the limelight as a public health problem, researchers recognize that these comorbidities specifically are accountable for the complexity and heterogeneity in the clinical outcome in patients with cardiomyopathies (Altay et al., 2017). The influence of comorbidities also extends to treatment modalities, particularly in patients with atrial fibrillation (AF) caused by cardiomyopathy. Recent studies have highlighted that cardiomyopathy is a strong predictor of arrhythmia recurrence following catheter ablation, which is a widespread treatment for AF. The risk of recurrence in patients with prior cardiomyopathy is considerably higher than in those without, which necessitates careful treatment of these patients. This link emphasizes the importance of cautious patient evaluation because it may guide clinicians toward the potential effectiveness of ablation and other therapies. By comprehending the influence of comorbidity on prognosis in arrhythmia, doctors can enhance management of complex treatment options and improve long-term prognosis in patients with cardiomyopathy (Thomas et al., 2016). In addition, the multi-dimensionality of comorbidities necessitates an integrated approach in managing cardiomyopathies. An interdisciplinary team for managing cardiomyopathies comprising cardiologists, endocrinologists, and nephrologists can ensure an integrated care strategy. This synergy becomes critical for the delivery of individualized treatment regimens not only for the management of idiopathic cardiomyopathy but also for the treatment of co-existing conditions like diabetes and renal impairment. Moreover, individualized interventions can maximize cardiovascular outcomes and optimize the quality of life in such patients. Emphasizing the importance of comorbidity control remains vital, as this can potentially lead to an improved prognosis for those who have to cope with the challenges presented by cardiomyopathies (Altay et al., 2017).

11.3. Symptoms and Diagnosis

Diagnosis of cardiomyopathies calls for a thorough familiarity with their diverse symptoms, either minor or perilous. Clinical presentation is nonspecific and, therefore, subject to misdiagnosis. Infiltrative cardiomyopathies, for example, such as cardiac sarcoidosis, may occur with fatigue, palpitations, or even symptoms of heart failure, making them difficult to diagnose in the early stages. Symptoms may be very diverse and may not occur in some patients, with one being grossly affected by extensive cardiac involvement. Healthcare professionals should recognize such symptoms, thus the importance of timely and accurate diagnosis. Failure to diagnose them early results in rates of morbidity and mortality due to cardiomyopathies, underscoring the importance of a high level of suspicion when seeing patients with unusual cardiac symptoms (Smyrnova et al., 2025). The diagnostic process of cardiomyopathy most commonly involves a combination of invasive tests, imaging studies, and clinical evaluation as indicated. Echocardiography is typically the initial imaging study ordered, and it provides essential information about ventricular shape and function. For example, in cardiac sarcoidosis, an echocardiogram may reveal evidence of ventricular dilation and valvular disease and is of paramount significance in making a diagnosis (Smyrnova et al., 2025). However, since echocardiography has limitations in some cases, more advanced methods like cardiac magnetic resonance imaging (MRI) and positron emission tomography (PET) can play essential roles in making more precise valuations. The newer modalities overcome the challenge of diagnosing conditions like cardiac sarcoidosis by demarcating areas of myocardial inflammation and enhancing the assessment of cardiac structure and function (Smyrnova et al., 2025).

Another traditional condition in the group of cardiomyopathies is arrhythmogenic right ventricular cardiomyopathy (ARVC), which has particular diagnostic challenges due to its expressivity variability and potential for asymptomatic presentation. Syncope and ventricular arrhythmias can manifest abruptly, particularly in young athletes, so that diagnosis before overt disease can be challenging. Right ventricular wall motion and morphology assessment using echocardiography remains part of the diagnostic criteria for ARVC. Still, evaluation can be difficult due to the intricate structure of the right ventricles. Therefore, clinicians should consider an integrated strategy with clinical history, family history, and imaging findings, stressing the importance of a multidisciplinary approach in accurate diagnosis and effective management of ARVC and other cardiomyopathies (Figure 11.9).

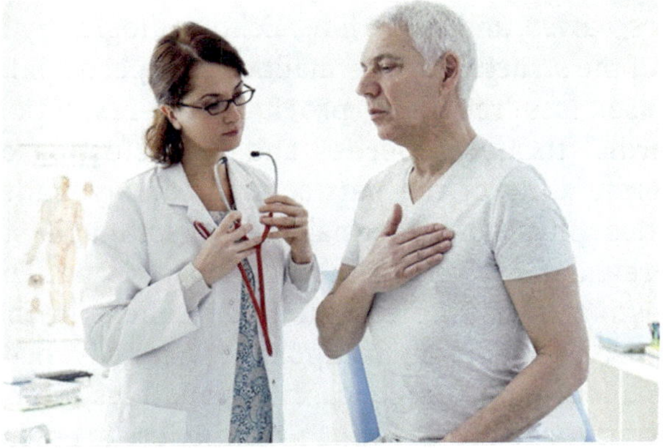

Figure 11.9. Diagnosis of cardiomyopathies.

Source: https://d2jx2rerrg6sh3.cloudfront.net/image-handler/picture/2017/8/shutterstock_174171521.jpg.

11.3.1. Common Symptoms Experienced by Patients

The presentation of cardiomyopathies is diverse, with patients having a broad spectrum of symptoms that have a significant impact on their quality of life. The most frequent symptom that many patients share is dyspnea, or breathlessness, which can occur with effort but also, occasionally, at rest. The symptom can be extreme in the case of DCM, where effective pumping of the heart is compromised. Patients may also exhibit fatigue and orthopnea, the latter being shortness of breath on lying down, indicative of fluid accumulation in the lungs. The symptoms are not only disabling but also create psychological distress and tension as patients cope with the limitations of their condition. The clinicians should identify these symptoms early to implement effective therapy interventions because the earlier intervention happens, the better the outcome, and this improves not just the survival but also the quality of life for the patients suffering from cardiomyopathy (Ljungman et al., 2023). Palpitations are also a notable symptom that patients of cardiomyopathy may have, and they manifest as abnormal beats or the feeling that the heart is pounding or racing. This symptom can be a reason for considerable distress among the patients, leading them to be more conscious of cardiac issues. These arrhythmias are often associated with certain types of cardiomyopathies like ARVC and HCM. Syncope or loss of consciousness is also experienced by some patients in these cases, which is caused by inadequate blood supply due to an abnormal heart rhythm. These symptoms must be tracked and controlled, as they can place patients at risk for more severe complications, including sudden cardiac death. As research continues to investigate the relationship between specific cardiomyopathies and their symptom presentations, clinicians can more fully individualize interventions to treat the physiology and psychology of managing patients

(Ljungman et al., 2023). In addition to dyspnea and palpitations, fatigue is a prominent symptom that is found in all types of cardiomyopathy in patients. Fatigue presents as an unusual tiredness, not just due to physical exertion but because the inability of the heart to supply adequate blood and oxygen makes it fail to meet the body's metabolic demands. Fatigue has the consequence of making a dramatic reduction in functional capacity, which has effects on activities of daily living. Fatigue becomes persistent despite proper rest, contributing to the psychological burden on patients who are made to feel helpless through their condition. Furthermore, gastrointestinal issues such as nausea or loss of appetite have also been encountered by some patients. They can indirectly be linked to heart failure and its overall impact on the body. Such multidimensional symptoms can help medical practitioners to develop combined patient management plans that not only address the physiological complications of cardiomyopathies but also promote the overall well-being of patients (Figure 11.10).

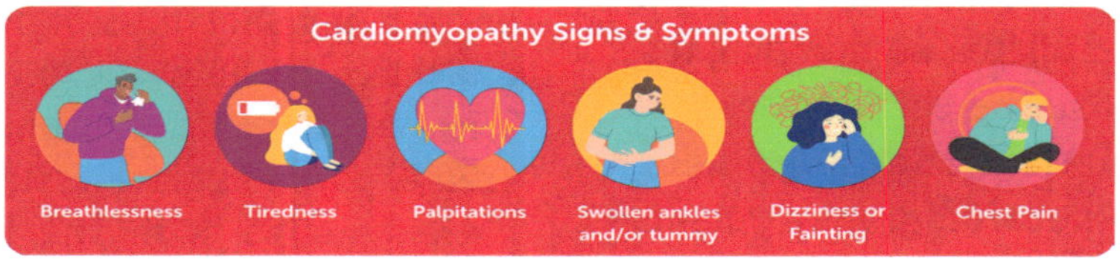

Figure 11.10. Cardiomyopathy signs and symptoms.

Source: https://www.cardiomyopathy.org/sites/default/files/images/2022-09/xChest,P20Pain.png.pagespeed.ic.zpIkQ-E8kk.webp.

11.3.2. Diagnostic Tests and Procedures

The diagnosis of cardiomyopathies relies to a great extent on a spectrum of diagnostic tests and investigations to accurately determine the structure and function of the heart. The commonly employed procedures are echocardiography, MRI, and ECG. Echocardiography is an initial modality that provides immediate images of the heart's chambers, valves, and blood flow. Echocardiography is an essential non-invasive investigation in the diagnosis of the structural abnormalities of hypertrophic, dilated, and restrictive cardiomyopathies. MRI, while used less frequently, provides high-resolution images that may offer information regarding myocardial tissue properties and the detection of inflammation or fibrosis, and hence aid in the understanding of the particular cardiomyopathy subtype. Through the use of these diagnostic modalities, physicians can make a correct diagnosis to inform treatment interventions and management regimens to obtain the best possible patient outcomes. Apart from imaging modalities, genetic testing is also an essential component in the diagnosis of specific cardiomyopathies, particularly those with a family component. With advances in molecular genetics, the detection of gene mutations underlying familial cardiomyopathies can be very clinically relevant. Genetic testing allows for risk stratification by enabling practitioners to assess familial inheritance and implement targeted surveillance in high-risk relatives. Nevertheless, the implication of genetic test findings can be complex, necessitating an interdisciplinary team of genetic counselors, cardiologists, and other specialists. Integration of genetic testing into the diagnostic process attempts to mark a paradigm shift towards an understanding of cardiomyopathies in a more personalized modality of treatment that honors individuals' genetic makeup and susceptibility. The clinical course of patients with cardiomyopathy is also highly diverse based on the subtype and associated comorbidities. Current studies emphasize the need for close monitoring and ongoing follow-up, since patients are likely to continue having a high risk of severe cardiovascular events despite symptomatic improvement with initial management. From (Arbustini et al., 2021), it has been observed that different cardiomyopathy subtypes present with varying patterns of complications, necessitating targeted patient management approaches. For instance, dilated cardiomyopathy patients may require a different medication regimen compared to restrictive cardiomyopathy patients. Thus, executing comprehensive diagnostic testing, together with continued monitoring, allows clinicians to adjust treatment regimens accordingly, delivering evidence-based care that is aligned with the individualized needs of each subject, ultimately improving overall health outcomes in the population with cardiomyopathy (Figure 11.11).

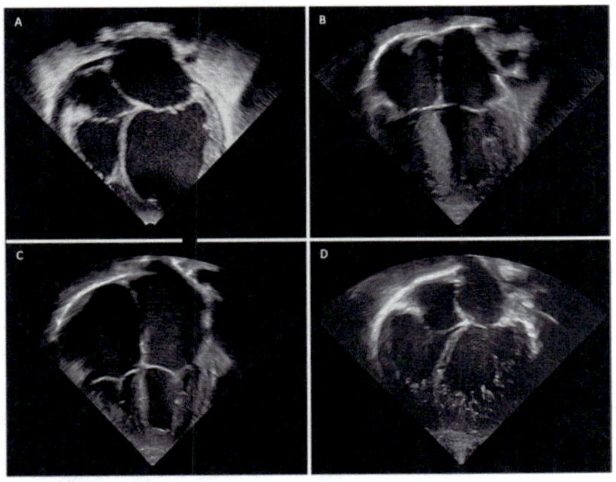

Figure 11.11. Echocardiographic images of cardiomyopathy phenotypes.

Source: https://www.frontiersin.org/files/Articles/708732/fped-09-708732-HTML/image_m/fped-09-708732-g001.jpg.

11.3.3. Importance of Early Detection

Early diagnosis of cardiomyopathies is essential for effective management and improved patient outcomes. Cardiomyopathies usually present with late or insidious symptoms, and therefore, treatment and diagnosis are often delayed. Since the clinical course of such diseases can lead to substantial morbidity, like heart failure and sudden cardiac death, early diagnosis is a must. An example of a 2-year-old child highlights the need for close follow-up in children. During routine surgery, intraoperative electrocardiographic abnormality suggested underlying cardiac disease, ultimately revealing hypertrophic cardiomyopathy in the postoperative phase. This highlights the significance of rigorous monitoring and early intervention strategies that can avert danger and enhance the prognosis of such affected patients. Therefore, awareness and education regarding signs and symptoms of cardiomyopathies are of utmost priority in facilitating early diagnosis among different patient groups, including children and adults. Moreover, technical improvements in diagnostic techniques, such as enhanced imaging modalities and biomarker examination, play a central role in the early diagnosis of cardiomyopathies. For example, routine echocardiography and screening for specific biomarkers, such as elevated troponin-T and brain natriuretic peptide, aid in the diagnosis of conditions such as myocarditis, particularly among infectious conditions such as COVID-19. Research has indicated that patients with secondary myocarditis occurring due to COVID-19 are at a much higher risk of requiring ventilatory support and increased rates of mortality. Identification of such cardiac complications is a direct indicator of the ability to provide early and targeted treatment interventions. Because early diagnosis has the ability to alter the trajectory of disease development radically, integration of these new diagnostic technologies into routine clinical practice is required to optimize the care of patients with cardiomyopathies. In conjunction with advancements in technology, clinicians must also utilize a proactive approach in surveillance of those with high risk populations, i.e., underlying cardiac disease or cardiomyopathy family history. Regular screening and follow-up testing can facilitate the detection of asymptomatic cases, and this, in turn, may prompt timely and proper treatment interventions. The recognition that underlying heart conditions exacerbate the effect of developing new complications, for instance, among COVID-19 patients, stresses the importance of early monitoring and personalized care interventions. Studies have found that patients with non-ischemic cardiomyopathy do much worse, highlighting the need for targeted action in the diagnosis and treatment of cardiomyopathies. Early diagnosis has the added benefit, beyond individual patient outcomes, of contributing to general understanding of the epidemiology and impact of these diseases on the health system as a whole and of guiding public health policy improvement.

11.4. Treatment Options

Management for cardiomyopathies varies widely, based on the patient and the type of cardiomyopathy. HCM points towards individualized patient care, where therapy is based on the degree of symptoms and sudden cardiac death risk factors. Non-dihydropyridine calcium channel blockers and beta-blockers are usually prescribed to diminish chest pain and dyspnea on exertion symptoms. In addition, newer drugs like disopyramide and myosin inhibitors of the heart are increasingly being employed to support better outcomes overall. The treatments are set to reduce left ventricular outflow obstruction and enhance cardiac function, reflecting the importance of personalized care highlighted in recent reviews (Cirillo et al., 2024). Interventional therapies also have a critical role in managing cardiomyopathies and often serve as an adjunct to medical therapy. For instance, septal reduction surgical treatments can be applied to patients with extreme obstructive HCM, significantly relieving symptoms and improving quality of life. Nonoperative methods, like alcohol septal ablation, offer an alternative intervention, particularly for patients who cannot withstand major surgery. In other cases, ICDs are reserved for patients who are at significant risk of malignant arrhythmias, underscoring the value of risk stratification in management. This spectrum of options underscores the necessity of determining each patient's clinical presentation and preferences to optimize management strategies for cardiomyopathies (Cirillo et al., 2024). The future of cardiomyopathy therapy looks bright, with ongoing advances in the investigation of new therapeutic paradigms. New gene therapy and emerging drug candidate products are leading clinical trials, which predict a shift toward more complex and targeted therapies. These emerging therapies are being studied for their risks and benefits with a focus on genetic etiologies of cardiomyopathies that promise to unveil the possibility of personalized treatment in the disease. Furthermore, collaboration between scientists and clinicians is essential to bring such information to the clinic. As the care environment of cardiomyopathy evolves further, patient-centeredness will remain a vital element in ensuring best outcomes for patients with this challenging complex of conditions (Cirillo et al., 2024) (Figure 11.12).

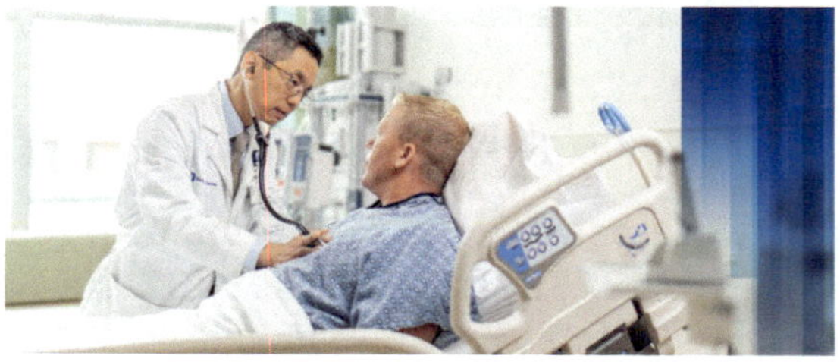

Figure 11.12. Cardiomyopathy treatment.

Source: https://www.dukehealth.org/sites/default/files/styles/hero_image_lg/public/treatment_detail/treatment_cardiomyopathy_1500x430.jpg?itok=UuggKTOb.

11.4.1. Medications and Their Roles

The role of drugs in the management of cardiomyopathies is significant in the improvement of patient outcomes and quality of life. Therapeutic interventions have been constructed, particularly in the symptomatic management of specific forms of cardiomyopathy, such as DCM. DCM, either as a result of genetic mutations or acquired origin, is characterized by decreased myocardial contractility and subsequent dilatation of the heart. Such drugs as ACE inhibitors, beta-blockers, and diuretics are prescribed on a regular basis to relieve heart failure symptoms and enhance cardiac function. By lowering preload and afterload, these drugs can ease a failing heart considerably, demonstrating the importance of drug treatment in managing the complexities of this disease. Furthermore, existing research attempts to identify genotype-specific therapies that may enable more personalized medication regimens, leading to improved patient prognosis and outcomes (Arnăutu et al., 2024). Apart from conventional pharmacological treatment, emerging advances indicate novel therapeutic strategies. The use of heart failure medications in association with genetic insight into the root cause of cardiomyopathies has transformed therapeutic strategy. For instance, the development of specific antisense oligonucleotides and gene therapies targeting the molecular causes of cardiomyopathy holds promise for future treatment protocols. These innovative treatments reflect the evolving nature of cardiomyopathy therapy, in which specific drugs have the potential to revolutionize patient outcomes. As research on the relationship between genetic predispositions and cardiomyopathy development continues, it is more evident that individualized approaches to medication control using genetic testing would have the potential to revolutionize treatment protocols in the forthcoming years (Arnăutu et al., 2024). Moreover, inclusion of non-pharmacological interventions as an adjunct to drugs forms an integral part of the holistic management of cardiomyopathies. Although drug treatment alleviates symptoms and slows disease progression, lifestyle modification and health education are essential for comprehensive patient care. Patients are encouraged to adopt heart-healthy habits, such as diet modification, exercise regimen, and smoking cessation, which work synergistically to increase the effectiveness of drugs administered. Moreover, awareness of treatment options, including the non-pharmacologic type, allows patients to join a partnership in their own care. The mutual relationship between medication adherence and life modification highlights the importance of proper educational material through which individuals can make informed decisions based on facts that can enhance therapeutic outcomes and overcome the incapacitating effects of cardiomyopathies (Figure 11.13).

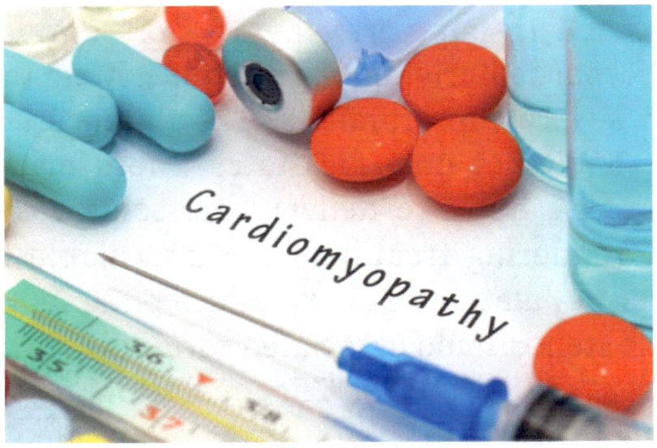

Figure 11.13. Role of drugs in the management of cardiomyopathies.

Source: https://belvoir-university-health.s3.amazonaws.com/media/2017/05/07225004/cardiomyopathy-graphic.jpg.

11.4.2. Surgical Interventions

Surgical interventions in the management of cardiomyopathies play a critical role in managing severe cardiac disorders that do not respond to medical intervention. Ventricular restoration, septal myectomy, and heart transplant are among the operations performed to alleviate symptoms and improve the quality of life of patients with various forms of cardiomyopathy. For instance, in hypertrophic cardiomyopathy, operative procedures such as septal myectomy can notably reduce obstruction to heart outflow. The surgery is critical in patients with marked symptoms because it can lead to a dramatic improvement in exercise tolerance and a lowering of the life-threatening risk of the disease. However, the decision to proceed to surgery is based on detailed evaluations with consideration of the patient's overall status, functional status, and likelihood of success with surgery. Additionally, expanding surgical therapy, transcatheter methods like TAVR are increasingly utilized in the treatment of patients with severe aortic stenosis, a disease oftentimes coupled with a broad range of cardiomyopathies and hence hastens symptomatology. According to the FinnValve registry analysis, TAVR has increased in popularity as a viable option to SAVR, particularly among the elderly or those with severe comorbidities. The findings show that TAVR not only facilitates a less invasive procedure but also delivers the same results, thus rendering treatment more available to a larger population of heart failure patients with aortic stenosis and associated cardiomyopathies (Jalava et al., 2021). The evolution of such surgical procedures is a growing recognition of their therapeutic potential to improve survival and functional capacity among high-risk populations. In addition, the integration of surgical principles with the advancements in personalized medicine could portend enhanced patient outcomes when addressing cardiomyopathy. With continuous development in imaging modalities, there is improved ability to tailor surgical strategy to the individual's own cardiac anatomy and disease pathology. To date, optimal knowledge of the pathophysiology of the underlying disease has been shown to lead to better surgery strategies and, by extension, different treatment paradigms. Such synergistic technologies result in extraordinary improvements in both preventing arrhythmias and improving the overall success of surgery, as demonstrated by the example of catheter ablation treatments for the management of atrial fibrillation (Calkins et al., 2017). As more is developed, the role of surgical procedures in the treatment of cardiomyopathies will also grow, and thus the importance of further studies to refine these treatments for patient-directed therapy cannot be overlooked.

11.4.3. Lifestyle Modifications and Management

Diet is an essential aspect of the care of cardiomyopathies, as it can significantly affect the disease's progression and the progression of complications. Among the most important recommendations for the patients is the use of a heart-healthy diet. Emphasizing the intake of fruits, vegetables, whole grains, and lean proteins, while reducing saturated fat, sodium, and sugar intake, not only aids in weight control but also in cholesterol and blood pressure management. Moderate alcohol use or abstinence is also typically advised because alcohol can exacerbate certain types of cardiomyopathies. These dietary changes, along with physical exercise, contribute to improved cardiovascular function and overall quality of life for individuals with this condition. Physical exercise, other than diet, forms the core component of the formula for lifestyle modification in the management of cardiomyopathy. Regular aerobic exercise is beneficial, as it conditions the heart muscle and increases blood flow. However, exercise regimens must be modified for every patient's capacity and the type of cardiomyopathy. Low-to-moderate intensity exercise, such as walking, swimming, or cycling, is typically advised in patients, with the avoidance of high-risk activities that involve a greater risk of injury or cardiovascular emergency. A supervised program would be required in most cases, particularly when the symptoms are more pronounced. Such scrupulous control of physical activity can enhance physical fitness and mental wellbeing equally, favoring an even lifestyle plan significant for long-term health. Another important consideration in changing lifestyle is control of psychosocial determinants, which have immediate impacts on cardiovascular well-being. Stress reduction practices such as mindfulness, yoga, and cognitive behavior therapy can reduce anxiety levels and enhance emotional resilience. This is particularly pertinent to individuals faced with the challenges presented by cardiomyopathies, as emotional health is immediately connected to physical consequences. Besides, genetic counseling would be helpful for families with disorders such as Carvajal syndrome since it supports the understanding of the inherited nature of specific cardiomyopathies and recommends lifestyle for family members carrying risk factors, as shown by findings of desmoplakin mutations and their impacts on family well-being. Coupling of complete lifestyle transformation with medical advice makes a strong foundation for the management of cardiomyopathies (Figure 11.14).

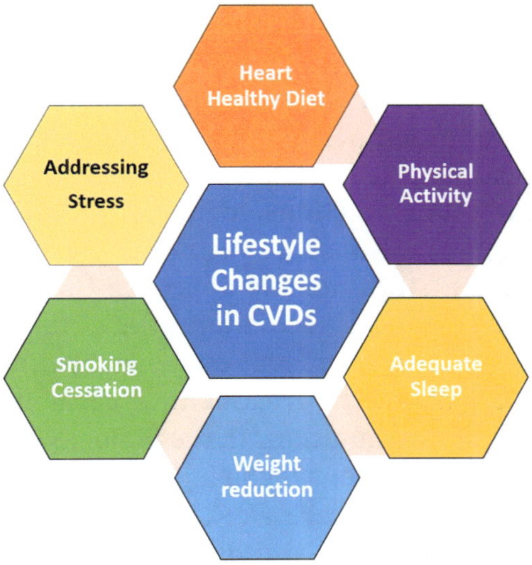

Figure 11.14. Lifestyle changes in cardiovascular disease.

Source: https://assets.cureus.com/uploads/figure/file/688742/lightbox_49d74ce022d111ee9a792dbb7719cd14-Lifestyle.png

SUMMARY

In summarizing cardiomyopathy research, it should be noted that the multiformity of cardiomyopathies needs to be appreciated. Every one of the subforms of cardiomyopathy, e.g., hypertrophic, dilated, restrictive, and arrhythmogenic right ventricular cardiomyopathy, is associated with specific characteristics and determinants of prognosis. Learning from the first European Cardiomyopathy Registry has significant findings, e.g., standard frequency of familial cardiomyopathy, to document the hereditary determinants that affect disease manifestation. Along with that, the differential patient outcomes for subtypes, in which patients with restrictive cardiomyopathy experience a significantly higher incidence of heart failure events, are indicative of subtype-stratified treatment approaches. The impact of such subtleties is revealed in clinical practice and even in future research, ultimately maximizing patient outcomes and treatment in this heterogeneous group of patients (Kaski et al., 2024). Apart from this, the impact that cardiovascular health exerts on other public health conditions cannot be overestimated, especially for interactivity-dependent diseases like COVID-19. Statistics show an alarming intersection between cardiomyopathy and hematological diseases in which patients with prior cardiac disease are most vulnerable in instances of viral pandemics. This point highlights the importance of holistic patient management, not only addressing the cardiomyopathy condition per se but also addressing overall health weaknesses in such patients. The research-based identified risk factors, such as incomplete immunization and past interventions that compromise immune reactions, highlight the importance of vigilant monitoring and preventive measures in the management of such patients (Piñana et al., 2024). Therefore, are treated by physicians who maintain a holistic approach in mind, considering overall health. Ultimately, understanding cardiomyopathies necessitates the development of novel treatments and diagnostic tools. In the future, research should focus on genetic testing and personalized treatment, which have the potential to contribute to the treatment of cardiomyopathy patients significantly. The high incidence of underlying genetic mutations in the majority of cardiomyopathies justifies the need for an expansion of routine management involving genetic testing and counseling. Moreover, multidisciplinary cooperation among healthcare workers, researchers, and institutions will play a pivotal role in the establishment of registries and data-sharing platforms that will further clarify the etiology and course of the diseases. The construction of a robust framework of clinical practice and research would not only increase the understanding of cardiomyopathies but also chart the path to enhancing outcomes and quality of life in patients afflicted with such life-altering illnesses (Kaski et al., 2024).

Cardiomyopathies represent a pleomorphic group of heart muscle diseases with structural and functional abnormalities of the heart capable of affecting the heart's ability to pump blood effectively. The classification of cardiomyopathies as several subtypes, such as hypertrophic, dilated, arrhythmogenic, and restrictive types, emphasizes the heterogeneity of these conditions. Each of the subtypes possesses distinctive pathophysiological features and differentiated clinical presentations. For instance, dilated cardiomyopathy is likely to be associated with heart failure and low ejection fraction, but hypertrophic cardiomyopathy may result in obstructive symptoms through thickening of the cardiac muscle. Aggregate clinical data indicate the usefulness of proper diagnosis because inappropriate treatment regimens and complications in patients can be established by misclassifying the conditions. In elderly people, cardiac disease shares common ground with cardiomyopathies, which also require aggressive screening and treatment in concert. For instance, research conducted in Muhimbili National Hospital raised issues that highlight hypertension as a prevalent comorbidity in elderly cardiac disease patients, in over 67% of the study population. Moreover, studies found that there was a high prevalence of patients with diastolic dysfunction and left ventricular hypertrophy, showing extreme remodeling patterns of the myocardium in chronic disease. All this must be identified as early as possible since cardiomyopathies are most likely to lead to severe complications like heart failure. Therefore, there must be systematic screening for cardiovascular diseases in geriatric patients even when they have other primary conditions. The histopathological changes of cardiomyopathies, i.e., the contribution of myocardial fibrosis, must be investigated further since they are the principal causes of harmful cardiac remodeling. Myocardial fibrosis, consisting of the accumulation of excess extracellular matrix protein, is an important event in heart failure pathogenesis. It is an initial reparative process that eventually leads to pathological fibrosis, arrhythmias, and diastolic dysfunction and therefore profoundly compromises cardiac function. Experiments indicate that although there is clearly mild fibrosis, it is invariably accompanied by adverse clinical outcomes. Advanced non-invasive imaging technologies are increasingly being used to image myocardial fibrosis to facilitate improved diagnosis and treatment of the disease. It is essential to know the epidemiology of myocardial fibrosis and its significance in all types of cardiomyopathies in the development of patient care and optimization of treatment strategies (Kisenge et al., 2011; de Boer et al., 2020).

A CLOSER LOOK

INDUCED PLURIPOTENT STEM (IPS) CELL DEVELOPMENT FROM DCM HEART

iPS cell derivation is one of the most promising regenerative medicine technologies. iPS cell is initiated by the epigenetic suppression of somatic cells by the Yamanaka factors, that is, the four transcription factors Oct4, Sox2, Klf4, and c-Myc. Advances in iPS cell reprogramming technology will enable the replacement of old or damaged cells with the patient's own rejuvenated cells; consequently, the clinical application of this technology holds promise for curing age-related degenerative diseases. Senescent or pathologic tissue, but not juvenile or healthy tissue, has relatively low reprogramming efficiency and thus will result in incomplete cell reprogramming. Our lab developed a novel reprogramming method for deriving iPS cells from somatic cells of the pathologic recipient heart, which is associated with severe heart failure in DCM.

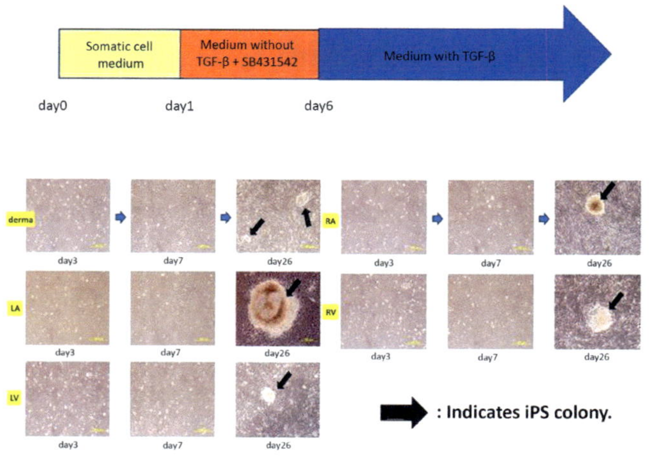

Figure 11.15. Gene transfection.

Source: https://cdnintech.com/media/chapter/76628/1512345123/media/F5.png.

For the gene transfection of iPS cell differentiation, in addition to the Yamanaka factors, GLIS1 and TET-1 were added. Transcription factors similar to Gli (Glis) belong to the Krüppel-like zinc-finger transcription factors, and three GLIS genes have been identified: GLIS1–3. Yoshioka et al. have shown that Yamanaka factor RNAs with Glis-1 RNA purified from an RNA-replicative vector provided high-efficiency reprogramming of aged adult human cells into iPS cells. Tet-1, a DNA demethylase, is involved in the differentiation of the inner cell mass at the stage of blastocyst and regulates the maintenance of ES cells through modification of the DNA methylation pattern. Olariu et al. discovered that TET1 can replace OCT4 in the reprogramming Yamanaka cocktail of iPS cells and that the control of the pluripotency genes is determined by DNA methylation. As Tet-1 has also been found to stimulate the expression of Dnmt3b in the transition phase to the epiblast stage, TET-1 was included in the last list of six genes that were utilized for transfection in our protocol.

Cardiac fibroblasts isolated from a donor heart expressed strongly α-smooth muscle actin (α-SMA), which is a usual marker of myofibroblasts. Myofibroblasts are located in a converging region of mesenchymal cells, which are induced by acute or chronic inflammation due to stimulation with TGF-β, Ang II, and cytokines. Notably, the myofibroblasts of our patient's heart tissue did not differentiate into human iPS cells by previous methods. Thus, the cell culture medium used for iPS cell induction was also produced in detail. TGF-β was eliminated from the cell culture medium for iPS cell induction, and selective TGF-β inhibitor SB431542 was introduced during the initial five days after transfection. Ultimately, through a combination of these techniques, we produced a very efficient system to induce human iPS cells from pathologic somatic cells (Figure 11.15).

References

1. Fortuni, F., Ciliberti, G., De Chiara, B., Conte, E., Franchin, L., Musella, F., Vitale, E., Piroli, F., Cangemi, S., Cornara, S., Magnesa, M., Spinelli, A., Geraci, G., Nardi, F., Gabrielli, D., Colivicchi, F., Grimaldi, M., & Oliva, F. (2024). Advancements and Applications of Artificial Intelligence in Cardiovascular Imaging: a Comprehensive Review. *European Heart Journal - Imaging Methods and Practice*, *2*(4). https://doi.org/10.1093/ehjimp/qyae136Aimo, A., Barison, A., Emdin, M., Keren, et al. (2022). *Restrictive Cardiomyopathy: Definition and Diagnosis.* https://core.ac.uk/download/566468098.pdf (accessed on 29th May 2025).

2. Alhadlaq, A., Alamri, O., Lazher, J., & Obeid, F. M. (2023). Does the Saudi population have awareness and perception regarding new treatment options other than medications for migraine? *Majmaah Journal of Health Sciences*. https://www.semanticscholar.org/paper/71cb89239546cadc926072a3cf2f51903e37a08d (accessed on 29th May 2025).

3. Allwood, R. (2024). A right ventricular bulge: A clinical dilemma in diagnosis. *Journal of Clinical Ultrasound: JCU*. https://www.semanticscholar.org/paper/065643a91b4cb5ab2f8915ab160d4fc020336840 (accessed on 29th May 2025).

4. Altay, H., & Pehlivanoglu, S. (2017). *Heart Failure with Preserved Ejection Fraction.* https://core.ac.uk/download/322429354.pdf (accessed on 29th May 2025).

5. Amr, A., Arbustini, E., Barb, I., Bellazzi, et al. (2014). *Atlas of the Clinical Genetics of Human Dilated Cardiomyopathy*. https://core.ac.uk/download/146821867.pdf (accessed on 29th May 2025).

6. Arbustini, E., Barriales-Villa, R., Biagini, E., Caforio, et al. (2021). Prospective follow-up in various subtypes of cardiomyopathies: Insights from the ESC EORP cardiomyopathy registry. *European Heart Journal – Quality of Care and Clinical Outcomes.* https://core.ac.uk/download/336585706.pdf (accessed on 29th May 2025).

7. Arenja, N., Hellige, J. G., Ricciardi, S. I., Schild, et al. (2019). *Current Pathophysiological and Genetic Aspects of Dilated Cardiomyopathy.* https://core.ac.uk/download/322440922.pdf (accessed on 29th May 2025).

8. Arnăutu, D., Cozma, D., Lala, I. R., Arnăutu, S., Tomescu, M., & Andor, M. (2024). Risk assessment and personalized treatment options in inherited dilated cardiomyopathies: A narrative review. *Biomedicines*, *12*. https://www.semanticscholar.org/paper/f7b347b629ff6ceeff34e2d48959224307725f33 (accessed on 29th May 2025).

9. Asselbergs, F. W., Boonstra, M. J., Bosman, L. P., Bourfiss, et al. (2021). Risk stratification and subclinical phenotyping of dilated and/or arrhythmogenic cardiomyopathy mutation-positive relatives: CVON eDETECT consortium. *Neth. Heart J.* https://core.ac.uk/download/519039731.pdf (accessed on 29th May 2025).

10. Babu, R., & Bembey, R. A. (2024). *Cardiomyopathy in a Nutshell: From Etiopathogenesis and Diagnosis to Treatment.* https://core.ac.uk/download/613230070.pdf (accessed on 29th May 2025).

11. Bai, X., Chen, M., Tang, Y., Liu, R., & Zhang, L. (2024). [Epidemiologic investigation of cardiac arrest and current research status on its risk factors analysis]. *Zhonghua Wei Zhong Bing Ji Jiu Yi Xue*, *36*(4), 445–448. https://www.semanticscholar.org/paper/dab6122b3338f773d98963e38af87d9933cd8191 (accessed on 29th May 2025).

12. Baldini, K., De Gregorio, M. G., Girolami, F., Olivotto, et al. (2020). *Comprehensive Risk Management in Arrhythmogenic Cardiomyopathy Associated with Autosomal Dominant Carvajal Syndrome.* https://core.ac.uk/download/351116833.pdf (accessed on 29th May 2025).

13. Biggins, S. W., Angeli, P., García-Tsao, G., Ginés, P., Ling, S. C., Nadim, M. K., Wong, F., et al. (2021). Diagnosis, evaluation, and management of ascites, spontaneous bacterial peritonitis and hepatorenal syndrome: 2021 practice guidance by the American Association for the Study of Liver Diseases. *Hepatology, 74*, 1014–1048. https://doi.org/10.1002/hep.31884 (accessed on 29th May 2025).

14. Burban, A., Pucyło, S., Sikora, A., Opolski, G., Grabowski, M., & Kołodzińska, A. (2023). Hypertrophic cardiomyopathy versus storage diseases with myocardial involvement. *International Journal of Molecular Sciences, 24*. https://www.semanticscholar.org/paper/2b2e053e87c06f0ab488f01effb92151b1bf6e5e (accessed on 29th May 2025).

15. Calkins, H., Cleland, J. G. F., Heist, E. K., Kowey, et al. (2017). *The Burden of Proof: The Current State of Atrial Fibrillation Prevention and Treatment Trials.* https://core.ac.uk/download/80696856.pdf (accessed on 29th May 2025).

16. Carro, T. (2012). *The Effects of Polychlorinated Biphenyls (PCBs) on Avian Cardiac Development.* https://core.ac.uk/download/56109538.pdf (accessed on 29th May 2025).

17. Chalapa, V., Sabitov, A. U., Sergeev, A. G., Itani, T., Kungurtseva, M. S., Sharova, A. A., Slautin, V., et al. (2024). Out-of-hospital infant mortality associated with herpesviruses. *Ural Medical Journal.* https://www.semanticscholar.org/paper/f1be9c9c3a4c6e2a264ceda89c14a8f6ff7c0fcf (accessed on 29th May 2025).

18. Ciarambino, T., Giordano, M., Menna, G., & Sansone, G. (2021). *Cardiomyopathies: An Overview.* https://core.ac.uk/download/534981528.pdf (accessed on 29th May 2025).

19. Cirillo, C., Perillo, A., Monda, E., Palmiero, G., Verrillo, F., Rubino, M., Diana, G., et al. (2024). Treatment options for hypertrophic obstructive cardiomyopathy: A patient-centric review. *Expert Review of Cardiovascular Therapy.* https://www.semanticscholar.org/paper/82413dce4de1bb958b4638fd7c82aa286243173f (accessed on 29th May 2025).

20. Cusano, A., Inclan, P. M., Jackson, T., Weiss, L. J., Barnes, R., Kinderknecht, J. J., Taylor, S. A., et al. (2024). Team approach: Diagnosis, management, and prevention of sudden cardiac arrest in the athlete. *JBJS Reviews, 12*. https://www.semanticscholar.org/paper/592e8730eb24678fda45fa5aa522bc217ed73a0f (accessed on 29th May 2025).

21. De Boer, R. A., Eijgenraam, T. R., & Silljé, H. H. W. (2020). *Current Understanding of Fibrosis in Genetic Cardiomyopathies.* https://core.ac.uk/download/519029512.pdf (accessed on 29th May 2025).

22. Duffy, G., Cheng, P., Yuan, N., He, B., Kwan, A. C., Shun-Shin, M., Alexander, K., et al. (2022). High-throughput precision phenotyping of left ventricular hypertrophy with cardiovascular deep learning. *JAMA Cardiology, 7*, 386. https://doi.org/10.1001/jamacardio.2021.6059 (accessed on 29th May 2025).

23. El Hadi, H., Freund, A., Desch, S., Thiele, H., & Majunke, N. (2023). Hypertrophic, dilated, and arrhythmogenic cardiomyopathy: Where are we? *Biomedicines, 11*. https://www.semanticscholar.org/paper/3d5ef713822258fa18af08ee1d51393f881bb1b7 (accessed on 29th May 2025).

24. Freeman, L. M., Huggins, G. S., Maron, M. S., Rush, et al. (2017). *Feline Hypertrophic Cardiomyopathy: A Spontaneous Large Animal Model of Human HCM.* https://core.ac.uk/download/323068173.pdf (accessed on 29th May 2025).

25. Gadelsayed, J., Wani, T., Rehman, S., & Tobias, J. D. (2024). Intraoperative ST segment depression during general anesthesia in a child: Early detection of hypertrophic cardiomyopathy. *Cardiology Research, 15*, 467–471. https://www.semanticscholar.org/paper/0831501d141a942a700492 83d0fd50f389f2c825 (accessed on 29th May 2025).

26. Ghazal, R., Wang, M., Liu, D., Tschumperlin, D. J., & Pereira, N. L. (2025). Cardiac fibrosis in the multi-omics era: Implications for heart failure. *Circulation Research, 136*, 773–802. https://www.semanticscholar.org/paper/9d2ff6d46b17fab5eaa9ee11d27d8765f418bda7 (accessed on 29th May 2025).

27. Haryanto, J. (2024). Short-term versus long-term portfolio management strategies and the selection of securities. *Advances in Management & Financial Reporting*. https://www.semanticscholar.org/paper/d42aef922574daaf06dda243312abc611945ada7 (accessed on 29th May 2025).

28. Heather, L. C., Gopal, K., Srnic, N., & Ussher, J. R. (2024). Redefining diabetic cardiomyopathy: Perturbations in substrate metabolism at the heart of its pathology. *Diabetes, 73*, 659–670. https://doi.org/10.2337/dbi23-0019 (accessed on 29th May 2025).

29. Jalava, M. P. (2021). *Aortic Stenosis and Heart Failure – Invasive Treatment and Prognosis*. https://core.ac.uk/download/481513310.pdf (accessed on 29th May 2025).

30. Kamath, S., Gomah, M. H. T., Stepman, G., DiMartino, P., & Adetula, I. (2023). COVID-19-associated acute myocarditis: Risk factors, clinical outcomes, and implications for early detection and management. *Cureus, 15*. https://www.semanticscholar.org/paper/beee5533e5a93f2b987ca3b5f1169ac458830517 (accessed on 29th May 2025).

31. Kaski, J., Norrish, G., Gimeno, B. J. R., Charron, P., Elliott, P., Tavazzi, L., Tendera, M., et al. (2024). Cardiomyopathies in children and adolescents: Aetiology, management, and outcomes in the European Society of Cardiology EURObservational Research Program Cardiomyopathy and Myocarditis Registry. *European Heart Journal, 45*, 1443–1454. https://www.semanticscholar.org/paper/2793c5d2a69cae22a54626be7c70d2ba689860a1 (accessed on 29th May 2025).

32. Kisenge, P. R. (2011). *Pattern of Cardiovascular Diseases Among Elderly Patients Admitted in Medical Wards at Muhimbili National Hospital Dar es Salaam Tanzania*. https://core.ac.uk/download/pdf/16666639.pdf (accessed on 29th May 2025).

33. Kitsiou, A., Caforio, A. L. P., Porta-Sanchez, A., Vahanian, A., Iung, B., Carrera, C., Szymanski, C., et al. (2013). *ESC Core Curriculum for the General Cardiologist (2013).* https://core.ac.uk/download/55756305.pdf (accessed on 29th May 2025).

34. Li, X., Li, C., Zhang, W., Wang, Y., Qian, P., & Huang, H. (2023). Inflammation and aging: Signaling pathways and intervention therapies. *Signal Transduction and Targeted Therapy, 8*. https://doi.org/10.1038/s41392-023-01502-8 (accessed on 29th May 2025).

35. Lindgren, M. (2020). *Familial Risks of Heart Failure in Sweden*. https://core.ac.uk/download/322707665.pdf (accessed on 29th May 2025).

36. Ljungman, C., Bollano, E., Rawshani, A., Nordberg, B. C., Dahlberg, P., Valeljung, I., Björkenstam, M., et al. (2023). Differences in phenotypes, symptoms, and survival in patients with

cardiomyopathy—A prospective observational study from the Sahlgrenska CardioMyoPathy center. *Frontiers in Cardiovascular Medicine, 10.* https://www.semanticscholar.org/paper/31eb5b66c3945c9751880b2462bc3d32e944e914 (accessed on 29th May 2025).

37. Lombardo, B., Mirra, B., Mazzaccara, C., Barretta, F., Frisso, G., & Scudiero, O. (2020). *Sudden Cardiac Death in Young Athletes: Literature Review of Molecular Basis.* https://core.ac.uk/download/323188263.pdf (accessed on 29th May 2025).

38. Naghavi, M., Ong, K. L., Aali, A., Ababneh, H., Abate, Y. H., Abbafati, C., Abbasgholizadeh, R., et al. (2024). Global burden of 288 causes of death and life expectancy decomposition in 204 countries and territories and 811 subnational locations, 1990–2021: A systematic analysis for the Global Burden of Disease Study 2021. *The Lancet, 403*, 2100–2132. https://doi.org/10.1016/s0140-6736(24)00367-2 (accessed on 29th May 2025).

39. Namkoong, J., & Minhas, K. (2025). A review of the common causes of acute coronary syndrome (ACS) in females, and the role of estrogen on its pathologies and risk factors. *Canadian Journal of Physiology and Pharmacology*. https://www.semanticscholar.org/paper/e665e7c7b785cf594bfd097e564698ff149bb735 (accessed on 29th May 2025).

40. Navarro, J., Jeewa, A., Fang, J., Lee, D. S., & Jean-St-Michel, E. (2024). Abstract 4134957: Survival and cardiac recovery in pediatric dilated cardiomyopathy: A long-term cohort study of risk factors, prognosis, and health outcomes followed into adulthood. *Circulation*. https://www.semanticscholar.org/paper/15d0f3f27bbf8e758cd447cd2204af9d5996ca54 (accessed on 29th May 2025).

41. Piñana, J., Vázquez, L., Heras, I., Aiello, T., López-Corral, L., Arroyo, I., Soler-Espejo, E., et al. (2024). Omicron SARS-CoV-2 infection management and outcomes in patients with hematologic disease and recipients of cell therapy. *Frontiers in Oncology, 14.* https://www.semanticscholar.org/paper/a46f892e55303cf182f0fff6dee3b978ee29a827 (accessed on 29th May 2025).

42. Rohde, S., Weber, W., Berlis, A., Urbach, H., Reimer, P., Schramm, P., German Society of Interventional Radiology and Minimally Invasive Therapy, et al. (2021). Acute endovascular stroke treatment in Germany in 2019. *Clinical Neuroradiology*, *31*, 11–19. https://www.semanticscholar.org/paper/aaa2fd54d2c27dabf5abd6667ef299724d4867e8 (accessed on 29th May 2025).

43. Sammani, A., Baas, A. F., Asselbergs, F. W., & te Riele, A. S. J. M. (2021). Diagnosis and risk prediction of dilated cardiomyopathy in the era of big data and genomics. *Journal of Clinical Medicine, 10,* 921–921. https://doi.org/10.3390/jcm10050921 (accessed on 29th May 2025).

44. Shields, R., Paterson, D., & Tamma, P. (2023). Navigating available treatment options for Carbapenem-resistant *Acinetobacter baumannii-calcoaceticus* complex infections. *Clinical Infectious Diseases, 76,* S179–S193. https://www.semanticscholar.org/paper/5e2746bbeaa59ba503c9204adbcd33cf3b43095e (accessed on 29th May 2025).

45. Smyrnova, G., Storozhchuk, Y., Kundina, V., Sakhno, T. K., Polishchuk, O. V., & Kuzevanova, M. V. (2025). Modern possibilities of radiological diagnostics of cardiac sarcoidosis. *Український Радіологічний та Онкологічний Журнал*. https://www.semanticscholar.org/paper/7e9cbde59e0bab837a674e26cf1dc180269322ba (accessed on 29th May 2025).

46. Stinson, L., Carter, S., Waldron, J., Stehlik, J., Godara, A., Sideris, K., Brinker, L., et al. (2023). Abstract 12278: A case of hereditary transthyretin amyloidosis caused by a rare mutation. *Circulation.*

https://www.semanticscholar.org/paper/d01d581e2539de0c064d3cd91d4eb775c3834a14 (accessed on 29th May 2025).

47. Taleb, Y., Memon, P., Jalbani, A., Al-Anazi, N., Al-Garni, A., AlTaweel, M., Khan, M. A., et al. (2025). Genotype–phenotype correlations in inherited cardiomyopathies, their role in clinical decision-making, and implications in personalized cardiac medicine in multi-omics as well as disease modeling eras. *Saudi Journal for Health Sciences*. https://www.semanticscholar.org/paper/2b00fd6cece62b04328b18c7fa5df2ca49c324a3 (accessed on 29th May 2025).

48. Thomas, K. (2016). *Catheter Ablation for Atrial Fibrillation: Predicting Recurrence*. https://core.ac.uk/download/61688478.pdf (accessed on 29th May 2025).

49. Wesół-Kucharska, D., Greczan, M., Witulska, K., Piekutowska-Abramczuk, D., Ciara, E., Kowalski, P., & Rokicki, D. (2021). Improvement of cardiomyopathy after ketogenic diet in a patient with Leigh syndrome caused by MTND5 mutation. Nutrients. https://www.semanticscholar.org/paper/4183bf2feff50bfdbc26458c501fe010316e0cff (accessed on 29th May 2025).

50. Zhou, D., Zhu, L., Li, S., Wu, W., Zhuang, B., Xu, J., Yang, W., et al. (2025). Prognosis and risk stratification in dilated cardiomyopathy with LVEF ≤35%: Cardiac MRI insights for better outcomes. *Circulation: Cardiovascular Imaging, 18*, e017246. https://www.semanticscholar.org/paper/37baef3503dad6330bf775719da76559a4bb3c59 (accessed on 29th May 2025).

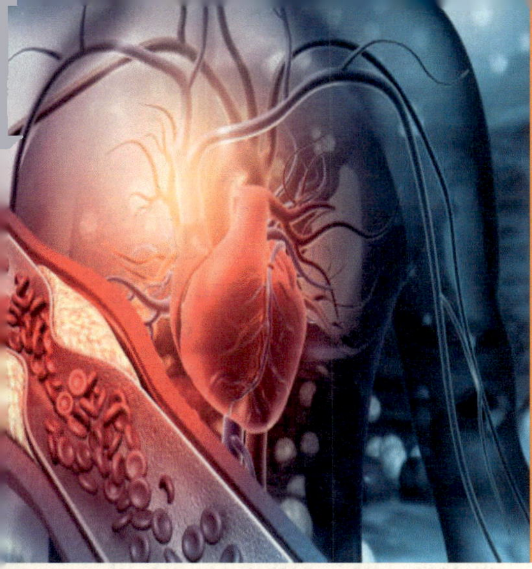

Chapter 12
VASCULAR DISORDERS

Contents

Introduction

Vascular illnesses encompass a wide range of diseases that attack the blood vessel network within the body, which consists of arteries, veins, and capillaries. There are numerous causes of vascular illnesses, ranging from genetic causes to lifestyle and environmental effects. One of the most common conditions is atherosclerosis, where plaques form in arteries, reducing blood circulation. Peripheral artery disease can also lead to pain and discomfort in limbs due to reduced circulation. Information regarding these disorders is highly crucial, as they can lead to serious complications like heart attacks, strokes, and chronic venous insufficiency. A comprehensive overview of vascular disease serves as the foundation of learning its etiology, risk factors, and probable treatments, thereby enabling healthcare practitioners and patients to cope with vascular illness rationally. With the rising vascular disease worldwide, particularly in an aging population, timely and accurate diagnosis is increasingly critical. The earliest possible detection can play a crucial role in preventing the progression of such disorders and minimizing associated health effects. Physicians routinely employ a combination of diagnostic tools such as Doppler ultrasound, angiography, and magnetic resonance imaging to examine vascular status with precision. Furthermore, guidelines from reputable organizations, including the ESC/EAS Guidelines, prioritize incorporating new scientific evidence into clinical reasoning to optimize patient treatment and care (François Mach et al., 2019). This also reinforces the importance of ongoing education in vascular health, with an affirmation of the necessity for clinicians to remain abreast of developments in diagnostic and therapeutic strategies. Aside from clinical assessment, vascular disorders are treated with a multidisciplinary approach that includes lifestyle modification, pharmacotherapy, and even surgical intervention. The patient is typically induced to adopt habits favorable for healthy hearts, such as a regular regimen of physical exercise, proper nutrition with low intake of saturated fats and cholesterol, and cessation from smoking to reduce vascular risk.

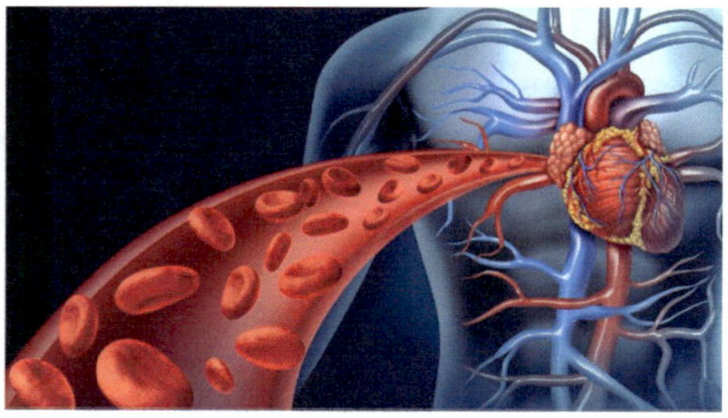

Figure 12.1. Vascular diseases.

Source: https://stgaccinwbsdevlrs01.blob.core.windows.net/newcorporatewbsite/blogs/october2023/detail-main-Vascular-Diseases.jpeg?w=3840&q=75.

Management strategies must also be aware of comorbidities, such as diabetes and hypertension, which will tend to exacerbate vascular complications. Groups like Research UK demand planning for dementia care, which demonstrates the intertwined connection of vascular health with other chronic illnesses (Livingston et al., 2020). By encouraging an integrated approach to vascular disease, clinicians are better positioned to address individual patients' needs, ultimately enhancing overall health outcomes and quality of life (Figure 12.1).

Definition of Vascular Disorders

Many conditions called vascular disorders can affect the blood vessels, which are the arteries, veins, and capillaries. They often result in significant problems for the heart and the rest of the body. The primary vascular disorders are arterial diseases, venous diseases and issues with the microcirculation: atherosclerosis and similar conditions cause the arteries to thicken and narrow, which decreases the flow of blood. At the same time, problems in the veins, such as varicose veins, happen when the valves do not work correctly, resulting in poor blood flow and swelling. Knowing these classifications is necessary since the causes of these conditions are not the same, so different approaches to treatment and care are needed for each patient. A significant part of vascular disorders is how various pathological processes work together in these diseases. Hypertension can cause hypertensive crises, which in turn can lead to problems in several organ systems. In a study examining pregnant women with gestosis, it was shown that different types of hemodynamics presented challenges in managing hypertensive conditions, such as hypertensive-hypodynamic dissociation, which emphasizes the complexity of vascular health (Sadchikov et al., 2021). Correctly understanding and diagnosing these mechanisms is necessary to provide the right therapies that fix hemodynamics and slow down the disease. Moreover, by assessing these conditions individually, healthcare providers can use effective treatments that significantly benefit patients. Recent research has revealed that vascular dysfunction can occur even in the absence of obstructive lesions, specifically in conditions like Ischemia with No Obstructive

Coronary Artery Disease (INOCA). INOCA exemplifies the broader complexity of vascular disorders, as it highlights mechanisms such as microvascular dysfunction and vasospasm that contribute to the symptoms of ischemic heart disease (Solovey, 2021). The results suggest that vascular disorders should now be understood as including changes that are not always blockages. Thus, a comprehensive approach to vascular disorders not only encompasses the identification of vascular abnormalities but also necessitates an understanding of the underlying physiological processes that may disrupt normal vascular function across different patient populations (Figure 12.2).

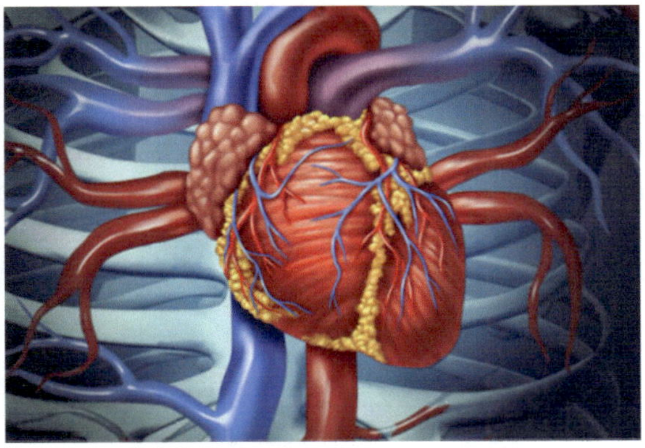

Figure 12.2. Understanding Vascular Disorders.

Source: https://daijiworld.ap-south-1.linodeobjects.com/Linode/images3/cardio_090724_1.jpg.

12.1. Types of Vascular Disorders

There are many vascular disorders, and most of them involve the blood vessels, which can change how blood flows and is delivered to different parts of the body. Atherosclerosis is a typical example, where plaques form in arteries, which can make the arteries narrow and increase the risk of heart attacks and strokes. Additionally, venous disorders such as deep vein thrombosis (DVT) provoke critical complications, where blood clots form in deep veins, typically in the legs, leading to symptoms such as swelling and pain, and potentially resulting in pulmonary embolism if a clot dislodges and travels to the lungs. Such vascular disorders highlight the importance of timely medical care to handle and prevent serious outcomes from problems with blood flow. Another significant category of vascular disorders involves peripheral artery disease (PAD), arising from atherosclerosis or other causes that impede blood flow to the limbs. PAD is usually recognized by leg pain during exercise, known as claudication, and it can become critical limb ischemia if not treated. Conditions affecting the veins, such as varicose veins and chronic venous insufficiency (CVI), also deserve attention. Varicose veins happen when veins become swollen and twisted, making them visible on the skin, and this often results in discomfort, while CVI means the blood does not return to the heart properly because of valve problems, which can cause swelling and changes in the skin. Understanding these disorders highlights the diverse nature of vascular conditions and the intricate systems in which they manifest (Shayor et al., 2024). Besides the types mentioned before, some vascular disorders are caused by hereditary factors or by conditions that develop over time. For example, Ehlers-Danlos syndrome, which is inherited, can damage connective tissues and cause the blood vessels to become weak and form aneurysms. Autoimmune diseases or infections can cause vasculitis, which is inflammation of the blood vessels, and this can seriously disrupt blood flow and cause damage to tissues. Furthermore, modern technological advancements in microfluidics and computational fluid dynamics (CFDs), serve as valuable tools for studying these disorders. Researchers use computer models to study blood flow and interactions in vessels, which helps them learn about diseases and create treatments for them. This approach underscores the importance of innovative methodologies in advancing the understanding and management of various vascular diseases (Harale et al., 2024).

12.1.1. Peripheral Artery Disease (PAD)

PAD is a severe vascular condition in which the arteries narrow and become smaller, preventing blood flow to the extremities, particularly the legs. It is primarily due to atherosclerosis, wherein fat accumulates along arterial walls, causing inflammation and vascular rigidity. The manifestations of PAD can range from exertional claudication—exercise-induced pain without an adequate blood supply—to more serious complications such as critical limb ischemia, which may result in loss of the extremity. Prompt diagnosis is critically important to recognize these symptoms because delayed treatment will severely limit mobility and quality of life. In addition, PAD is also a valuable marker for systemic atherosclerosis, and a patient with PAD is at greater risk for coronary artery disease and cerebrovascular events. Hence, a patient with PAD needs a comprehensive cardiovascular evaluation to avoid these associated risks. PAD diagnosis is typically established by combining clinical assessment and non-invasive testing. Clinicians can use the ankle-brachial index (ABI), which compares the blood pressure of a patient's ankle with that of the arm to test for blockages in arteries. Other imaging techniques, such as angiography or ultrasound, can also be used to visualize arterial blockages. Lifestyle changes and medications are both used in treating PAD. Cessation of smoking, diet changes, and exercise regimens under supervision are crucial components of disease management and can largely alleviate symptoms. In established disease, surgical intervention in the form of angioplasty or bypass grafting may be needed to restore normal blood flow. Aggressive management is justified because not only does PAD have an impact on physical ability, but it also has psychological dimensions due to apprehension of associated complications and dependency. The high degree of overlap between PAD and other vascular illnesses, such as spontaneous coronary artery dissection (SCAD), highlights the multi-factorial etiology of vascular diseases. Emerging evidence demonstrates that while PAD is traditionally linked with atherosclerotic pathophysiology, illnesses such as SCAD also present unique challenges in diagnosis and management, particularly in specific groups of individuals like young women. Studies have shown that most patients with PAD have recurrent cardiovascular events and even systemic arteriopathies like fibromuscular dysplasia that complicate their clinical presentations (Halvorsen et al., 2022). Awareness of such complexities allows more effective treatment and enhanced understanding of patient risk. Discussion of PAD in the broader context of vascular disease emphasizes the importance of multifaceted care strategies, encouraging advancement in patient education as well as multidisciplinary treatment options (Hayes et al., 2018) (Figure 12.3).

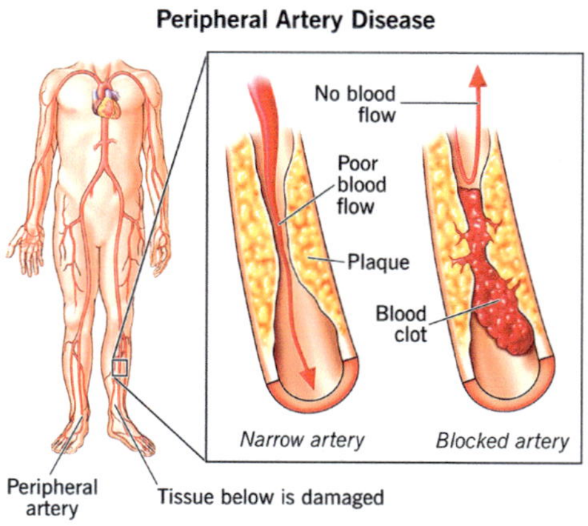

Figure 12.3. Peripheral artery disease hurts blood flow in your leg arteries because of plaque buildup.

Source: https://my.clevelandclinic.org/-/scassets/images/org/health/articles/17357-peripheral-arterial-disease-illustration-2.

12.1.2. Aneurysms

Aneurysms are a serious condition in vascular diseases, with the classic description being an abnormal dilatation of the vessels. Aneurysms are most likely to occur in arteries and may arise due to numerous different causes of etiology, including genetic predisposition, hypertension, atherosclerosis, or trauma. Presentation is varied based on the location and size of the aneurysm. Symptoms can vary from as innocuous as a mild headache to as ominous as acute severe pain and potential rupture. A ruptured aneurysm can cause catastrophic, life-threatening hemorrhage, making identification and control at early stages pertinent. Additionally, developments in imaging technology, such as magnetic resonance angiography and computed tomography angiography, have enhanced the ability of medical professionals to identify aneurysms at earlier stages, thereby providing improved prognosis to patients with vascular health. The impact of aneurysms is not just the direct health implications, but also affects the entire healthcare setting economically and psychologically. Patients are typically left with extreme anxiety and doubt regarding their future, necessitating an integrated approach to the patient involving psychological and emotional concerns. In addition, the cost of treatment, including potential surgeries and follow-up surveillance, is an added burden not only on patients but also on healthcare systems. Preventive measures, such as lifestyle modifications to regulate blood pressure and cholesterol, can be key in the prevention of aneurysm occurrence, a cost-saving measure for minimizing the load of intervention and treatment on healthcare services, given that risk factors relate to systemic disorders prevalent in disease conditions like pseudoxanthoma elasticum, which is related to enhanced susceptibility to aneurysm development, as noted in the literature (Azi et al., 2024). Aneurysm treatment most commonly demands a multimodal approach, combining various specialties of medicine to optimize the patient. For those who are asymptomatic, intervention could be as simple as cautious monitoring; for those in complex or urgent cases, it could require surgery. Technical improvements in the minimally invasive pathway, such as endovascular aneurysm repair (EVAR), have simplified therapy with the ability for faster recovery and hospitalization time. Secondly, the application of genetic testing for individuals at risk of inherited disease is increasingly coming into focus, helping to refine preventive measures and surveillance programs. As there is expanding awareness of vascular diseases, including aneurysms, there is more development of innovative methods such as artificial intelligence in risk assessment and personalized treatment regimens, further enhancing diagnosis and management capabilities in modern vascular practice (N/A, 2021) (Figure 12.4).

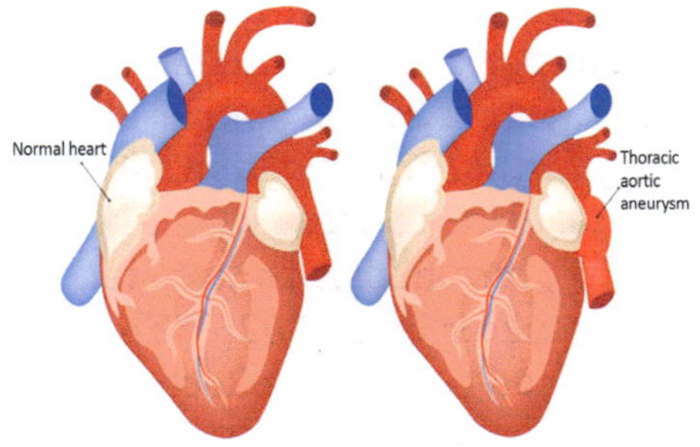

Figure 12.4. Aneurysms.

Source: https://media.istockphoto.com/id/1152385628/vector/heart-anatomy-and-types-of-heart-disease-vector-illustration.jpg?s=612x612&w=0&k=20&c=T_ih_RjGFInKhXGLQiSQZ0JCgL4EdgP-T92E5q7vkg0=.

12.1.3. Venous Thromboembolism (VTE)

Because VTE is both difficult to treat and occurs often, it is a major vascular disorder. Characterized primarily by deep vein thrombosis (DVT) and pulmonary embolism (PE), VTE poses significant health risks, including potential mortality and long-term morbidity. Yearly, millions of people around the world are affected by VTE, and experts believe that around 10 million cases are diagnosed each year. The disease commonly shows up with swelling, pain, and tenderness in the affected area or, in PE, with chest pain and trouble breathing. Spotting the condition early is crucial, but many people remain undiagnosed, highlighting the need for increased awareness among both doctors and patients. Several recent studies have found that psychiatric disorders and VTE may influence each other in both directions. It is becoming clear that people with chronic vascular conditions, for example, portal vein thrombosis, may also have mental health issues, which can make their treatment more difficult. A significant case shows this relationship: a 38-year-old woman had psychotic symptoms 12 years after being diagnosed with portal vein thrombosis, demonstrating the link between blood vessels and mental health. The pathophysiological mechanisms underlying this relationship remain poorly understood, warranting further investigation into the ways psychological disturbances may influence, or be influenced by, thrombosis and related vascular disorders (Boukdir et al., 2025). These studies are essential for designing effective treatment plans for people who are affected. Additionally, specific anatomical abnormalities, such as May-Thurner syndrome (MTS), can precipitate the development of VTE, particularly in female patients. MTS causes the left iliac vein to be squeezed, which raises the risk of DVT and can lead to pulmonary embolism. Because MTS is often not recognized, there is a strong need for healthcare workers in acute settings to be more aware of it. Prompt recognition and management of MTS help patients and also make doctors consider other possible causes for DVT-like symptoms. As reflected in a clinical case, recognizing MTS as a differential diagnosis can lead to life-saving interventions through appropriate anticoagulation and ongoing monitoring (Krishnan et al., 2024). In this way, addressing both anatomical and psychological factors is essential in the holistic management of VTE and its related syndromes (Figure 12.5).

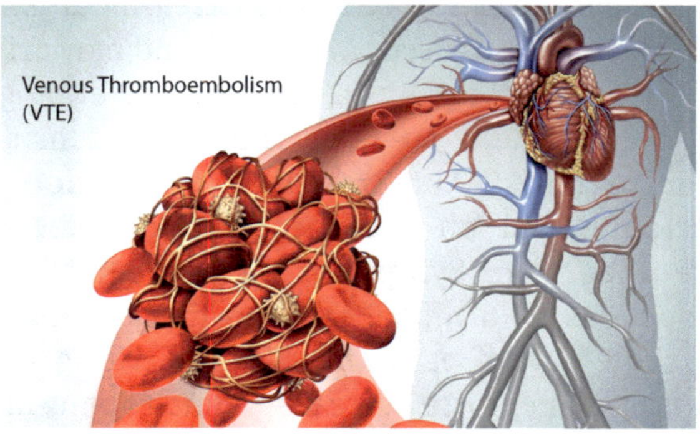

Figure 12.5. Venous thromboembolism (VTE).

Source: https://vegasvascular.com/wp-content/uploads/2023/05/Venous-thromboembolism-VTE.png.

12.2. Causes and Risk Factors

The pathogenesis of vascular disease is a multifactorial convergence of numerous causes and risk factors, which cumulatively give rise to the vascular disease. The most critical among them is the development of atherosclerosis, a process involving the laying down of plaques in the arterial walls. This can lead to occlusion of the arteries and eventually result in serious consequences such as heart attacks and strokes. Additionally, genetic vulnerability also determines a person's susceptibility to vascular disease. Genetic factors can either affect lipid metabolism, blood pressure regulation, and the inflammatory process to worsen the risk when combined with other lifestyle determinants. Understanding the interactive causes is essential to the planning of specific prevention strategies and curative interventions to reduce the burden of vascular disease. In addition to the inherent danger, various lifestyle determinants also have an important function to play in the development of vascular diseases. Smoking, for instance, is a accepted risk factor that accelerates plaque formation by promoting damage to the endothelium and by causing inflammation. Moreover, food consumption, such as excessive intake of saturated fats and sugars, can also have a significant contribution to the gain in weight and an increase in levels of cholesterol, both leading to obesity and cardiovascular disease. Furthermore, physical inactivity contributes to the risk, as physical inactivity is associated with poor cardiovascular function and an increased likelihood of hypertension. All together, these lifestyle factors emphasize the need for public health interventions that promote healthy lifestyles and aim to reduce the incidence of vascular disease in the population. Obesity is a notable risk factor for vascular disease and a significant topic of discussion in health discussions today. Increased body weight has been found to lead to detrimental changes in vascular function, including increased arterial stiffness and impaired endothelial function. Notably, the function of perivascular adipose tissue (PVAT) is also being given more prominence in this regard; PVAT that surrounds blood vessels has been found to possess both defensive and detrimental properties depending on its metabolic state. Pankova (2024) hypothesizes that obesity negatively affects the anticontractile activity of PVAT, ultimately leading to enhanced vascular contractility. This mechanism can cause hypertension and other vascular complications, reiterating the need for effective therapies directed toward weight control as an integral part of preventing the development and progression of vascular disease.

12.2.1. Genetic Predisposition

Having a specific genetic makeup is very important in the development and progression of vascular disorders, especially those that are cardiovascular diseases. These disorders, which may be affected by genetics and the environment, include hypertension, atherosclerosis, and thrombosis. Studies have found that those with a family history of vascular disorders are more likely to be affected, which suggests a strong hereditary link. Mendelian disorders, which happen due to a single gene mutation, form the basis of our knowledge about genetic predisposition. Because such disorders usually have predictable inheritance patterns, they can be spotted early and managed properly, which highlights the value of genetic testing in healthcare. The ability to assess a family history can facilitate risk stratification, thereby affecting management guidelines in populations at risk for these conditions (Whelton et al., 2017; Wilde et al., 2022). New genetic testing methods, such as whole-exome and whole-genome sequencing, have made it easier to study the genetic causes of vascular disorders. They make it possible to look at many genetic variants at once, which helps find possible genetic causes of various heart diseases. In particular, polygenic risk scores, which combine many minor genetic effects, are now commonly used to predict who might get these disorders. It has been found that such scores can predict the risk of common cardiovascular diseases such as coronary artery disease and aneurysms. Furthermore, understanding the interplay between genetic predispositions and lifestyle factors can enhance the precision of risk assessments, guiding preventive strategies tailored to individual patients or populations (Whelton et al., 2017; Wilde et al., 2022). It is also necessary to realize that environmental factors can alter the risk of vascular disorders based on someone's genes. Eating habits, exercise, and smoking can strongly impact the way genes related to heart health work. It shows that genes alone are not always enough to cause a disease; the environment must be considered as well. Studies indicate that individuals who have specific genetic changes for vascular disorders can lower their risk by changing their lifestyle. So, helping people understand the risks of heredity and inspiring them to adopt healthy habits is important for managing and avoiding vascular disorders. This comprehensive approach reinforces the need for integrative strategies in cardiovascular care, encompassing genetic insights and lifestyle interventions (Whelton et al., 2017; Wilde et al., 2022) (Figure 12.6)

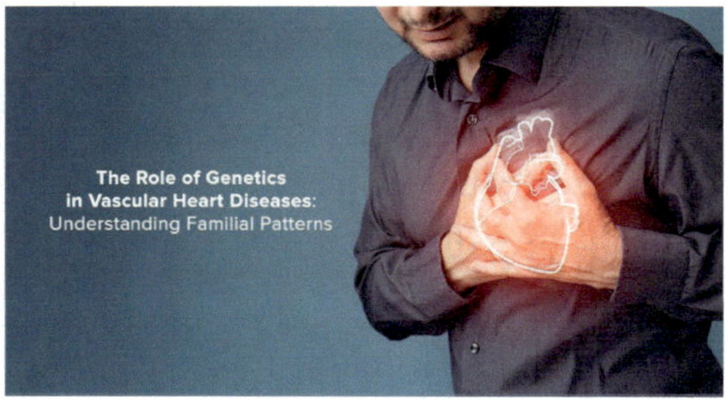

Figure 12.6. The role of genetics in vascular heart diseases: understanding familial patterns.

Source: https://www.eternalhospital.com/uploadedfiles/gallery/1708329554_1300-x-700_The-Role-of-Genetics-in-Vascular-Heart-Diseases.jpg.

12.2.2. Lifestyle Factors (Diet, Exercise, Smoking)

The cross-talk between lifestyle factors and vascular disease points to the central role of diet, physical activity, and smoking in determining cardiovascular health. A proper diet of fruits, vegetables, whole grains, and lean meat sustains maximum vascular function. Diets rich in saturated fat, sugars, and salt, conversely, have been presented as disease causes for hypertension and atherosclerosis.

The interaction between these diet habits and cardiovascular diseases is significant because it might trigger or complicate existing conditions or develop new ones. To explain this, individuals with large intakes of processed food might be more susceptible to plaque buildup in arterial walls. As such, dietary modification is of utmost importance not merely to increase the well-being of blood vessels but also to diminish the risk of chronic disease, which in turn further improves quality of life. In addition to effects on diet, daily physical activity is an essential way of life when battling vascular disease. Regular exercise enhances cardiovascular health by improving circulation, reducing pressure within the blood, and optimizing blood lipids. Studies have indicated that sedentary life is related to increased risks of vascular complications, suggesting that physical inactivity is etiologically vital in the causation of vascular diseases. Incorporation of moderate to vigorous exercise routines into daily life has beneficial effects on endothelial function, thus reducing risks for vascular disease. In addition, exercise has some unique psychological benefits, which may ease stress that often precedes prolonged illness. Therefore, the development of the culture of regular exercise could be the most effective method of reducing the prevalence of vascular disease among the population. Smoking remains one of the most dangerous lifestyle factors affecting vascular health. Toxic substances contained in tobacco smoke can cause extensive vascular injury and the development of atherosclerosis and other cardiovascular diseases. Not only does smoking continue the constriction of vessels, but it is also harmful to the flow of blood and tends to increase the susceptibility to blood clotting, creating a classic combination for potential vascular complications. Hypothetical connections between exposure to secondhand smoke and vascular dysfunction also justify the regulation of secondhand smoke in terms of public health policies. The importance of quitting smoking cannot be overemphasized, as evidence indicates that even small reductions in the rate of smoking can lead to significant improvements in health. Counteracting smoking in public health measures is crucial because its elimination will, in turn, lower the burden of vascular diseases on society and eventually promote overall well-being.

12.2.3. Comorbid Conditions (Diabetes, Hypertension)

The presence of comorbid conditions, i.e., diabetes and hypertension, significantly impairs the progress and prognosis of vascular diseases. The two metabolic diseases have been noted to co-occur with high frequency among patients, elevating the risks of cardiovascular events and other forms of complications. Diabetes and hypertension patients most often have similar pathophysiological features, such as insulin resistance and endothelial dysfunction, that contribute to deteriorating vascular function. Together, the combination aggravates the development of vascular disease, associated with enhanced morbidity and mortality compared to patients who possess either disease independently. Treatment of these diseases needs an integrated, multidisciplinary strategy, treating not only the individual clinical symptoms but also the underlying causes for vascular dysfunction. The deleterious action of diabetes and hypertension doesn't limit itself to basic cardiovascular complications. For instance, both conditions immensely raise the risk for chronic kidney disease, creating a vicious cycle that further strains vascular systems. The oxidative stress and the systemic inflammation experienced by diabetic and hypertensive patients may lead to extreme structural and functional alterations in blood vessels. As such, the risk for sudden vascular events such as myocardial infarction or stroke is significantly raised. Additionally, the collective impact of these conditions is more likely to cause a significant decline in the quality of life, and thus, early diagnosis and aggressive management strategies are warranted. The clinicians ought to be vigilant in the recognition of patients at risk because timely interventions have the possibility of minimising complications and improving patient outcomes. The symptomatic treatment of both diabetes and hypertension has overlapping tendencies, thus offering an opportunity for co-ordinated management strategies. Recent advances in pharmacotherapy, such as SGLT inhibitors and GLP-1 receptor agonists, have not only demonstrated potential in glycemia control but also in blood pressure lowering and cardiovascular health improvement. The medications can permit a two-way management of those comorbidities that tend to occur together. It is worth noting that diet and exercise, as lifestyle modifications, are of central significance in countering the effects of these comorbidities. A treatment strategy should encompass these elements, as patient education and reinforcement of the necessity to comply with therapies must continue. As the biology of diabetes, hypertension, and vascular disease becomes better understood, the development of novel and effective treatment modalities will be central to advancing patient care and reducing the burden of vascular disease associated with these comorbidities (Haseeb et al., 2024; Hezam et al., 2024) (Figure 12.7).

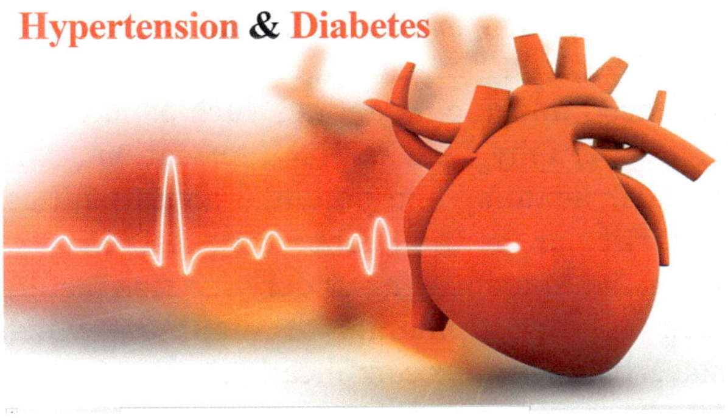

Figure 12.7. Hypertension and diabetes.

Source: https://i0.wp.com/thelecc.com/wp-content/uploads/2018/09/1.png?fit=973%2C549&ssl=1.

12.3. Symptoms and Diagnosis

The variety of symptoms of vascular disease may rely quite significantly on the underlying pathology and which regions of the vascular system are involved. Characteristic presentations typically include pain, swelling, and alterations in the skin that may indicate compromised circulation. For instance, conditions such as venous insufficiency may present with leg edema and varicose veins, and peripheral artery disease presenting as claudication, i.e., exertional pain due to inadequate blood supply. In addition, such acute conditions as stroke may present abruptly with neurological deficits, i.e., hemiplegia or aphasia. A thorough understanding of these symptoms is necessary for accurate diagnosis and early treatment since delayed diagnosis can lead to severe complications and reduced quality of life in patients with vascular diseases, hence the importance of symptomatic understanding among physicians. Vascular disease is most often a multi-faceted challenge to diagnose due to the overlapping symptoms with other illnesses. A thorough history and physical examination are the initial steps in the diagnostic workup. Routine practice is that clinicians may apply non-invasive techniques such as Doppler ultrasonography to quantify blood flow and identify obstructions. Advanced imaging modalities such as MRI and CT angiography yield helpful information about vascular anatomy and potential abnormalities. Of particular mention, laboratory tests may be beneficial in identifying underlying risk factors such as hyperlipidemia or diabetes, which exacerbate vascular complications. Diagnosis of the said disorders is made even more challenging by overlapping presentations of heterogeneous diseases, necessitating rigorous, systematic workup to establish proper management and treatment plans tailored to each patient's needs, as described in neuropsychiatric presentations of vascular disease literature (Jayasinghe et al., 2025). In vascular illnesses, the use of biomarkers has been one of the potential methods for the enhancement of diagnostic accuracy. Recent research evidence indicates that some biomarkers derived from extracellular vesicles may be used to distinguish between various cognitive illnesses and therefore shed light on the pathophysiologic mechanisms that influence treatment outcomes (Taha et al., 2024). Using a meta-analytical approach, studies have shown that general extracellular vesicle biomarkers provide more clear-cut diagnostic paths than those that are context-specific within the central nervous system. Implications of these findings point towards the need to work on adaptive diagnostic criteria based on biomarker analysis, most importantly in complex cases where traditional methods may generate ambiguous results. With ongoing research, these advances promise to significantly improve diagnostic sensitivity and thus guide more effective therapeutic interventions for numerous vascular disorders.

12.3.1. Common Symptoms Associated with Vascular Disorders

Vascular disease encompasses a broad range of conditions that can seriously impact an individual's health and well-being. Common symptoms of these conditions are usually associated with poor blood circulation, which could present itself as pain, heaviness, or fatigue within afflicted areas. PAD, for instance, is generally accompanied by intermittent claudication, which refers to leg cramps or leg ache upon exertion. Additionally, vascular disease can lead to additional complications in the form of chronic wounds or non-healing ulcers, particularly in diabetics or individuals with circulatory issues. These symptoms not only disable physical movement but also lead to mental anguish and lower overall health and quality of life. Chronic pain is also a frequent symptom of vascular disease, particularly with conditions such as Ehlers–Danlos syndrome. This inheritable connective tissue condition is usually characterized by joint hypermobility and tissue friability, resulting in repeated pain that may affect daily living and emotional well-being. Ehlers–Danlos syndrome patients rank chronic pain as one of the most disabling aspects of their disease, which affects their ability to socialize and engage in family relationships.

The psychic strain of having chronic pain is an added bodily symptom, and in addition to this, comes frustration and helplessness. With the cumulative effect of symptoms on different fronts, integrated management guidelines taking physical as well as psychic aspects of vascular disease into consideration become an immediate necessity (Inmaculada-Concepción Palomo-Toucedo et al., 2024). Dyslipidemia, typically asymptomatic, is full of perils that are intrinsically linked with vascular health. This abnormality, which is defined by an increased level of lipids, is a central factor in the development of atherosclerosis and goes on to cause serious complications such as coronary artery disease, cerebrovascular accidents, and peripheral vascular diseases. The manifestations are typically evident only when serious complications arise, such as myocardial infarction due to widespread vascular degeneration. Due to this hidden onset, early intervention and detection are essential. Moreover, the awareness of the psychological and physiological consequences of dyslipidemia highlights the need for integrative management strategies combining traditional practices, like Ayurveda, with conventional medicine. The detection of similar symptoms between vascular disorders enables clinicians to predict complications better and tailor management programs for better outcomes (Gopan et al., 2024) (Figure 12.8).

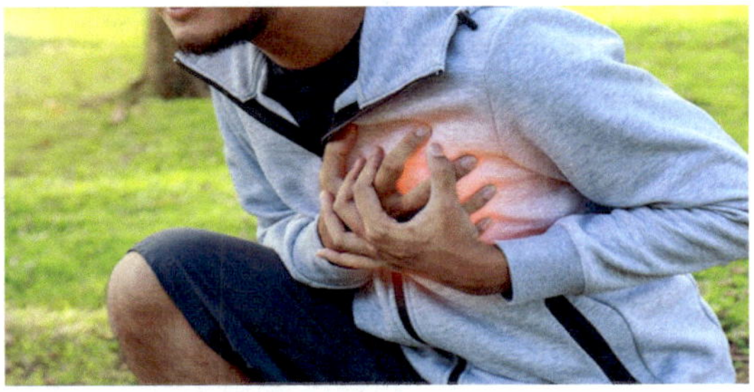

Figure 12.8. Symptoms of vascular disorders.

Source: https://c.ndtvimg.com/2022-12/7j5qbje8_heart-attack_625x300_06_December_22.jpg?downsize=773:435.

12.3.2. Diagnostic Tests (Ultrasound, Angiography)

Diagnostic imaging plays a crucial role in the management of vascular disease, that is, in the correct diagnosis of diseases such as peripheral vascular disease (PVD). Of the diagnostic modalities available, Doppler ultrasound (DUS) and computed tomography angiography (CTA) are two of the most beneficial due to their capability to visualize vascular anatomy and assess blood flow hemodynamics. DUS is advantageous because it is non-invasive, provides real-time imaging, and is inexpensive, making it suitable for initial tests. It can detect gross hemodynamic changes and abnormalities like stenosis or occlusion. In patients of all ages, DUS is an effective first-line tool, with advantages of safety and convenience, particularly in pediatric patients where damage caused by radiation is a problem (Sehar et al., 2025). Supplementing DUS, CTA provides high-quality images that allow for a detailed. Anatomical assessment. of complicated vascular diseases. For elderly patients who frequently suffer from severe atherosclerosis and other complex vascular diseases, this imaging method is especially beneficial. The accuracy of CTA is crucial for surgical planning because it allows physicians to see nearby anatomical structures in addition to blood circulation, which is crucial for selecting the best surgical procedure. Evidence has established that CTA significantly improves diagnostic accuracy in the identification of life-threatening lesions and therefore improves patient outcomes. For example, a comparative analysis revealed that although DUS successfully identified vascular abnormalities, CTA confirmed findings with higher specificity, particularly in complicated cases (Cantador et al., 2024). Utilization of both DUS and CTA in clinical practice illustrates the efficacy of applying a multimodal approach in diagnosing vascular disease. By integrating the strengths of each modality, practitioners can optimize diagnostic strategies and tailor treatment protocols to individual patient needs. For instance, DUS can be utilized as the preferred initial screening modality because of its convenience, while CTA is used as final diagnosis or surgical planning when called for. The complementary nature of these imaging modalities emphasizes the need for ongoing research for further optimization of their application in varying age groups and patient populations. This dual use of ultrasound and angiography enables full comprehension of vascular pathology, finally resulting in overall management of the patient in vascular disease (Cantador et al., 2024; Sehar et al., 2025) (Figure 12.9).

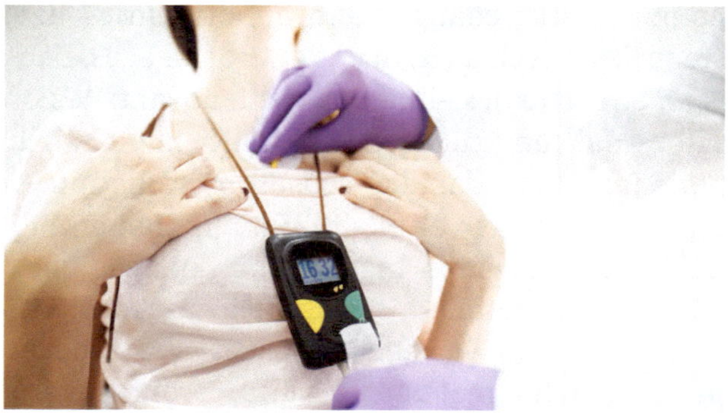

Figure 12.9. Diagnostic testing of vascular disorders.

Source: https://bswh-p-001-delivery.sitecorecontenthub.cloud/api/public/content/fc58de7fd271477c98b4420a90a38724?v=08b9d43c.

12.3.3. Importance of Early Detection

The early diagnosis of vascular illnesses cannot be overemphasized. Early diagnosis of vascular illnesses such as atherosclerosis, aneurysms, and peripheral artery disease is essential for effective treatment and control of the disease. Early diagnosis allows for the timely treatment of the illnesses by medical practitioners before complications can set in, thereby preventing severe health effects, including heart attack and strokes, which are commonly associated with advanced vascular illness. It also assists in decreasing healthcare costs, as early treatment is generally less expensive than the management of acute events caused by late-stage vascular disease. By utilizing screening tools and risk factor assessment, clinicians can identify patients at high risk and apply preventive interventions, complementing the critical role played by early detection in improving patient outcomes and quality of life. In addition to reducing morbidity and mortality, early detection fosters collaboration among the patients and healthcare providers. When patients participate in their treatment, once they identify the hazards and the necessity for periodic check-ups, they are more prone to adhere to recommended lifestyle changes and treatment regimens. This engagement comprises educational interventions that educate patients to notice signs and symptoms that are indicative of vascular disease so that they can seek consultation from a physician early enough. Further, the engagement is supported by up-to-date clinical guidelines identifying the importance of early treatment (Visseren et al., 2021). By fostering a culture of shared responsibility, patients and healthcare providers can collaborate to achieve improved vascular health outcomes, thereby enhancing outcomes related to vascular disease. A second highly significant aspect of early detection is its impact on mental health and quality of life. Patients can be severely emotionally disturbed while having undiagnosed vascular disease, eventually resulting in anxiety and depression. Through early diagnosis and on-time treatment, patients can relax, reducing the burden of fear and creating a positive attitude towards their health process. Additionally, cognitive health management is also most crucial, especially in the case of elders, wherein vascular disorders are linked with conditions like dementia and delirium (Livingston et al., 2020). By actively managing vascular health, medical systems not only minimize bodily threats to health but also improve mental health, illustrating how early detection stands at the heart of whole-patient care and quality of life.

12.4. Treatment Options

Effective therapeutic measures for vascular disorders have improved considerably, embracing both conservative and surgical approaches to cater to the needs of patients. Conservative treatment usually involves lifestyle changes, including dietary restrictions and increased physical exercise, combined with pharmacological interventions through the use of venoactive drugs. Research has proven that micronized purified flavonoid fraction can alleviate symptoms of chronic venous disease by enhancing venous tone as well as decreasing edema. These nonoperative interventions are aimed at supporting quality of life in patients and halting disease progression. Furthermore, the use of elastic compression stockings is firmly established as a treatment for the management of chronic venous insufficiency, with external reinforcement of the venous system, thus preventing such complications as edema and venous skin changes. Surgical interventions provide a more interventionist method of treatment for more established vascular disease. Endovenous laser ablation and radiofrequency ablation are some of the more noted procedures now, as less invasive means to cure varicose veins. The European Society for Vascular Surgery emphasizes these treatments due to their safety profile, efficacy, and lower recurrence rates compared to traditional surgery. Furthermore, endovenous thermal ablation treatments consist of the sealing of defective veins with heat, which leads to symptom relief and improved venous function. In decision-making, care must be taken to weigh the potential benefits of novel technologies against patient-specific conditions, confirming the necessity for individualized treatment regimens in vascular therapy. When utilizing traditional modes of treatment, novel therapies like ultrasound-guided foam sclerotherapy and cyanoacrylate adhesive closure hold much promise in the management of venous disease. The procedures minimize recovery time while effectively managing symptomatology of chronic venous insufficiency and superficial venous reflux. Ultrasound-guided foam sclerotherapy allows for direct treatment of affected veins with a sclerosing agent, causing occlusion of the vein and eventual removal by the body. Current guidelines emphasize the importance of matching decision-making with evidence-based practice, ensuring that clinicians and patients work together to determine the most appropriate intervention. The incorporation of these novel therapies into the treatment armamentarium for vascular disease is an indicator of a shift toward more patient-centered, streamlined care paradigms for the specialty of vascular health, as delineated in contemporary clinical guidelines (Al-Khayri et al., 2022; Maeseneer et al., 2022) (Figure 12.10).

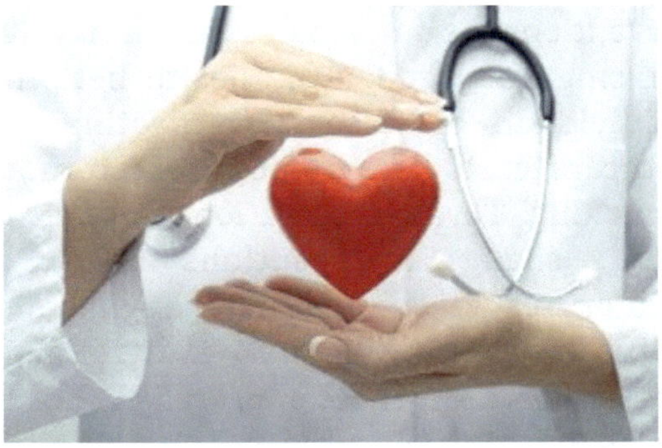

Figure 12.10. Treatment options for vascular disease.

Source: https://www.cvmus.com/sites/default/files/2015/02/455237505-300x200.jpg.

12.4.1. Lifestyle Modifications

Life modification plays a key role in the prevention and control of vascular disease. These modifications encompass various health-related behaviors, including diet, exercise, and smoking. For instance, consumption of a Mediterranean-type diet rich in fruits, vegetables, whole grains, and healthy fats has been associated with reduced rates of vascular disease (ESC Guidelines). Also, regular physical exercise not only promotes cardiovascular well-being but also enhances quality of life. Such lifestyle choices become crucial in ensuring improved blood circulation and reduced hypertension, mandatory factors for the handling of existing vascular situations. By initiating such changes, health care professionals are more likely to help patients develop long-term habits that prevent them from even acquiring severe vascular complications. In addition, the role of smoking cessation cannot be emphasized too highly in the discourse regarding vascular health. The harms of tobacco extend far and wide, affecting virtually all organs throughout the body, as well as complicating and worsening pre-existing vascular disease. Evidence repeatedly shows that smoking cessation is associated with significant improvements in vascular function and a reduction in cardiovascular events. Health interventions for smoking cessation have been promising not just for the health betterment of individuals but also for mitigating public healthcare costs of chronic diseases induced by smoking. Through cessation programs and lifestyle change interventions, health care providers can facilitate life-changing health modifications in high-risk individuals for vascular disorders. These efforts align effectively with advice that encourages overall strategies in patient care, respecting the interdependence of vascular health outcomes and lifestyle behavior. Psychosocial factors also influence the effectiveness of lifestyle modification as a means of vascular disorder control. The mental and emotional condition of patients can impact their ability to adopt and maintain healthier behaviors. For instance, stress management abilities such as mindfulness, yoga, and counseling can enhance lifestyle change adherence. Supportive social systems, such as family and community resources, can also facilitate the patient in making and sustaining these changes. Treatment of the psychological dynamics of the health behavior change can make the environment more conducive for individuals to seek to improve their vascular well-being. Ultimately, an integrative approach bringing together both lifestyle modifications as well as psychosocial interventions not only increases the well-being of the individual but also constitutes part of evidence-based practice aiming to reduce the effects of vascular disease on society in general (Livingston et al., 2020; Visseren et al., 2021) (Figure 12.11).

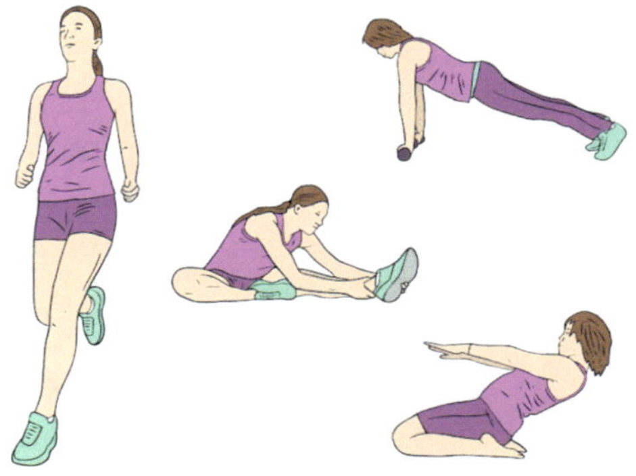

Figure 12.11. Best Exercises for Peripheral Artery Disease (PAD).

Source: https://www.drsumitkapadia.com/wp-content/uploads/2024/10/PAD-Exercises.webp.

12.4.2. Medications (Anticoagulants, Statins)

Medications such as anticoagulants and statins play a vital role in the management of vascular diseases, with a significant impact on the outcomes of the patient. Anticoagulants, warfarin, and the more recently developed direct oral anticoagulants are employed to prevent the development of thrombus, thus minimizing risk factors for illnesses such as deep vein thrombosis and pulmonary embolism. These medications work by inhibiting multiple aspects of the coagulation cascade, which ultimately reduces the risk of blood clots leading to severe vascular complications. Given that they are responsible for providing a guarantee that blood will still flow and that ischemic events will not take place, anticoagulants are considered essential in patients with a history of vascular issues, highlighting their vital role in contemporary treatment plans. Statins, on the other hand, function primarily to lower lipids but also have a clear-cut profile of pleiotropic effects on which their efficacy in vascular disease management is based. Statins can do this through the inhibition of HMG-CoA reductase, which inhibits the synthesis of cholesterol and enhances the liver's uptake of LDL and lowers overall cardiovascular risk. Their additional advantages, however, have increasingly been uncovered by research, such as improving endothelial function and having anti-inflammatory effects. For instance, studies have confirmed that statins modulate the CCL2/CCR2 signaling pathway, a central player in inflammation and atherogenesis. This multi-target action not only assists in cholesterol management but also contributes to vascular health on various fronts (Gholamalizadeh et al., 2024). Anticoagulant and statin co-administration can be highly beneficial for the treatment of patients with vascular disorders, particularly with associated comorbidities such as diabetes. Statins have been recognized for their capacity not only to stabilize atherosclerotic plaques but also to enhance the global endothelial response to vascular injury. This is especially useful in diabetic patients, who will most likely experience heightened cardiovascular risk through twin pathophysiologic abnormalities of both lipid metabolism and coagulation pathways (Mosina, 2025). Thus, the adjunctive administration of anticoagulants and statins likely has a synergistic effect, in effect lowering the risk of harmful cardiovascular events by multiple, redundant mechanisms. Overall, the strategy of using these drugs validates the general strategic notion of treating vascular disease as an all-encompassing process with special utility in the creation of personalized, multifactorial treatment strategies in modern healthcare (Figure 12.12).

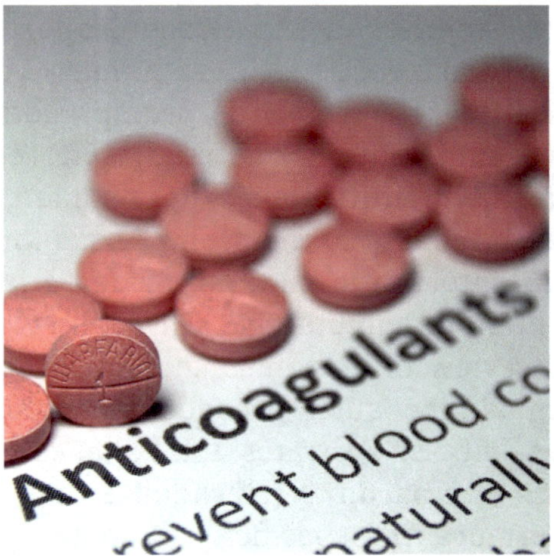

Figure 12.12. Anticoagulants.

Source: https://www.stoptheclot.org/wp-content/uploads/2017/11/Anticoag_SQ.jpg.

12.4.3. Surgical Interventions (Bypass Surgery, Stenting)

Surgery, particularly bypass surgery and stenting, plays a significant part in vascular disease treatment. Bypass surgery is the process of bypassing a pathway for blood flow to circumvent blocked or constricted arteries to restore an adequate supply of blood to affected tissues. It is typically suggested for disorders such as atherosclerosis and critical limb ischemia. In comparison, stenting is a less invasive method where an artery is maintained open through the insertion of a tubular device into the artery, typically with angioplasty. Whether one intervention is used over the other depends on several factors, including the patient's overall health, the location and extent of the vascular blockage, and the specific anatomy of the blood vessels involved. Evidence indicates that prompt initiation of surgical care has a significant impact on patient outcomes. For example, extremity vascular injuries, which are usually due to trauma, may require primary repair such as bypass or ligation to promote limb salvage. In a multicenter audit of 120 patients with extremity vascular injuries, a significant proportion of these patients received these primary repairs, highlighting the value of prompt action in surgical intervention. The study referred to a median intervention time of approximately 169 minutes, pointing to the prompt need for early surgical intervention in limb preservation and prevention of amputations. Through evidence-based review of outcomes, medical specialists can maximize such procedures to achieve higher limb salvage rates and enhance patient care in trauma units (Hurndall et al., 2024). Furthermore, the specificity of some vascular injuries underscores the need for specialized surgical techniques, such as endovascular therapy.

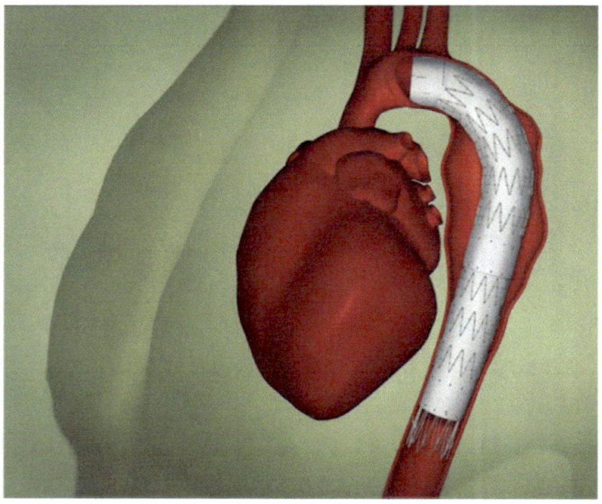

Figure 12.13. Thoracic endovascular aortic repair (TEVAR).

Source: https://ufhealth.org/sites/default/files/media/health-topics/tevar-figure-2.jpg.

Transcatheter techniques, for example, thoracic endovascular aortic repair (TEVAR), have become essential in the treatment of catastrophic injury to the aorta, particularly traumatic. With most of these operations under severe stress and in diverse anatomical settings, the results of stress after the procedure underscore the need for strict monitoring and ongoing national studies. For instance, the post-procedure mortality rate in a recent UK audit was 8%, reflecting both the hazards involved and the overwhelming requirement for surgical expertise and control of resources. Alongside such innovations, evidence-based practice included in the protocol for management of surgery for vascular disease also needs to be present to improve patient safety and the quality of care (Hurndall et al., 2024) (Figure 12.13).

12.5. Prevention Strategies

Effective prevention planning leads to controlling the increasing incidence of vascular diseases, primarily against ischemic stroke and atrial fibrillation (AF). Preventive planning regarding control of risk factors such as hypertension, diabetes, and dyslipidemia forms the foundation of any prevention. Public health programs for ensuring proper awareness about lifestyle modification in the form of increased physical activity, an appropriate diet, and refraining from smoking are a must in preventing these risk factors. Moreover, the adoption of evidence-based interventions such as anticoagulation can significantly reduce the occurrence of thromboembolic events in AF, which, when left untreated, has severe health implications for patients in the form of increased vulnerability to strokes and associated morbidities (Manolis et al., 2024). Promoting compliance with these preventive measures can reinforce outcomes for those at risk and enhance the overall efficacy of stroke prevention programs. The significance of anticoagulants in ischemic stroke prevention underscores the need for timely and proper interventions in preventive care. Anticoagulants are especially significant in primary and secondary prevention, and they significantly reduce the risk for stroke in patients with conditions predisposing them to stroke, such as atrial fibrillation, antiphospholipid antibody syndrome, and other vasculopathies (Manolis et al., 2024). Because the optimal time for anticoagulant treatment might vary depending on the patient's unique circumstances, medical practitioners need to understand the nuances of such therapies. Moreover, routine practices that deliver tailored treatment and regular follow-ups can play a role in enhancing compliance and health among patients. By giving appropriate antithrombotic therapy and education about their importance to patients, clinicians can dramatically reduce the incidence of disabling strokes and improve the quality of life in those at risk. Patient awareness and education in the community are key components of effective prevention schemes for vascular disease. Encouraging individuals to go for regular health check-ups can facilitate the early detection of risk factors to allow interventions to be done in good time for the prevention of strokes. As an additional measure, conducting education campaigns to educate individuals on TIAs signs and symptoms can allow them to consult doctors in time, thereby reducing the risk of major events (Measar et al., 2024). Effective interaction among the healthcare workers and patients is also central to enforcing compliance with prescribed lifestyle changes and treatment regimes. By promoting prevention through sensitization and education, communities can collectively strive towards a radical reduction of the burden of vascular disorders, leading to improved public health outcomes.

12.5.1. Healthy Lifestyle Choices

Healthy lifestyle practices play an essential role in the prevention and control of vascular disease. With regular physical activity, one of the leading causes of better vascular function is ensured, as physical activity ensures weight control, lowers blood pressure, and enhances blood flow. Research indicates that even mild exercise, like walking or cycling, is more than enough to substantially reduce the risk of developing diseases like hypertension and atherosclerosis. Further, when exercise is coupled with other healthy behaviors—such as a wholesome diet full of fruits, vegetables, and whole grains—there are synergistic benefits that add strength to cardiovascular health. These dietary modifications not only improve vascular function but also quality of life, emphasizing the importance of a multifaceted approach to the prevention of vascular disease (Visseren et al., 2021). Diet plays a vital role in the development of vascular health since it influences blood pressure and cholesterol levels directly. Dietary intake that is high in saturated fat and sugar promotes vascular disease, while one that is high in omega-3 fatty acids, antioxidants, and fiber promotes vascular integrity. The Mediterranean diet, for instance, is high in healthy fats, lean protein, and abundant plant foods, which offer significant benefits in preventing cardiovascular disease. Adequate hydration is also less understood but significantly contributes to the optimum vascular function. Consumption of sufficient quantities of water and regulation of sodium intake can curb dangers posed by high blood pressure, demonstrating the position played by food in the healthy way of life of vascular disorders (Livingston et al., 2020). Together with choices concerning diet and exercise, psychosocial factors also contribute significantly to the development and management of vascular health. Stress management techniques, such as yoga and mindfulness, have also been associated with lowering blood pressure and improved cardiovascular health. Furthermore, abstention from unhealthy behaviors like smoking and alcohol consumption is crucial since both tend to impair vascular function severely and lead to a high risk for vascular disease. Social support systems play a crucial role in reinforcing healthy habits, as individuals with support systems around them are more likely to adopt and maintain healthy lifestyle habits. Lastly, the management of both the physiological and psychosocial dimensions of health presents a general package for reducing the prevalence of vascular diseases and enhancing outcomes of health among populations (Livingston et al., 2020) (Figure 12.14).

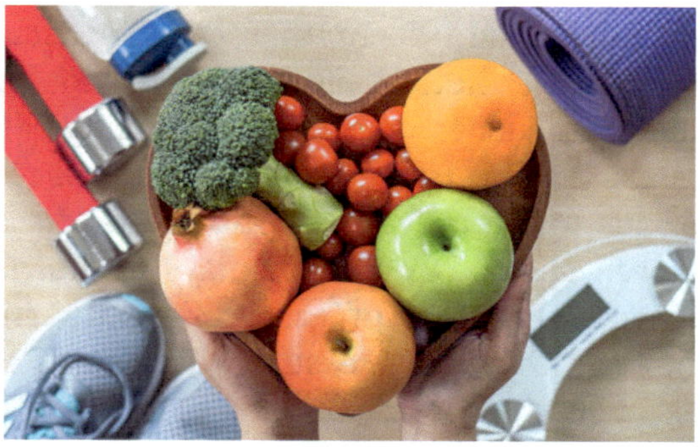

Figure 12.14. Healthy lifestyle choices for better vascular health.

Source: https://www.nps.org.au/assets/_750x468_crop_center-center_75_none/GettyImages-953674568.jpg.

12.5.2. Regular Health Screenings

Regular health checks constitute a foundation of preventive medicine, in particular towards vascular disease. The checks make it possible to identify probable vascular disease, such as hypertension, chronic kidney disease, and venous thrombosis, which can arise as a result of poor blood circulation. Prioritizing regular checks enables doctors to diagnose risk factors and vascular defects at early stages, prior to becoming a full-blown disease. With its advanced venous and arterial network in organs like the kidneys, it is crucial to monitor these systems closely. Consistent with the literature, renal vascular formations are responsible for generating severe clinical effects through disruptions in these formations, including chronic renal failure, and as such, constant health checkups as part of an effective public health plan (Akbaev et al., 2025). Moreover, regular medical screening provides access to advanced methods of diagnosis that enhance the accuracy of measurements. Angiography, ultrasound diagnostics, and MRI are among the techniques that play a major role in imaging and evaluating vascular integrity. Such equipment provides reliable information regarding the anatomical and topographic features of vascular structures, thus enabling health workers to detect changes representing vascular diseases in their early stages. Continuous evaluation and interaction between various vascular systems are needed to uncover latent pathologies. Highlighting the importance of detection in the screening process can significantly reduce morbidity and mortality due to vascular diseases and thus justify concerted health programs that advocate for regular screenings (Akbaev et al., 2025). In the health sector, the promotion of regular screening is essential, especially as age and lifestyle-related vascular disorders have been on the rise. Such programs promoting healthcare providers and the population at large regarding the need for such screenings can lead to improved health outcomes.

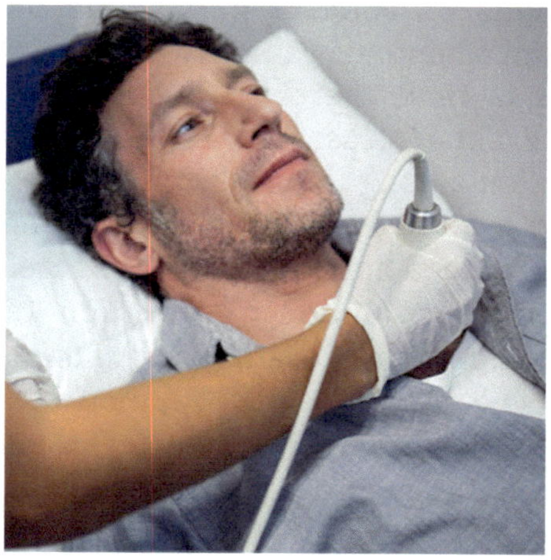

Figure 12.15. Vascular screening.

Source: https://www.summahealth.org/-/media/project/summahealth/website/page-content/flourish/4_30a_fl_vascularscreen_400x400.webp?la=en&h=400&w=400&hash=DB2F82BF3CD96C52FBF5B879932A9258.

A few of these programs could include adding routine screening programs for populations with a higher risk of vascular complications as part of the routine health programs. Strategic deployment of multi-dimensional screening measures, like in oral cancer assessment, can serve to identify vascular disease more efficiently and at earlier stages. Normalizing conventional health screening within healthcare systems has the potential to consolidate positive health control and thereby mitigate the long-term public health burden of vascular disease (Figure 12.15).

12.5.3. Education and Awareness Programs

Education and awareness programs are central interventions in the management of vascular disorders, impacting prevention and care strategies to a large extent. By raising public awareness of such conditions, education and awareness programs aim at educating people with the information necessary on risk factors, symptoms, and the importance of early diagnosis and treatment. For example, awareness programs for those at increased risk, including those with a family history of cardiovascular disorders, can bring about changes in behavior that support the preservation of vascular well-being. In addition, workshops that present lifestyle changes—dietary changes, exercise programs, and giving up smoking—can enable individuals to be in control of their health. Evidence indicates that extensive educational programs strongly increase health behavior scores among participants, leading to better health outcomes and reduced risks from vascular disorders (Sharifi et al., 2024). In addition to improving the health of individuals, awareness programs also play a critical role in building community resilience against vascular disorders. Communities benefit from efforts that integrate local health challenges with particular educational programs. With the co-operation of health professionals, schools, and civic organizations, these programs can adapt material to suit the specific needs of differing populations. For example, by combining cultural considerations and materials rendered available to such groups, participation rates among diverse groups may be enhanced. Socio-economic status barriers and language barriers, for example, could be overcome through tailored programming that maximizes access by such populations to essential information regarding vascular disorders. Increased social consciousness encourages personal responsibility and requires systemic changes in the availability of healthcare and healthcare resources toward creating a healthier and better-informed population. Additionally, the success of the awareness and educational programs can be measured by the extent to which they increase understanding of related health issues and ailments. Interventions for the management of co-morbidities associated with vascular disorders, such as diabetes and hypertension, can enhance participants' knowledge and attitudes towards disease management. For instance, educational interventions designed to modify lifestyles can enhance participants' knowledge regarding how lifestyle modification can decrease the risk of development of vascular disorders. Results of systematic research have shown a tremendous increase in knowledge and positive attitudes after exposure to such programs (Nelson et al., 2024). Observations indicate the importance of continued support and financing of education programs because not only do they enhance health literacy, but also prevent and effectively control vascular diseases both separately and at the community level.

SUMMARY

Finally, the study of vascular disorders highlights the intricate interaction of various risk factors and their role in the health of patients. From a meticulous investigation of the same, vascular disorders are not found to be singular incidents but interconnected variables that may ultimately lead to significant complications like dementia and other neurological conditions. The systematic critical review of recent research suggests that interventions such as Androgen Deprivation Therapy (ADT) do pose a risk for cognitive impairment. The findings from systematic reviews unequivocally point towards the necessity of further research into the development of interventions to effectively counteract the risks and enhance patient outcomes. As healthcare continues to develop, solving the intricacy of vascular diseases will be required to advance clinical practice as well as improve patient education and care. More so, the application of health-related quality of life (HRQL) assessments when dealing with vascular diseases cannot be overemphasized. Tools such as the SF-36, as well as PROMIS-29, provide rich data about the physical and emotional health of patients battling such illnesses. One key discovery is that patients' experiences of vascular disease are greater than mere physiological symptomatology, encompassing emotional and psychological components impacting their overall quality of life. Through the assumption of these standardized measures, clinicians can better quantify patient needs, tailor treatments, and ultimately improve health outcomes. Elucidation of the relationship between HRQL and traditional clinical endpoints can guide interventions that affect both the physiological and psychosocial aspects of patient care, in harmony with contemporary practices in holistic health care. Finally, research priorities need to be directed towards the convergence of vascular diseases with prevalent health disorders because comorbidities seriously complicate treatment and management protocols. The inclusion of evidence indicating that illnesses such as depression and dementia can be caused by vascular compromise is at the center of the need for a multidisciplinary approach in medicine. Integrative treatments that bring together cardiology, neurology, and mental health will provide more effective patient management. By learning more about these associations, scientists can determine underlying mechanisms and inform public health policy that supports preventive strategies. In essence, understanding vascular disease is a collective effort towards reconciling personal experience and general health patterns so that healthcare decisions in the future are in balance.

In the etiology of vascular illnesses, a sophisticated knowledge of the molecular pathways is crucial. Several such genes, crucially critical in the pathophysiology of such illnesses, have been implicated by recent research. Six of them, for instance, CLEC1B and GPR146, were the subject of sleep deprivation research that found them to play a role in critical biological processes such as DNA repair as well as immune response. These genes exhibit differential expression patterns that correlate with immune scores, which suggests their use as biomarkers for vascular dysfunction-related diseases. Research on these genes sheds light on the complex relationship between genetic elements and vascular health, which may be employed to create more accurate therapeutic interventions (Chen et al., 2025). Puncture management during hemodialysis is also an essential aspect of patient treatment for vascular access complications. Efficient techniques must be used to minimize complications and yield the most favorable outcomes for patients treated through arteriovenous fistula (AVF). To this end, an integration of systematic review evidence and clinical guidelines has yielded salient points for use while the puncture is being carried out. These include the timing of initial puncture, pre-puncture evaluation, and post-procedure management.

By employing evidence-based practices, medical professionals can ensure the maximum safety and efficacy of vascular access procedures and, consequently, directly impact patients' general treatment outcomes (Zhang et al., 2025). Lastly, the integration of immune response considerations into vascular disorder management is a vital field of research. Immune pathway dysregulation can worsen vascular diseases and, therefore, the study of the relevant genes is pertinent not just for diagnosis but also for therapeutic targets. Identification of some genes with immune pathways provides opportunities for designing treatments tailored to an individual patient's unique genetic background. Because the current literature increasingly emphasizes the relationship between immune function and vascular health, knowledge of such interactions is crucial to furthering clinical practice and optimizing patient prognosis with vascular disease (Chen et al., 2025).

A CLOSER LOOK

COMPLICATIONS OF VASCULAR DISORDERS

Complications secondary to vascular disease can have significant implications for patient outcome, particularly in patients with connective tissue disorders such as Ehlers-Danlos syndrome (EDS) and Marfan syndrome (MFS). Both of these conditions predispose them to catastrophic vascular events like aneurysms and dissections. In a recent study, it was identified that a high percentage of patients with such vascular connective tissue diseases experienced adverse vascular events, highlighting the fact that routine imaging follow-up is critical for the early detection and management of complications. What is surprising about the study is the emphasis on employing standardized imaging protocols for monitoring arterial diameter growth, as disease progression heterogeneity hinders effective monitoring of patients. Therefore, reducing the risk of vascular diseases in individuals with such demographics requires the implementation of well-documented guidelines for imaging modalities and surveillance intervals. Aside from connective tissue disorders, vascular complications have also been prevalent in metabolic disorders like diabetes. Diabetic patients present with high susceptibility to macrovascular and microvascular complications, where their risk mainly stems from the onset of advanced glycation end-products (AGEs) (Walter et al., 2024).

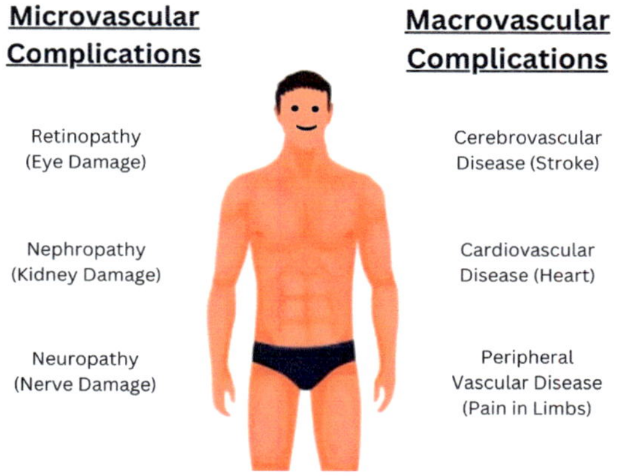

Figure 12.16. Types of Vascular Complications.

Source: https://aasayurveda.com/wp-content/uploads/2023/04/Microvascular-Complications.webp.

High levels of AGE have been associated with the formation of vascular complications in diabetic patients and have proved to be strongly correlated with poor vascular status at high levels of AGE. Another study assessing serum AGE levels showed that complicated diabetics had very high levels of AGE when compared to uncomplicated diabetics. This suggests that monitoring of AGE levels in patients can be a critical indicator of vascular health and risk stratification, ultimately providing for more goal-directed treatment approaches in the therapy of vascular disease (Kato et al., 2024). In addition to the physical health consequences, the effects of vascular complications extend to more general psychological and economic influences on the patient and the healthcare system.

The recurrent threat of vascular events can lead to anxiety, depression, and decreased quality of life, which mandates that health care practitioners adopt holistic care strategies that address both the patients' physical and psychological needs. The cost to the medical system associated with frequent visits, imaging tests, and potential interventions also imposes a significant strain on health resources. Therefore, an integrated strategy that incorporates preventive care, psychological therapy, and economical use of resources is the key to addressing the complexity of vascular disease and complications (Figure 12.16).

References

1. Akbaev, S., Lechiev, Z. U., & Kafarov, E. (2025). Topographic-anatomical relationships of the arterial and venous beds of the kidneys. *City Healthcare*. https://www.semanticscholar.org/paper/82a07c569faab082f19fb5f08fd8868ee663a2ce (accessed on 29th May 2025).
2. Al-Khayri, J. M., Sahana, G. R., Nagella, P., Joseph, B. V., Alessa, F. M., & Al-Mssallem, M. Q. (2022). Flavonoids as Potential Anti-Inflammatory Molecules: A review. *Molecules*, *27*(9), 2901. https://doi.org/10.3390/molecules27092901Althumairy, A., Alyami, J. M. H., Alyami, A. M., Al Abduljabbar, R. M., Alfawaz, N. M., & Khbrani, A. H. (2024). Oral cancer screening in geriatrics: Importance, tools, and outcomes. *Journal of Healthcare Sciences*. https://www.semanticscholar.org/paper/ac06ca6d05d50ce6d90c3ecebd9a37644c14d718 (accessed on 29th May 2025).
3. Azi, C. I., Carsrud, N. D. V., DelGiodice, M. J., Egli, et al. (2024). The multisystem impact of *Pseudoxanthoma elasticum* (PXE): Systemic manifestations, multidisciplinary management, and diagnostic and therapeutic advances. *Eur. J. Med. Health Res.* https://core.ac.uk/download/621451766.pdf (accessed on 29th May 2025).
4. Boukdir, A., Ballouk, H., Khallouk, A., Rhaouti, A., Bahetta, S., & Toufiq, J. (2025). Psychosis and venous thromboembolism: A clinical analysis and literature review. *Scholars Journal of Medical Case Reports*. https://www.semanticscholar.org/paper/a11342d345f86a1853837dc33cea964fbeb93b2c (accessed on 29th May 2025).
5. Burley, N., Dy, P. S., Kalantri, S., & Razzaq, K. (2021). Aortic thrombosis and acute limb ischemia secondary to COVID hypercoagulability. *Cureus*. https://doi.org/10.7759/cureus.16171 (accessed on 29th May 2025).
6. Cantador, A. A., & Guillaumon, A. T. (2024). Comparison between vascular Doppler ultrasound and contrast exams in chronic peripheral arterial disease. *Jornal Vascular Brasileiro*, *23*. https://www.semanticscholar.org/paper/07a6f4085854a0827550005408b1175173bda26d (accessed on 29th May 2025).
7. Chen, J., Hou, J., Chen, X., Fan, W., & Sun, P. (2025). Identifying key genes for neurobehavioral disorders caused by long-term sleep deprivation. *Current Analytical Chemistry*. https://www.semanticscholar.org/paper/226aaea61497554fdc3e4ec669387aa3c0f2d43c (accessed on 29th May 2025).
8. De Maeseneer, M., Kakkos, S. K., Aherne, T., Bækgaard, N., Black, S., Blomgren, L., Giannoukas, A., et al. (2022). Editor's choice – European Society for Vascular Surgery (ESVS) 2022 clinical practice guidelines on the management of chronic venous disease of the lower limbs. *European Journal of Vascular and Endovascular Surgery*, *63*, 184–267. https://doi.org/10.1016/j.ejvs.2021.12.024 (accessed on 29th May 2025).
9. Gholamalizadeh, H., Ensan, B., Karav, S., Jamialahmadi, T., & Sahebkar, A. (2024). Regulatory effects of statins on CCL2/CCR2 axis in cardiovascular diseases: New insight into pleiotropic effects of statins. *Journal of Inflammation (London, England)*, *21*. https://www.semanticscholar.org/paper/c2fe1c9005bf48f7e54f64d95219a8e2845c6ff6 (accessed on 29th May 2025).
10. Gopan, Y., & Kamath, S. T. (2024). *Ayurvedic Management of Dyslipidemia – A Conceptual Analysis*. https://www.semanticscholar.org/paper/2e998fd21bde767571efc777c786e40318e6c2f1 (accessed on 29th May 2025).

11. Hachinski, V., Krishnamoorthy, E., Kuey, L., & Kirmayer, L. J. (2023). Brain health and mental health: Common vascular risk factors and practical implications. *Alzheimer's & Dementia, 19*, 4248–4251. https://www.semanticscholar.org/paper/9d17d81df2715e72c4eea6e06363000fb37ddfe0 (accessed on 29th May 2025).

12. Halvorsen, S., Mehilli, J., Cassese, S., Hall, T. S., Abdelhamid, M., Barbato, E., De Hert, S., et al. (2022). 2022 ESC guidelines on cardiovascular assessment and management of patients undergoing non-cardiac surgery. *European Heart Journal, 43*, 3826–3924. https://doi.org/10.1093/eurheartj/ehac270 (accessed on 29th May 2025).

13. Han, J., Yoon, I., & Jeon, H. J. (2024). Microfluidic system-based quantitative analysis of platelet function through speckle size measurement. *Biomolecules, 14*. https://www.semanticscholar.org/paper/a26c86b0fea0fde3dcd2887ff05c30b2b337bd9f (accessed on 29th May 2025).

14. Harale, A. M., Bairagi, V. K., Boonchieng, E., & Bachute, M. (2024). Nodules detection in lungs CT images using improved YOLOv5 and classification of types of nodules by CNN-SVM. *IEEE Access, 12*, 140456–140471. https://www.semanticscholar.org/paper/038a12f507da9ac44aabea02120a900b0210a8e7 (accessed on 29th May 2025).

15. Haseeb, S., Qureshi, M. A., Ahmed, O., Munir, S., Siddiqui, T., Gehres, E., Zaman, M., et al. (2024). Abstract 4145052: Impact of postprocedural delirium on inpatient outcomes in transcatheter aortic valve replacement patients: A retrospective propensity matched analysis. *Circulation*. https://www.semanticscholar.org/paper/062fc2b217a04e240ba97ff0fb7b25e8bf1cab8a (accessed on 29th May 2025).

16. Hayes, S. N., Kim, E., Saw, J., Adlam, D., Arslanian-Engoren, C., Economy, K. E., Ganesh, S. K., et al. (2018). Spontaneous coronary artery dissection: Current state of the science: A scientific statement from the American Heart Association. *Circulation, 137*. https://doi.org/10.1161/cir.0000000000000564 (accessed on 29th May 2025).

17. Hezam, A. A. M., Shaghdar, H. B. M., & Chen, L. (2024). The connection between hypertension and diabetes and their role in heart and kidney disease development. *Journal of Research in Medical Sciences: The Official Journal of Isfahan University of Medical Sciences, 29*. https://www.semanticscholar.org/paper/fb456f8beed4d28639be950191349f3f2dfcbd77 (accessed on 29th May 2025).

18. Hinojosa-González, D., Zafar, A., Saffati, G., Kronstedt, S., Zlatev, D. V., & Khera, M. (2024). Androgen deprivation therapy for prostate cancer and neurocognitive disorders: A systematic review and meta-analysis. *Prostate Cancer and Prostatic Diseases*. https://www.semanticscholar.org/paper/3f978ad93f995d7c90257de8290b67f69d87542d (accessed on 29th May 2025).

19. Hurndall, K. H., Leatherby, R., Tai, N., Davenport, R., & Glasgow, S. (2024). O64: Aortic trauma in the UK (UK): Vascular interventions and surgery in trauma audit (VISTA). *British Journal of Surgery*. https://www.semanticscholar.org/paper/b78893ae1ddb18a19b3f584a9b2386964ea08e33 (accessed on 29th May 2025).

20. Jayasinghe, M., Rashidi, F., Gadelmawla, A., Rissardo, J. P., Rashidi, M., Elendu, C. C., Caprara, A. L. F., et al. (2025). Neurological manifestations of systemic lupus erythematosus: A comprehensive review. *Cureus, 17*. https://www.semanticscholar.org/paper/08cc8ddf8bd527cc26f1e309bbd6273d7b63df55 (accessed on 29th May 2025).

21. Kato, S., Matsumura, T., Sugawa, H., & Nagai, R. (2024). Correlation between serum advanced glycation end-products and vascular complications in patient with type 2 diabetes. *Scientific*

Reports, 14. https://www.semanticscholar.org/paper/9a5b17c7a1c154ac9fe8edda64a8b1b8e78415c0 (accessed on 29th May 2025).

22. Kirsten, N., Mohr, N., Gensel, F., Alhumam, A., Bruning, G., & Augustin, M. (2021). Population-based epidemiologic study in venous diseases in Germany – Prevalence, comorbidity, and medical needs in a cohort of 19,104 workers. *Vascular Health and Risk Management, 17,* 679–687. https://www.semanticscholar.org/paper/2a67e42ef2eee086eba22ecc01a22a57aafe2da7 (accessed on 29th May 2025).

23. Krishnan, A., & Desai, P. (2024). Venous thromboembolism (VTE) in May-Thurner syndrome: Decision-making related to long-term anticoagulation. *Cureus, 16.* https://www.semanticscholar.org/paper/1d14faaf90740dc6539d034f0fba669509fce142 (accessed on 29th May 2025).

24. Kulkarni, C. A., Joshi, R., Katariya, I., & Palekar, T. J. (2024). A scoping review of influence of lifestyle factors on menstrual disorders in menstruating women. *The Scientific Temper.* https://www.semanticscholar.org/paper/c236c74dc67c53ddee7a4967bf8890613884dbc5 (accessed on 29th May 2025).

25. Liegl, G., Fischer, F. H., Martin, C. N., Rönnefarth, M., Blumrich, A., Ahmadi, M., Boldt, L. H., et al. (2024). Converting PROMIS®-29 v2.0 profile data to SF-36 physical and mental component summary scores in patients with cardiovascular disorders. *Health and Quality of Life Outcomes, 22.* https://www.semanticscholar.org/paper/44b1bab0cc7e5370cf4bdb45d108b249cbfed128 (accessed on 29th May 2025).

26. Lin, H. J., Chen, C. H., Su, M. W., Lin, C. W., Cheng, Y. W., Tang, S. C., & Jeng, J. (2023). Modifiable vascular risk factors contribute to stroke in 1080 *NOTCH3 R544C* carriers in Taiwan Biobank. *International Journal of Stroke, 19*, 105–113. https://www.semanticscholar.org/paper/3def312f9eedeabc3329b5d422ff0a5ef2457375 (accessed on 29th May 2025).

27. Livingston, G., Huntley, J., Sommerlad, A., Ames, D., Ballard, C., Banerjee, S., Brayne, C., et al. (2020). Dementia prevention, intervention, and care: 2020 report of the Lancet Commission. *The Lancet, 396*, 413–446. https://doi.org/10.1016/s0140-6736(20)30367-6 (accessed on 29th May 2025).

28. Mach, F., Baigent, C., Catapano, A. L., Koskinas, K. C., Casula, M., Badimón, L., Chapman, M. J., et al. (2019). 2019 ESC/EAS guidelines for the management of dyslipidemias: Lipid modification to reduce cardiovascular risk. *European Heart Journal, 41*, 111–188. https://doi.org/10.1093/eurheartj/ehz455 (accessed on 29th May 2025).

29. Manolis, A., Manolis, T. A., & Manolis, A. (2024). Current strategies for atrial fibrillation prevention and management: Taming the commonest cardiac arrhythmia. *Current Vascular Pharmacology.* https://www.semanticscholar.org/paper/146afe9df3dec2d27d5da379398db667be40b6fa (accessed on 29th May 2025).

30. Measar, M., & Alyahawi, A. (2024). The anticoagulation strategies for management and prevention of stroke in neurological practice. *Universal Journal of Pharmaceutical Research.* https://www.semanticscholar.org/paper/a48e8404b248f58f4a26e1bb8131b1ce689dd0c1 (accessed on 29th May 2025).

31. Mosina, A. A. (2025). Pleiotropic effects of statins in the framework of pharmacotherapy of metabolic disorders. *Bulletin "Biomedicine and Sociology."* https://www.semanticscholar.org/paper/71636a0b4a74c7e08150ca239fdce11a06aad7d3 (accessed on 29th May 2025).

32. N/A. (2021). *New Insight Into Cerebrovascular Diseases.* https://core.ac.uk/download/478129871.pdf (accessed on 29th May 2025).

33. Nelson, A. V., Desai, S., Rajashekharayya, C. K., Rathod, L., & Bhatangunaki, H. (2024). A study to evaluate the effectiveness of planned educational program on knowledge and attitude regarding psychosocial problems of eating disorders among adolescent girls studying in selected P.U colleges at Vijayapur. *International Journal of Community Medicine and Public Health.* https://www.semanticscholar.org/paper/d4f5454062c33c43f14106c74702a36aa4d03626 (accessed on 29th May 2025).

34. Neuenschwander, J., Sebastian, T., Barco, S., Spirk, D., & Kucher, N. (2022). A novel management strategy for treatment of pelvic venous disorders utilizing a clinical screening score and non-invasive imaging. *VASA. Zeitschrift für Gefäßkrankheiten.* https://www.semanticscholar.org/paper/13e2c4004e51ba000b985bfd8d8df35da426ef5e (accessed on 29th May 2025).

35. Oyinloye, O. D., Abiona, O. A., & Abiona, S. O. (2024). The impact of lifestyle factors on reproductive performance in the general population in Ede Local Government Area, Osun State. *International Journal of Research and Innovation in Social Science.* https://www.semanticscholar.org/paper/78047e880ec2944360c8ffd9a827604fcc05a321 (accessed on 29th May 2025).

36. Palomo-Toucedo, I. C., Reina-Bueno, M., Munuera-Martínez, P. V., Vázquez-Bautista, M. Del. C., Domínguez-Maldonado, G., & Leon-Larios, F. (2024). Self-perception of physical problems in patients with non-vascular type of Ehlers–Danlos syndrome: A qualitative study. *Healthcare, 12.* https://www.semanticscholar.org/paper/d8c64a2485f948364b9b32254c91fc9408849b5d (accessed on 29th May 2025).

37. Pankova, M. N. (2024). Obesity and anticontractile effects of adipose tissue in the regulation of aortic tone. *Timiryazev Biological Journal.* https://www.semanticscholar.org/paper/10fdaf6269b719d5e668dcb3404c707be7214f0d (accessed on 29th May 2025).

38. Sadchikov, D., & Elyutin, D. V. (2021). Peculiarities of hemodynamics in gestosis. *Kazan Medical Journal.* https://www.semanticscholar.org/paper/6df9d27cdd3017adf496b962d1753c3ab2600574 (accessed on 29th May 2025).

39. Sehar, A., Ashraf, R., Fatima, M., Akhtar, U., Saeed, F., & Sibtain, M. (2025). Comparison between Doppler ultrasound and computed tomography angiography in the diagnosis of peripheral vascular disease in different age groups. *Insights–Journal of Health and Rehabilitation.* https://www.semanticscholar.org/paper/7c503052297088435260ed124547da245aab3ca6 (accessed on 29th May 2025).

40. Sharifi, E., Ghelbash, Z., Karami, A., & Musarezaie, A. (2024). Effects of a comprehensive educational program on health behaviors and awareness of HIV, hepatitis B, and hepatitis C in men with substance use disorders. *Middle East Current Psychiatry.* https://www.semanticscholar.org/paper/4143bbc5832d63ddb9ffd6ac4ce7ed85febaf4d0 (accessed on 29th May 2025).

41. Shayor, A. A., Kabir, M. E., Rifath, M. S. A., Rashid, A., & Oh, K. W. (2024). A synergistic overview between microfluidics and numerical research for vascular flow and pathological investigations. *Sensors (Basel, Switzerland), 24.* https://www.semanticscholar.org/paper/a38d422a28eceab5d485aaadf43f5d1edd1e3269 (accessed on 29th May 2025).

42. Solovey, S. P. (2021). Angina without obstructive lesion coronary arteries (Part 1). Pathophysiological aspects of development. *Emergency Cardiology and Cardiovascular Risks*. https://www.semanticscholar.org/paper/ea9de8814eeab51fda52ff43682842fa4a2d78af (accessed on 29th May 2025).

43. Stacy, M. R. (2022). Molecular imaging of lower extremity peripheral arterial disease: An emerging field in nuclear medicine. *Frontiers in Medicine, 8*. https://doi.org/10.3389/fmed.2021.793975 (accessed on 29th May 2025).

44. Taha, H. B., Yacoub, F., Morris, A., & Birnbaum, A. (2024). Extracellular vesicles for the diagnosis of Alzheimer's disease and related dementias: A diagnostic accuracy meta-analysis. *Alzheimer's & Dementia, 20*. https://www.semanticscholar.org/paper/e095a23c638a717244339206263d578cfb9d5c04 (accessed on 29th May 2025).

45. Visseren, F. L. J., Mach, F., Smulders, Y. M., Carballo, D., Koskinas, K. C., Bäck, M., Bénétos, A., et al. (2021). 2021 ESC guidelines on cardiovascular disease prevention in clinical practice. *European Heart Journal, 42*, 3227–3337. https://doi.org/10.1093/eurheartj/ehab484 (accessed on 29th May 2025).

46. Walter, C., Leinweber, M. E., Mlekusch, I., Assadian, A., & Hofmann, A. (2024). Temporal pattern analysis of ultrasound surveillance data in vascular connective tissue disorders. *Diagnostics, 14*. https://www.semanticscholar.org/paper/b45da35995b66ec9baf86d409887108947befcf8 (accessed on 29th May 2025).

47. Whelton, P. K., Carey, R. M., Aronow, W. S., Casey, D. E., Collins, K. J., Himmelfarb, C. D., DePalma, S. M., et al. (2017). 2017 ACC/AHA/AAPA/ABC/ACPM/AGS/APhA/ASH/ASPC/NMA/PCNA guideline for the prevention, detection, evaluation, and management of high blood pressure in adults: A report of the American College of Cardiology/American Heart Association Task Force on Clinical Practice Guidelines. *Hypertension, 71*. https://doi.org/10.1161/hyp.0000000000000065 (accessed on 29th May 2025).

48. Wilde, A. A. M., Semsarian, C., Márquez, M. F., Sepehri, S. A., Ackerman, M. J., Ashley, E. A., Sternick, E. B., et al. (2022). European Heart Rhythm Association (EHRA)/Heart Rhythm Society (HRS)/Asia Pacific Heart Rhythm Society (APHRS)/Latin American Heart Rhythm Society (LAHRS) expert consensus statement on the state of genetic testing for cardiac diseases. *Heart Rhythm, 19*, e1–e60. https://doi.org/10.1016/j.hrthm.2022.03.1225 (accessed on 29th May 2025).

49. Zhang, X., Liu, J., Wang, J., Ma, T., & Zhang, H. (2025). Summary of the best evidence for puncture management during the early stage of autologous arteriovenous fistula in maintenance hemodialysis patients. *Journal of Clinical and Nursing Research*. https://www.semanticscholar.org/paper/40adcd7f71385a5c09f075f24cfe4610bb79aa54 (accessed on 29th May 2025).

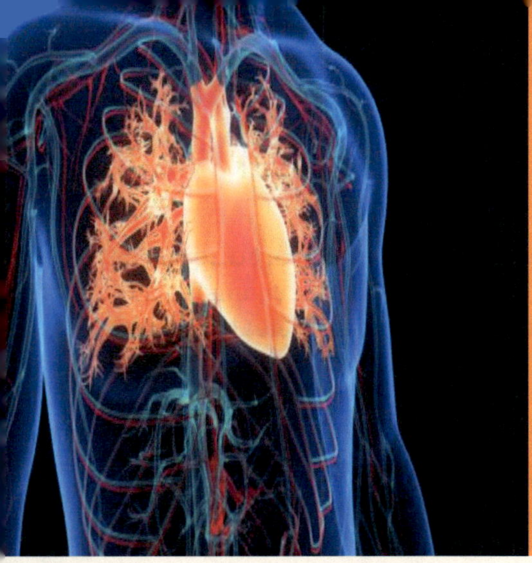

Chapter 13

PULMONARY HEART DISEASE

Contents

Introduction

Pulmonary heart disease, or cor pulmonale, is a severe condition where the right ventricle is enlarged and fails as a result of pulmonary hypertension. It usually develops from chronic respiratory disease, including chronic obstructive pulmonary disease (COPD) and pulmonary hypertension, resulting in decreased oxygenation of the blood. The condition is not only prognostic of significant morbidity and mortality but also reflective of severe issues in the treatment and management. With over 11% of pulmonary artery hypertension (PAH) conditions being related to congenital heart disease, patient outcomes are grave, and united efforts are needed in the optimization of understanding and intervention strategies in such cases (Wu et al., 2024). The complexity of pulmonary heart disease necessitates multi-dimensional analysis in the course of its research because different etiologic factors necessitate personalized therapeutic programs. Recent research has highlighted the importance of evidence-based therapy, particularly with proprietary Chinese medicines, which have been proven to possess promise in the management of chronic pulmonary heart disease (CPHD). A systematic review reported that, during the past decade, there has been a discouraging downward trend in published evidence for treatment effectiveness, pointing to the imperative of large-scale clinical studies (Wu et al., 2024). Most trials have focused on symptomatic treatment, with an acute lack of effort on overall outcome measures, including quality of life and extended prognosis. The diversified approaches to management and therapy of pulmonary heart disease reflect the pressing need for well-regimented guidelines and uniform practice patterns. Current evidence suggests that a blend of both local and modern therapeutic maneuvers is likely to lead to better clinical outcomes. For instance, physical exercise therapy is helpful when used in addition to traditional pharmacotherapy in enhancing functional capacity, thereby improving the quality of life in patients (Pratiwi et al., 2023). To design an effective management paradigm for pulmonary heart disease, further research must be conducted to identify promising therapeutic avenues and confirm that clinical practice is underpinned by strong evidence supporting outstanding patient outcomes (Figure 13.1).

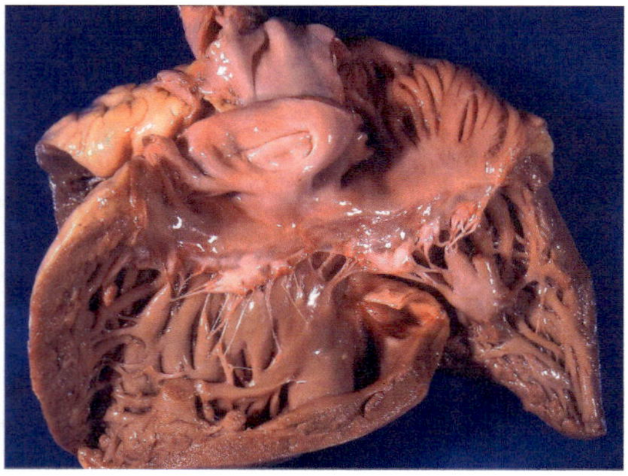

Figure 13.1. Pulmonary heart disease.

Source: https://upload.wikimedia.org/wikipedia/commons/9/93/Heart_-_cor_pulmonale-_right_ventricular_hypertrophy_%284351912426%29.jpg.

Definition of Pulmonary Heart Disease

It is crucial to know pulmonary heart disease, or cor pulmonale, in realizing its mechanisms and clinical implications. Pulmonary heart disease occurs through the transformation of the right ventricle of the heart, which is both enlarged and weakened by chronic lung disease. COPD is one of the leading precipitating causes of pulmonary heart disease because ongoing hypoxia raises pulmonary artery pressure, which overloads the right heart. The progressive nature of this association soon results in right ventricular failure if not attended to. Thus, believing in the definition of pulmonary heart disease as a complication of respiratory diseases is vital for early detection and treatment that would have a very positive effect on patients' health status. Diagnosis of pulmonary heart disease calls for a detailed assessment of the patient's clinical history and current health status. The clinicians utilize a range of diagnostic examinations, such as echocardiograms, to evaluate the structure and function of the right ventricle and the pulmonary artery pressures. It also aids in understanding the nature of the exacerbation, such as those explained in COPD exacerbations, to determine the onset and course of pulmonary heart diseases. The acute worsening of respiratory symptoms must be ascribed to potential right heart stress, emphasizing the importance of thorough evaluation of those with chronic pulmonary disease. On top of that, adding objective measures, such as blood counts and other biomarkers, enhances diagnostic accuracy, facilitating an individualized management approach for those with pulmonary heart disease (MacLeod et al., 2021). The complexity of pulmonary heart disease persists in pulmonary heart disease treatment and management. Traditional approaches are symptom-oriented in addressing the ancillary symptoms of the underlying lung disease with retention of global cardiac support. Future research suggests the need for disease-specific therapy that intervenes against the involved inflammatory pathways driving the disease progression. Available evidence suggests that starting pharmacologic treatments and lifestyle interventions will effectively cure pulmonary heart disease and its complications. Second, treating comorbid disease, such as heart failure, establishes an integrative strategy that reduces the overall disease burden (Palazzuoli et al., 2021). Understanding their interaction becomes critical in developing treatment plans that improve patient quality of life and reduce the likelihood of adverse outcomes (Figure 13.2).

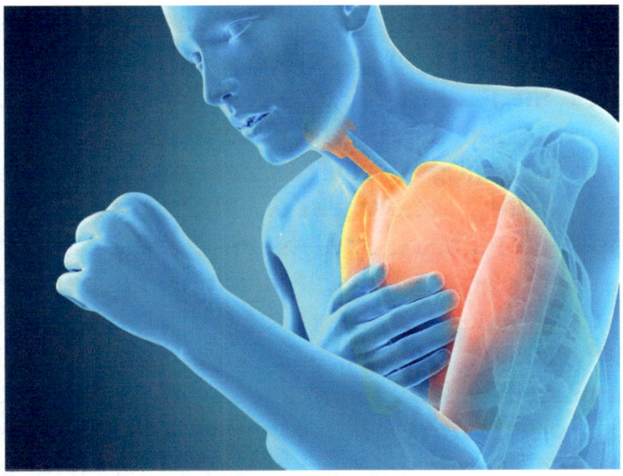

Figure 13.2. Understanding Pulmonary Heart Disease.

Source: https://www.heart.org/en/-/media/Images/News/2018/October-2018/1002CACCOPD_SC.jpg?sc_lang=en.

13.1. Anatomy and Physiology of the Heart

The anatomy and physiology of the heart provide a foundation to understand various cardiovascular diseases, such as pulmonary heart disease, which is specifically aimed at the right side of the heart. The heart consists of four chambers: the left and right atria and the left and right ventricles, with valves allowing blood flow in one direction. Blood returns to the right atrium, passes through the tricuspid valve to the right ventricle, and is pumped out to the lungs in the pulmonary arteries. This pathway is necessary for oxygenation, where carbon dioxide can be expelled and oxygen taken in. Interference with this cycle, whether from structural malformations or functional malformations, may lead to elevated right heart pressure and stress that results in pulmonary heart disease, whereby the right ventricle is exposed to elevated workload owing to dysfunctional pulmonary circulation (Grech et al., 1999). The physiological aspects of the operation of the heart, that is, the cardiac cycle, play a significant role in achieving efficient circulation. At systole, the heart muscle contracts to pump blood out of the ventricles; in diastole, the muscles relax to allow the chambers to fill with blood. Such a rhythm of contraction and relaxation is required for optimal blood flow and pressure regulation in the body. Blood diseases such as pulmonary hypertension result in heightened pulmonary arterial resistance, and this results in right ventricular hypertrophy as the heart tries to overcome high pressures. The resulting alterations in heart function and structure reflect the significance of appreciating anatomical relationships in the heart since their disregard can trigger or worsen pulmonary heart diseases (Kitsiou et al., 2013). In addition, the interrelationship between the heart's anatomy and physiology reflects the essential interaction among different cardiovascular components. Not only does the right heart circulate deoxygenated blood to the lungs, but it is also reliant upon pulmonary veins and arteries, which are involved in gas exchange and overall cardiovascular function. When the right ventricle gets overwhelmed, this reflects a systemic issue that may include pulmonary disease, having secondary effects such as right-sided heart failure. A detailed understanding of the anatomy of the heart allows medical specialists to diagnose and treat pulmonary heart disease successfully, tailoring interventions to address the associated physiological dysfunctions along with any resultant anatomical abnormalities. Such an integrated approach enhances the quality of care and optimizes patient outcomes because it recognizes the heart's critical role of sustaining life through adequate circulation (Grech et al., 1999) (Figure 13.3).

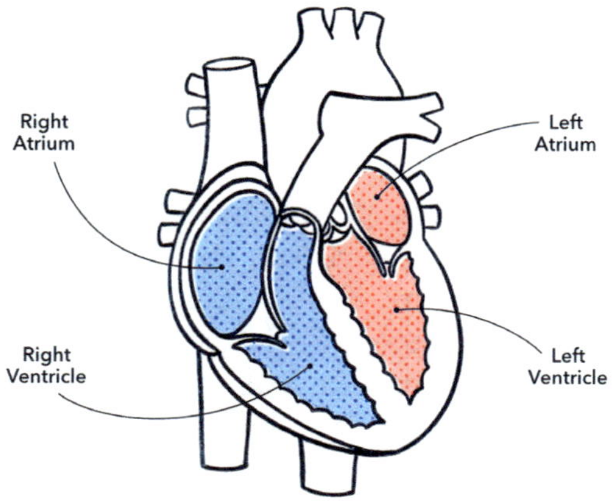

Figure 13.3. Anatomy and physiology of the human heart.

Source: https://www.pocketprep.com/wp-content/uploads/2021/03/Anatomy-and-Physiology-of-the-Human-Heart_post-image-inline.jpg.

13.1.1. Structure of the Heart

The structure of the heart is a highly structured system that includes four chambers: the right atrium, the left atrium, the right ventricle, and the left ventricle. All of these work together, receiving and pumping blood throughout the body. The right atrium receives deoxygenated blood from the body via the superior and inferior vena cavae. It relays it to the right ventricle, which ejects the blood to the lungs via the pulmonary arteries to be oxygenated. The left heart, by contrast, receives oxygen-rich blood from the lungs via the pulmonary veins to allow the left atrium to fill before relaying to the left ventricle. The thick muscular walls of the ventricles are crucial in generating the pressure required to pump blood adequately, which is a fundamental aspect of cardiac structure necessary for maintaining systemic circulation with the accompaniment of pulmonary heart disease. Both the function and structure of the heart may be significantly altered in patients with pulmonary heart disease. This state typically follows chronic overloading of the pulmonary circulation from continuous pressure, which causes right ventricular hypertrophy as it attempts to compensate for the increased resistance to blood flow. Ultimately, the long-term strain can cause right heart failure, disrupting the heart's normal anatomical structure. Not only does this disrupt the right ventricles' proper pumping, but it may even affect the left heart due to the interdependence of the right and left ventricles. Accurate understanding of such structural changes is vital in the development of effective treatment modalities since they highlight the associations between pulmonary circulation and cardiac dysfunction. According to the ISUOG guidelines, these congenital and acquired abnormalities are discussed, which enhances the overall treatment of such cardiovascular complications, thereby enhancing outcomes for patients (Carvalho et al., 2023).

Monitoring structural heart integrity using sensoring is crucial when monitoring persons at risk of pulmonary heart disease. Methods such as echocardiography are a focus of the assessment of cardiac structure, facilitating imaging of dimensions of chambers, thickness of walls, and blood flow dynamics. Non-invasive imaging techniques further contribute to diagnostic capability, providing clues about the presence of structural abnormalities that could result in cardiovascular sequelae in patients. Preventive screening is promoted to identify conditions such as right ventricular dilation or wall motion abnormalities that, if detected early, could steer particular interventions. As outlined in recent guidelines of practice, the use of echocardiographic assessment as part of routine prenatal screening represents a growing acknowledgment of the importance of structural analysis in facilitating an appreciation of risk associated with cardiac malformations and eventually lowering the burden of pulmonary heart disease in affected individuals (Vahanian et al., 2021) (Figure 13.4).

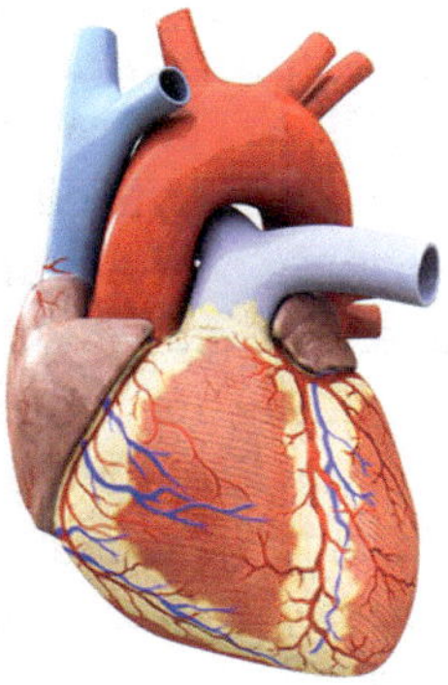

Figure 13.4. Structure of the Heart.

Source: https://onlinesciencenotes.com/wp-content/uploads/2017/09/heart-human.jpg.

13.1.2. Function of the Right Ventricle

The right ventricle is responsible for moving deoxygenated blood from the heart to the lungs to get oxygen. The chamber receives blood from the right atrium and pumps it into the pulmonary arteries through the pulmonary valve by contracting. In healthy conditions, the right ventricle operates under lower pressure compared to the left ventricle, which works with oxygenated blood that will make its way into systemic circulation. Under pathologic conditions such as pulmonary heart disease, the right ventricle may experience a higher workload from elevated pulmonary pressure. This high blood pressure condition can lead to right ventricular hypertrophy, weakening its effectiveness and, at times, progressing to right-sided heart failure if not treated, highlighting the significance of this chamber in achieving quality cardiopulmonary function. Novel evidence has been putting a focus on genetic factors affecting the right ventricle's proper functioning, particularly in individuals suffering from diseases like diabetes. A recent report found diabetes to be a major independent genetic risk factor for elevated pulmonary pressure and reduced right ventricular function.

Through the use of integrated electronic health records, scientists found a significant association between genetic susceptibility to diabetes and worsening right ventricular load stress. This emphasizes the importance of specific interventions targeting these genetic risks, as treating diabetes can positively affect right ventricular function and general pulmonary health. Identification of these correlations allows healthcare professionals to adopt a more personalized strategy in the treatment of pulmonary heart disease and in taking preventive actions according to the genetic make-up of the patient (Bagheri et al., 2023). Therapeutic advances have also been seen to be beneficial in improving right ventricular function, particularly among heart failure patients. For instance, sacubitril/valsartan therapy has been empirically linked to enhanced right ventricular performance and reduced pulmonary hypertension. Clinical meta-analyses indicate that therapies using this agent consistently increase measures such as tricuspid annular plane systolic excursion and tricuspid annular peak systolic velocity, markers of right ventricular efficiency. Furthermore, these treatments transfer essential benefits to the right ventricle and entire heart anatomy, suggesting a complicated interaction between the left and right chamber while under therapy. Thus, the role of the right ventricle is even more pivotal in pulmonary heart disease, where, with specific therapies, functional improvement is possible and can reverse the heart failure process (Zhang et al., 2022) (Figure 13.5).

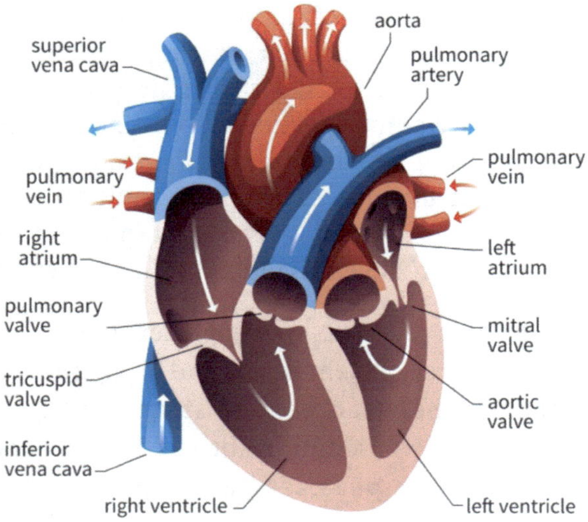

Figure 13.5. The Function of the Heart Ventricles.

Source: https://www.thoughtco.com/thmb/iyctF-drsw6xgSR-ruu7h9AC4Tw=/1500x0/filters:no_upscale():max_bytes(150000):strip_icc()/heart_cross-section-57ed79845f9b586c3512474e.jpg

13.1.3. Role of the Pulmonary Circulation

Pulmonary circulation is a vital component of the cardiovascular system, providing unique physiological functions that are vital for overall cardiovascular well-being. The deoxygenated blood is circulated from the right heart to the lungs by this circuit and subjected to the exchange of gases. Carbon dioxide is exhaled in the lungs, and oxygen is absorbed into the circulation, so oxygenated blood can be made for return to the left heart to be pumped to the body. Dysfunction or failure of this circuit may lead to pulmonary heart disease (cor pulmonale), an etiologically diverse condition of increased pulmonary artery pressure, including chronic obstructive pulmonary disease (COPD) and pulmonary hypertension. It is essential to know the fundamental role of pulmonary circulation in comprehending how such conditions develop and how the heart function gets impacted in turn, thereby justifying the interdependence of pulmonary and cardiac wellness. The relationship between pulmonary circulation and the heart is also compounded by all the risk factors that make people susceptible to pulmonary heart disease. In regions such as China, where cardiovascular disease is a leading cause of death, these connections must be recognized. Hypertension, high cholesterol, diabetes, and other metabolic syndromes overburden pulmonary circulation, ultimately leading to right ventricular failure (The Writing Committee of the Report on Cardiovascular in China et al., 2023). When lung vessels are damaged or blocked, it causes an extra workload on the right ventricle, making its job to pump blood increasingly complex. Preventive measures that can prevent risk factors become obligatory in order to counteract the extra workload on the pulmonary and cardiovascular systems. These measures can initiate awareness and timely intervention in high-risk patients for developing these interdependent pathologies. Advances in our understanding of pulmonary circulation also necessitate a thorough examination of the pathology of pulmonary heart disease, specifically sudden cardiac death. While as intricate as the etiology of sudden cardiac death is, recent correlations have been found to pulmonary hypertension and its associated effects on the cardiac configurations. There are new diagnostic measures in place that allow improved detection of underlying conditions in SCD (Basso et al., 2017). Knowing this is important because pathologists and cardiovascular healthcare professionals collaborate to generate guidelines that will standardize diagnosis and improve patient outcomes. Multidisciplinary groups with cardiologists, geneticists, and pathologists are required to evolve to undertake the effective screening and prevention measures with a focus not only on treatment but also on identifying emerging patterns of diseases that affect both pulmonary circulation and overall cardiac health (Figure 13.6).

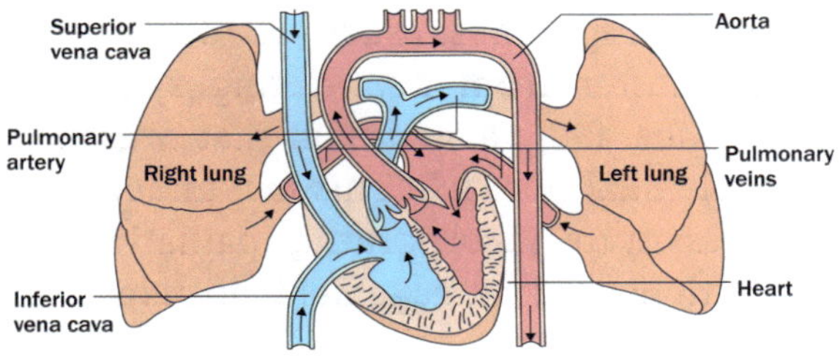

Figure 13.6. Pulmonary circulation.

Source: https://encrypted-tbn0.gstatic.com/images?q=tbn:ANd9GcTTzDO_2zTnNf3CzewnNQ6PADmuiBPcF9AgKw&s.

13.2. Causes of Pulmonary Heart Disease

Among the many determinants of pulmonary heart disease, a major one is COPD. COPD is characterized by chronic airflow limitation secondary to inflammatory changes in the lungs, typically following prolonged exposure to noxious gases and particles such as tobacco smoke and ambient air pollution. The resultant chronic inflammation will cause vascular changes and eventually pulmonary hypertension, a rise in pulmonary arterial pressure. The right ventricle of the heart labors to pump blood against this augmented pressure, leading to progressive right heart failure. Furthermore, studies illustrate the presence of severe pulmonary heart disease in approximately 15%–20% of COPD patients, emphasizing the intense interdependence of lung function and cardiovascular health. Intervention is critically required on account of both conditions' influence on patients' quality of life as well as on healthcare utilization. The other common etiology of pulmonary heart disease is pulmonary embolism, where a blood clot, typically originating in the deep veins of the legs, becomes lodged in the pulmonary arteries. This acute increase in pulmonary vascular resistance can lead to sudden occlusion of pulmonary arteries and dramatically change heart function. The right heart has to work harder to provide sufficient blood flow, and chronically this increased stress will result in right ventricular failure or hypertrophy. Those patients at risk, including those with recent surgery, immobility, or certain coagulopathies, are most susceptible to pulmonary embolism. The frequency of repeated embolic events necessitates ongoing medical surveillance and treatment, with an increased emphasis placed on preventive therapy among individuals predisposed. In the face of delayed diagnosis and treatment, the prognosis is fatal, thus highlighting the intimate relationship between thromboembolic disease and pulmonary heart disease. Finally, sleep apnea, particularly obstructive sleep apnea (OSA), is increasingly recognized as an inciting cause in the development of pulmonary heart disease. OSA leads to repetitive episodes of apnea during sleep, resulting in cyclical hypoxia and increased negative intrathoracic pressure. High pulmonary circulation pressure is caused by pulmonary vasoconstriction as a result of this physiological alteration. Subjects with untreated or inadequately managed sleep apnea may eventually experience extensive right ventricular dysfunction and strain. Research indicates that OSA patients are at risk of developing pulmonary hypertension, contributing to cardiac morbidity. Hence, it is essential to look for sleep apnea symptoms and signs among high-risk populations, such as obese patients or those with a family history of sleep apnea. Treatment of sleep apnea with lifestyle modifications or continuous positive airway pressure (CPAP) can decrease the risk of later cardiac complications to a significant level, thus implicating the link between respiratory disturbances and cardiovascular stability.

13.2.1. Chronic Obstructive Pulmonary Disease (COPD)

COPD is a progressively developing inflammatory

lung disease that significantly affects the respiratory status of patients, in most instances resulting in severe systemic manifestations like the formation of pulmonary heart disease. It is characterized by chronic airflow limitation and predominantly results from cigarette smoke and air pollution exposure. The condition, in its progression, destroys lung tissue, leading to impaired gas exchange. This inefficiency leads to hypoxemia and hypercapnia, which in turn can cause stress on the right ventricle of the heart and ultimately result in pulmonary hypertension and right-sided heart failure. This condition is most often referred to as cor pulmonale. Understanding the interaction between COPD and pulmonary heart disease is crucial for effective management and treatment, highlighting the importance of holistic care for the patient (American Thoracic Society et al., 1388). In addition, systemic manifestations of COPD are typically superimposed by inflammatory processes, and in particular, by high serum biomarkers. Serum highly sensitive C-reactive protein (hs-CRP) at elevated levels has been reported to be significantly higher in patients with COPD. It may serve as a potential biomarker for disease severity and progression. For instance, in a clinical investigation of patients with chronic obstructive pulmonary disease who had been exposed to sulfur mustard, there was a robust inverse correlation between hs-CRP and forced expiratory volume in one second (FEV1), proving the systemic inflammation that is present in COPD. Systemic inflammation suggests more than simply an impact on pulmonary function; it suggests an effect on cardiovascular status as well, complicating the clinical picture in a patient with COPD. With advanced disease, clinicians need to be watchful for the heightened risk of pulmonary heart disease in such patients (Boland et al., 2013). In addition, COPD management needs to be holistic and involves both respiratory and cardiovascular care to optimize patient outcomes. Existing national guidelines support comprehensive palliative care that addresses the physical as well as psychosocial aspects of life-limiting illness such as COPD. Most patients suffer from debilitating symptoms like dyspnea, fatigue, and pain that drastically limit their quality of life. This fact underscores the necessity of incorporating palliative care interventions and management of respiratory health to maximize the delivery of care. Intervention strategies need to be developed by multidisciplinary teams in a collaborative effort to address the specific issues besetting COPD patients, most importantly those involving the efficient management of accompanying pulmonary heart disease. Further studies must be conducted to identify optimal practice in models of care that integrate respiratory care with palliative care effectively, offering practical support for this high-risk patient group (Boland et al., 2013) (Figure 13.7).

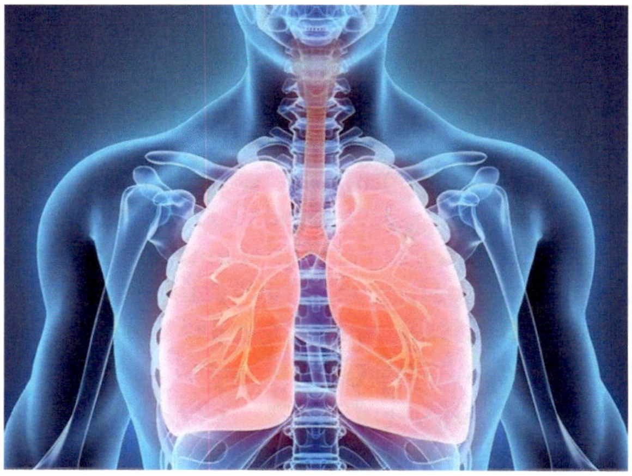

Figure 13.7. Chronic obstructive pulmonary disease (COPD).

Source: https://montgomerypulmonary.com/wp-content/uploads/2020/10/COPD.jpg.

13.2.2. Pulmonary Hypertension (PH)

The intricacies of PH significantly influence its identification and therapy within the overall context of pulmonary heart disease. Elevated pulmonary arterial pressure is what characterizes PH, and it could arise from a variety of etiologies, including left heart disease, chronic lung disease, and congenital cardiac defects. In every case, the challenges are different, particularly when therapy options are considered. For instance, PAH-CHD is separated into distinct groups, which consist of Eisenmenger syndrome and those with severe shunt lesions. Consequences of such a separation are critical to prognosis prediction and the management direction of paradigms because such patients can be managed using personalized therapeutic approaches depending on the etiology of their PH (AbdelMassih et al., 2025). Recognition of these dynamics emphasizes the need for an integrated diagnostic approach to optimize results in pulmonary heart disease patients. The most serious concern with pulmonary hypertension management is its chronic nature, particularly for PE survivors. Literature indicates that survivors of PE are at high risk of long-term cardiovascular morbidity, including pulmonary hypertension and heart failure. The findings of a new meta-analysis emphasize this correlation, commenting that the history of PE is associated with significantly higher hospitalization rates and active cardiovascular comorbidities when compared to the general population (Aurangzeb et al., 2024). This emphasizes the requirement of long-term monitoring and individualized care protocols in these patients. Such preemptive measures can identify the onset of PH early on, making it possible for interventions that can improve the quality of life for patients as well as avert the long-term condition of pulmonary heart disease. The increasing prevalence of pulmonary hypertension further underlines the need for interprofessional care. Treatment of PH is ideally best managed with joint effort from cardiologists, pulmonologists, and family healthcare doctors to ensure an all-encompassing care plan. This is particularly relevant in distinguishing the various forms of pulmonary arterial hypertension and respective therapeutic interventions. An example is the distinction between idiopathic PAH and hereditary or secondary etiologies by underlying disease, which can direct treatment and prognostication. An extensive understanding of mechanisms for various PH classes permits improved strategies in fighting pulmonary heart disease progression, ultimately resulting in a better patient outcome. Therefore, a uniform approach based on current evidence and tailored to the patient is the solution to address the sophisticated challenge of pulmonary hypertension (Figure 13.8).

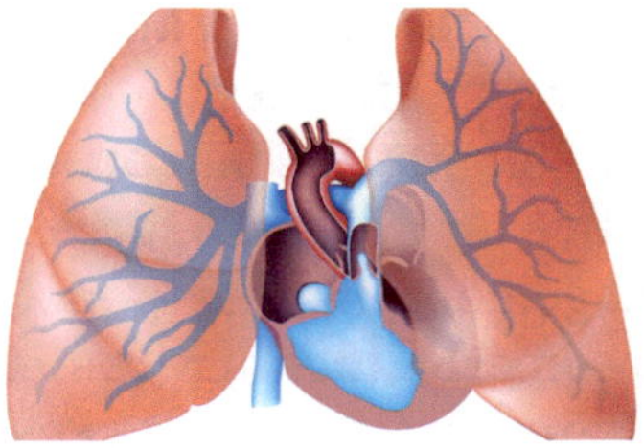

Figure 13.8. Pulmonary hypertension.

Source: https://myheart.net/wp-content/uploads/2020/09/dreamstimelarge_27276044-e1602801088207.jpg.

13.2.3. Congenital Heart Defects (CHD)

The significance of CHD would be lost in comparisons of pulmonary heart disease. CHD is a term covering many structural cardiac abnormalities that occur at birth, the most common of which is a ventricular septal defect (VSD). These defects have the potential to disrupt normal heart and lung blood flow and lead to problems such as increased pulmonary blood flow and elevated pulmonary vasculature pressures. As a result, patients with untreated CHD are at greater risk for developing pulmonary heart disease with right ventricular hypertrophy and ultimate heart failure. Interestingly, the birth prevalence of VSD by surgical method is 0.83 per 1,000 live births, again highlighting the scope of congenital heart disease in children and advocating the importance of early diagnosis and surgery in preventing long-term pulmonary sequelae (Grech et al.,

1997). Even though the surgical management of congenital heart disease has improved, the long-term consequence of such conditions persists in adulthood and exert a significant influence on patient outcomes. Over time, patients with CHD are saddled with comorbid conditions that have a direct impact on their cardiovascular system. Studies show that CHD adults are nearly twice as susceptible to developing any comorbidity as non-CHD individuals, with personal vulnerabilities to cardiovascular and non-cardiovascular diseases (Agarwal et al., 2019). This highlights the importance of taking an integrative approach to surveillance and health management in this population since unattended comorbidities may complicate underlying cardiac conditions or result in pulmonary heart disease. Therefore, healthcare professionals must identify the individual clinical requirements of such patients, which they must treat in accordance as they develop into adults. Since the nature of congenital heart defects is complex and they carry long-term consequences, a multidisciplinary management strategy is required to manage such patients effectively. Coordination of cardiologists, pulmonologists, and primary care providers is paramount in providing maximum benefit to the patient. Such cooperation can guarantee early detection and management of such complications as pulmonary hypertension and heart failure that may arise in CHD patients. Not only does this early-in-time measure acknowledge cardiovascular well-being as a significant component, but it also manages non-cardiovascular issues that accompany it, thereby improving the overall quality of life of these individuals. By acknowledging and treating the intricate interaction between pulmonary heart disease and congenital heart disease, clinicians can design efficient interventions that improve patient outcomes and maintain longevity, significantly impacting individuals with the repercussions of congenital heart disease (Agarwal et al., 2019) (Figure 13.9).

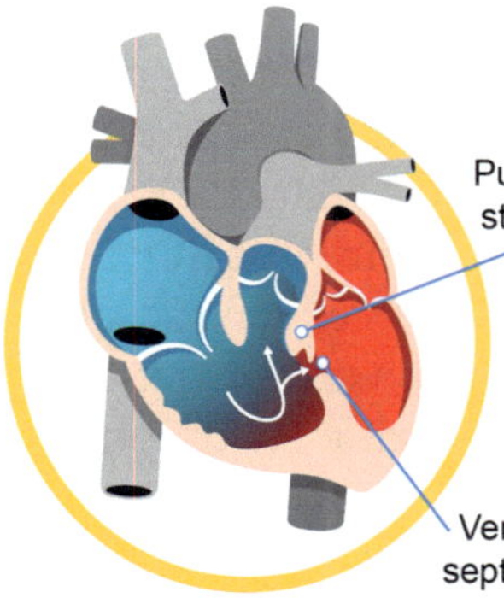

Figure 13.9. Congenital heart defects (CHD).

Source: https://www.pantai.com.my/images/pantaihospitalmalaysialibraries/specialties/cardiology/congenital_heart_defect_banner_1.png?sfvrsn=2c680c1c_7.

13.3. Symptoms and Diagnosis

The clinical presentation of pulmonary heart disease or cor pulmonale typically results from secondary chronic pulmonary hypertension, which significantly impairs right ventricular function. The patient may present with shortness of breath, weakness, and dyspnea on exertion. Edema in the extremities may result from fluid overload and impaired cardiac output. As the disease progresses, such signs may intensify, leading to complications of right-sided heart failure. The practitioners need to be observant about the insidious nature of such signs, as their slow onset might lead to misdiagnosis or delayed intervention. Familiarity with such manifestations is essential for early intervention, as timely detection can improve patient outcomes and quality of life. Diagnosis of pulmonary heart disease is established through a multi-faceted approach that includes clinical assessment and use of several diagnostic modalities. Initial evaluation generally includes a diligent history and physical examination, followed by imaging tests such as echocardiography to assess right ventricular size and function. Augmented by chest X-ray and arterial blood gas determination, additional tests may provide helpful information about the degree of respiratory impairment. The diagnostic process is crucial, above all in distinguishing cor pulmonale from other cardiac conditions, which may present with identical symptoms. Techniques such as the Padua Prediction Score serve to offer valuable tools for determining the risk of venous thromboembolism, particularly in hospitalized patients, such as those with pulmonary heart disease, thereby enhancing diagnosis accuracy and affecting treatment strategies (Zhang et al., 2024). In comorbid illness, differential diagnosis becomes more complex due to the interaction between heart failure and COPD. Common risk factors and overlapping symptoms usually compound the actual pathology, and hence, differential diagnosis becomes challenging. The literature now emphasizes the utilization of transthoracic echocardiography, a speedy and cost-effective modality, for identifying heart failure in COPD patients. This imaging technique is not only valuable for the diagnosis of heart failure but also plays a vital role in observing disease progression and response to therapy. Enhanced diagnostic abilities are required to optimize patient management techniques, especially in combined pulmonary heart disease with other cardiovascular illnesses (Sycheva et al., 2024). Correct diagnosis is the cornerstone of the decrease in morbidity and mortality of such interrelated diseases.

13.3.1. Common Symptoms of Pulmonary Heart Disease

The symptomatology of pulmonary heart disease, or cor pulmonale, is typically accompanied by a cluster of common symptoms that are indicative of the underlying strain on the heart caused by pulmonary disorders. Shortness of breath, particularly on exertion, resulting from reduced oxygenation as a consequence of impaired blood flow through the lungs, is most frequently reported among patients. As the disease progresses, this dyspnea is also noted at rest, most critically reflecting growing right ventricular overload. In addition to respiratory distress, patients also typically develop fatigue, a source of significant interference with their overall quality of life. They become extremely fatigued even with very mild exertion, driven by the heart's decreased efficiency in being able to pump against the elevated pressures in the pulmonary arteries (Jacobson et al., 2023). Early detection of these symptoms is crucial for late intervention and management. Cyanosis, or blue coloration of the skin and mucous membranes, is another salient symptom of pulmonary heart disease caused by low levels of oxygen in the blood. This can occur when pulmonary hypertension places extra work on the right side of the heart and leads to ineffective oxygen exchange in the lungs. In addition, peripheral edema may result as fluid accumulates in the extremities due to compromised cardiac function. Ankle or leg swelling is what patients usually suffer from, as the heart is unable to control blood volume properly. Such symptoms, besides pointing out the complexity of pulmonary heart disease, also point out the necessity of comprehensive diagnosis and treatment strategies in responding to pulmonary as well as cardiac dysfunction (Blanco et al., 2023). Physicians must be attentive to such signs because they are an indication of acute and chronic cardiovascular status changes. Additionally, the dynamics of pulmonary diseases and heart function can complicate symptoms in presentation. For instance, COPD patients may develop exacerbations that reveal underlying cardiac impairment, i.e., chronic heart failure (CHF). It has been found through research that COPD patients and CHF comorbidities have severe dyspnea at rest and during exertion, making diagnosis and treatment of these co-existing conditions difficult (Jacobson et al., 2023). Medics need to differentiate between such overlapping symptoms to individualize appropriate treatment therapies with a focus on both pulmonary disease and cardiac disease elements effectively. This is why knowledge of common symptoms triggered by pulmonary heart disease is essential not only for the diagnosis, but also for designing targeted interventions and therapies (Blanco et al., 2023). Eventually, it enhances patient outcomes through the provision of holistic care strategies (Figure 13.10).

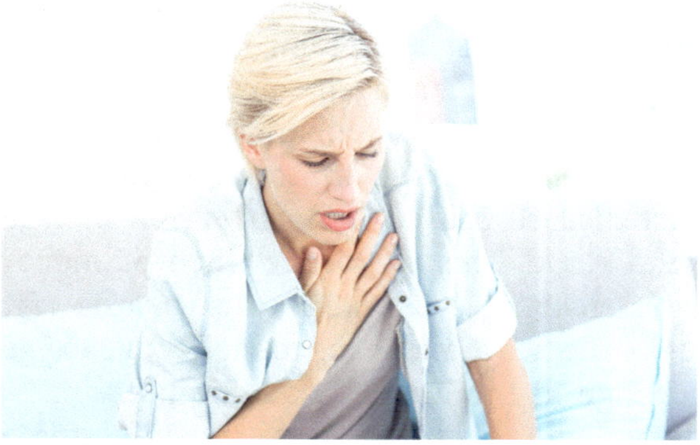

Figure 13.10. Symptoms of pulmonary heart disease.

Source: https://www.visitcompletecare.com/attachment/shutterstock_274015055-1/.

13.3.2. Diagnostic Tests and Procedures

Diagnosis of cor pulmonale, also known as pulmonary heart disease, is a rigorous one with a series of diagnostic interventions and tests. The initial step is a diligent clinical history and physical examination, which are critical to ascertain the occurrence of symptoms like dyspnea, cyanosis, or edema. Diagnostic imaging, including chest X-rays and echocardiography, is most crucial to visualize the heart and the pulmonary vasculature.

Chest X-rays help detect enlargements or structural changes in the heart, and echocardiograms provide valuable details about the function of the hearts and valves. These investigations set the stage for more in-depth investigation, allowing clinicians to assess the degree of pulmonary involvement and to rule out other conditions that might mimic pulmonary heart disease (Kitsiou et al., 2013). Following initial assessments, higher-level interventions are employed to establish the diagnosis and interpret underlying mechanisms.

Right heart catheterization is an absolute diagnostic test; it directly measures pulmonary artery pressures and cardiac output, and thus safely establishes the diagnosis of pulmonary hypertension. It is essential in distinguishing among various groups of pulmonary disease, which overlap in clinical presentation. Apart from this, lab tests like arterial blood gases and biomarkers can be performed to assess oxygenation and identify underlying respiratory pathology responsible for pulmonary heart disease. Comprehensive assessment using these diagnostic tests can guide the appropriate therapeutic interventions based on the underlying disease mechanisms identified (Abbott et al., 2020).

Integration of findings on diagnostics leads to a structured treatment protocol for pulmonary heart disease. Since the response to therapy varies greatly depending on the etiology, understanding the etiology is essential to appropriate care. Treatment for pulmonary arterial hypertension, for instance, will vary when secondary to left heart disease versus a diagnosis based on COPD. Additionally, surveillance through follow-up echocardiogram or exercise test must be performed to assess disease course and response to therapy. Such procedures and diagnostic multilayered practices not only enable targeted treatments but also improve patient outcomes through earlier interventions before the onset of significant morbidity (Abbott et al., 2020) (Figure 13.11).

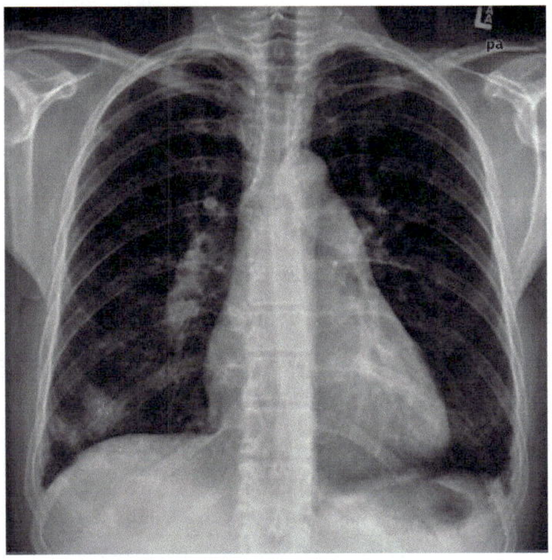

Figure 13.11. Chest X-Ray for the diagnosis of pulmonary heart disease.

Source: https://www.bhf.org.uk/-/media/images/information-support/tests/chest-x-ray/normal-chest-x-ray-620x400.jpg?h=400&w=620&rev=d9cfde6ea0a249649d60284ae972f2da&hash=116C2CF5D2AA30EC9CDCAE7712897203.

13.3.3. Importance of Early Detection

Early detection of pulmonary heart disease (PHD) is critical for improving patient life expectancy and survival. Because PHD is typically asymptomatic early in the course of the disease, patients do not see the healthcare provider until advanced complications have ensued. Early detection allows intervention, which can avoid the necessity of having to treat advanced disease and severe complications such as right ventricular failure. Moreover, screening regularly and educating patients on PHD risk factors are central in creating awareness and encouraging active health practices. Placing early detection through frequent health checks and symptom monitoring at the forefront can lay the groundwork for better management approaches, which then lead to enhanced patient quality of life as well as health outcomes. Yet another critical aspect of early detection is its ability to facilitate individualized care plans. When pulmonary heart disease is diagnosed earlier, doctors can maximize treatment regimens, taking into consideration the specific needs and physiological condition of each patient. For instance, the application of new imaging techniques and diagnostic equipment can contribute to the understanding of the pathophysiological mechanisms of the diseases and support decision-making for treatments. Moreover, patients with specific cardiac abnormalities can be maintained in close observation for any indications of_timer. Pourghasemi et al. (2025) determines how congenital heart conditions, potentially leading to PHD, are diagnosed without clear symptoms, further supporting regular screening programs. Individualized treatment of this nature not only provides a foundation for an improved targeted therapeutic process but also empowers the patient with active participation in the care process.

The result would be monumental, leading to severe health outcomes and fatality in pulmonary heart disease patients. Delayed diagnosis leaves only a limited field of therapy and higher mortality. An example is patients with complications from Fontan who may develop chronic health issues from the effects of poor circulation and extra workload on the heart. López et al. (2024) illustrate the way early intervention would prevent such complications, emphasizing the importance of vigilant follow-up treatment and strict monitoring in modified Fontan physiology patients. Emphasizing the importance given to early detection, medical practitioners can advocate for extensive screening guidelines and educational courses that highlight the value of early diagnosis and treatment in the general public health context. Finally, early diagnosis acts as a door to enhancing health outcomes and guaranteeing the sustainability of quality care for patients with pulmonary heart disease.

13.4. Treatment Options

Management of pulmonary heart disease, particularly in cases such as chronic thromboembolic pulmonary hypertension (CTEPH), requires a strategy that is reflective and incorporates recent advances in both medical and operative therapy. CTEPH results from unresolved thromboembolic pulmonary artery occlusion, causing elevated pulmonary artery pressure and, consequently, right heart failure. The therapeutic landscape has revolutionized, with pulmonary endarterectomy as a widely accepted surgery that has demonstrated significant progress in patient outcomes. Balloon pulmonary angioplasty is also gaining favor as a valuable interventional therapy in individuals who are deemed inoperable and represents the diversity in treatment modality choices. Medical therapies, such as the pulmonary vasodilator riociguat, have expanded inoperable patients' treatment options and represent the trend toward personalized medicine in the management of multicomponent disease associated with CTEPH (Chang et al., 2025). In addition to surgical and percutaneous therapy for pulmonary heart disease, concomitant conditions such as tricuspid valve disease need to be addressed to manage overall. Tricuspid valve disease is likely to be accompanied by pulmonary hypertension and may exacerbate right heart failure, thus complicating the clinical course. In the past, therapy was only medical or surgical. The development of new technology in transcatheter tricuspid valve therapeutics has created new avenues for patients who otherwise had very few long-term treatment options. Given the complexity of tricuspid valve disease, these minimally invasive treatments become more relevant since they may be tailored to the patient's anatomy and pathology. This range of treatment contributes to the enhancement of quality of care and, as a result, survival rates in patients with pulmonary heart disease (Davidson et al., 2024). Overall, management of pulmonary heart disease needs to be a holistic one that includes the use of several therapeutic interventions. An entire treatment regimen not only addresses the direct cause, such as CTEPH or tricuspid valve incompetence, but also aims to address patient-related variables, including comorbidities, risk stratification, and global health status. The advances in transcatheter and surgical treatments emphasize the requirement for flexibility in treatment protocols to yield tailored options that can address the unique problems presented by individual patients. Moreover, studies in new emerging medical therapies support the requirement for continuous evaluation and implementation of new therapy modalities to enhance patient outcomes. Lastly, the objective is to provide an integrative approach to treating acute symptoms and chronic health problems for pulmonary heart disease patients (Figure 13.12).

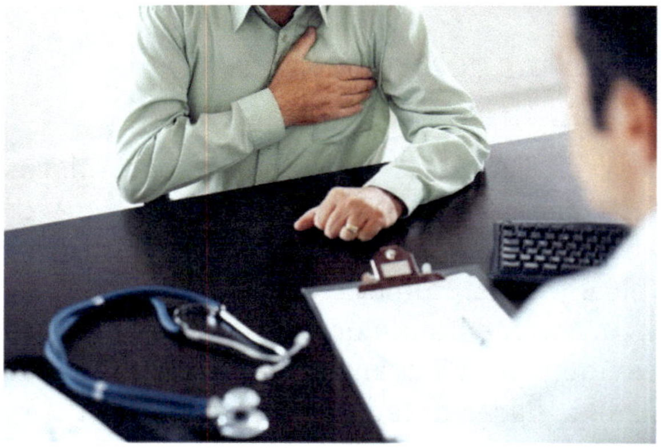

Figure 13.12. Treatment of pulmonary heart disease.

Source: https://globalnews.ca/wp-content/uploads/2023/06/GettyImages-157592738.jpeg?quality=85&strip=all&w=1200.

13.4.1. Medications for Managing Symptoms

The therapy for pulmonary heart disease in most instances needs to be multidimensional, particularly as far as the pharmacologic therapy intended for controlling symptoms and improving patient outcomes is concerned. Medications such as diuretics are essential for managing fluid overload, which is a common complication in the event of right heart failure. Furosemide uniquely allows the relief of pulmonary congestion by enabling renal excretion of sodium and water and therefore the mitigation of symptoms such as edema and dyspnea. In the case of secondary cardiovascular defect, as illustrated by DLs experience, careful titration of diuretics will prevent heart failure intensifications and enhance daily functioning. Still, prescribers need to be cautious of possible electrolyte imbalances, particularly when used in conjunction with other medications that affect renal function or fluid status, indicating the necessity of individualized treatment protocols. Together with diuretics, beta-agonists, and bronchodilators significantly contribute to alleviating respiratory symptoms for pulmonary heart disease. They are relaxants of airway smooth muscle, thereby enhancing airflow and relieving wheezing and dyspnea. Short-acting preparations can provide instant relief, while long-acting preparations might be employed in chronic control to make it easier for patients to engage in normal activities. Furthermore, encouraging patients to adopt pulmonary prophylactic measures, such as adhering to the possible administration of inhaled corticosteroids, may reduce chronic symptoms. Although, the pharmacodynamic patterns of these medications are well established, incorporation into a worldwide treatment regimen has to be done on an individual patient-by-patient basis, as seen with heterogeneity of DLs response to the drug. Finally, it should be emphasized that pharmacologically dependent treatment cannot be the sole regimen for treating pulmonary heart disease, since adjunct treatments can complement treatment efficacy. One of the areas where oxygen therapy is very crucial in improving oxygenation in hypoxemic patients. Oxygen therapy is also non-invasive and may lead to significant improvements in quality of life, which may help in maintaining functional independence in patients. Education of patients regarding appropriate use of medications, changes in lifestyle, and referring a patient for an additional medical workup is also as significant. As exemplified in all patient cases, like DL, the benefit of meticulous symptom management must be weighed against possible side effects to optimize treatment. Patient-specific consideration leads to enhanced health outcomes, with attention to individualized care regimens being essential in the treatment of pulmonary heart disease (Figure 13.13).

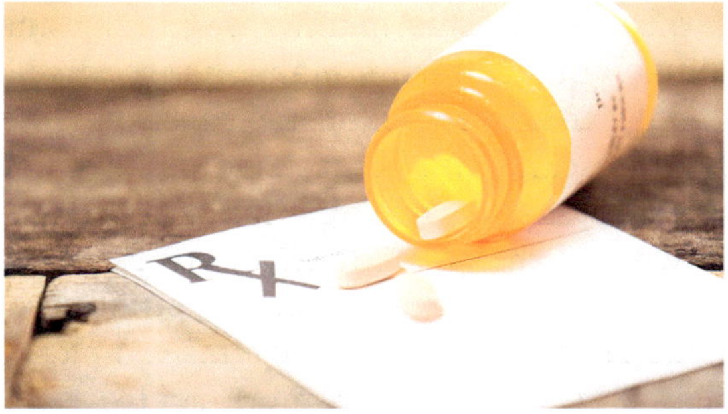

Figure 13.13. Medication for pulmonary heart disease.

Source: https://www.heart.org/-/media/Images/Health-Topics/High-Blood-Pressure/pill-bottle-knocked-over.jpg?sc_lang=en&hash=F249124BD801ECA7EFF0908B56AD0D96.

13.4.2. Surgical Interventions

In pulmonary heart disease, surgery is also crucial in managing advanced stages of the disease when conservative methods could be insufficient. Surgical intervention can range from corrective surgical operations for pre-existing structural defects to more intensive surgical procedures for relieving right ventricular stress or repairing damaged pulmonary vasculature. Surgery such as pulmonary endarterectomy, in which chronic clots are removed from the pulmonary arteries, has proven effective in patients with chronic thromboembolic pulmonary hypertension. Not only do the surgeries fix hemodynamics, but they also improve the general quality of life for pulmonary heart disease patients, avoiding the threat of morbidity due to advanced right heart failure. Moreover, the role played by catheter ablation in the management of atrial fibrillation (AF) offers an applicable factor in the broad canopy of surgical interventions for pulmonary heart disease. As AF is a prevalent condition among those suffering from chronic pulmonary hypertension, ablative procedures have joined the fold as viable choices to maximize outcomes. The methodological and technological innovations in ablation are a testimony to growing respect for the mechanisms maintaining arrhythmias brought on by pulmonary heart disease. Although there remain obstacles, e.g., the need for large-scale clinical trials to validate long-term success, catheter ablation is a promising pathway to the prevention of AF recurrence and ultimately to the augmentation of cardiac function in patients affected by this complication (Calkins et al., 2017). In more acute settings, surgical interventions become the last resort for patients with severe PE and right ventricular failure. Although thrombolytic therapy is usually the first line of intervention, surgical interventions in the form of embolectomy remain highly relevant for those patients that cannot tolerate thrombolytics or with extreme clinical presentation. These interventions are essential in restoring appropriate pulmonary perfusion and decreasing right ventricular afterload, which are essential in preventing cardiogenic shock and potential mortality. Understanding the complexities of pulmonary embolism and an aggressive multidisciplinary surgical management is essential to optimize outcomes in these critically ill patients. The urgency of proper risk stratification and immediate surgical treatment underscores the importance of interprofessional teamwork among a variety of healthcare providers in addressing this essential global health problem (Bellis et al., 2018).

13.4.3. Lifestyle Modifications and Rehabilitation

The management of pulmonary heart disease, or cor pulmonale, involves an integrated approach that includes simple lifestyle modifications and rehabilitation measures. These measures not only relieve symptoms of the disease but also enhance the quality of life in patients. Essential lifestyle modifications like exercise, diet, and stopping smoking are primary features of rehabilitation. Exercise particularly increases cardiovascular conditioning, increases lung volume, and improves blood flow—necessities in patients with pulmonary heart disease. Moreover, sweating out a healthy diet rich in antioxidants and low in saturated fats can be an excellent helper in controlling underlying conditions like hypertension and atherosclerosis, thereby reducing the strain on the heart and lungs. As aging has been linked with poor outcomes of cardiovascular health, these modifications will hamper the rate of progression of the diseases and encourage healthier aging (Li et al., 2025). Patient education is also an essential element in the framework of lifestyle modification and rehabilitation. Informing individuals about their disease empowers them to make healthy decisions for themselves. Educational programs should include knowledge on recognizing early signs of deterioration, understanding the importance of treatment adherence, and implementing healthy lifestyle changes. Given that patient compliance is generally based on patients' knowledge of the disease and required treatment, tailored educational interventions are most effective for improving outcomes in patients. Moreover, collaboration from health care workers, such as nurses, can extend the efficacy of education interventions. Nurses play a pivotal role in developing self-management skills, psychological well-being management, and behavioral change support facilitation needed to manage pulmonary heart disease (Alazmi et al., 2024). Provision of psychological interventions as part of rehabilitation services is also pivotal for pulmonary heart disease patients. Depression and anxiety are prevalent among chronic diseases and have a significant impact on treatment adherence and overall health. Stress relief using mindfulness-based stress reduction, cognitive-behavioral therapy, and support groups can provide patients with the coping skills they require, generally enhancing their quality of life. In addition, exercise programs tailored to each patient's strengths and weaknesses can optimize physical rehabilitation. By bridging the gap between physical health and emotional support, rehabilitation programs can offer holistic care that addresses the physiological as well as psychological needs of pulmonary heart disease management. By so doing, patients are better able to engage in their rehabilitation process, with improved outcomes and management over their illness (Alazmi et al., 2024) (Figure 13.14).

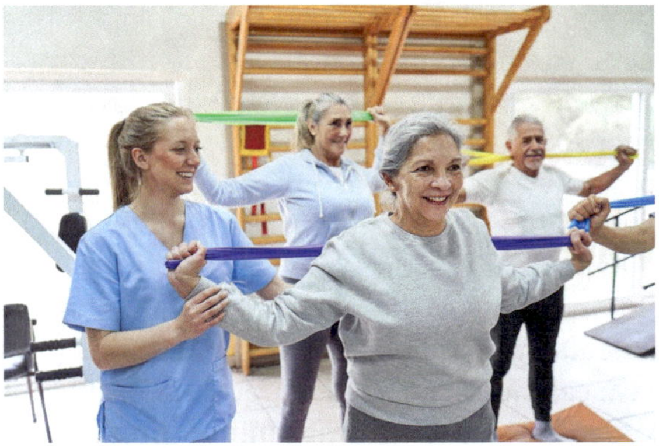

Figure 13.14. Rehabilitation.

Source: https://blog.rehabselect.net/hs-fs/hubfs/cardiac-rehab-blog-post.jpg?width=900&height=600&name=cardiac-rehab-blog-post.jpg.

SUMMARY

In examining the complexity of pulmonary heart disease, it is evident that early diagnosis and the immediate response play a critical role in maximizing the survival of patients. As indicated by the recent research, particularly for patients who present with comorbid respiratory conditions like COVID-19, the interdependence between cardiac parameters and lung involvement is deep. Specific measurements, such as the pulmonary artery to ascending aorta diameter ratio, provide essential indicators of the disease process and underscore the need for comprehensive imaging techniques in managing heart health. This interaction between pulmonary pathology and cardiovascular dynamics underscores the need for interdisciplinary approaches to addressing the complexities of pulmonary heart disease and for maximizing therapeutic interventions against adverse outcomes, particularly among high-risk populations (Rouzrokh et al., 2024). Furthermore, the heterogeneity of diseases under the broad spectrum of pulmonary heart disease necessitates customized treatment protocols to adapt to the unique presentation of each patient. The functional echocardiographic findings present evidence not only of anatomical dysfunction but also of functional derangement that makes clinical management difficult. The findings validate that without proper hemodynamic evaluation, life-threatening conditions such as congenital cardiac abnormalities are left undiagnosed, thus emphasizing the role played by advanced imaging in enabling early intervention. The addition of such technologies to standard assessment protocols in neonatal and intensive care units can revolutionize care for hemodynamically unstable or respiratory distress patients, so that all underlying cardiovascular issues are addressed appropriately (Torres et al., 2024). In sum, collective experience derived from present literature and clinical practice supports the overall message that pulmonary heart disease is not an independent disease but a spectrum of interdependent disease states. The synergy between imaging modalities and careful patient observation of cardiac and pulmonary state can powerfully affect the recognition and management of these multistreamed interactions. With an increasing number of healthcare professionals understanding the significance of early diagnosis and personalized treatment plans, the potential for improved patient outcomes in pulmonary heart disease increases continuously. With continued research and cooperation with specialists, a greater understanding of this disorder can be achieved, and eventually, new solutions that favor patient care in various healthcare settings (Rouzrokh et al., 2024; Torres et al., 2024).

In examining the critical characteristics of pulmonary heart disease, it is essential to realize the interaction of pulmonary disease and cardiovascular impact. Pulmonary heart disease, characterized by right-sided heart failure from chronic pressure overload or reduced oxygenation, often occurs secondary to chronic respiratory disease such as COPD or interstitial lung disease. The complexities of these interlinked conditions require a multidisciplinary management strategy that addresses not only the pulmonary but also the cardiovascular expressions. Of particular relevance, the associated symptoms of dyspnea and fatigue have significant impacts on patients' quality of life, requiring individualized approaches to management with pharmacological and non-pharmacological measures directed towards alleviation of suffering and enhancement of well-being. Moreover, extensive epidemiologic research has shown an unprecedented prevalence of pulmonary heart disease, where early detection and intervention have been necessitated. A review of meta-analyses of large clinical trials and observational studies elucidates risk factors such as smoking, obesity, and genetic influences that precipitate the development and occurrence of the disease. New re-evaluations, like the FDA's recent critical evaluation of cardiovascular endpoints in trials like the RECORD trial, underscore the necessity to clarify these types of associations. These types of regulatory results improve our knowledge of patient outcomes and guide clinical practices in treating comorbidities that are associated with pulmonary heart disease, thereby improving patient care. Apart from this, this highlights the need for advancement in clinical research to clarify the long-term consequences of curative interventions on pulmonary and cardiac health to reduce morbidity and mortality rates among patients. Finally, the integration of palliative and supportive care into the treatment model for pulmonary heart disease is pivotal in caring for the patient's comprehensive needs. With the recognition of disabling pain and discomfort symptoms observed in patients, especially in advanced pulmonary disease, palliative care is now being recommended as part of the management of all life-limiting illness patients, including chronic lung disease. Experience has shown that skilled palliative care teams may greatly optimize symptom treatment, enhance quality of life, and enable more efficient communication of end-of-life wants. Ongoing research continues to evaluate the effects of various models of service delivery and interventions, as well as the significance of collaborative care models bringing palliative care services together with respiratory specialties to offer comprehensive patient care for pulmonary heart disease and its related conditions (Bigelow et al., 2013; Boland et al., 2013).

A CLOSER LOOK

COMPLICATIONS ASSOCIATED WITH PULMONARY HEART DISEASE

Complications of pulmonary heart disease are serious, impacting morbidity and mortality among affected individuals. The heart, subjected to the chronic pulmonary pressures, experiences dysfunction that can lead to right heart failure, arrhythmias, and sudden cardiac death. The interaction between pulmonary hypertension and right ventricular hypertrophy exacerbates the complication, with the heart struggling to pump blood efficiently with elevated vascular resistance. Thereafter, individuals with pulmonary heart disease go on to develop disabling symptomatology of fatigue, intolerance to exercise, and dyspnea that significantly impact their quality of life. It becomes essential to discover the predictors of such complications, including background cardiovascular comorbidities and specific surgical factors, in an attempt to establish effective management strategies to prevent such unfavorable outcomes, as has been illustrated through findings reached from studies on similar issues (Li et al., 2025).

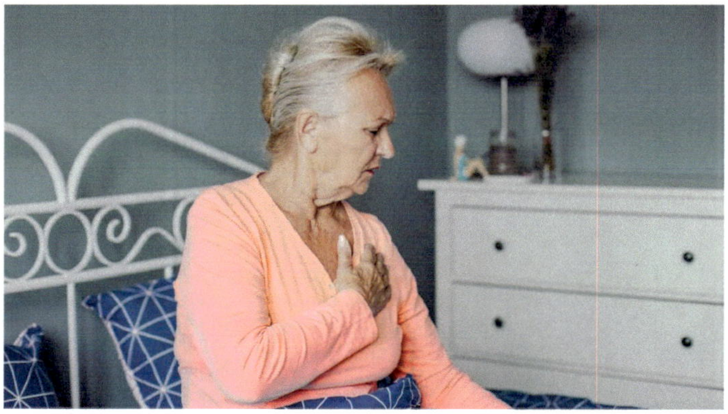

Figure 13.15. Complications Associated with Pulmonary Heart Disease.

Source: https://i0.wp.com/post.medicalnewstoday.com/wp-content/uploads/sites/3/2021/05/Senior-woman-suffering-from-chest-paim-1296x728-header-1024x575.jpg?w=1155&h=1528.

Besides, treatment of pulmonary heart disease complications is typically multifaceted, consisting of a combination of pharmacologic and interventional therapies. For instance, the use of pulmonary vasodilators has been found to show promising outcomes in symptom relief and hemodynamic improvement among patients with advanced disease. Nonetheless, these interventions must be tailored about patient profiles in an individualized manner, taking into account comorbid conditions such as ischemic heart disease or diabetes, which add complexity to pulmonary heart disease. According to research, the assessment of patients at risk using surgical stress scores and basic physiological assessment can permit early intervention, which can enhance outcomes for surgery as well as reduce hospitalization (Li et al., 2025). This signals the need for an immediate, organized system to stratify and deal with pulmonary heart disease complications effectively, particularly since the number of persons afflicted continues to rise among the aged population. Longitudinal studies illustrate that asymptomatic mitral regurgitation (MR), a condition widely related to pulmonary heart disease, bears significant long-term complications for patients in terms of their survival rates. In a cohort of such patients, almost 47% had MR-related complications, such as new-onset heart failure or pulmonary hypertension, within 10 years, much more than in matched control subjects. This points to the multifactorial nature of pulmonary heart disease, wherein innocuous-appearing structural changes can initiate a domino effect of deleterious health outcomes. Long-term disease management programs are therefore essential to monitor and manage these complications efficiently. They must also reassess the timing of any potential surgical treatments to optimize outcomes and improve survival among asymptomatic patients presenting with such complications, necessitating a paradigm shift in the clinical management of pulmonary heart disease overall (Figure 13.15).

References

1. Reinero, C., Visser, L. C., Kellihan, H. B., Masseau, I., Rozanski, E., Clercx, C., Williams, K., Abbott, J., Borgarelli, M., & Scansen, B. A. (2020). ACVIM consensus statement guidelines for the diagnosis, classification, treatment, and monitoring of pulmonary hypertension in dogs. *Journal of Veterinary Internal Medicine*, *34*(2), 549–573. https://doi.org/10.1111/jvim.15725AbdelMassih, A., AlAli, A., Nasr, E., Hanafy, E., & AlRamsi, M. (2025). Group D of pulmonary arterial hypertension and its relationship to congenital heart disease: Is there a non-invasive way to predict the unpredictable? *Global Cardiology Science and Practice*. https://www.semanticscholar.org/paper/7da968f8e76f24218913d4784858fbf7d35858e1 (accessed on 29th May 2025).

2. Acar, L., Behrendt, C., Baldus, S., Falk, V., Smetak, N., Nzomo, M. M., Marschall, U., et al. (2024). Prognostic impact of disease-related complications in asymptomatic mitral regurgitation: A health insurance claims analysis. *Clinical Research in Cardiology: Official Journal of the German Cardiac Society*. https://www.semanticscholar.org/paper/533feffa3e6de9b9d51ede687363868050b221fc (accessed on 29th May 2025).

3. Agarwal, A., Broberg, C. S., Dudley, R. A., Foster, et al. (2019). Age- and lesion-related comorbidity burden among US adults with congenital heart disease: A population-based study. *J. Am. Heart Assoc.* https://core.ac.uk/download/323079618.pdf (accessed on 29th May 2025).

4. Alazmi, A. H. S., Khiriy, S. A., Khiriy, M. A., Alabdulaal, F. A., Aldossry, K. M. H., Alshammari, K. R., Al Otaibi, R. H. S., et al. (2024). Comprehensive nursing care in coronary heart disease: Biochemical markers, strategies, challenges, and evidence-based approaches for effective patient management and outcomes. *Egyptian Journal of Chemistry*. https://www.semanticscholar.org/paper/e21c08a469bc71eb58194d5177f1d3157ba79961 (accessed on 29th May 2025).

5. Asnaashari, A., Attaran, D., Attaran, D., Ghanei, M., Ghobadi, M. H., Ayatollahi, H., et al. (2009). Highly sensitive C-reactive protein levels in Iranian patients with pulmonary complication of sulfur mustard poisoning and its correlation with severity of airway diseases. *Human and Experimental Toxicology 28*(12) 739–745. https://core.ac.uk/download/11684426.pdf (accessed on 29th May 2025).

6. Aurangzeb, L., Tayyab, M., Umar, Z., Ahmad, Z., Khan, M. S., Hunain, M., Sana, U., et al. (2024). The association between pulmonary embolism and long-term cardiovascular disease progression: A meta-analysis of heart failure, pulmonary hypertension, and hospitalization rates. *Indus Journal of Bioscience Research*. https://www.semanticscholar.org/paper/35674677aff6f10cd17dd430fa989e2487e911b5 (accessed on 29th May 2025).

7. Babu-Narayan, S. V., Ernst, S., Mantziari, L., Suman-Horduna, et al. (2013). *Advanced Ablation Strategies for Management of Post-Surgical Atrial Arrhythmias.* https://core.ac.uk/download/77002709.pdf (accessed on 29th May 2025).

8. Bagheri, M., Agrawal, V., Annis, J., Shi, M., Ferguson, J., Freiberg, M., Mosley, J., et al. (2023). Genetics of pulmonary pressure and right ventricle stress identify diabetes as a causal risk factor. *Journal of the American Heart Association: Cardiovascular and Cerebrovascular Disease, 12*. https://www.semanticscholar.org/paper/444b639e200e3d96a2dbb4773140ac1fc96b3b9d (accessed on 29th May 2025).

9. Basso, C., Aguilera, B., Banner, J., Cohle, S., D'Amati, G., Gouveia, R., Gioia, C., et al. (2017). Guidelines for autopsy investigation of sudden cardiac death: 2017 update from the Association for European cardiovascular pathology. *Virchows Archiv.*, *471*, 691–705. https://www.semanticscholar.org/paper/29fde51340974d8ac13bed62116986e7b84143a7 (accessed on 29th May 2025).

10. Bigelow, R., Burns, S., Dickerson, S., Hafley, et al. (2013). Methodology of a reevaluation of cardiovascular outcomes in the RECORD trial: Study design and conduct. *Am. Heart J.* https://core.ac.uk/download/42359786.pdf (accessed on 29th May 2025).

11. Blanco, I., Hernández-González, F., Garcia, A. R., Torres-Castro, R., & Barberà, J. (2023). Management of pulmonary hypertension associated with chronic lung disease. *Seminars in Respiratory and Critical Care Medicine*, *44*, 826–839. https://www.semanticscholar.org/paper/f90c1fec4cbbcce8a153d8916423d06dddfbf7cd (accessed on 29th May 2025).

12. Boland, J., Martin, J., Ross, J. R., Ross, et al. (2013). Palliative care for people with non-malignant lung disease: Summary of current evidence and future direction. https://core.ac.uk/download/151156967.pdf (accessed on 29th May 2025).

13. Calkins, H., Cleland, J. G. F., Heist, E. K., Kowey, et al. (2017). *The Burden of Proof: The Current State of Atrial Fibrillation Prevention and Treatment Trials.* https://core.ac.uk/download/80696856.pdf (accessed on 29th May 2025).

14. Carvalho, J. S., Axt-Fliedner, R., Chaoui, R., Copel, J. A., Cuneo, B. F., Goff, D. A., Gordin, K. L., et al. (2023). ISUOG practice guidelines (updated): Fetal cardiac screening. *Ultrasound in Obstetrics and Gynecology*, *61*, 788–803. https://doi.org/10.1002/uog.26224 (accessed on 29th May 2025).

15. Chang, S. A., Yang, J. H., Jung, D. S., & Kim, N. H. (2025). Recent advances in chronic thromboembolic pulmonary hypertension: Expanding the disease concept and treatment options. *Korean Circulation Journal.* https://www.semanticscholar.org/paper/9be24cd73aeb79a4ffe4e6b0f8dcb063d3895f30 (accessed on 29th May 2025).

16. Daliento, L., & Folino, A. F. (2005). *Arrhythmias After Tetralogy of Fallot Repair.* https://core.ac.uk/download/pdf/86430.pdf (accessed on 29th May 2025).

17. Davidson, L. J., Tang, G., Ho, E. C., Fudim, M., Frisoli, T., Camaj, A., Bowers, M. T., et al. (2024). The tricuspid valve: A review of pathology, imaging, and current treatment options: A scientific statement from the American Heart Association. *Circulation.* https://www.semanticscholar.org/paper/972eac2464eb8e98522ae57a5582e5e8f6e187ac (accessed on 29th May 2025).

18. De Bellis, A., D'Abramo, M., Frati, G., Greco, et al. (2018). *Surgical Embolectomy for Acute Massive Pulmonary Embolism: State of the Art.* https://core.ac.uk/download/188822613.pdf (accessed on 29th May 2025).

19. Dhakal, B., & Pokharel, B. (2024). Coronary artery disease (CAD) demystified – Causes, symptoms & treatment. *The American Journal of Patient Health Info.* https://www.semanticscholar.org/paper/743740c3c9e419e7767cc47ab5202ae6c8855976 (accessed on 29th May 2025).

20. Dori, Y., Mazurek, J., Birati, E., & Smith, C. L. (2023). Ascites in animals with right heart failure: Correlation with lymphatic dysfunction. *Journal of the American Heart Association: Cardiovascular and Cerebrovascular Disease, 12.* https://www.semanticscholar.org/paper/bc77afe3fee026206b0dd0cfd13e5c17f6ab685d (accessed on 29th May 2025).

21. Grech, V. E. (1997). *Changing Trends in Surgery for Ventricular Septal Defect in Malta.* https://core.ac.uk/download/46601969.pdf (accessed on 29th May 2025).

22. Grech, V. E., & Savona-Ventura, C. (1999). *Concepts in Cardiology: A Historical Perspective.* https://core.ac.uk/download/46602848.pdf (accessed on 29th May 2025).

23. Huang, S. L., Xin, H. Y., Wang, X. Y., Feng, G. G., Wu, F. Q., Feng, Z. P., Xing, Z., et al. (2023). Recent advances on the molecular mechanism and clinical trials of venous thromboembolism. *Journal of Inflammation Research, 16*, 6167–6178. https://www.semanticscholar.org/paper/a3a0b67bfe1f24de7523fd18634a03156dc2d67c (accessed on 29th May 2025).

24. Jacobson, P., Lind, L., & Persson, H. (2023). Applying the Rome proposal on exacerbations of chronic obstructive pulmonary disease: Does comorbid chronic heart failure matter? *International Journal of Chronic Obstructive Pulmonary Disease, 18*, 2055–2064. https://www.semanticscholar.org/paper/e8b61849f6e723f2eb45e93238b92570932e34f7 (accessed on 29th May 2025).

25. Jiandani, M., Jain, K. B., & Lohakare, P. K. (2024). Perception and impact of long-term oxygen therapy on the functioning and quality of life of patients with chronic respiratory disease: A mixed-method study. *Cureus, 16*. https://www.semanticscholar.org/paper/f432164e9f958714af66dd2dc63f8538c933a8d3 (accessed on 29th May 2025).

26. Kitsiou, A., Caforio, A. L. P., Porta-Sanchez, A., Vahanian, A., Iung, B., Carrera, C., Szymanski, C., et al. (2013). *ESC Core Curriculum for the General Cardiologist (2013).* https://core.ac.uk/download/55756305.pdf (accessed on 29th May 2025).

27. Li, Q., Zhang, H., Xiao, N., Liang, G., Lin, Y., Yang, X., Yang, J., et al. (2025). Aging and lifestyle modifications for preventing aging-related diseases. *FASEB Journal: Official Publication of the Federation of American Societies for Experimental Biology, 39*(9), e70575. https://www.semanticscholar.org/paper/88824116cc0ccc3370bbfd5797218ab6302270a3 (accessed on 29th May 2025).

28. Li, Y., Wang, B., Tsang, L., Zou, M., Yu, L., Xia, S., & Wu, W. J. (2025). Predictive value of physiological capacity and surgical stress scores for perioperative complications in radical resection for colorectal cancer: A propensity-matched analysis. *American Journal of Translational Research, 17*(1), 254–266. https://www.semanticscholar.org/paper/ea3e0704c2ff8ed63d046854830302cd7a50dbf9 (accessed on 29th May 2025).

29. Liu, R., Yuan, T. Y., Wang, R., Gong, D., Wang, S. B., Du, G., & Fang, L. (2023). Insights into endothelin receptors in pulmonary hypertension. *International Journal of Molecular Sciences, 24*. https://www.semanticscholar.org/paper/08f7e67b5111ee6373da588262ba10fb0a61e6c9 (accessed on 29th May 2025).

30. MacLeod, M., Papi, A., Contoli, M., Beghé, B., Celli, B., Wedzicha, J., & Fabbri, L. (2021). Chronic obstructive pulmonary disease exacerbation fundamentals: Diagnosis, treatment, prevention and disease impact. *Respirology, 26*, 532–551. https://www.semanticscholar.org/paper/0187176d51ec18d56c6dabb6a5c443a84bc3ba31 (accessed on 29th May 2025).

31. Malakan, R. E., & Hijazi, Z. (2024). Transcatheter pulmonary flow restrictors: Current trends and future perspectives. *Catheterization and Cardiovascular Interventions: Official Journal of the Society for Cardiac Angiography & Interventions.* https://www.semanticscholar.org/paper/e7f57e4237ce16ada11e257aa9dbecb0d0d477d1 (accessed on 29th May 2025).

32. Marepalli, G. S., Kollu, P. K., & Inavolu, M. D. (2024). Early detection of chronic obstructive pulmonary disease in respiratory audio signals using CNN and LSTM models. In *2024 IEEE International Conference on Contemporary Computing and Communications (InC4)*, *1*, 1–6. https://www.semanticscholar.org/paper/a4219b6c0fe2fa7462d6ed153d23d0352087511c (accessed on 29th May 2025).

33. Medina, A. R., Hammerness, P., Ihyembe, D., Plummer, S., Diekroger, E. A., & Fogler, J. M. (2024). Complex ADHD challenging case: Managing co-occurring attention-deficit hyperactivity disorder and congenital heart disease with a limited medication formulary: A case from Mexico. *Journal of Developmental and Behavioral Pediatrics: JDBP*, *45*(3), e271–e273. https://www.semanticscholar.org/paper/dec1d5a555a006b78bf8cef13e310dc479415a56 (accessed on 29th May 2025).

34. Nora, M. E., Murni, I., Nugroho, S., & Noormanto, N. (2022). Predictors of heart failure in children with congenital heart disease. *Pediatrica Indonesiana*. https://www.semanticscholar.org/paper/cdb559eecb7d923cc5c38bd27c593e4c14eb2f12 (accessed on 29th May 2025).

35. Palazzuoli, A., & Mullens, W. (2021). Cardiac congestion assessed by natriuretic peptides oversimplifies the definition and treatment of heart failure. *ESC Heart Failure*, *8*, 3453–3457. https://www.semanticscholar.org/paper/17d528ff59bf4ec40eb7c96d0068c2cb89c8918e (accessed on 29th May 2025).

36. Peters, A. E., Clare, R. M., Chiswell, K., Harrington, J., Kelsey, A., Hernandez, A. F., Felker, G., et al. (2024). Implications of trial eligibility in patients with heart failure with mildly reduced or preserved ejection fraction. *ESC Heart Failure*, *11*, 2813–2824. https://www.semanticscholar.org/paper/0733995325ca462081df02e3690f5ea0028fa058 (accessed on 29th May 2025).

37. Peterson, J. K., Clarke, S., Gelb, B. D., Kasparian, N. A., Kazazian, V., Pieciak, K., Pike, N. A., et al. (2024). Trisomy 21 and congenital heart disease: Impact on health and functional outcomes from birth through adolescence: A scientific statement from the American Heart Association. *Journal of the American Heart Association: Cardiovascular and Cerebrovascular Disease*, *13*. https://www.semanticscholar.org/paper/75ceacade7ee523041798c7931c2aedc231a792f (accessed on 29th May 2025).

38. Pourghasemi, Z., Norouzi, N., Safari, N., Khakpour, H., Keypoori, D., Shams, F., Abdous, A., et al. (2025). Prevalence of congenital heart diseases in dogs in Tehran, Iran: A retrospective study from 2013 to 2023. *Veterinary Medicine International*, *2025*. https://www.semanticscholar.org/paper/5908a5108f23c5ea72edde4cc6cb29de63cea027 (accessed on 29th May 2025).

39. Pratiwi, I. K., Martini, H., Tjahjono, C. T., Anjarwani, S., & Handari, S. D. (2023). The effect of exercise training as adjuvant treatment on functional capacity in congenital heart disease with negative Vaso reactivity test pulmonary hypertension patient at Saiful Anwar Hospital Malang. *Heart Science Journal*. https://www.semanticscholar.org/paper/ea4278c4625ddd8f38834413642af62b5730efc1 (accessed on 29th May 2025).

40. Rouzrokh, P., Rezaee, M., Mohammadipour, Z., Tavana, S., Khaheshi, I., Sheikhy, A., & Faghihi, L. T. (2024). The association of radiologic right heart strain indices with the severity of pulmonary parenchymal involvement and prognosis in patients with COVID-19. *Journal of Cardiovascular and Thoracic Research*, *16*, 171–178. https://www.semanticscholar.org/paper/67eca8db248419347fd94a42a42642cc6cb8b3c4 (accessed on 29th May 2025).

41. Silva, L. D. E., Reyes, L. F., Muñoz, B. K. I., Ávalos, N. J. A., Durán, L. L. P., & Regalado, V. E. E. (2024). Long-term follow-up in patients with modified Fontan: Assessing outcomes, complications, and management strategies for single-ventricle survivors. *International Journal of Medical Science and Clinical Research Studies*. https://www.semanticscholar.org/paper/ca39833eede98c3ddbe42d805bb0c5cd9f45dd07 (accessed on 29th May 2025).

42. Sycheva, T. V., & Perelman, J. (2024). Diagnosis of heart failure in patients with chronic obstructive pulmonary disease. *Bulletin Physiology and Pathology of Respiration*. https://www.semanticscholar.org/paper/83c49dab9698fd372e3b229d3e776fb1b59458f0 (accessed on 29th May 2025).

43. Szydlowski, S., Szydlowski, S., Luliak, M., & Luliak, M. (2020). Prevention of disease-related mortality from chronic non-communicable diseases. *Journal Name Not Provided*, *11*, 28–33. https://www.semanticscholar.org/paper/751febd36d5fc740667af49710b4444eaa72e9b3 (accessed on 29th May 2025).

44. Tarras, E., Singh, I., Kreiger, J., & Joseph, P. (2025). Exercise pulmonary hypertension and beyond: Insights in exercise pathophysiology in pulmonary arterial hypertension (PAH) from invasive cardiopulmonary exercise testing. *Journal of Clinical Medicine*, *14*. https://www.semanticscholar.org/paper/12e34ba276d5ae5596b88d918384fab67c765899 (accessed on 29th May 2025).

45. The Writing Committee of the Report on Cardiovascular in China, Sheng-Shou Hu. (2023). Report on cardiovascular health and diseases in China 2021: An updated summary. *Journal of Geriatric Cardiology: JGC*, *20*(6), 399–430. https://www.semanticscholar.org/paper/b3da8bacf180f6e35d727cc389a5a67cf39fb90d (accessed on 29th May 2025).

46. Torres, R., & Torres, T. (2024). A Brazilian neonatal unit's experience with functional echocardiography and diagnostic findings in congenital heart disease. *Medical Research Archives*. https://www.semanticscholar.org/paper/0929370005a75ba29c5e1c52b419808a8d3dc632 (accessed on 29th May 2025).

47. Vahanian, A., Beyersdorf, F., Praz, F., Milojevic, M., Baldus, S., Bauersachs, J., Capodanno, D., et al. (2021). 2021 ESC/EACTS guidelines for the management of valvular heart disease. *European Heart Journal*, *43*, 561–632. https://doi.org/10.1093/eurheartj/ehab395 (accessed on 29th May 2025).

48. Wang, L., Li, Y., Zhang, R., Liu, H., & Chen, L. (2024). Clinical features and risk factors for recurrence of idiopathic pulmonary hemosiderosis in children. *BMC Pulmonary Medicine*, *24*. https://www.semanticscholar.org/paper/b64ac415a5b314e901456ed60765a63f9da3f529 (accessed on 29th May 2025).

49. Wu, W. J., Zhang, C. D., Sun, Y., Li, X., Li, X. Y., & Zhu, M. J. (2024). [Analysis of evidence map of clinical research on Chinese patent medicines in treatment of chronic pulmonary heart disease]. *Zhongguo Zhong Yao Za Zhi = Zhongguo Zhongyao Zazhi = China Journal of Chinese Materia Medica*, *49*(19), 5354–5364. https://www.semanticscholar.org/paper/19890d8b196ea6e3d0062981f84ba7f150683d70 (accessed on 29th May 2025).

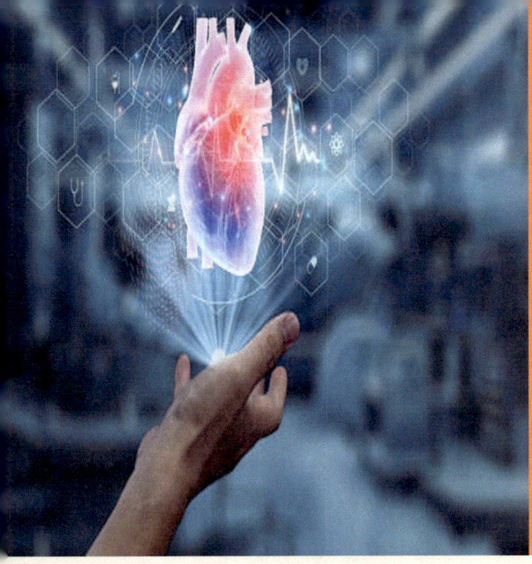

Chapter 14

DISEASES OF THE PERICARDIUM

Contents

Introduction

The two-layered pericardial sac that encloses the heart has a vital role in cardiac protection and function. The pericardium has vital and critical role in reducing frictional forces during heart operation by lubricating the heart, and it also governs the location of the heart in the thoracic cavity. Pericardial diseases can result in profound complications that affect overall cardiovascular health. Pericarditis, pericardial effusion, and constrictive pericarditis disrupt the normal functioning of this protective sac, often producing a lot of pain and necessitating the intervention of a physician. The growing awareness of these conditions highlights the significance of clinicians considering pericardial disease in the differential diagnosis of chest pain and other cardiac-related presenting complaints, thus enhancing patient care and outcomes in clinical practice. Pericardial disease presentation may be variable and thus difficult to diagnose. Pericardial disease typically presents as pleuritic, sharp, well-defined chest pain radiating to the shoulder or the neck, requiring a detailed differential diagnosis. The symptoms usually overlap with other cardiac and non-cardiac disease, including acute myocardial infarction and respiratory diseases. Moreover, progression from mild distress to life-threatening conditions, such as cardiac tamponade secondary to massive pericardial effusion, demands prompt response to presentation. For their optimal management, clinicians must exercise diligence in finding the nuance of presentation and employing correct diagnostic tools to confirm their impression, as outlined by existing clinical guidelines and best practices (Ponikowski et al., 2016).

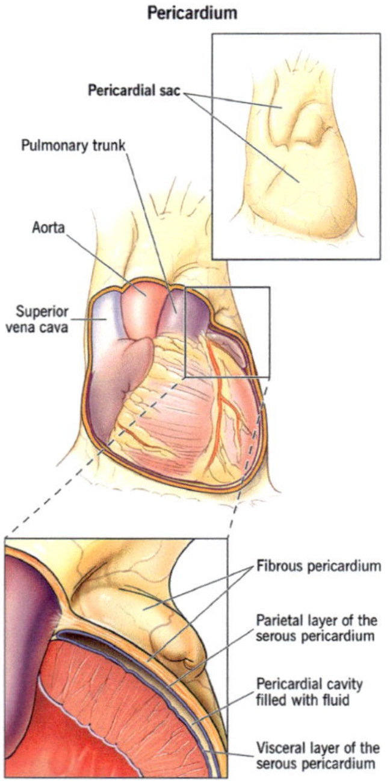

Figure 14.1. Your pericardium has two main layers that surround your heart. The inner layer (serous pericardium) is itself made of two layers with pericardial fluid in between.

Source: https://my.clevelandclinic.org/-/scassets/images/org/health/articles/23561-pericardium.

Integration of contemporary guidelines in clinical settings greatly enhances the treatment of pericardial conditions. The medical practitioners are urged to familiarize themselves with available guidelines that aim at early detection and intervention strategies based on specific patient needs. It not only aids in accurate diagnosis but also ensures that treatments do not contradict existing health authority guidelines. Moreover, education about evolving diagnostic techniques and therapeutic interventions is also required for providing the best patient care. With the evolution of medicine and medical science, new developments and findings take place continuously, and it becomes essential to remain updated with the latest information so that quality healthcare in the form of pericardial diseases can be ensured (Adler et al., 2015) (Figure 14.1).

Definition of the Pericardium

The pericardium is a double-layered fibrous sac covering the heart, and it is of utmost relevance in maintaining cardiac function and health. It is a structure composed of an outer fibrous layer and an inner layer of serous membrane, again dividing into the parietal and visceral pericardium. The fibrous layer provides mechanical protection, protecting the heart from trauma and infection. In contrast, the serous layer secretes pericardial fluid, which is a lubricant employed to reduce friction between the heart and the surrounding tissues during the cardiac cycle. It is essential to know the definition and anatomy of the pericardium because numerous diseases can directly involve this tissue, leading to serious cardiovascular complications. When speaking of the diseases of the pericardium, it is of fundamental significance to know its function as concerns the mechanics of the heart. The pericardium provides the most favorable pressure and positional stability of the heart within the thoracic cavity. Various pathological conditions can arise, like pericarditis, pericardial effusion, and constrictive pericarditis. Pericarditis refers to inflammation of the pericardial sac caused usually by viral infections, autoimmune disorders, or postoperative illness. Contrarily, pericardial effusion refers to a pathological accumulation of fluid within the pericardial space, which can lead to cardiac tamponade, a life-threatening situation where the functioning capacity of the heart is compromised. These conditions are of high risk and require comprehensive evaluation and care procedures to ensure patient health and safety. Moreover, the role of the pericardium extends beyond its structural function, as it also governs the inflammatory response and overall cardiovascular function. Notably, deposition of epicardial adipose tissue (EAT) around the heart has been blamed for many cardiovascular diseases, which highlights how pericardial anatomy is related to overall health. Recent research points to the importance of EAT as a primary imaging biomarker, particularly under low-dose computed tomography (LDCT) for cardiovascular risk stratification. Pericardial pathophysiology and diseases associated with it not only contribute to diagnosis but to the development of therapeutic targeting strategies as well, thereby supporting the clinical relevance of careful studies in this area (Hoskins et al., 2022; Liu et al., 2024). Through further investigation into the pericardium's definition and role, clinicians can enhance patient outcomes and achieve effective interventions in pericardial diseases (Figure 14.2).

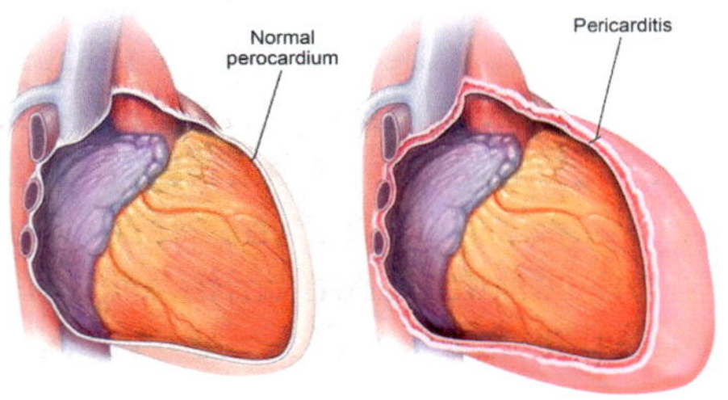

Figure 14.2. Pericarditis.

Source: https://i.ytimg.com/vi/ChdeYvBqC8Y/hq720.jpg?sqp=-oaymwEhCK4FEIIDSFryq4qpAxMIARUAAAAAGAElAADIQj0AgKJD&rs=AOn4CLAQC7YztPisK3wtz5_bQpIb_zdyzA.

14.1. Anatomy and Physiology of the Pericardium

The pericardium, a two-layered sac encasing the heart, plays a vital role in maintaining cardiac integrity and protecting the heart from infection and trauma. The pericardium consists of an outer fibrous layer and an inner serous layer. It functions to position the heart within the mediastinum and to restrict excessive movement of the heart with exercise. The fibrous layer contains dense connective tissue that provides the structural support, and the serous layer is further divided into the visceral and parietal layers so that the smooth movement between the heart and nearby structures is facilitated. This configuration reduces friction and permits the heart to expand and contract during the cardiac cycle, allowing the heart to function effectively despite the constant demands of circulation. These anatomical features highlight the pericardium's significant contribution to homeostasis and maintenance of cardiac well-being. The physiological functions of the pericardium extend beyond mechanical support; it is incredibly influential on hemodynamics and plays a crucial role in cardiac function. The pericardial space contains a small quantity of pericardial fluid that acts as a lubricant, reducing friction as the heart beats. This fluid also serves to cushion the heart from external pressures and trauma, which is highly crucial during physical exercise or trauma. Additionally, the pericardial sac also assists in regulating intracardiac pressure, essentially acting to coordinate the heart's volume and pressure relationships. Implications arise with some pericardial disorders, such as pericarditis and pericardial effusion, where pericardial structure and function changes can lead to compromised cardiac output. The intricate relationship between the pericardium's anatomy and its physiological functions cannot be overestimated, as both are essential to understanding the potential impact of disease on the overall health of the heart. In the presence of disease affecting the pericardium, the importance of a comprehensive understanding of its physiology and anatomy is amplified. Condition like constrictive pericarditis, in which the pericardium becomes rigid and obstructs filling of the heart, demonstrates a mechanism by which impaired structural integrity has significant hemodynamic consequences. Similarly, pericardial effusion may create a challenge whereby accumulation of excess fluid obstructs cardiac enlargement and leads to cardiac tamponade—a severe, life-threatening situation. In the realm of patient treatment, particularly in the fields of anesthetic and surgical care, understanding pericardial disease is crucial in planning effective perioperative patient management. Multidisciplinary intervention is typically required, all working together across cardiology, surgery, and critical care to ensure the optimal outcome for the patient. The understanding of the complex interaction between the anatomy and physiology of the pericardium enables clinicians to meet the challenges posed by these conditions with success (Correia et al., 2019) (Figure 14.3).

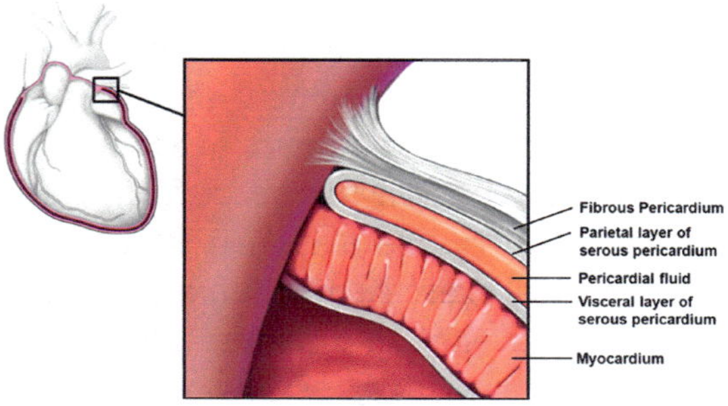

Figure 14.3. Anatomy of the normal pericardium.

Source: https://www.clevelandclinicmeded.com/medicalpubs/diseasemanagement/cardiology/pericardial-disease/images/figure-1.jpg.

14.1.1. Structure of the Pericardium

The pericardium, being a fibrous and serous sac enveloping the heart, consists of two layers known as the fibrous pericardium and the serous pericardium. The fibrous pericardium is an outer cover protecting the heart. It provides structural support and attaches the heart to its position inside the mediastinum such that it is not inappropriately displaced on exercise. This outer layer is firm, which is fitting given the heart's high functional needs, particularly regarding contractility and volume changes. The inner layer, or serous pericardium, is then further divided into the parietal and visceral layers, the latter of which is directly adhered to the myocardium. This arrangement is an essential component in reducing the friction of heartbeats and allowing smooth cardiac movement, emphasizing the importance of the structural integrity of the pericardium in maintaining effective cardiovascular performance. Besides its protective role, the pericardium is marked by unique immunological features, specifically with the addition of serosa-associated lymphoid clusters. These pericardial lymphoid tissues have a very significant role to play in their immune function, protecting the heart from infection and organizing immune response when invoked. Recent studies have indicated that the lymphoid population consists primarily of small and medium-sized lymphocytes and cells resembling plasma cells, which are crucial in the formation of antibodies. These facts suggest the dynamic nature of the pericardial structure not just as a mechanical barrier but also as an active participant in the cardiovascular immune environment, which is crucial in the context of pericardial disease (Verba et al., 2024). It is essential to have a vision of the intricate structure of the pericardium while examining pericardium diseases such as pericarditis or pericardial effusion. Pericardial layer disturbances may result in inflammation, infection, or fluid accumulation, substantially affecting cardiac function. For example, inflammation can adversely affect the pericardium's mechanical function and lymphatic drainage conductance, leading to excessive fluid accumulation that might hamper cardiac dynamics. Owing to the dual role of the pericardium as a structural support and immune activity location, any anatomical or pathological alteration in its anatomy impacts global cardiovascular health severely. It is hence imperative to recognize the complex structural components of the pericardium as the bedrock for determining the etiology and pathophysiology of pericardial diseases (Samsudin et al., 2024) (Figure 14.4).

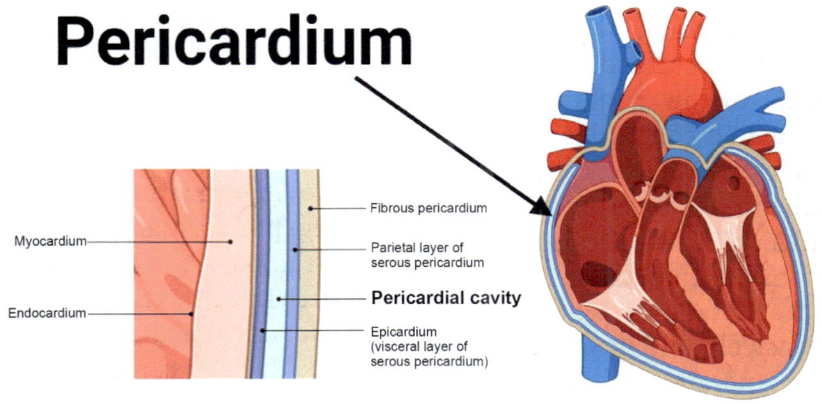

Figure 14.4. Structure of the pericardium.

Source: https://microbenotes.com/wp-content/uploads/2023/08/Pericardium.jpg.

14.1.2. Functions of the Pericardium

The pericardium, or the fibrous double-walled sac that covers the heart, serves several functions that are vital to cardiovascular health. Perhaps most significantly, it constitutes a protective covering that shields the heart from infection and trauma to the body. This structural protection is most important in the case of illnesses such as pericarditis, where inflammation can arise from a variety of etiologies. Also contained within the pericardium is a limited amount of circulating serous fluid, which facilitates smooth cardiac movement with the heart's cyclic contractions and relaxations. It is this lubrication that serves to decrease friction, thereby enabling efficient heart movement, essential to overall cardiovascular operation. Also, the pericardium possesses an active immunological role, positioned at the center of a growing focus on unmasking inflammatory cardiac conditions, making it essential beyond structural function (Aronow et al., 2019). Another crucial function of the pericardium is its influence on hemodynamics. Pericardial sac pressure can influence cardiac output and filling mechanics. Constrictive pericarditis, for instance, results in a rigid pericardial casing that restricts myocardial enlargement during diastole, which, ultimately, alters ventricular filling and reduces stroke volume. The pericardium, therefore, not only limiting but actively participates in the regulation of cardiac function, thereby underscoring its role in disease and health. In this capacity, pericardial volume alterations may exert significant influences on cardiac biomechanics. This indicates the need for a precise understanding of pericardial functions in determining clinical reactions to various pericardial diseases, where treatment may be directed at compensating for the pericardial restriction on cardiac efficiency (Alvarez et al., 2011). The function of the pericardium also involves its role in systemic physiological reaction and adaptation. As the body regulates fluid balance and adjusts to the physical demands, the pericardium acts in tandem with these adjustments, varying the volume of the pericardial effusion as needed. Under pathological states, however, such adaptive mechanisms become particularly significant, where excess fluid accumulation, or pericardial effusion, can result. An understanding of these processes is essential to the management of pericardial disease-related conditions because early treatment will spare the complications, such as cardiac tamponade, from arising due to unrestrained effusion. The multifunctional functions of the pericardium thus form a complex mosaic, the details of which need to be explored extensively within the context of cardiac wellness and disease regulation, with justification for ongoing research into pericardial pathology being a requirement for treatment advancements (Aronow et al., 2019) (Figure 14.5).

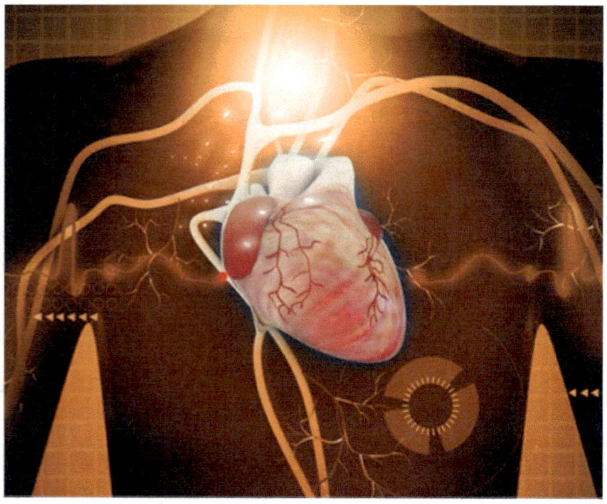

Figure 14.5. Functions of the Pericardium.

Source: https://acupunctureismylife.com/wp-content/uploads/2020/08/The-Functions-of-the-Pericardium.png.

14.1.3. Relationship with Surrounding Cardiac Structures

The double-layered fibrous sac surrounding the heart, the pericardium, plays a significant role in association with adjacent cardiac structures. The model of anatomy plays a vital role in functional integrity and in pathologic conditions that may be derived from the pericardial cavity. The pericardium houses the heart and provides a protective shield of its elastic nature, such that the heart may move freely during the relaxation and contraction period. Interestingly, the health of the pericardium can reflect the functional status of overlying structures, such as the myocardium and coronary arteries. During pericardial disease, e.g., pericarditis or effusion, it can significantly alter the biomechanics of these structures, modulating cardiac function and even aggravating systemic disease such as cardiovascular disease. Hence, awareness of such a relationship is imperative in formulating an optimal management strategy for cardiovascular pathology. Additionally, the intricate relationship between the pericardium and adjacent structures extends to the effect of adipose tissue surrounding the heart. Recent evidence explains how dysfunctional pericardial adipose tissue can exert detrimental consequences on the myocardium, significantly affecting cardiovascular disease pathogenesis. Essentially, when adipose tissue is dysfunctional, local tissue milieus become pro-inflammatory and insulin-resistant, influencing adjacent cardiac tissue. These adipokine factors could have the potential to enhance the pericardial disease-associated inflammatory milieu and enhance risk factors for T2DM. The cross-talk between pericardial adipose tissue and cardiac structures highlights the intricacy of cardiac pathology and the importance of considering these cross-talks while formulating therapeutic strategies (Chait et al., 2020). In the environment of the extracellular matrix, the pericardium illustrates a significant interconnection with surrounding cardiac tissue through its composition of collagen. Collagens are important structural proteins that contribute to the mechanical strength and stability of the pericardium and the heart in general. This extracellular matrix integrity is substantial in order to accommodate normal function of the myocardium, particularly in disease conditions such as fibrosis or hypertrophy. When pericardial disease exists, changes in collagen architecture can have a direct effect on cardiac compliance and contractility, with a consequent cascade of harmful effects on cardiac function. In addition, the ability to change collagenous structure through engineering and biochemical techniques opens up promising avenues for future therapeutic interventions toward the restoration of function. As further research continues to evolve in this area, it will be most crucial to be aware of the relationship between pericardial collagen dynamics and neighboring cardiac structures to treat pericardial diseases effectively (Sorushanova et al., 2018).

14.2. Types of Pericardial Diseases

The pericardium, which is a double-layered sac enveloping the heart, is prone to many diseases, each having characteristic pathological features and clinical importance. The most prevalent type of pericardial disease is pericarditis, an inflammatory condition of the pericardium. Pericarditis may be acute or chronic and is usually caused by viral infections, autoimmune responses, or post-operative causes. Acute pericarditis is typically marked by sudden chest pain and may be accompanied by pericardial effusion, where there is accumulation of fluid in the pericardial space. Chronic forms, if they follow acute episodes, may lead to progressive fibrosis and constriction and later compromise the heart's functional capacity. These distinctions are crucial for successful diagnosis and treatment, supporting the need to identify different clinical presentations about pericarditis. Pericardial effusion represents a second large category of pericardial disease and is characterized by the abnormal accumulation of fluid in the pericardial space. Many etiologies, including malignancy, infection, or systemic disease such as kidney failure or hypothyroidism may produce pericardial effusion. Effusion size, rate of accumulation, and underlying etiology play a crucial role in determining the course of the disease. In severe cases, rapid fluid buildup can lead to cardiac tamponade, a potentially life-threatening situation where pressure on the heart prevents it from pumping effectively. Diagnosis typically involves the use of echocardiography, which allows for visualization of fluid volumes and examination of hemodynamic stability. Immediate intervention, either through pericardiocentesis or surgical drainage, must be employed to prevent the risks associated with this life-threatening condition. Constrictive pericarditis is yet another serious form of pericardial disease that manifests as thickening and scarring of the pericardial sac consequent to a process of chronic inflammation or pericardial effusion. This leads to a rigid pericardium that obstructs the diastolic filling of the heart, ultimately leading to signs of heart failure such as dyspnea and edema. Clinically, patients may have presentation features such as elevated jugular venous pressure and pericardial knock, an early low-pitched murmur that is characteristic of constricted filling. Clinically, diagnosis is most reliant on imaging procedures such as echocardiography and magnetic resonance imaging that demonstrate the thickened pericardium and assess ventricular function. Therapy choice is generally surgery, including pericardiectomy, which can profoundly impact patient outcomes. It is essential to appreciate the nuances of constrictive pericarditis for optimal treatment and quality-of-life enhancement in patients with it (Figure 14.6).

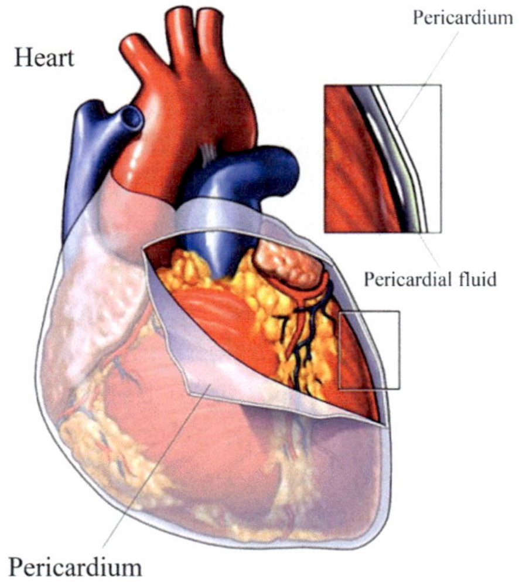

Figure 14.6. Pericardium.

Source: https://www.cardiosurgeon.co.uk/wp-content/uploads/2021/01/Pericardium.png.

14.2.1. Acute Pericarditis

Acute pericarditis is a pericardial inflammation and a grave clinical syndrome with numerous etiologic varieties and consequences on the health of the patient. Given the variety of etiologies and the complex nature of diagnosis and therapy, pericarditis may be caused by autoimmune disorders, infections, or secondary symptoms of systemic diseases. Clinically, acute pericarditis is characterized by intense signs such as severe chest pain, which spreads to the neck or shoulder, and dyspnea and fever. The burden of acute idiopathic recurrent pericarditis is high, with an estimated 27.7 per 100,000 individuals affected, emphasizing the public health significance of understanding this disease and effective control of the condition (Murkamilov et al., 2024). Consequently, treatment and early diagnosis are crucial to prevent complications like pericardial effusion or cardiac tamponade, which have a serious impact on prognosis and therapeutic success. The investigation for acute pericarditis is based predominantly on detailed clinical examination, both physical and laboratory, and advanced imaging techniques, the most crucial of which are echocardiography. This diagnostic center is essential because it allows for the assessment of pericardial effusion, which can be a complicating factor of the clinical presentation and needs urgent treatment. When diagnosed early, management of acute pericarditis often entails the use of corticosteroids and non-steroidal anti-inflammatory drugs (NSAIDs) to quiet inflammation and alleviate symptoms. Importantly, inflammatory marker tracking, along with patient symptomatology, plays a vital role in measuring response to therapy. Where conservative management fails, other treatments such as drainage of effusion may be required to minimize the occurrence of harmful complications (Murkamilov et al., 2024).

The multifactorial etiology of acute pericarditis, therefore, necessitates a multi-faceted treatment and long-term care strategy. Pathophysiology in acute pericarditis is complex, with interwoven molecular and systemic mechanisms reaching far beyond cardiac significance. Since acute pericarditis can result in heart failure, identification of the associated hemodynamic changes is significant, since the disease not only affects the pericardium but also results in a multisystemic response. The intricate association of inflammation with cardiac function suggests that treatment should not just focus on relieving pericarditis symptoms but also on considering the ramifications for cardiac health. As chronic inflammation was found to induce heart failure syndromes, additional studies would be necessary to characterize the pathophysiology of acute pericarditis and potential progression to chronic diseases. In addition, new advances in therapeutic management that treat concurrently the systemic consequences might enhance the outcome of patients. As such, a more integrative approach for heart disease must be adopted for future strategies in treating acute pericarditis (Figure 14.7).

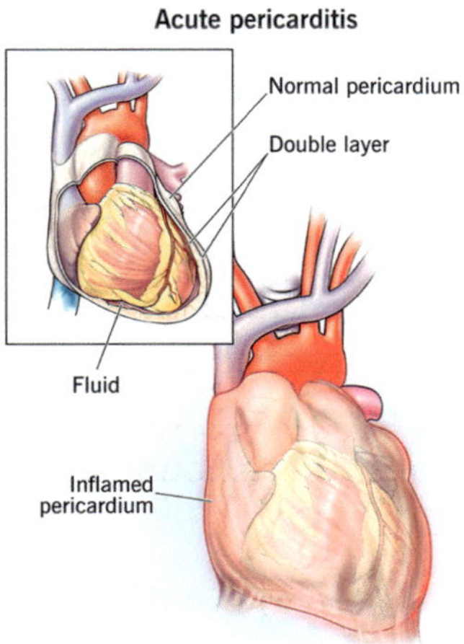

Figure 14.7. Acute pericarditis.

Source: https://my.clevelandclinic.org/-/scassets/images/org/health/articles/22918-acute-pericarditis.

14.2.2. Pericardial Effusion

In understanding the clinical significance of pericardial effusion in pericardial disorders, it is essential to understand its inherent anatomical and physiological characteristics. The pericardium is a two-walled covering sac around the heart, which is usually filled with a minute amount of fluid—approximately 20–50 mL—to allow for lubrication of the heart's motion. However, pericardial effusion represents pathological accumulation of excess fluid within this sac due to various pathogenic processes, including infection, malignancy, or inflammation. Beyond its structural function, the pericardium also has active immunological activity that is engaged in the pathophysiologic process of related cardiac illnesses like pericarditis and myocarditis. This complexity underscores the importance of accurate diagnosis of pericardial effusion as a precursor to successful disease care and management and treatment strategies (Aronow et al., 2019). The etiologic conditions responsible for causing pericardial effusion may be varied, covering the range of acute and chronic illness. Infectious causes, such as viral or bacterial infections, and non-infectious causes, such as autoimmune disease or malignancy, are some of the frequent causative agents. In addition, fluid accumulation may be transudative, exudative, or sanguineous depending on the fundamental mechanism of fluid accumulation. Of note, as in planning the management of pericardial effusion, the clinical context and patient history should also be taken into account to plan an appropriate treatment strategy. Diagnostic equipment such as echocardiography is valuable when evaluating pericardial effusion, allowing clinicians to quantify the size of the effusion and its potential hemodynamic impact on cardiac function.

This knowledge is useful when creating interprofessional care strategies for patient management (Al-Razik et al., 2022). Untreated pericardial effusion carries grave clinical ramifications, which can lead to cardiac tamponade, a potentially deadly syndrome in which increased pressure surrounding the heart inhibits its normal filling and ejection. Pericardial effusion patients may be symptomatic with chest discomfort, dyspnea, and evidence of hemodynamic compromise, for which urgent medical evaluation is warranted. Management of these effusions not only involves addressing the root etiology, but in certain situations, therapeutic intervention in the form of pericardiocentesis needs to be initiated to bring relief and restore normal cardiac function. Ideal patient outcomes demand an interdisciplinary approach, with emphasis placed upon communication among health professionals—primary care physicians, cardiologists, and surgeons—towards coordination of care. Lastly, recognition and early treatment of pericardial effusion can significantly enhance prognosis and quality of life in involved patients (Aronow et al., 2019) (Figure 14.8).

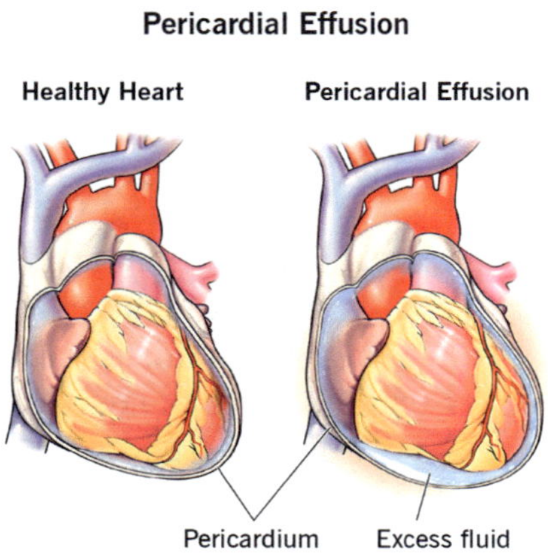

Figure 14.8. Pericardial effusion.

Source: https://my.clevelandclinic.org/-/scassets/images/org/health/articles/17351-pericardial-effusion.

14.2.3. Constrictive Pericarditis

Constrictive pericarditis is an ominous pathological transformation of the pericardium, with fibrosis and thickening of the pericardial sac. Constrictive pericarditis causes the pericardium to lose its elasticity, a condition necessary for the heart to expand during diastole. Because the heart cannot be filled adequately due to this limited space, patients with this condition typically manifest signs of heart failure like fatigue, dyspnea, and edema.

Furthermore, the etiology of constrictive pericarditis is also possibly multifactorial and ranges from infectious origins to post-operative change following cardiac surgery. Understanding these pathways is vital for improving diagnostic and therapeutic interventions, as clinical presentation often mimics other forms of heart disease, thereby making the evaluation process more complex (Aronow et al., 2019). The treatment of constrictive pericarditis should be careful, multidisciplinary, recognizing the need for both medical and surgical interventions. Medical therapy may be palliative but has been found not to change the active fibrotic process. Hence, surgery, particularly pericardiectomy, has emerged as the definitive therapy, to remove the contractile pericardial layer to provide proper filling pressures. Studies show that patients undergoing the procedure maintain a 10-year survival rate of almost 50%, where timely intervention is of paramount importance (Al-Razik et al., 2022).

While there is potential with surgery, careful monitoring of patients to prevent postoperative complications and adequate follow-up care are crucial considerations, which emphasizes the need for a multidisciplinary approach between healthcare professionals in treating this severe condition effectively. In assessing constrictive pericarditis patients' outcomes and quality of life, it is clear that the prognosis is greatly affected by early treatment and diagnosis. Since this condition tends to be long-lasting, the long-term issues gradually worsen, negatively affecting common daily functions and overall well-being. As noted, there should be collaboration among cardiologists, surgeons, and physical rehabilitation experts to fully utilize the potential for patient outcomes and recovery (Al-Razik et al., 2022). Not only does such an extensive approach address the short-term physiological fluctuations posed by constrictive pericarditis, but it also touches on the emotional and psychological well-being of patients with this disabling condition. Lastly, ongoing research and clinical trials into emerging medical treatments and new surgical strategies can further refine management techniques and perhaps enhance survival rates for those who have pericardial diseases, such as constrictive pericarditis (Figure 14.9).

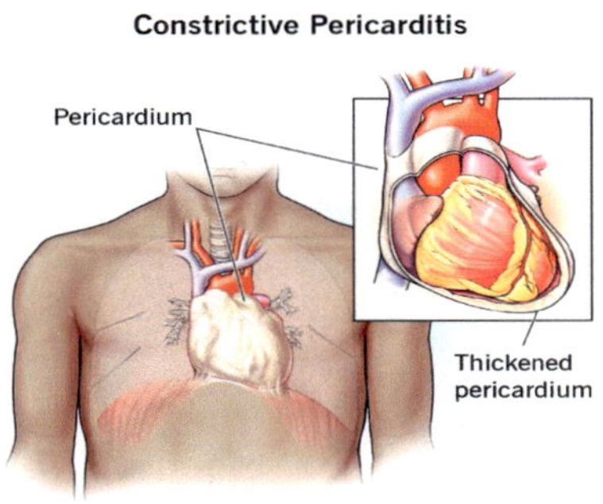

Figure 14.9. Constrictive pericarditis.

Source: https://my.clevelandclinic.org/-/scassets/images/org/health/articles/22373-constructive-pericarditis.

14.3. Causes of Pericardial Diseases

The etiology of pericardial diseases is multifaceted, including a variety of infectious, inflammatory, and non-infectious causes. Among the determinants affecting them, viral infections are notably frequent, and Coxsackievirus and echovirus are often implicated viruses. The etiologic agents can cause acute pericarditis, an intense inflammation of the pericardium, with chest pain and hemodynamic alterations. In addition, both fungal and bacterial causes are capable of initiating pericardial effusion and cardiac tamponade, which are associated with an excess of fluid in the pericardial sac.

Although infection is usually the immediate factor, autoimmune diseases such as systemic lupus erythematosus and rheumatoid arthritis also play a vital role in inducing pericardial diseases through the production of chronic inflammation and fibrosis. Recognition of these diverse etiologies is essential to diagnose and develop effective treatment protocols for affected patients accurately. Pericardial disease, except for infectious etiology, may occur secondary to non-infectious diseases such as malignancies, renal failure, and post-myocardial infarction syndromes. Neoplastic illness may lead to direct pericardial infiltration or induce effusions secondary to cancer therapy. Likewise, chronic renal failure patients may develop uremic pericarditis due to the accumulation of toxic metabolites. Post-myocardial infarction may trigger a particular form of pericarditis, called Dresslers syndrome, which is an autoimmune reaction following cardiac injury. Diuretic therapy in heart disease patients can amplify these fluid imbalances and lead to an increased risk of pericardial effusion. Therefore, understanding these associations in managing and preventing pericardial disease complications is crucial, particularly for patients with underlying cardiovascular conditions (Poelgeest et al., 2023). Lifestyle and environmental factors are also responsible for the development of pericardial disease. The COVID-19 pandemic, as reported by current studies, has altered people's habits and diet, which may exacerbate existing health issues like cardiovascular disease. Specific populations revealed higher rates of obesity and poor dietary habits during isolation, which are associated with a higher incidence of cardiovascular comorbidities like pericarditis. Furthermore, psychosocial stressors during the pandemic might contribute to the pathogenesis of inflammatory processes in vulnerable patients. As suggested by recent evidence, synergy between lifestyle choices, systemic health, and infection reflects the multifactorial nature of pericardial disease. Targeted nutritional supplements and public health interventions can be effective in minimizing pericardial disease-associated risk factors and overall cardiovascular wellness during disasters (2 et al., 2023) (Figure 14.10).

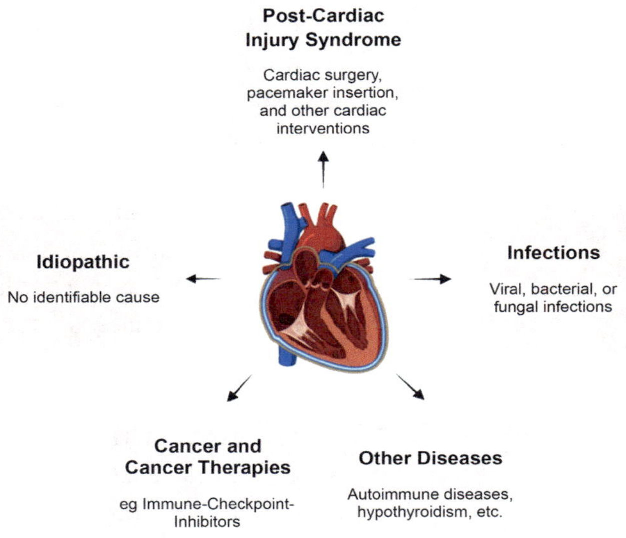

Figure 14.10. Causes of pericardial diseases.

Source: https://ucsfhealthcardiology.ucsf.edu/sites/ucsfhealthcardiology.ucsf.edu/files/inline-images/Screenshot%202024-07-30%20at%206.02.05%20PM_0.png.

14.3.1. Infectious Agents

Infectious agents play a crucial role in pericardial disease pathogenesis, particularly pericarditis and effusion disease. Pericarditis caused by coxsackievirus and echovirus viral infections ranks among the highest in acute pericarditis. These pathogens are capable of stimulating violent immune reactions, resulting in inflammation and fluid buildup in the pericardial space. Also, bacterial infections—most often tuberculosis, pneumonia, and staphylococcal infections—can be responsible for both effusion and constrictive pericarditis. The multicriteria role of such infectious agents necessitates timely and proper diagnosis to optimize treatment and prevent grave sequelae. For instance, acute accumulation of pericardial effusion can lead to critical hemodynamic impairment, which underscores the necessity to be aware of the infectious etiology of these fluid collections (Bacalbasa et al., 2020). In addition to viral and bacterial infections, fungal and parasitic illnesses are increasingly being recognized as potential causes of pericardial disease. Fungal infections, particularly those due to endemic mycoses such as histoplasmosis and coccidioidomycosis, can produce extensive pericardial effusion. The infections may be insidiously acquired rather than being typical bacterial pathogens, so early diagnosis and treatment are problematic. Parasitic infestation, as by Trypanosoma cruzi, can lead to Chagas disease, with associated inflammation of the heart and resulting pericardial disease. The variety of infections between causes of pericardial disorders makes the clinical scenario for experts to handle more difficult, particularly in endemic regions where specific pathogens are more prevalent (Haritha et al., 2019). Diagnosis and treatment of pericardial diseases demand a thorough understanding of the causative infectious agents, whose unique characteristics dictate both clinical presentation and therapeutic approach. Diagnostic imaging such as echocardiography is significant in the identification of pericardial effusion and assessment of severity, especially in the setting of infectious disease. The evaluation protocols should include serological tests and imaging studies to determine the causative contagious etiology. Follow-up treatment regimens may involve antimicrobial therapy that is targeted to the cause of the pathogen, from antiviral medications to antibiotics, depending on the causative agent. By using a well-organized and informed approach to the diagnosis and treatment of causative infections that lead to pericardial disease, patients can be assisted by healthcare providers and the risk for severe complications minimized (Bacalbasa et al., 2020) (Figure 14.11).

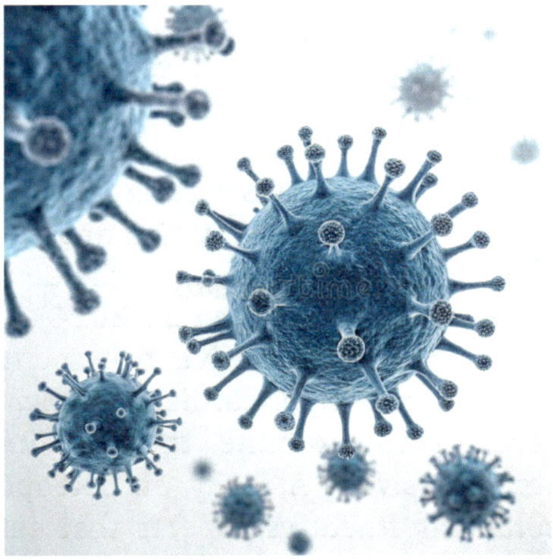

Figure 14.11. Infectious agents.

Source: https://thumbs.dreamstime.com/b/microscopic-view-infectious-agents-isolated-white-background-microscopic-view-infectious-agents-isolated-white-365926643.jpg.

14.3.2. Autoimmune Disorders

The relationship between autoimmune and pericardial diseases is a good representation of the intricate relationship between cardiovascular health and the immune system. Autoimmune diseases such as systemic lupus erythematosus and rheumatoid arthritis have been shown to impact the pericardium, leading to conditions like pericarditis—an inflammation of the pericardial sac. The malfunction of the immune system in these disorders can lead to a perpetual state of inflammation, which can predispose one to cardiac complications. A deregulated immune response not only causes tissue damage in peripheral organs but can also spill over to have an impact on the heart and surrounding structures. The complexity of this interaction underlines the need for continued research into the pathways of autoimmune-induced cardiovascular pathology and the development of targeted therapies for treating both autoimmune disease and its impact on cardiac health. Moreover, pathophysiologic mechanisms linking autoimmune diseases with pericardial disease are multifactorial, including genetic predisposition and environmental elements. Some autoantibodies can contribute to the development of pericardial effusion, represented by the accumulation of fluid within the pericardial cavity. Such effusions can significantly impair cardiac performance, leading to symptoms such as chest discomfort and shortness of breath. On a related note, autoimmune illnesses like multiple sclerosis highlight how systemic inflammation predisposes patients to increased cardiovascular morbidity. Still more recent evidence suggests that the persistent inflammatory milieu characteristic of autoimmune illnesses plays a central role in pericardial disease pathogenesis (Francesco, 2024). Clarifying the complex relationship is the key to devising holistic treatment plans that consider both autoimmune and cardiovascular factors. Finally, significant correlations have also been demonstrated between thyroid and skin autoimmune diseases and their cardiac counterparts. For instance, epidemiological studies have documented correlations between illnesses like vitiligo and autoimmune thyroid disease with potential health effects on the cardiovascular system. Autoimmune thyroid diseases (AITDs), in particular, are involved in modulating heart function, possibly through mechanisms mediated through thyroid hormone action on cardiac tissue. The bidirectional associations between many autoimmune conditions form an intricate scenario for diagnosis and management, particularly when pericardial disease is involved (Chen et al., 2024). As physicians face more patients with comorbid autoimmune and cardiac disease, comprehension of these correlations becomes essential to offering multifaceted care that considers the patients' general well-being and quality of life (Figure 14.12).

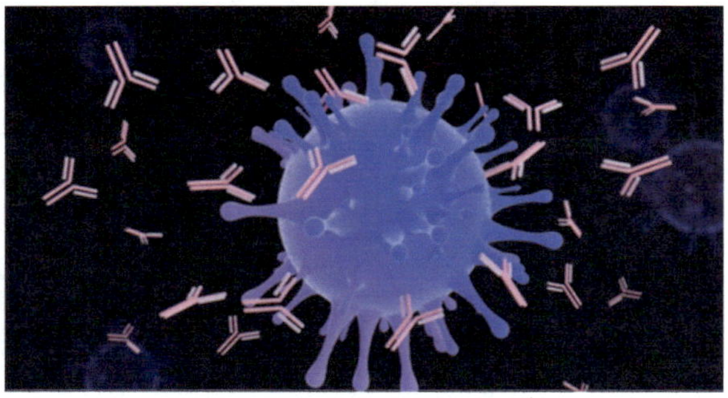

Figure 14.12. Autoimmune diseases.

Source: https://images.contentstack.io/v3/assets/blt324fd0a04af716e6/blte2a9081f701888f2/64cb36bd4bfeb1d3de86059c/Floating_antibodies.jpeg?fit=crop&width=480&height=256.

14.3.3. Trauma and Surgical Complications

Trauma and surgical complications are fundamental considerations in the case of pericardial diseases, particularly when managing conditions like pericarditis and tamponade. Trauma can lead to direct insults to the pericardium, destroying its functional and structural integrity and giving rise to complications like infection and effusion. Surgical interventions, whether emergent or elective, also have built-in risks. The treatment plan usually depends on the severity of the underlying disorder and concomitant trauma. Where surgery is inevitable, the nature of the approach—conventional open or minimal-invasive procedures—greatly influences the occurrence of complications. The understanding of these dynamics is crucial for clinicians to pre-empt risks and optimize outcomes in patients. Recent studies emphasize the necessity for better surgical methods to reduce traumatic injury and pericardial disease complications. For instance, robotic pancreatic resection with vascular resection has become a legitimate option. It has delivered similar outcomes to traditional methods but with potentially less risk of conversion and blood loss. The studies indicate that surgery time may be surprisingly longer, which may correlate with increased postoperative complications. By observing the results of minimally invasive procedures, one can see that despite some studies observing higher complication rates with radical approaches, survival is still in favor overall. When it comes to the management of pericardial diseases, this contradiction necessitates a careful evaluation of each patient's clinical situation and surgical history as crucial components of the decision-making process (Ferrara et al., 2024). Under the scenario of conservative treatment and surgery of traumatic pericardial complications, it is crucial to examine the outcome of patients extensively. A study on osteoporotic thoracolumbar fractures reports that surgical intervention has a tendency to be more invasive and has a greater rate of complications, such as surgical site infections or mechanical failure. The findings reveal that while conservative treatment poses less danger, the invasive options yield better improvement in pain control and mobility for more severe conditions. Thus, the severity of patient conditions as defined by the present classification remains a good indicator of the interventions needed. This observation indicates the need for clinicians to effectively consider the advantages and limitations while developing treatment modalities for patients with pericardial disease, particularly in the context of injury or complication (Ullrich et al., 2023).

14.4. Symptoms and Diagnosis

The clinical presentation of pericardial disease is very heterogeneous, making accurate diagnosis a demanding task for doctors. Repeated symptoms of the pericardium include chest pain, dyspnea, and palpitations. The chest pain is said to be sharp and pleuritic, aggravated by deep inspiration or coughing. In some cases, symptoms can be insidious, i.e., fatigue or a minimal diminution in tolerance to exercise. As symptoms of pericardial disease can be similar to other cardiac and respiratory diseases, history and clinical examination play a role. Moreover, acute presentation, i.e., angina, can be misleading. With the possibility of non-specificity of the symptoms, doctors must employ an evidence-based approach for differentiating pericardial disease from other thoracic diseases, hence the need for a balanced method of diagnosis. To achieve a definitive diagnosis of pericardial disorders, medical professionals typically utilize a range of imaging modalities in combination with clinical assessment. A chest X-ray may be initially performed; however, the latter is typically nonspecific to show pericardial disease. Referral to advanced imaging modalities such as computed tomography (CT) and magnetic resonance imaging (MRI) is needed for pericardium visualization and evaluation of accompanying structures like the heart and great vessels. Multimodal diagnostic strategies allow practitioners to build a better representation of the status of the patient. For example, in cases of congenital pericardial agenesis or pericardial cysts, advanced imaging can point out the relevant anatomical structures that are used in surgical plans and intervention. Notably, the application of imaging is accentuated by the inherent complexity of these pathologies, which tends to undermine the efficacy of primary evaluations. In addition, the etiology of pericardial disease also converges with imaging and clinical findings to further limit the diagnosis. Differentiation between various types of pericardial disease, including pericarditis, effusion, or constrictive pericarditis, is made on the identification of symptoms and correlating it with imaging studies. For instance, recognition of abnormal pericardial structures, i.e., agenesis or cysts, is important for planning treatment, especially when surgery is needed. As observed in clinical experience, congenital malformations can lead to extraordinary surgical challenges, thus stressing the importance of accurate diagnostic assessment before intervention (Badgett et al., 2024). In addition, pericardial illnesses can be associated with other cardiac ailments, making the diagnostic picture more complex. Therefore, a thorough appreciation of symptoms and sound diagnostic practices is absolutely necessary to ensure successful management of pericardial illnesses, ultimately improving the outcomes of patients (Figure 14.13).

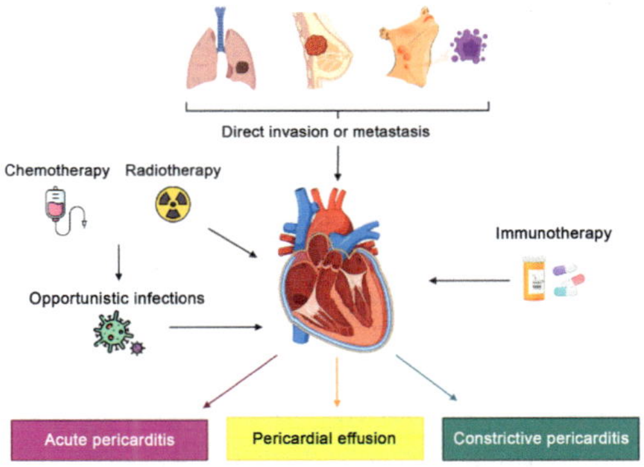

Figure 14.13. Clinical manifestations of pericardial disease.

Source: https://www.mdpi.com/cancers/cancers-16-03466/article_deploy/html/images/cancers-16-03466-g001.png.

14.4.1. Common Symptoms Associated with Pericardial Diseases

The symptomatic spectrum of pericardial

illnesses is broad, reflecting the spectrum of etiologies that can affect the pericardium. The most common clinical manifestation is chest pain, typically sharp and pleuritic in character, always exacerbated by deep breathing or coughing. As with acute pericarditis, the cause of the pain is an inflammation of the pericardial sac. Additionally, patients may develop dyspnea, shortness of breath, particularly with exertion, and present with fatigue and malaise. Although these may be acute presentations, chronic disease may be presented insidiously with resulting worsening heart failure symptoms as the disease evolves. This symptomatology complexity usually demands a full clinical evaluation to differentiate pericardial diseases from other cardiovascular illnesses, ultimately affecting patient care and outcomes within healthcare, a concern heightened by studies on cardiovascular disease prevalence and mortality trends (Morgan et al., 2024). In addition to the common symptoms of chest pain and dyspnea, patients with pericardial diseases may exhibit pericardial effusion, which can lead to typical findings of hypotension and muffled heart sounds. The combination of these three symptoms, defined as Beck's triad, is particularly found in cardiac tamponade. This condition can be life-threatening because of the excess amount of fluid accumulating in the pericardial space. Also, patients may have pulsus paradoxus, decreasing blood pressure with inspiration, further obscuring the presentation clinically. Detection of such vital signs is crucial to offer early intervention because uncorrected cardiac tamponade can be followed by severe hemodynamic instability. Medical practitioners must be vigilant during inspection of such signs because they are primarily markers of severity and clinical significance of the pericardial diseases in favor of a proper diagnostic technique and treatment approach (Al-Attar et al., 2024). Furthermore, psychosocial disturbances typically occur after physical symptoms of pericardial diseases, affecting patients' general state and well-being. The chronic pain of these conditions, along with potentially imposed lifestyle restrictions, can induce more anxiety and depression. The psychological burden can worsen the perception of pain and render treatment nonadherence difficult, which justifies the need for a multidisciplinary approach in the management of pericardial disease patients. It is vital to grasp the relationship between physical symptoms and psychosocial processes in developing integrated care plans that not only cure the medical condition but also address the emotional and psychological demands of patients. Establishing an environment where clinicians are aware of these facets, the result of healthcare can be significantly improved, and treatment of pericardial diseases may be made holistic and patient-centered (Morgan et al., 2024) (Figure 14.14).

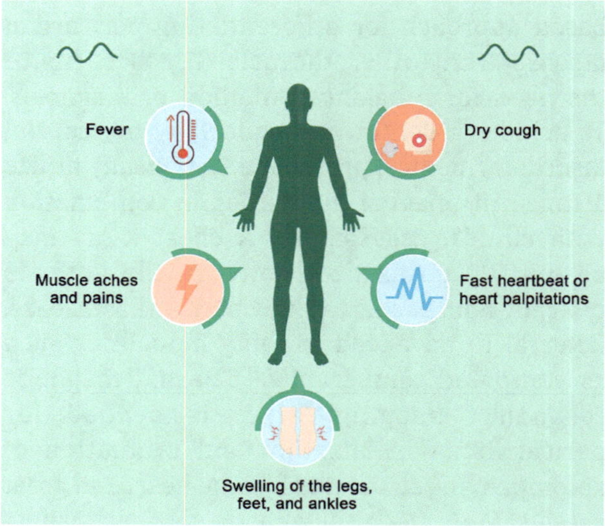

Figure 14.14. Symptoms associated with pericardial diseases.

Source: https://images.everydayhealth.com/images/seo-graphic-content-initiative/eh-symptoms-of-pericarditis-1080x1080-seo-graphics-gs.png?w=1110.

14.4.2. Diagnostic Imaging Techniques

Diagnostic imaging modalities are critically

important for the diagnosis and treatment of pericardial illnesses, providing clinicians with basic information about the status of the cardiovascular system. Among all modalities, CMR is exceptional in that it allows for detailed anatomical and functional assessment of the pericardium. CMR has particularly been renowned for its multiplanar imaging and characterization of tissue, allowing detailed evaluation of diseases such as pericarditis, pericardial effusion, and constrictive pericarditis. Its non-invasive nature and absence of ionizing radiation also contribute to its utility in routine clinical practice. Clinicians need to understand the various imaging sequences utilized in CMR so that they can interpret the findings meaningfully and correlate them with the clinical presentation of patients, ultimately determining management (Wang et al., 2022).

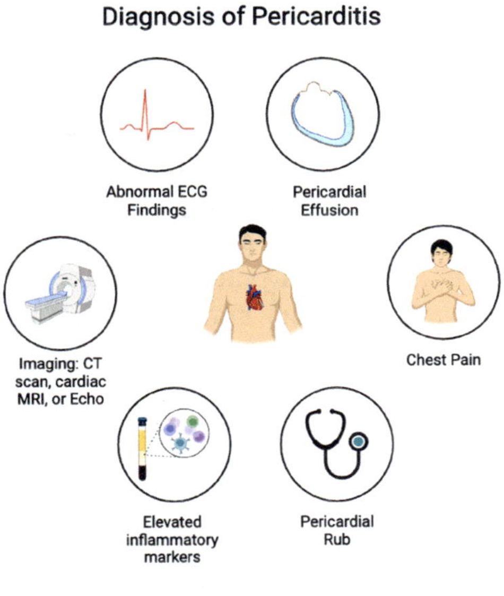

Figure 14.15. Diagnosis of pericarditis.

Source: https://ucsfhealthcardiology.ucsf.edu/sites/ucsfhealthcardiology.ucsf.edu/files/inline-images/Screenshot%202024-07-29%20at%204.28.49%20PM_0.png.

The incorporation of CMR in the diagnostic pathways thus underscores the significance of imaging in addressing pericardial diseases. Aside from CMR, echocardiography remains a cornerstone in the diagnosis of pericardial diseases due mainly to its availability and real-time imaging. This imaging modality is most appropriate in pericardial effusion evaluation, where physicians cannot only visualize the presence of fluid but also assess the hemodynamic effect of the effusion. Besides, echocardiography can be helpful to identify signs of cardiac tamponade and to evaluate ventricular size and function, both of which are relevant in the management of patients with large effusions. However, while echocardiography is extremely widespread, imaging limitations in some individuals or body habitus can necessitate the use of complementary imaging techniques. Lastly, combining echocardiography with more recent technologies such as CMR can provide a global image of pericardial disease, opening the door to improved treatment strategies (García-Pavía et al., 2021). Enhanced imaging technologies have also opened diagnostic avenues for some diseases, such as cardiac amyloidosis, which may be associated with pericardial disease. Cardiac amyloidosis is characterized by the deposition of amyloid fibrils within myocardial tissue, which evokes a range of effects duplicating or exacerbating pericardial disease. Newer literature has indicated that sophisticated imaging modalities, not only CMR but also positron emission tomography (PET), play significant roles in the diagnosis of cardiac amyloidosis. These modalities enable the detection of amyloid deposits and distinguish among the various forms of the disease—hereditary versus acquired. Thus, the joint usage of these advanced imaging technologies enhances the ability of clinicians to diagnose and treat advanced cardiac illnesses, such as amyloid-associated pericardial disease, and closes the gap between diagnostic capability and clinical management (García-Pavía et al., 2021) (Figure 14.15).

14.4.3. Laboratory Tests and Biomarkers

Diagnosis and management of pericardial diseases also increasingly rely on novel laboratory tests and biomarkers. The pericardium is a double-layered sac enclosing the heart that is an essential structure for the function of the heart and potentially involved in a wide range of pathological processes, such as inflammation and effusion. Laboratory investigations, including measurement of biomarkers, provide valuable information about the mechanisms of pericardial diseases. For instance, elevated levels of B-type natriuretic peptide (BNP) and NT-proBNP are also used in the clinical setting as a diagnostic indicator of heart failure, which is a complication of or can occur concurrently with pericardial illness. As these markers reflect the hemodynamic burden on the heart, their evaluation enhances the clinician's evaluation of cardiac issues that may result as a direct consequence of pericardial disease, highlighting the importance of integrative diagnostic approaches. Novel biomarkers such soluble ST2 and galectin-3, in addition to BNP monitoring, alert physicians to the possibility of adverse cardiac outcomes by indicating pathologic cardiac remodeling. They are instrumental in chronic heart failure, where fibrosis and long-term inflammation can occur in conjunction with pericardial disease. The clinical value of these biomarkers lies in their ability to provide complementary information on cardiac structure and function beyond traditional assessment. Clinical utility for these tests necessitates their integration into everyday practice, backed up by firm guidelines that govern their diagnostic and prognostic use in patients whose symptoms are suggestive of pericardial disease. Hence, an informed understanding of biomarker dynamics is indispensable in the optimization of therapy plans so that individualized treatment of each patient is possible. Furthermore, the interpretation of laboratory tests must be put in the background of the overall image of patient populations, particularly in the context of geriatric populations. As the pericardium undergoes age-related changes, the incidence of conditions such as acute pericarditis and cardiac tamponade increases, and hence, rigorous examination of the available clinical information becomes necessary. In elderly patients, traditional biomarkers may fluctuate based on inherent physiological alterations and therefore impact the pericardial disease diagnosis and treatment. An interdisciplinary approach by integrating biomarker evaluation with clinical evaluation and imaging methods can significantly assist in managing such disorders. Through the systematic analysis of laboratory findings in addition to patient history and symptoms, medical professionals can develop more efficient management plans to counteract the complexities involved with pericardial diseases, ultimately enhancing patient outcomes as a whole.

14.5. Treatment Options

Pericardial disease management also varies widely based on the precise disease diagnosed. For instance, in pericarditis, NSAIDs and corticosteroids are routinely used to reduce pain and prevent inflammation. Other drugs, such as colchicine, can be added in recurrent or chronic cases to prevent recurrence. Besides, more serious presentations, such as constrictive pericarditis, typically necessitate surgery, most often in the guise of pericardiectomy, which entails removal of the fibrotic pericardium. The operation has proven to be successful for symptom alleviation and restoration of cardiac function (Fernández Colino et al., 2019). All the treatment approaches emphasize the importance of addressing the disease symptoms as well as the underlying pathologic mechanisms behind pericardial diseases. In more complicated cases, such as pericardial effusion, the therapeutic approach may include medical as well as invasive management. While minor effusions are treated conservatively with observation and symptomatic care, symptomatic or extensive effusions typically require drainage. It may be performed through pericardiocentesis, when fluid from the pericardial space is aspirated with a needle, which gives quick relief of symptoms (Bressan et al., 2015). A more targeted intervention, like the surgical implantation of a pericardial window, would be required in cases when effusions do recur. This is for continuous drainage of fluid while maintaining the anatomical arrangement of the pericardium, illustrating the complexity and tailored management of pericardial disease. In addition, advances in medical technology have led to new therapeutic interventions for pericardial disease, particularly for stenting and grafting. There has also been an investigation into the use of elastin-like recombinamers (ELRs) in enhancing coronary stent performance, applicable if pericardial effusion is in some way related to coronary artery disease (Fernández Colino et al., 2019). Similarly, the use of decellularized bovine pericardium as a membrane for guided tissue regeneration is a sign of growing interest in regenerative approaches, which can be used to augment healing and restore function (Bressan et al., 2015). These new approaches represent a shift towards more sophisticated and biomimetic treatment modalities, with improved prospects for superior patient outcomes in pericardial illness. Hence, further research into such novel therapies is pivotal to the evolving world of the management of pericardial diseases (Figure 14.16).

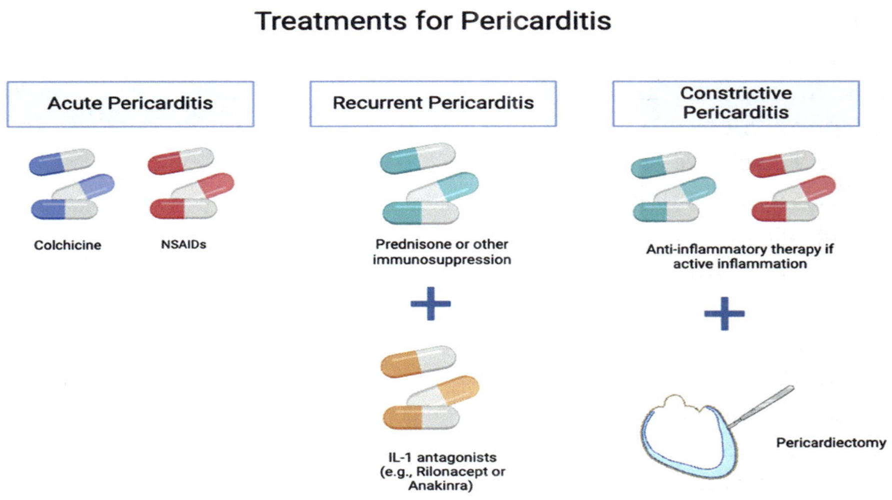

Figure 14.16. Treatment for pericarditis.

Source: https://ucsfhealthcardiology.ucsf.edu/sites/ucsfhealthcardiology.ucsf.edu/files/inline-images/Screenshot%202024-07-30%20at%206.06.04%20PM.png.

14.5.1. Medical Management

Effective medical management of pericardial diseases necessitates a careful understanding of the pathophysiology involved and the clinical presentation—ideally, treatment endeavors to address both the etiology and the symptoms that cause pericardial effusions. Medical treatment is commonly NSAIDs and corticosteroids in cases of inflammatory etiologies, such as autoimmune diseases.

The decision to initiate such treatments is, however, dependent on various factors like the general health of the patients, effusion volume, and presence of any underlying illnesses. Individualized management may be warranted in some pericardial diseases, emphasizing that one size does not fit all. Most specifically in chronically asymptomatic patients, conservative management with close monitoring may be the sole requirement, as the prognosis for idiopathic effusions is very favorable (Lazaros et al., 2021). Therefore, tailored therapy regimens are crucial to improving outcomes for patients with pericardial illness. Pericardial effusion management is often an invasive procedure beyond medical therapy, especially in hemodynamically unstable or in cardiac tamponade-presenting patients. In such situations, invasive interventions in the form of pericardiocentesis or pericardial window formation are valuable procedures. These interventions allow for concomitant diagnostic and therapeutic approaches with immediate heart decompression. The choice of intervention is based on the effusion size, etiology, and the patient's clinical status. In addition, effective management involves a multimodal approach, with cardiologists, radiologists, and surgical units coordinating to develop an effective treatment plan. The growing knowledge base for pericardial diseases highlights the necessity of prompt intervention to prevent risks and complications from large effusions, particularly those that are malignant or overt inflammatory causes (Tuck et al., 2019). As such, early procedure and medical treatment are the hallmark of patient management in this field. Research into the medical management of pericardial disease is always required as knowledge of the disease advances with clinical practice and technological advancements. Existing literature suggests that determining patients' risk factors and health status is the key to achieving optimal results from treatment. With evolving advice based on continuous evidence, health care professionals must remain aware of the disparate presentation and prognostic implications of differing pericardial illnesses. For instance, recurrent small idiopathic effusions are often benign and require little management, but larger symptomatic deposits require more energetic treatment interventions. Also, knowledge of the intricate interplay between pericardial illness and worldwide cardiac performance makes the clinician most effective in therapy. As science unravels the complexities of pericardial disease, the intersection of contemporary diagnostic and therapeutic modalities will continue to optimize patient management and outcomes (Tuck et al., 2019; Lazaros et al., 2021) (Figure 14.17).

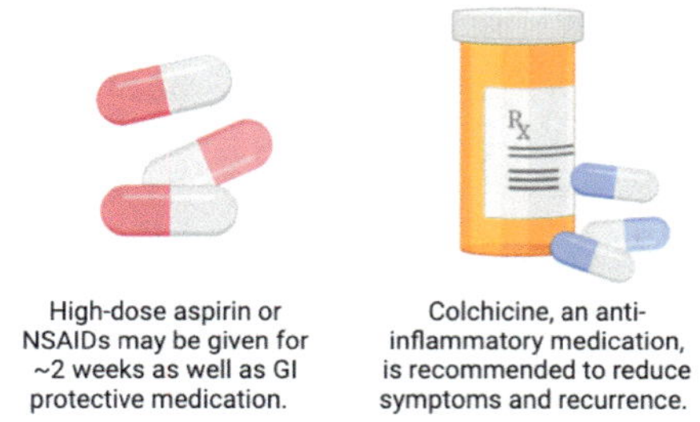

Figure 14.17. Medical management of pericardial diseases.

Source: https://ucsfhealthcardiology.ucsf.edu/sites/ucsfhealthcardiology.ucsf.edu/files/inline-images/Screenshot%202024-07-30%20at%206.05.15%20PM.png.

14.5.2. Surgical Interventions

Surgical interventions are critical in the management of several pericardial diseases, particularly where conservative treatment is not effective in controlling symptoms or addressing the causative factors. Pericardiocentesis is one of the surgical interventions usually applied as the initial surgical intervention for alleviation of symptoms accompanying pericardial effusion, which may lead to cardiac tamponade. In this procedure, a needle is threaded into the pericardial space to drain excess fluid, thereby restoring heart function to normal. Further interventions can also be needed for recurrent effusions that persist despite drainage, such as a pericardial window or pericardiectomy. A pericardial window is the formation of a window in the pericardium to enable continuous drainage. At the same time, pericardiectomy is the surgical resection of the pericardium itself, and it could alleviate symptoms in patients with constrictive pericarditis or other long-standing conditions secondary to pericardial thickening and fibrosis. The outcome of the operation for pericardial disease typically hinges on the cause of the disease and the time of operation. For instance, constrictive pericarditis patients can be given considerable relief in symptoms and improvement in cardiac output following pericardiectomy. All complications are not reversible by surgery, however, as infections, bleeding, or damage to neighboring structures can result. Preoperative evaluation, including imaging, must be practical in order to tailor the surgical approach. In concomitant cardiovascular patients, careful perioperative management is warranted, particularly if surgical resection is required. Similarly, in other such conditions, as observed for example in surgery for cancer of the pancreas, adjuvant treatment is used to maximize the survival rate; the efficient use of surgical procedures for pericardial diseases can significantly enhance the quality of life of the patients (Dam et al., 2023). Moreover, advances in minimally invasive surgical techniques have expanded the options for treating pericardial disease. Techniques like video-assisted thoracoscopy (VATS) enable surgeons to perform interventions with reduced risks and recovery times compared to open conventional methods. These techniques are priceless for addressing challenging situations, particularly in patients with recurrent pericardial effusion or drug-resistant traditional treatments. The integration of these innovations with well-performed perioperative care significantly enhances the outcomes of patients, as in surgical interventions for other specialties (Nogueira et al., 2023). Continued investigation into the cost-effectiveness and long-term consequences of these surgeries is needed to maximize treatment protocols in clinical settings. Lastly, appropriate utilization of surgical options presents an advantageous choice for further improving the care of pericardial ailments with improved patient prognosis and quality of life.

14.5.3. Lifestyle Modifications and Supportive Care

Treatment of pericardial diseases is often extensive in terms of lifestyle modification and a robust supportive care system. Those that are diagnosed with pericardial diseases, such as pericarditis or pericardial effusion, may present with a variety of symptoms, such as chest pain and fatigue. Getting patients to make healthier lifestyle decisions—like taking part in regular exercise, eating a balanced diet that is low in processed foods, and balancing stress levels—will help them in terms of their overall well-being. Along with this, proper patient education regarding the need for these changes is vital, as this allows people to take responsibility for their health and make good decisions. The inclusion of supportive care, including routine follow-ups and counseling, can alleviate the psychological impact of chronic diseases, thereby enhancing the quality of life for patients with pericardial disease. A very vital component of supportive care in managing pericardial diseases is addressing the modifiable risk factors for the diseases. Interestingly, studies have also determined that habits of life, such as poor eating, physical inactivity, and drug use, may precipitate or exacerbate such diseases. For example, individuals who consume excessive alcohol or tobacco have elevated chances of co-existing cardiovascular conditions, which complicate pericardial diseases. Through the execution of specific interventions aimed at reducing such behaviors, medical professionals can not only better control symptoms but also prevent possible complications. Additionally, frequent evaluation of lifestyle choices, together with education on the consequences of poor lifestyle choices, can establish a culture of wellness among patients and thus enhance adherence to lifestyle changes. Lastly, the role of interdisciplinary care teams in providing lifestyle interventions and supportive care in pericardial disease patients cannot be overstressed. Through the involvement of cardiologists, nutritionists, psychological specialists, and physical therapists in the process, a multidisciplinary model can be employed. Through this all-encompassing approach, individualized intervention is facilitated, addressing the unique needs of each patient and, therefore, can promote long-term lifestyle interventions that yield improved health outcomes. Moreover, engaging patients in group therapy or support groups could serve to provide a sense of belonging and dispel feelings of isolation that so frequently accompany chronic disease. It is imperative that the healthcare systems pay attention and start integrating these as an integral part of their treatment protocols, as it might significantly enhance the effectiveness of care for patients suffering from pericardial diseases (Figure 14.18).

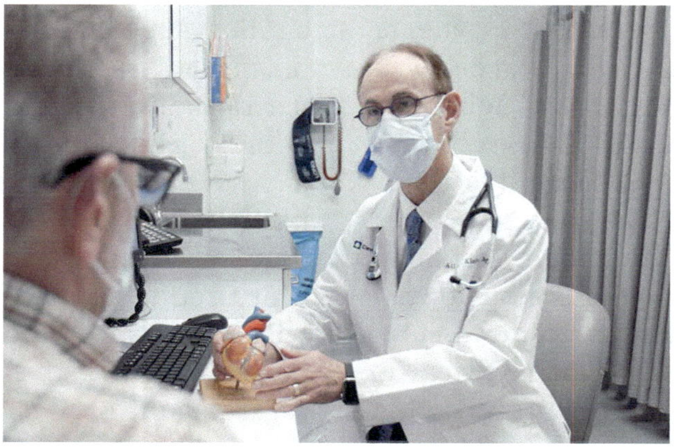

Figure 14.18. Supportive care in managing pericardial diseases.

Source: https://my.clevelandclinic.org/-/scassets/images/org/care-pages/hvti/carepage-pericardial-disease-feature.jpg.

SUMMARY

Diseases of the pericardium present with subtle complications that necessitate a multidisciplinary insight into their physiological significance and therapeutic modalities. As highlighted in the discussion, the diseases may range from pericarditis to effusion and constriction, each with specific clinical manifestations. Medical science, particularly tissue engineering science, has unveiled promising avenues for intervention. For instance, the application of bovine pericardium as a scaffold material categorically indicates the potential for improved outcomes in cardiac surgery, particularly the management of congenital heart disease. Notably, evidence suggests that the mechanical properties and biocompatibility of such scaffolds are significantly influenced by different decellularization processes, suggesting that personalized approaches will enhance surgical efficacy for pericardial disease treatment (N/A, 2024). Therefore, continued research on this topic is needed to refine surgical techniques further and improve overall results of patient care. By examining the immune mechanisms at work with the pericardium, it can be observed that this organ is more than a home for the heart; it is an integral part of the cardiovascular system's immune function. Greater awareness of the structure of the pericardium, particularly its lymphoid component, has serious implications for pathology as well as potential curative strategies. Research has demonstrated that the lymphoid component of the pericardium is dynamic during the process of ontogenesis, contributing to the organ's immunological capabilities (Verba et al., 2024). Thus, further development of our knowledge of these interactions not only informs clinicians about potential vulnerabilities in pericardial integrity but also sets forth new paths for the augmentation of immune responses in pericardial disease patients. The interaction of insights from immunological research with clinical practice can potentially develop plans for new treatment paradigms. Also, the multifactorial pathogenesis of pericardial diseases underscores the significance of cooperative research as well as clinical care by a multidisciplinary team. Increased development in diagnostic methods, as well as continued study of cellular and molecular mechanisms, will be the key to improving targeted therapy development. Integration of knowledge involving tissue engineering, immunology, and cardiology will lead to more efficient pericardial disease management strategies. As recent studies on scaffolding materials and uses in cardiac surgery demonstrate, innovation in treatment technologies has the potential to improve patient outcomes (N/A, 2024). In the end, creating a multifaceted approach to learning about and treating pericardial disease will serve to further enhance the area, giving hope for healthier and more fulfilling lives for victims.

The pericardium, which is a fibrous sac containing the heart, is crucial to heart function and integrity. Pericardial diseases such as pericarditis, pericardial effusion, and constrictive pericarditis create a variety of clinical issues and presentations. Pericarditis is inflammation of the pericardial layers, typically causing severe chest pain that may be exacerbated by respiration or positional movements. In contrast, pericardial effusion is the most frequent condition, wherein there is accumulation of fluid in the pericardial space with resultant hemodynamic compromise and cardiac tamponade, a physical emergency requiring prompt treatment. Their identification is paramount for appropriate management and treatment planning, since they can quickly evolve into serious complications. Diagnosis of pericardial disease depends upon diligent history-taking, physical examination, and advanced imaging. Diagnostic imaging, including echocardiography, is an essential aspect of pericardial effusion assessment, while CMR can provide sophisticated assessments of both pericardium and myocardium in challenging cases. Laboratory tests also identify underlying etiologies, including autoimmune disorders, infections, and malignancies, that are responsible for causing pericardial inflammation. Integration of such diagnostic technologies, in addition to enhancing the specificity of disease detection, directs future therapeutic interventions. Understanding the pathophysiology of pericardial diseases enhances clinical practice and allows for the development of more specific interventions. The management of pericardial disease is multifaceted, consisting of both medical and surgical intervention. Pericarditis is managed using NSAIDs and corticosteroids, which decrease inflammation and pain. In cases where the pericardial effusion is significant, interventions can include pericardiocentesis to relieve pressure on the heart and alleviate symptoms. To reduce the restriction to the heart's filling, surgical treatment such as pericardiectomy would be necessary for chronic conditions like constrictive pericarditis. Moreover, developments in cardiac interventional procedures and new materials—like new stent technology—could play a part in the treatment of complications of pericardial disease, emphasizing the importance of ongoing research and development in the treatment of these conditions (Cappuzzo et al., 2009; Fernández Colino et al., 2019).

A CLOSER LOOK

COMPLICATIONS OF PERICARDIAL DISEASES

The complications of pericardial diseases are an important clinical issue as they result in significant morbidity and mortality. Pericarditis, for example, may progress to constrictive pericarditis with the pericardium becoming rigid and restrictive to diastolic filling of the heart. Such progression may manifest as signs of heart failure, such as dyspnea, fatigue, and edema, and therefore requires early diagnosis and treatment. In addition, effusion of the pericardium, or fluid buildup in the pericardial sac, can lead to cardiac tamponade, a fatal condition that necessitates urgent intervention. The excess fluid compresses the heart, leading to decreased cardiac output and shock. These complications are crucial for doctors to understand, as they highlight the urgent need for early corrective therapies to mitigate adverse effects. The other significant issue with pericardial disease is susceptibility to recurring symptoms and complications. In idiopathic or viral pericarditis, patients may experience recurrent attacks, which affect their quality of life. These recurrences not only aggravate physical symptoms but may also lead to psychological problems. In addition, autoimmune patients such as those with lupus erythematosus are also at a greater risk of developing chronic pericardial disease that might complicate the treatment of their underlying disease. The simplicity of pericardial diseases, therefore, demands a comprehensive treatment approach that is appropriate to cure physical and psychological conditions. Improved management practices and ongoing research are needed to minimize these complexities and maximize overall patient outcomes, an aspect that highlights the need for maintaining caution in clinical practice. In general, the complications of pericardial disease point to the intricate interplay between the pericardium and cardiac function. The treatment of these complications involves symptomatic relief, along with intervention to address the causative etiology, which can range from infectious to inflammatory. For instance, tuberculous or bacterial pericarditis can complicate the treatment plans if not diagnosed and treated with proper therapy in time. Moreover, the effect of these diseases extends beyond the immediate cardiac issue and impacts associated systems and overall health. Hence, an interdisciplinary approach is crucial for optimal management of patients with pericardial disease, fostering collaboration among cardiologists, primary care physicians, and infectious disease and rheumatology experts. Thus, periodic research and monitoring of complications of pericardial disease need to be done to enhance clinical outcomes and patient care (Figure 14.19).

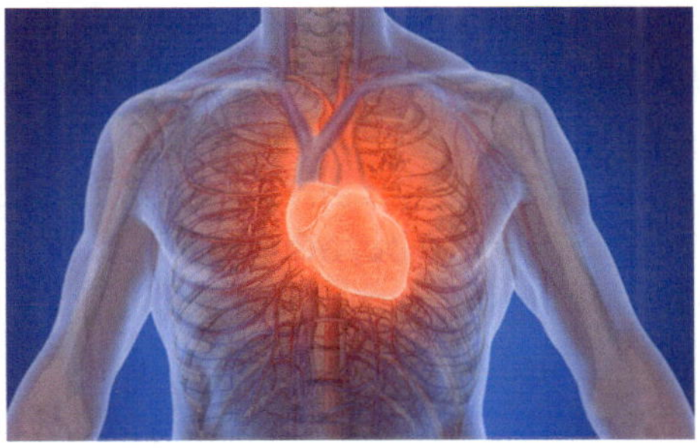

Figure 14.19. Complications of Pericardial Diseases.

Source: https://www.acep.org/siteassets/sites/peer-old-donotuse/media/podcast-images/article-images/cardiactamponade-800x495.jpg.

References

1. Abd Al-Razik, A. H., Elsaka, O., Gamil, M. A., Ghazali, et al. (2022). *A Review on Pericardial Effusion*. https://core.ac.uk/download/621125337.pdf (accessed on 29th May 2025).
2. Elsaka, O., Noureldean, M. A., M, A. G., M, T. G., H, A. a. A., & Hisham, D. (2022a). ETIOLOGY, INVESTIGATIONS, AND TREATMENT IN CASES OF CONSTRICTIVE PERICARDITIS. *Zenodo (CERN European Organization for Nuclear Research)*. https://doi.org/10.5281/zenodo.7640514Adler, Y., Charron, P., Imazio, M., Badano, L. P., Barón-Esquivias, G., Bogaert, J., Brucato, A., et al. (2015). 2015 ESC Guidelines for the diagnosis and management of pericardial diseases. *European Heart Journal, 36*, 2921–2964. https://doi.org/10.1093/eurheartj/ehv318 (accessed on 29th May 2025).
3. Al-Attar, M., Butterworth, S., & McKay, L. (2024). A quantitative and qualitative analysis of patient group narratives suggests common biopsychosocial red flags of undiagnosed rare disease. *Orphanet Journal of Rare Diseases, 19*. https://www.semanticscholar.org/paper/898fe4844d95b854b2fd968b95987fc718cecad3 (accessed on 29th May 2025).
4. Alvarez, L., Riera, J. M. A., Bourges, J. Y., & Garcia, P., et al. (2011). Relationship between fiber orientation and tensile strength of natural collagen membranes for heart valve leaflets. *Anales de Mecánica de la Fractura*. https://core.ac.uk/download/148661384.pdf (accessed on 29th May 2025).
5. Aronow, W. S., Athar, A., & Dhaduk, K. (2019). *Pericardial Diseases in Elderly Patients*. https://core.ac.uk/download/322444678.pdf (accessed on 29th May 2025).
6. Bacalbasa, N., Bratu, O. G., Diaconu, C. C., Manea, et al. (2020). *Diagnosis and Management of Pericardial Effusion*. https://core.ac.uk/download/345454068.pdf (accessed on 29th May 2025).
7. Badgett, C., Winegarner, A., & Hayward, G. (2024). Hybrid coronary revascularization in congenital pericardial absence: A case report. *The American Journal of Case Reports, 25*. https://www.semanticscholar.org/paper/1f554975e88b97e88e819518ff5825fb41a6678d (accessed on 29th May 2025).
8. Bressan, E., De Benedictis, G. M., Ferroni, L., Finotti, et al. (2015). Decellularization and delipidation protocols of bovine bone and pericardium for bone grafting and guided bone regeneration procedures. *PLoS One*. https://core.ac.uk/download/53520971.pdf (accessed on 29th May 2025).
9. Cappuzzo, B. (2009). *The Translation of Chinese Medical Terms into English: Linguistic Considerations on the Language of TCM*. https://core.ac.uk/download/53257559.pdf (accessed on 29th May 2025).
10. Ceusters, W., Dhaen, C., Kumar, A., Smith, et al. (2004). Mistakes in medical ontologies: Where do they come from and how can they be detected? *Stud. Health Technol. Inform*. https://core.ac.uk/download/131212600.pdf (accessed on 29th May 2025).
11. Chait, A., & Den. H. L. J. (2020). Adipose tissue distribution, inflammation and its metabolic consequences, including diabetes and cardiovascular disease. *Frontiers in Cardiovascular Medicine, 7*. https://doi.org/10.3389/fcvm.2020.00022 (accessed on 29th May 2025).
12. Chen, Y., Zhang, Y., Liu, W., Huang, X., Luo, X., & Wang, H. (2024). The causal relationship between vitiligo and autoimmune thyroid diseases: A bidirectional two-sample Mendelian randomization analysis. *Skin Research and Technology, 30*. https://www.semanticscholar.org/

paper/02e7fab72ac68098e3787a5714b2b4aef7effdbc (accessed on 29th May 2025).

13. Correia, M. (2019). *Anesthesia for Patients with Pericardial Disease.* https://core.ac.uk/download/322442858.pdf (accessed on 29th May 2025).

14. Dam, J. L., Verkolf, E., Dekker, E., Bonsing, B., Bratlie, S., Brosens, L., Busch, O., et al. (2023). Perioperative or adjuvant mFOLFIRINOX for resectable pancreatic cancer (PREOPANC-3): Study protocol for a multicenter randomized controlled trial. *BMC Cancer, 23.* https://www.semanticscholar.org/paper/0a3a717488a97803432fc76abf4783b2d91b292d (accessed on 29th May 2025).

15. De Francesco, M. D. (2024). Herpesviridae, neurodegenerative disorders and autoimmune diseases: What is the relationship between them? *Viruses, 16.* https://www.semanticscholar.org/paper/a285063e3f326b7a330ee8c711081f4cbda721f6 (accessed on 29th May 2025).

16. Diana, D., Cardillo, I., Polizzi, V., & Musumeci, F. (2021). 544 Two cases of constrictive pericarditis temporally associated with mRNA-1273 COVID-19 vaccination. *European Heart Journal Supplements, 23.* https://doi.org/10.1093/eurheartj/suab142.014 (accessed on 29th May 2025).

17. Fernández, C. A., Jockenhoevel, S., Mela, P., Moreira, et al. (2019). Layer-by-layer biofabrication of coronary covered stents with clickable elastin-like recombinamers. *European Polymer Journal.* https://core.ac.uk/download/286693421.pdf (accessed on 29th May 2025).

18. Ferrara, V. Z., Martinino, A., Toti, F., Schilirò, D., Pinto, F., Giovinazzo, F., & On Behalf of the Smageics Group. (2024). Robotic vascular resection in pancreatic ductal adenocarcinoma: A systematic review. *Journal of Clinical Medicine, 13.* https://www.semanticscholar.org/paper/1306c0b1ea0ef4e0ee9c94888d6eacd6214c9e18 (accessed on 29th May 2025).

19. García Sánchez, M. D. (2015). *Ébola in TChM: Diagnosis, Principles of Treatment and Economical Analysis.* https://core.ac.uk/download/62906573.pdf (accessed on 29th May 2025).

20. García-Pavía, P., Rapezzi, C., Adler, Y., Arad, M., Basso, C., Brucato, A., Burazor, I., et al. (2021). Diagnosis and treatment of cardiac amyloidosis: A position statement of the ESC Working Group on Myocardial and Pericardial Diseases. *European Heart Journal.* https://www.semanticscholar.org/paper/b2f288c0925b2f6649e3777b353e6f825c47963e (accessed on 29th May 2025).

21. Gerosa, G., & Iop, L. (2015). Guided tissue regeneration in heart valve replacement: From preclinical research to first-in-human trials. *Biomed Res. Int.* https://core.ac.uk/download/53532873.pdf (accessed on 29th May 2025).

22. Haritha, G. S. (2019). *Pericardial Effusion in Dogs.* https://core.ac.uk/download/322444782.pdf (accessed on 29th May 2025).

23. Herbella, F. A. M., Patti, M. G., & Takassi, G. F. (2013). Anatomic variations in the surgical anatomy of the thoracic esophagus and its surrounding structures. *Arq. Bras. Cir. Dig.* https://core.ac.uk/download/37711184.pdf (accessed on 29th May 2025).

24. Hoskins, E. (2022). *Tissue-Engineered Living Pulmonary Valve for Young Adult Patients.* https://core.ac.uk/download/539558805.pdf (accessed on 29th May 2025).

25. Jois, G. S., Kulkarni, M. M., Eshwari, K., Kunder, M. A., & Shivashankar, K. N. (2024). IJCM_161A: Lifestyle related risk behavior among hypertensive fishermen: Baseline characteristics of an interventional study. *Indian Journal of Community Medicine: Official Publication of Indian*

Association of Preventive & Social Medicine, 49, S47–S47. https://www.semanticscholar.org/paper/e3c19d75ebcde961acc2184c91edb6cbba61e810 (accessed on 29th May 2025).

26. Lazaros, G., Vlachopoulos, C., Lazarou, E., Tousoulis, D., & Tsioufis, C. (2021). Contemporary management of pericardial effusion. *Panminerva Medica*. https://www.semanticscholar.org/paper/497a420a5cb1b1729f72b99c5cfbecfdc79ef82d (accessed on 29th May 2025).
27. Lim, R., Yeo, S., Barratt, J., & Rizk, D. V. (2024). An update on current therapeutic options in IgA nephropathy. *Journal of Clinical Medicine, 13.* https://www.semanticscholar.org/paper/1cfdedd9924677042b06983e29e8dcc0f7346c72 (accessed on 29th May 2025).
28. Liu, L. (2024). *Anatomy-Aided Deep Learning for Medical Image Segmentation with Application to Epicardial Adipose Tissue.* https://core.ac.uk/download/621168078.pdf (accessed on 29th May 2025).
29. Lyon, A. R., López-Fernández, T., Couch, L. S., Asteggiano, R., Aznar, M. C., Bergler-Klein, J., Boriani, G., et al. (2022). 2022 ESC guidelines on cardio-oncology developed in collaboration with the European Hematology Association (EHA), the European Society for Therapeutic Radiology and Oncology (ESTRO) and the International Cardio-Oncology Society (IC-OS). *European Heart Journal, 43*, 4229–4361. https://doi.org/10.1093/eurheartj/ehac244 (accessed on 29th May 2025).
30. M., 2., N., 1., T. P., 3., of Hygiene, and Epidemiology, Medical, I. Milas, 1., et al. (2023). Eating behavior of the Croatian working population during the COVID-19 pandemic. *The European Journal of Public Health, 33.* https://www.semanticscholar.org/paper/a6057d4c2b81d7f8ef2875fea4e366130331e5f1 (accessed on 29th May 2025).
31. Morgan, M., Yellapu, V., Short, D., & Ruggeri, C. (2024). Trends in in-hospital mortality in patients admitted with cardiovascular diseases in the United States with demographics and risk factors of all cardiovascular in-hospital mortality: Analysis of the 2021 National Inpatient Sample Database. *Cureus, 16.* https://www.semanticscholar.org/paper/2724eec5f8b28e3b2836d70282cbfc5c261d4f63 (accessed on 29th May 2025).
32. Murkamilov, I., Aitbaev, K., Raimzhanov, Z., Duisheeva, G., Hakimov, Sh., Ymankulov, D., Yusupova, Z., et al. (2024). Pericarditis: Causes, mechanisms of development, variants of course and therapeutic approaches in modern conditions. *Bulletin of Science and Practice.* https://www.semanticscholar.org/paper/b3e56ea3b981ed0f341c9660c2653613d1bdf437 (accessed on 29th May 2025).
33. Nazarov, N. N., Madazimov, M. M., Makhmudov, A. L., Turgunboev, A. A., & Nazirdzhonov, I. K. N. (2024). Combination of pericardial celomic cyst and thymus cyst. *Hirurg (Surgeon).* https://www.semanticscholar.org/paper/c70b4b0f1614b1114559c6755b1c5d8301daf0ba (accessed on 29th May 2025).
34. Nogueira, A., Barreto, J., Moura, F., Luchiari, B., Abuhab, A., Bonilha, I., Nadruz, W., et al. (2023). Comparative effectiveness and cost-effectiveness of cardioprotective glucose-lowering therapies for type 2 diabetes in Brazil: A Bayesian network model. *Health Economics Review, 13.* https://www.semanticscholar.org/paper/8138a95537f0a26b76453f162fc32aab4bb16b9f (accessed on 29th May 2025).
35. Oostendorp, J. Y., Sluckin, T., Han-Geurts, I., Dieren, S., Schouten, R., & on behalf of The Italian Surgical Societies Working Group. (2023). Treatment of hemorrhoids: Rubber band ligation or sclerotherapy (THROS)? Study protocol for a multicenter, non-inferiority, randomized

controlled trial. *Trials, 24.* https://www.semanticscholar.org/paper/268433ada733a4d8cd112339ab061399fb1ffc30 (accessed on 29th May 2025).

36. Pinto, L. M., Regatieri, C. V. S., Rigueiro, M. P., & Tavares, et al. (2008). Uso de pericárdio suíno no recobrimento de implantes de drenagem de glaucoma: Um estudo experimental. https://core.ac.uk/download/37707944.pdf (accessed on 29th May 2025).
37. Poelgeest, E. P., Handoko, M. L., Muller, M., Velde, N., & On behalf of the EUGMS Task Finish Group on Fall-Risk Drugs. (2023). Diuretics, SGLT2 inhibitors and falls in older heart failure patients: To prescribe or to deprescribe? A clinical review. *European Geriatric Medicine, 14,* 659–674. https://www.semanticscholar.org/paper/61e97a2b96498a5ec0c10520b4ad18307c5cb5c4 (accessed on 29th May 2025).
38. Ponikowski, P., Voors, A. A., Anker, S. D., Bueno, H., Cleland, J. G. F., Coats, A. J. S., Falk, V., et al. (2016). 2016 ESC Guidelines for the diagnosis and treatment of acute and chronic heart failure. *European Heart Journal, 37,* 2129–2200. https://doi.org/10.1093/eurheartj/ehw128 (accessed on 29th May 2025).
39. Samsudin, E. Z., Yasin, S. M., Ruslan, N. H., Abdullah, N. N., Noor, A. F. A., & Hair, A. F. A. (2024). Socioeconomic impacts of airborne and droplet-borne infectious diseases on industries: A systematic review. *BMC Infectious Diseases, 24.* https://www.semanticscholar.org/paper/6a326cbb4f2c90dabc465886722f7807e960b57d (accessed on 29th May 2025).
40. Sel, K., Osman, D., Zare, F., Shahrbabak, S. M., Brattain, L., Hahn, J. O., Inan, O. T., et al. (2024). Building digital twins for cardiovascular health: From principles to clinical impact. *Journal of the American Heart Association: Cardiovascular and Cerebrovascular Disease, 13.* https://www.semanticscholar.org/paper/7d237c65a8f0f8b3e4a95a440b7bb2336607d704 (accessed on 29th May 2025).
41. Severino, P., D'Amato, A., Prosperi, S., Dei Cas, A., Mattioli, A., Cevese, A., Novo, G., et al. (2022). Do the current guidelines for heart failure diagnosis and treatment fit with clinical complexity? *Journal of Clinical Medicine, 11.* https://www.semanticscholar.org/paper/25016c811cf4b178de5fa51ebf6c56703a8dc2f1 (accessed on 29th May 2025).
42. Sorushanova, A., Delgado, L. M., Wu, Z., Shologu, N., Kshirsagar, A., Raghunath, R., Mullen, A. M., et al. (2018). The collagen suprafamily: From biosynthesis to advanced biomaterial development. *Advanced Materials, 31.* https://doi.org/10.1002/adma.201801651 (accessed on 29th May 2025).
43. Tuck, B. C., & Townsley, M. M. (2019). Clinical update in pericardial diseases. *Journal of Cardiothoracic and Vascular Anesthesia, 33*(1), 184–199. https://www.semanticscholar.org/paper/a4550d8eb64f80287e00948f85f4f1fdacc034f9 (accessed on 29th May 2025).
44. Ullrich, B., Schenk, P., Scheyerer, M., Bäumlein, M., Katscher, S., Schnake, K., Zimmermann, V., et al. (2023). Georg Schmorl Prize of the German Spine Society (DWG) 2022: Current treatment for inpatients with osteoporotic thoracolumbar fractures—Results of the EOFTT study. *European Spine Journal.* https://www.semanticscholar.org/paper/33a4b5530f0728c46848652528a973c407b6d99a (accessed on 29th May 2025).
45. Vetrani, C., Di Nisio, A., Paschou, S., Barrea, L., Muscogiuri, G., Graziadio, C., Savastano, S., et al. (2022). From gut microbiota through low-grade inflammation to obesity: Key players and potential targets. *Nutrients, 14.* https://www.semanticscholar.org/paper/c0b654848b8c5212e5b9d33855cc365aa1e51c84 (accessed on 29th May 2025).

46. Wang, T. K. M., Ayoub, C., Chetrit, M., Kwon, D. H., Jellis, C., Cremer, P. C., Bolen, M. A., et al. (2022). Cardiac magnetic resonance imaging techniques and applications for pericardial diseases. *Circulation: Cardiovascular Imaging, 15*, e014283. https://www.semanticscholar.org/paper/af90cc4f8bf60a1a7da1322f7594275789165c0e (accessed on 29th May 2025).

47. Wu, A. H. B. (2012). *Biomarkers Beyond the Natriuretic Peptides for Chronic Heart Failure: Galectin-3 and Soluble ST2.* https://core.ac.uk/download/323074780.pdf (accessed on 29th May 2025).

48. Zykova, A. S., Opravin, A. S., & Soloviev, A. (2024). Periodontitis as a risk factor for cardiovascular disease development: Systematic review. *Parodontologiya*. https://www.semanticscholar.org/paper/db931c9def920a6be65ff21fc04d683fc636a87e (accessed on 29th May 2025).

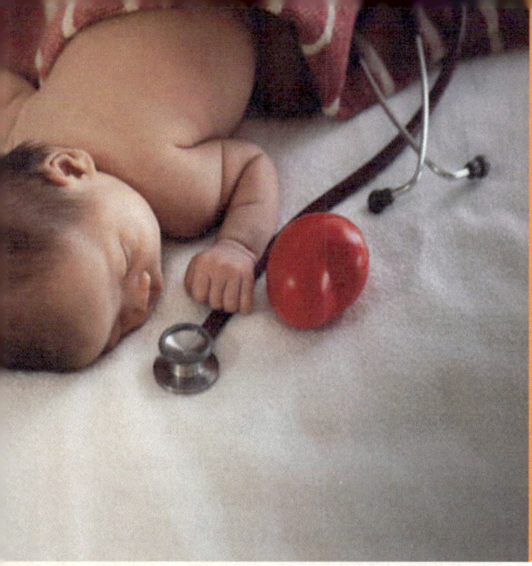

Chapter 15

CRITICAL HEART DISEASE IN INFANTS AND CHILDREN

Contents

Introduction

Child and infant critical heart disease is a significant public health issue due to its contribution to the morbidity and mortality among the youngest age groups. Congenital cardiac malformations are the most frequent category of birth defect among infants and encompass a large category of structural heart abnormalities. Spooky as it sounds, of these malformations, a quarter are critical congenital heart disease (CCHD), for which surgical or catheter intervention is necessary during the first year of life. With early diagnosis, early treatment and detection are crucial to maximize outcomes for affected children. The medical field recognizes that enhancing screening practices at the neonatal level is crucial for the early identification of cases that would otherwise remain clinically undetected, which is why it emphasizes the need for ongoing research and development in this field (Gadekar et al., 2013). The adoption of pulse oximetry screening is a welcome step towards the early detection of CCHD, and it steps up to the plate where the complex conditions present a challenge in a straightforward manner.

Through the adoption of pulse oximetry for clinically normal newborns within the initial hours of life, healthcare workers can achieve an objective basis of comparison for oxygen saturation levels. These screening examinations are essential in that a reading of below 90% for SpO2 requires additional diagnostic evaluation, such as echocardiography, which detects significant abnormalities. This new methodology aims to cover the absence of earlier diagnosis, which would reduce the incidence of severe complications from undiagnosed heart disease. The current studies highlight the effectiveness and beneficial role of this non-invasive screening process towards the improvement of the prognosis of CCHD infants and the delivery of overall pediatric cardiac care (Gadekar et al., 2013). When assessing the broader implications of infant and pediatric critical heart disease, one must consider that other illnesses in children, such as bronchiolitis, are potentially associated with heart disease and may occur in conjunction with it. High Flow Nasal Cannula (HFNC) is a newly proven method of supportive care in the case of bronchiolitis with the potential to alter outcomes by stopping disease progression. It is this that underscores the complexity of pediatric medicine, where minor consideration of treatment methods has to be addressed. The disparity in the management of acute respiratory illnesses and cardiac defects attests to the need for a multi-professional practice in addressing the health of the infant and child. Increased awareness and targeted investigation of CCHD and other affected conditions will eventually result in improvement in care provision and alleviate healthcare systems worldwide of some of the burden (Figure 15.1).

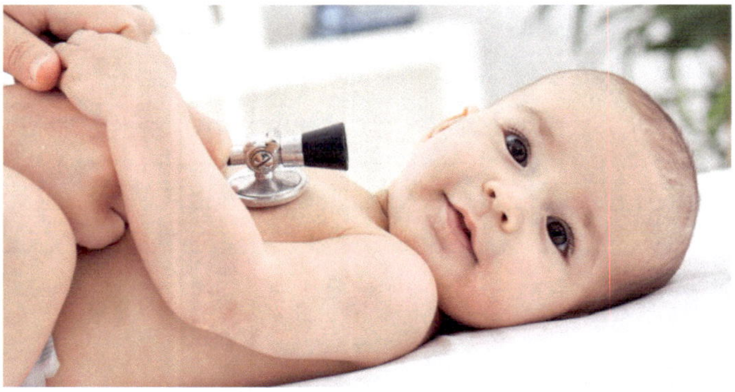

Figure 15.1. Congenital heart disease.

Source: https://dvl2h13awlxkt.cloudfront.net/assets/general-images/Knowledge/_1200x630_crop_center-center_82_none/congenital-heart-disease.jpg?mtime=1601442687.

15.1. Types of Critical Heart Disease (CHDs)

The geography of critical congenital heart disease in children and infants is characterized by various CHDs that need special medical attention. Tetralogy of Fallot (ToF) is one of the most common critical congenital heart diseases. A combination of four specific heart defects, ToF results in reduced lung blood flow, causing cyanosis or blue complexion. Early recognition and treatment are necessary because untreated ToF can lead to extreme complications as well as an increased risk of morbidity. Other essential conditions include pulmonary atresia and transposition of the great arteries, each with its treatment methods and surgical approaches that need to be utilized so that the best outcomes are obtained for affected infants. Knowledge about the manifestations of critical heart disease in this population can direct appropriate preventive strategies and also clinical maneuvers. Total anomalous pulmonary venous return (TAPVR) is another significant type of critical congenital heart disease in which the pulmonary veins do not connect normally to the left atrium. Instead, they connect to one of the other heart chambers or a blood vessel, and this leads to extreme oxygen saturation issues. This typically occurs in the neonatal period, with manifestations ranging from respiratory distress to cyanosis shortly after birth.

The need for urgent surgery for TAPVR patients highlights the importance of early diagnosis and the critical role played by pulse oximetry screening in the identification of such defects. Procedures adopted by health organizations, including the American Academy of Pediatrics, ensure early diagnosis, which is critical in ensuring proper disease management, as in the case of TAPVR (Martinez-Sarria et al., 2023). This highlights the need for continuous improvements in screening processes as well as doctor training to maximize the detection of serious heart diseases in infants. Finally, hypoplastic left heart syndrome (HLHS) is one of the most serious forms of severe congenital heart disease. It causes underdevelopment of the left side of the heart, thus impairing its ability to pump blood to the body. HLHS is commonly identified prenatally by imaging or in the first few months of life and must be treated early. Although there are surgical options to improve the prognosis of affected individuals, including staged surgical repair, the attendant complexity and risk with these procedures underscore the challenge healthcare providers have. Emotional and psychological effects of a HLHS diagnosis on families can be extensive, thus the need for holistic care models that reflect not only the medical aspect of treatment but also the familial one. As studies continue to explore family experiences following such diagnoses, more information can be available to improve care models (Martinez-Sarria et al., 2023) (Figure 15.2).

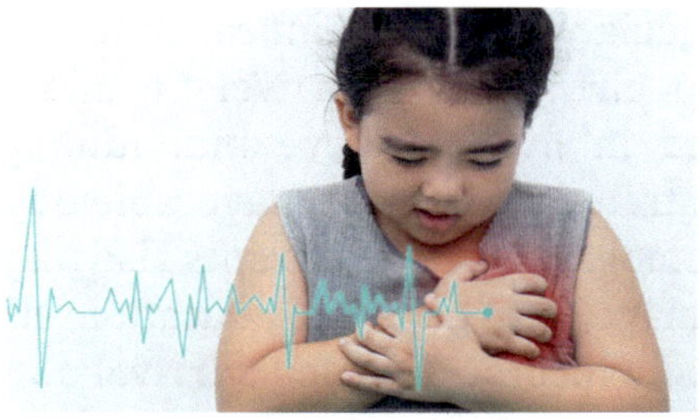

Figure 15.2. Types of critical heart disease (CHD).

Source: https://www.netmeds.com/images/cms/wysiwyg/blog/2023/04/1681368852_Heart-Disease-In-Children_898x450.jpg.

15.1.1. Congenital Heart Defects (CHDs)

CHDs are an excellent pediatric health issue that, in most instances, causes extreme morbidity and mortality. Abnormal or structural heart defects are molded in fetal existence and differ enormously in type and severity, leading to the predicted destiny for the afflicted infant. As defined, CHD is the most significant cause of death of congenital handicap and affects approximately 1% of live births (Akah et al., 2025). The effects of such defects extend beyond acute medical complications; children with CHDs frequently require long-term medical care, including surgery, medication, and frequent specialist review. This complex interface of medical treatments and physiological deficiencies adds a significant load on the medical system as well as family members, suggesting the necessity of robust early treatment and diagnosis models to realize an optimum outcome. Survival rate in infant cases of critical congenital heart defects (CCHDs) has increased significantly after enhancing the process of medical treatment and surgery. Current evidence indicates that one-year survival in CCHDs is 85.8% and five years is approximately 83.7% (Forestieri et al., 2024). These follow with high variability by defect categories—infants with univentricular function have significantly lower survival than those with biventricular function. Clinical predictors like preterm birth, low birth weight, and defects detected in number have individually been demonstrated to predict unfavorable outcomes. Sociodemographic determinants also play a role in the image, with maternal education, ethnicity, and family income affecting survival outcomes. It is thus essential to create awareness and intervene on such determinants to maximize the care of children with CHDs. Early detection of congenital heart defects will avoid their long-term consequences and enhance survivors' quality of life. Effective screening campaigns, including pulse oximetry and targeted echocardiography, have been necessary for the identification of affected newborns within the early timeframe following birth. This allows for early medical and surgical interventions, which are predictors of improved survival and outcomes in development (Akah et al., 2025). Further, there has been growing awareness of the importance of holistic care models involving medical as well as psychological and social support to families.

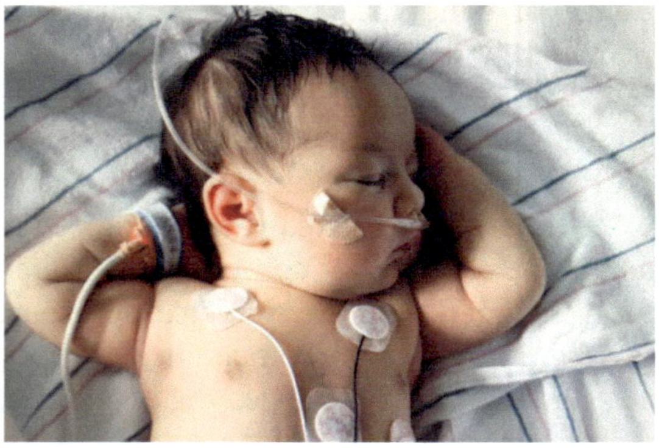

Figure 15.3. Congenital heart defects (CHD).

Source: https://www.heart.org/-/media/Images/Health-Topics/Congenital-Heart-Defects/Survivor-photos/Sloan-in-hospital.jpg?h=533&w=800&sc_lang=en.

These models will serve to address the overall requirements of children with CHDs, establishing a support milieu fostering enhanced recovery and addressing lifelong care needs. In the developing domain of pediatric cardiology, maintaining the importance of early detection and universal care will remain crucial in the management of affected children and families (Figure 15.3).

15.1.2. Acquired Heart Conditions

Congenitally acquired heart disease in children and infants is a significant clinical issue since it develops after birth and can alter a child's cardiovascular profile and development. They predominantly arise due to infection, inflammation, or environmental trauma and lead to conditions like rheumatic heart disease or myocarditis. They are particularly frustrating in the sense that they will not happen until adulthood, thereby raising problems with early treatment and diagnosis. The index of suspicion, therefore, must be heightened among physicians, especially in high-risk populations, such as individuals with a history of past viral infections or autoimmune illnesses. Knowledge of the etiologic determinants that influence acquired heart disease is fundamental in devising proper interventions to counteract its spread and impact on the health of children. Of interest in the management of acquired heart disease is a knowledge of its potential neurodevelopmental effects. Experience indicates that congenital heart disease, which in many cases goes undetected and yet accompanies acquired disease, has been cited to cause delays in developmental milestones in their gross motor abilities. According to the neurodevelopmental evaluation of children with congenital heart disease, there were some impairments, particularly in the gross motor skill component, supporting the hypothesis that the development of motor skills might be affected by heart disease (Vagha et al., 2023). Thus, the clinicians must treat not just the physiological presentation of heart disease but also the implications for neurocognitive development because early intervention will have a strong effect on long-term outcomes in such children. Additionally, treatment of acquired heart disease may need to be a multidisciplinary effort involving cardiology, neurology, and developmental pediatrics to be able to provide optimal care. New monitoring technologies, such as non-invasive optical monitoring, have been explored to quantify cerebral hemodynamics in real-time for the application of critical congenital heart disease (Winston et al., 2024). The technology can potentially identify instances of neurological vulnerability shortly following birth and offer a window of opportunity for possible intervention. These total care interventions are tailored to compensate for physical and mental health in infected children, thus improving their quality of life and growth cycles in the context of heart disease. Intervention in acquired heart diseases within an interdisciplinary framework not only improves immediate health outcomes but also guarantees long-term health because these children grow up in ensuing years (Figure 15.4).

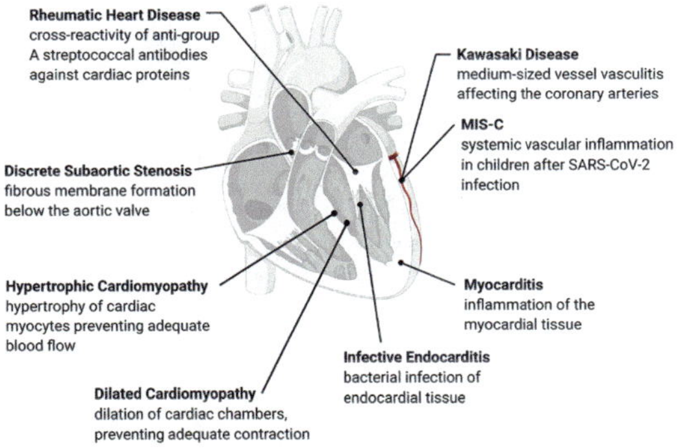

Figure 15.4. Overview of acquired pediatric heart disease.

Source: https://www.frontiersin.org/files/Articles/701224/fcvm-08-701224-HTML/image_m/fcvm-08-701224-g001.jpg.

15.1.3. Cardiomyopathy

Cardiomyopathy is a severe category of heart disease with significant implications for infants and children, posing daunting challenges for pediatric medicine. It initially impacts the myocardium, decreasing its ability to pump blood. The pathophysiology of cardiomyopathy includes several genetic and environmental causes leading to structural and functional abnormalities of the heart muscle. For instance, hypertrophic cardiomyopathy most commonly presents as an inherited disease of thickening of the heart wall with resulting obstruction to blood flow and arrhythmias. However, dilated cardiomyopathy, which is a dilatation of the chambers of the heart, is relatively caused by multifactorial etiologies like viral infections or toxins. Significantly, early diagnosis and detection in children of cardiomyopathy is fundamental to effective treatment and improved prognosis, and it is therefore vital that medical professionals remain vigilant to signs and symptoms that may signal this debilitating condition. Clinical presentation of cardiomyopathy in pediatric patients can be multifarious and tends to pose a challenge to the diagnostic process. Common presentations include fatigue, dyspnea, and syncope, although in infants, the presentation may be more subtle with difficulty feeding and failure to thrive. Such presentations can easily be confused with other less severe conditions, leading to delays in diagnosis and management. Because there is a risk of such children deteriorating quite quickly, prompt treatment is vital. Several diagnostic methods, such as echocardiography and cardiac MRI, may be employed to evaluate myocardial structure and function, thus guiding therapy. Highly specialized therapeutic approaches, including pharmacologic treatment and surgery, are in the pipeline. Besides, multidisciplinary treatment teams are crucial because of the complex interaction between the medical, psychological, and developmental complications of children with cardiomyopathy, particularly during times of essential growth. Research in cardiomyopathy has uncovered valuable insight into the biochemical and genetic mechanisms of the disease that may be the foundation for future therapy. Recent research suggests that numerous forms of genetic mutations can predispose children to various forms of cardiomyopathy and has prompted researchers to emphasize the importance of family screening and genetic counseling. Further, novel therapies targeting molecular targets of cardiomyopathy pathology are showing promise in clinical trials, and promise more targeted treatments for patients based on their genetic background. Greater awareness of associated syndromes, such as the J-wave syndromes, such as Brugada syndrome and early repolarization syndrome, also demonstrates the multimodality nature of cardiovascular risk in such patients (Zeppenfeld et al., 2022). Continuous interaction between cardiologists, geneticists, and other specialists is crucial during the development of knowledge and management of cardiomyopathy, ultimately leading to enhanced survival and quality of life among involved children (Antzelevitch et al., 2016) (Figure 15.5).

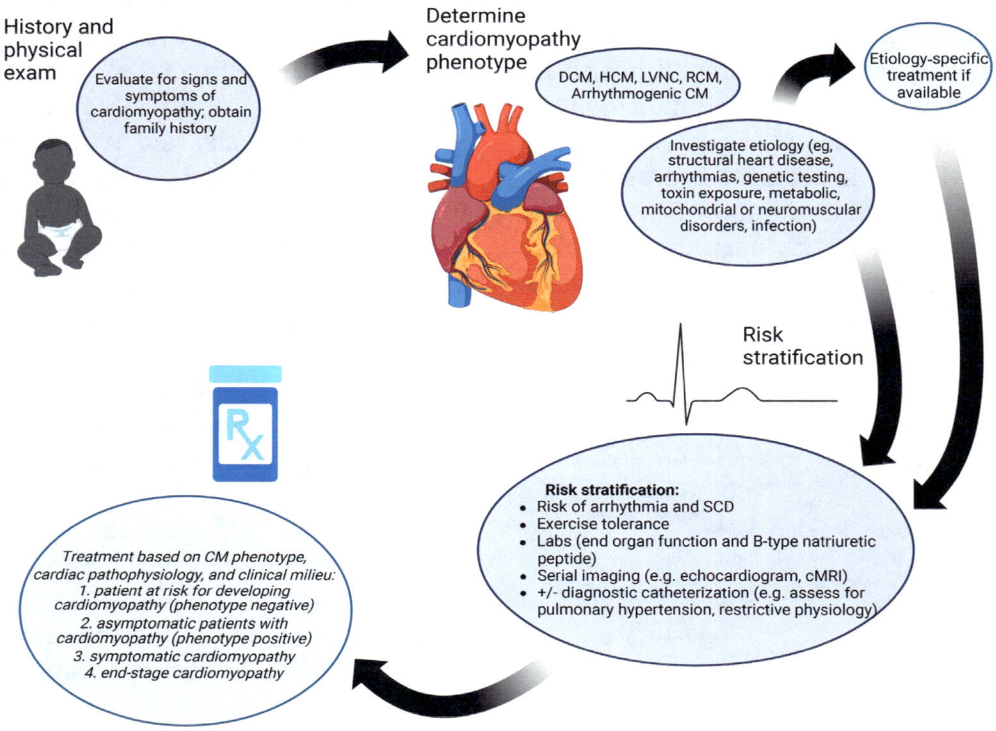

Figure 15.5. Overview of cardiomyopathy in children.

Source: https://www.ahajournals.org/cms/10.1161/CIR.0000000000001151/asset/e6028249-2b0c-43a6-b027-cb3615bf4960/assets/graphic/cir.0000000000001151.fig01.jpg.

15.2. Symptoms and Diagnosis

Critical heart disease in infants and children typically presents with a range of symptoms that can be quite dissimilar based on the illness. Presentations include cyanosis, or blue discoloration of the skin, most notably of the extremities and lips; intolerance to feeding that is manifested by fatigability; and tachypnea, or rapid breathing. Infants and children may have signs of distress, such as sweating with feeding or exertion. These signs often prompt a closer look when parents or guardians observe unusual changes in behavior or physical appearance. Accurate identification of these signs is crucial as they alert healthcare providers to perform a good screening for underlying cardiac defects, which need careful observation and prompt intervention in serious situations. Diagnosis of congenital heart disease involves several tools and techniques, beginning with a good clinical evaluation. Health care professionals use auscultation to detect abnormal heart sounds such as murmurs, which can indicate underlying structural heart disease. Non-invasive imaging, for example, echocardiography, plays an important role in visualizing the anatomy and function of the heart so that clinicians can diagnose conditions such as septal defects or valve disease. In some instances, advanced diagnostic methods, for example, MRI and cardiac catheterization, can be employed. The employment of these modalities is essential in providing a correct diagnosis, enabling proper management interventions to be initiated early in the course of the patient's treatment. The integration of palliative care into the diagnosis and management of infants with critical heart disease has been increasingly embraced over the past few years, signaling a shift towards integrated patient care. Preemptive palliative care can decrease maternal stress and enhance family relationships significantly in such severe conditions as single-ventricle disease. Research has established that systematic evaluation and psychosocial intervention not only improve maternal mental health outcomes but also facilitate better communication among families (Aiyagari et al., 2018). Because of the complexity that comes with congenital heart disease, early diagnosis followed by extensive palliative care procedures has the potential to improve parental adjustment mechanisms as well as family well-being, and thus underscores the importance of a multidisciplinary approach to managing such sensitive cases (Figure 15.6).

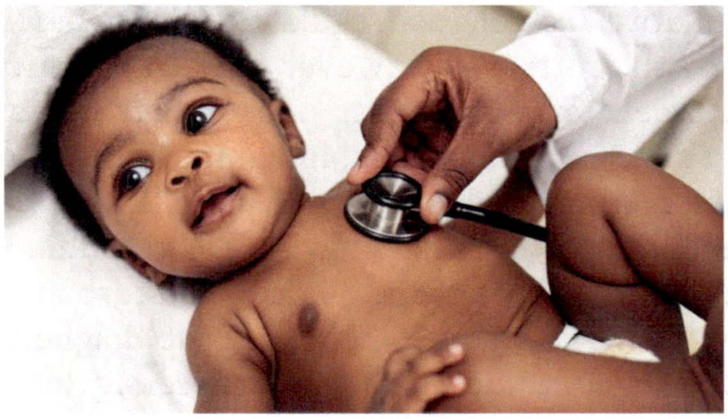

Figure 15.6. Baby heart examination.

Source: https://www.cdc.gov/heart-defects/media/images/baby_heart_exam.jpg.

15.2.1. Common Symptoms in Infants and Children

The development of typical symptoms in children and infants is essential for early detection of serious heart disease. Children and infants are particularly vulnerable because their symptoms may often be nonspecific and readily mimicked by other illnesses. Typical signs are poor feeding, breathing difficulties, lethargy, and irritability. The signs may be due to heart conditions such as a congenital heart defect that impairs normal circulation of blood and oxygen supply. Parents and caregivers must watch for changes in behavior, such as more than normal crying or fatigue, as these may be warning signs for underlying heart issues. Prompt treatment of such life-threatening heart conditions can have a significant effect on long-term health for affected children, emphasizing the importance of medical and parental awareness. With respiratory distress, children with severe heart ailments usually present with signs of poor development and growth, which may manifest as failure to thrive. This is quite apparent in cases of hypoplastic left heart syndrome, where failure of the heart to pump blood effectively hinders nutrient uptake. Moreover, these children will also have symptoms such as sweating during feeding or tachypnea, which are red flags and must be investigated.

Pediatricians conduct regular checks to assess growth patterns; however, the correlation between growth deficits and cardiac defects needs to be recognized. Most importantly, RSV infection has added layers of complexity, with severe forms in infants having the potential to result in long-term respiratory disturbances that could complicate heart disease diagnosis. These complexities highlight the necessity for an integrated approach during evaluations. By the time symptoms of critical heart disease manifest, they can be complicated during ordinary illness, further complicating diagnostic procedures. Diseases like RSV-caused bronchiolitis will complicate the pre-existing cardiac conditions and cause additional morbidity in the target population, including pre-existing cases of infants with cardiac conditions (King et al., 2017). Therefore, healthcare providers must consider both the chronic and acute implications while assessing infants and children presenting with respiratory complaints. Careful assessment of how cardiovascular health relates to infection is paramount to ensure proper treatment. Additionally, the parents' contribution towards screening for such symptoms cannot be stressed too much as early identification of atypical behaviors and health patterns can initiate timely medical evaluation, thus improving management and outcomes in infants and children with heart disease (King et al., 2017) (Figure 15.7).

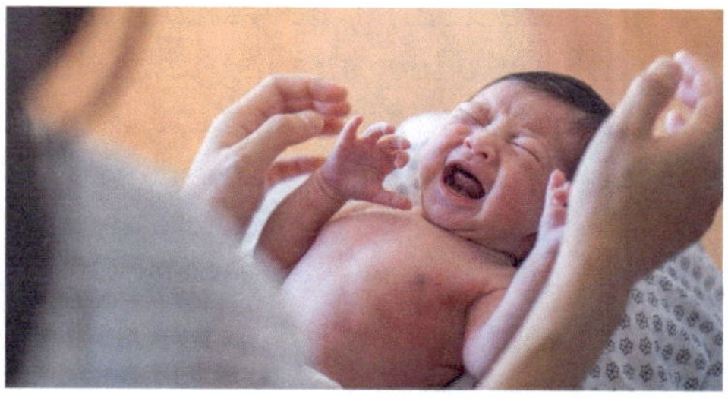

Figure 15.7. Common symptoms in infants and children.

Source: https://static.cdntap.com/tap-assets-prod/wp-content/uploads/sites/12/2021/01/newborn-baby-crying.jpg?width=700&quality=95.

15.2.2. Diagnostic Tools and Techniques

Accurate diagnosis of heart disease in infants and children is essential to manage and treat them accordingly. The most significant diagnostic tests among them are echocardiograms, which produce detailed images of heart function and structure by using ultrasound waves. An echocardiogram is a non-surgical procedure that allows clinicians to view congenital defects and assess cardiac function in real time. Additionally, echocardiography is particularly valuable in the pediatric setting, as it can be performed with very minimal distress to the child. With the development of 3D echocardiography, the diagnostic capabilities have further improved for more precise examination of complex heart defects. In summary, the technique is an essential tool in an enlarged diagnostic arsenal that plays a significant role in the timely and precise management of pediatric heart disease (Priori et al., 2015). Apart from echocardiography, electrocardiography (ECG) is as critical in the diagnosis of heart diseases in the younger population. ECG provides vital information regarding the electrical activity of the heart, and this will reveal arrhythmias that are suggestive of functional or structural underlying abnormalities. In infants, it is challenging to get an accurate ECG because of size and movement considerations; however, advances in technology have paved the way for the use of pediatric-specific equipment and electrodes, thereby making it more accurate and accessible. The addition of wearable technology is also revolutionizing this field by allowing continuous monitoring of heart rhythm, thereby enabling early detection of potential cardiac complications. With these new applications, the integration of traditional and newer diagnostic techniques has the potential to offer comprehensive information on the cardiac health of children and to authenticate the requirement for intervention at early stages (Islam et al., 2015). Non-invasive imaging technologies such as MRI and CT scans have begun to play increasingly significant roles in the diagnosis of serious heart disease in infants and children. MRI offers excellent anatomical detail without the radiation exposure of CT scans, and for this reason, MRI is particularly well-suited for use in children. With advances in technology on cardiac MRI, accurate evaluation of cardiac morphology and function so crucial for the assessment of congenital heart disease is now feasible. Conversely, CT angiography provides rapid assessment of vascular anatomy, making it an asset in acute settings. In addition to conventional modalities, these more recent imaging techniques are also a component of a comprehensive diagnostic strategy that allows physicians to develop effective treatment regimens based on a thorough understanding of each child's unique circumstances (Priori et al., 2015) (Figure 15.8).

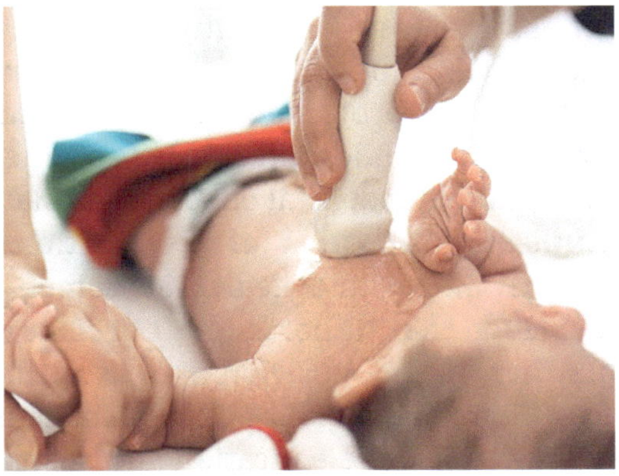

Figure 15.8. Pediatric echocardiography.

Source: https://storage.googleapis.com/jacksonh/1/Pediatric_Echocardiography-Advanced-Imaging.jpg.

15.2.3. Importance of Family History in Diagnosis

Family medical history plays a crucial role in the diagnosis of heart diseases, particularly in infants and children. The prevalence of CHDs is also linked with genetic influences, and it can be utilized to offer important information Family medical history to health care practitioners through careful assessment of family medical history. As clinicians obtain this information, they can identify a pattern of cardiac issues that may signify underlying genetic risks, enabling early detection and early intervention. For instance, if there is a history of congenital malformations or early childhood cardiovascular diseases, pediatricians can be more vigorous and watchful with investigations, providing a better prognosis to the child. Such thinking becomes even more critical with respect to subsequent children being born, since the familial traits leading to heart disease are likely to recur and thus monitoring such children uninterruptedly has to be followed. Moreover, integrating family medical history into the diagnosis is not all about discovering congenital defects. Even conditions that accompany cardiac conditions might be included, such as asthma or eczema, which occur in families with a history of atopy. An example case with accompanying conditions demonstrates how understanding a child's family medical history would contribute to complete management plans. In such a case, those children presenting symptoms of respiratory illness along with heart abnormalities must be screened not just for cardiac malformation but also for other likely allergic diseases that can complicate their condition. As demonstrated by the results regarding atopic diseases in families, such an integrated strategy guarantees complete care, thereby lowering the risks of misdiagnosis and fostering a comprehensive treatment plan that addresses all aspects of the child's health (Formosa et al., 2008). When considering preventive care, information about family history also impacts long-term health strategies. For families with a risk of severe heart disease, health experts can recommend early lifestyle changes and screenings that are especially designed to the genetic predispositions of the child. Being proactive in this manner can be important since lifestyle modification at an early stage significantly impacts overall cardiovascular health. Additionally, parents with a background of allergic diseases such as asthma should be educated on how the ailments and potential cardiovascular complications interplay, as seen in clinical studies concerning the application of emollients to prevent eczema (BEEP study team et al., 2020). Through this process, physicians empower families to be knowledgeable about information and tangible steps that can drive improved outcomes for children who are vulnerable to severe heart diseases. Lastly, consideration of the family history in diagnostics not only enhances near-care but also offers a supportive groundwork for long-term health and well-being (Figure 15.9).

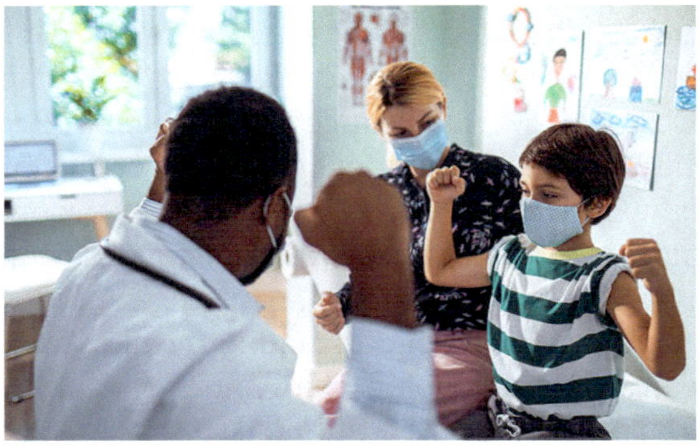

Figure 15.9. Family history and heart disease in children.

Source: https://www.uhhospitals.org/-/media/images/blog/2021/02/family-history-and-heart-disease-in-children_blog-mainarticleimage.jpg?h=450&w=720&la=en&hash=5D9D9BC6601181F37DA2F25790FC4A81.

15.3. Risk Factors

The pathophysiology of risk factors for critical heart disease in infants and children illustrates a multifactorial interaction of environmental, genetic, and socioeconomic variables. It has been shown through research that congenital heart disease tends to have a hereditary etiology and is due to several types of chromosomal anomalies. However, one should not underestimate the influence of environmental factors in pregnancy like exposure to drugs, infection, or teratogens. In addition, maternal conditions of diabetes and obesity further contribute to the risks of congenital heart diseases. Early detection and treatment are crucial as the identification of these risks helps develop focused management that can improve patient outcomes. Identification of such risk factors recognizes the necessity of full prenatal care and ongoing surveillance of vulnerable children to provide early intervention and support to families with these conditions. Aside from genetic and environmental determinants, socioeconomic status affects health outcomes in children with critical heart disease to a great extent. Research indicates that economically disadvantaged children, particularly Hispanic children, have poorer outcomes when diagnosed with congenital heart conditions such as hypoplastic left heart syndrome. It was demonstrated in one study that higher maternal education and private health insurance significantly lowered the risks of adverse outcomes in these groups, emphasizing the protective effect provided by higher socioeconomic status. More specifically, it was found that maternal education explained a significant proportion of the relationship between ethnicity and health outcomes and emphasized the importance of removing inequalities in the provision of healthcare services. Therefore, there is a need to implement policies that raise the education and economic resources of pregnant women and families residing in poor communities so that equitable access to care is promoted. Aside from that, early childhood lifestyle behaviors and choices are significant modifiable risk factors that influence lifetime cardiac health. For instance, childhood obesity, a known risk factor for long-term cardiovascular disease, is primarily due to improper diet, physical inactivity, and other lifestyle factors. As suggested in existing literature, most of these trends are shaped by family and community settings, which can encourage healthy habits or lead to risk factors such as Type II Diabetes Mellitus. Early onset of such conditions predisposes them to complications in later life, including cardiac diseases. Screening of infant and early childhood risk factors is crucial, and the risk of developing severe heart diseases can be significantly reduced with early interventions like a healthy diet and exercise. There must be joint action to educate families about the significance of such life choices towards preventing long-term health complications (Figure 15.10).

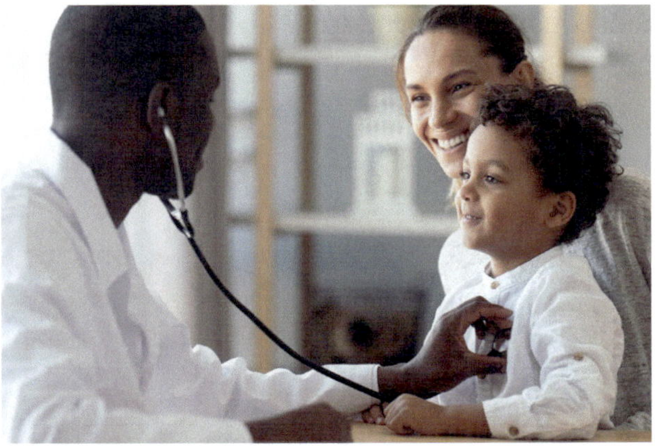

Figure 15.10. Examination of critical heart disease risk factors in children.

Source: https://emi.parkview.com/media/Image/Dashboard_952_heart_defects_8_22.jpg.

15.3.1. Genetic Predispositions

Genetic predispositions form the core of critical heart disease pathogenesis in infants and children, especially when considered within familial and environmental contexts. Research has indicated that CHD occurs in approximately 1% of live births, yet the etiology remains unknown; most cases appear to be due to complex gene-environment interactions (GxEs) (Al Ghadeer et al., 2024). This complexity renders it imperative that one identifies the individual genetic factors, such as mutations of specific genes that predispose a child to CHD. For instance, patients who have a pedigree history of congenital malformations among the family members are generally subject to an increased risk, revealing that hereditary factors may contribute significantly to the occurrence of such conditions. Detection and identification of these predispositions can facilitate interventions and screenings in high-risk groups, thereby decreasing the incidence of critical heart diseases in at-risk infants. Contributing to the genetic and environmental role in this regard, maternal health conditions such as diabetes mellitus have been found to exert remarkable influences on fetal development. Infants of diabetic mothers have a shared elevated overall risk of congenital anomalies, namely CHDs (Al Ghadeer et al., 2024). The relationship describes a robust GxE process where the intrauterine milieu engages with the genetic makeup of the infants to condition cardiac anomalies. Further, research has established that specific genetic pathways, such as haploinsufficiency of Notch1, engage in an adverse interaction with maternal diabetes to increase CHD probability. This forms a causality web that is worthy of unraveling, since understanding these interactions will allow for better screening procedures and targeted interventions for vulnerable babies. The genetic predispositions carry more than mere identification implications, directing clinical interventions and policy interventions to limit the occurrence of severe heart diseases. Genetic assessments and tests need to be integrated into prenatal health care, particularly in populations with identified risk factors, such as the mother's diabetes (Choudhury et al., 2024). Proper education of healthcare professionals to identify likely genetic markers can make early interventions possible that can restrict the severity and prevalence of congenital heart defects. Developing comprehensive guidelines for managing pregnancy at hereditary risk can empower both families and healthcare systems. As further investigation continues to elucidate the variables of genetic predisposition, such information must be translated into effective healthcare policies with a focus on early detection and prevention of essential heart disease in high-risk populations.

15.3.2. Environmental Influences

Environmental influences play a vital part in the pathogenesis of critical heart disease in children and newborns. Cardiovascular outcomes in the neonate are primarily influenced by maternal well-being, prenatal exposure to toxins, and socio-economic status. Research shows that maternal stress, mood disorders, and an adverse lifestyle during pregnancy can have long-term effects on the ontogenesis of a child's autonomic nervous system (ANS), potentially leading to cardiac issues. The ANS, which regulates the body's processes, including heart rate, is particularly vulnerable during pregnancy due to its active development and susceptibility to external influences. Siegel et al. (2021) underscore the interface between genetics and the environment in constructing the functional capacity of the ANS and point out the significance of specialized interventions addressing these factors in utero as a strategy for the avoidance of complications. Additional contributing to these issues are the health care and environmental inequalities experienced by differing socio-economic groups. Lower socio-economic status is often associated with disadvantage under the system, or a lack of access to prenatal exams, healthy foods, and secure shelter. Differences in exposure to toxins and pollutants also have potential impacts on the risk of congenital heart defects and other cardiovascular illnesses in youth. Evidence shows that the social environment, like resources available at the community level and supporting systems, plays a key role in influencing health outcomes. For instance, communities with high discrimination and socio-economic deprivation have higher infant mortality and morbidity rates with cardiovascular disease. Vadivelu (2021) emphasizes the importance of understanding environmental adversity with cumulative consequences for health, thereby highlighting the imperative requirement for policies aimed at promoting environmental and health equity. The intricate interplay between the environment and serious heart disease in children is translated into the early childhood development framework. Adverse experiences during pregnancy have been found to reshape the developing trajectory of the cardiovascular system to lead to long-term health. Additionally, postnatal influences such as exposure to environmental tobacco smoke in infancy or poor nutrition during child-rearing years also tend to affect heart health. The developing heart is highly sensitive to its environment, with there being indications that poor maternal lifestyle can have biological consequences for children.

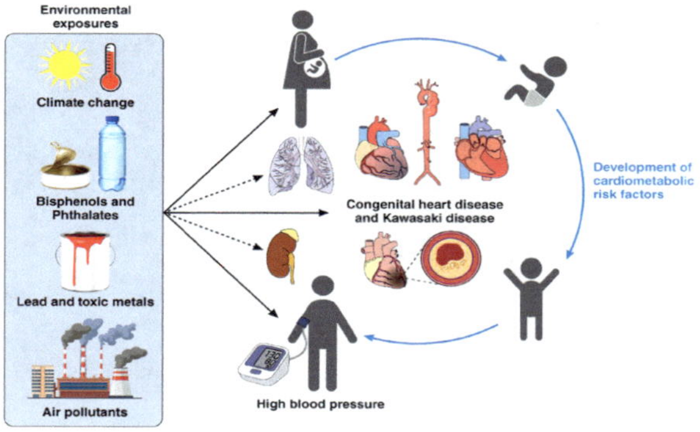

Figure 15.11. Environmental exposures, including climate change, airborne pollution, lead, and endocrine-disrupting chemicals, such as phenols and phthalates, influence multiple cardiovascular health outcomes, including congenital structural heart disease, Kawasaki disease, arterial hypertension, and atherosclerosis, across the life course from fetal life and beyond.

Source: https://www.ahajournals.org/cms/10.1161/CIR.0000000000001234/asset/bf4761f5-b42b-4682-b0d8-8ac08e24a69a/assets/graphic/cir.0000000000001234.fig01.jpg.

Recurrent exposure to adversity, including financial insecurity and psychosocial stressors, can cause alterations in physiology that risk-hinder young individuals from becoming vulnerable to heart disease in adulthood. Thus, environmental factors need to be addressed for the prevention and treatment of critical heart disease in infants and children, with a greater emphasis on the importance of general health and social interventions (Figure 15.11).

15.3.3. Maternal Health During Pregnancy

Mother's health in pregnancy is a significant factor that can have a powerful effect on the health of the offspring in adult life, down to childhood heart disease. Intrauterine conditions, as decided by maternal nutrition, stress, and pre-existing medical conditions, are of critical importance for fetal development. Maternal obesity, for instance, correlates with an increased incidence of congenital heart abnormalities in newborn infants. Pregnant females with conditions such as hypertension or diabetes are also at a higher risk of having children with serious cardiovascular conditions. Therefore, general prenatal care is crucial for maximizing the mother's health, as it minimizes such risks and leads to improvements in critical heart disease outcomes. Breastfeeding behavior is also a vital factor in dictating the pathways of children's health. Research indicates that longer periods of breastfeeding correlate with decreased levels of obesity and resulting cardiovascular disease in children as they grow. The protective effects of breast milk, particularly when prolonged for six months, are due to its unique properties that promote healthy growth trajectories. Hugely breastfed infants are less likely to be subject to excessive weight gain, a precursor of developing heart disease. Therefore, encouraging breastfeeding is not merely about infant nutrition but also serves as a protective factor for significant health issues, including heart disease, in the future (Beilin et al., 2014). Secondly, understanding the composition of human milk and its relationship with neonatal development is critical in the fight against maternal health during pregnancy. Maternal nutritional and metabolic status directly influences the quality of breast milk, which subsequently contributes to the health condition of the infant. For instance, newborn babies of mothers with poor nutritional status can lack essential fatty acids and nutrients required for cardiovascular health. Therefore, considering all the dimensions of maternal health, from nutrition to stress care, is crucial in ensuring not only the short-term well-being of the child but also the prevention of long-term conditions like heart disease. Such a multifaceted approach to maternal health gives way to targeted interventions that enhance both maternal and child health outcomes (Morrow et al., 2012) (Figure 15.12).

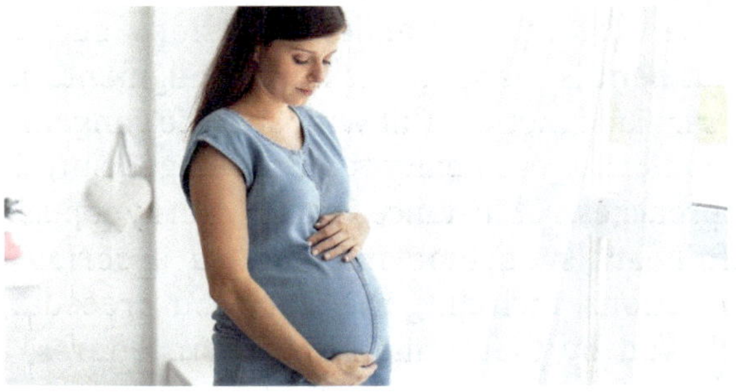

Figure 15.12. Maternal health during pregnancy.

Source: https://orthocarebhopal.in/wp-content/uploads/2021/10/pregnant-woman-in-nursey-1024x536-1.jpg.

15.4. Treatment Options

Treatment of severe heart disease in children and infants comprises of elements that usually need to be blended in the form of medical interventions, particularly formulated for the nature of the congenital flaw. Ideally, the condition is to be diagnosed early, and following that, pharmacological interventions can be initiated to manage symptoms and stabilize the patient's condition. Pharmacologic agents such as prostaglandins are beneficial in maintaining ductal patency with ductus arteriosus-dependent circulations to ensure more effective circulation until surgical planning. Diuretics are also commonly used to manage heart failure symptoms, substantially reducing fluid overload and improving the quality of life of the affected infants. These early medical interventions are critical in optimizing outcomes before further advanced surgical procedures are initiated, thus proving the importance of early medical intervention for cases of critical heart disease. Surgery remains the cornerstone of management for most forms of critical congenital heart disease. From palliative treatments, such as balloon atrial septostomy for hemodynamic augmentation, to reparative operations aimed at the correction of anatomic lesions, surgical treatment is mapped out for the augmentation of cardiac function. But with specific congenital lesions, the complexity requires staged surgical approaches. For instance, infants with hypoplastic left heart syndrome might need a series of operations, including the Norwood procedure, followed by Glenn and Fontan procedures, to sequentially reconstruct the circuits of blood flow and ensure adequate perfusion. The timing optimization of these procedures is critical in that anatomical and physiological maturity in the child significantly affects the success of surgical outcomes. Hence, an efficient treatment plan by a multi-disciplinary team is imperative to manage such challenging cases. The disparity in the outcomes of treatment for children with critical heart disease testifies to the impact of socioeconomic determinants on access to healthcare. It has been discovered that racial and ethnic minority groups, particularly Hispanic infants, are at greater risk of unfavorable outcomes owing to barriers in access to timely and proper care (Baer et al., 2018). Faced with such disparities, it is of the utmost importance that, besides focusing on the medical needs, the socioeconomic determinants hindering access to life-saving care be addressed. Public health interventions in ensuring fair access to care can make preventive interventions available and facilitate early treatment and diagnosis with the view to improving the results of treatment. Educational interventions that make families and healthcare providers aware of the potential risks of delayed treatment or inadequate provision may significantly alter the care dynamics in these high-risk groups so that there is a more level playing field of addressing critical congenital heart disease in the pediatric population (N/A, 2009) (Figure 15.13).

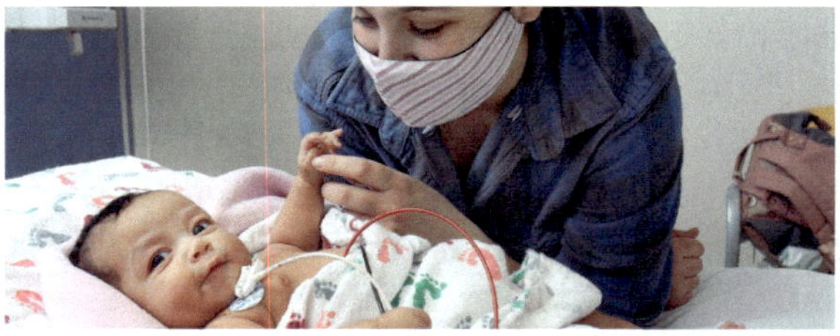

Figure 15.13. Treatment for critical heart disease in infants.

Source: https://www.hopkinsmedicine.org/-/media/images/health/1_-conditions/childrens-health/pediatric-cardiology-hero-johns-hopkins.jpg?h=500&iar=0&mh=500&mw=1300&w=1297&hash=727D8B565CD770B08808C8D895D6A600.

15.4.1. Medical Management and Medications

Medical management of severe heart disease in infants and children is a multi-modal approach, with drugs for physiological stabilization and support of vital organ function. In particular, the application of prostaglandin E1 (PGE1) is essential to maintain ductal patency in neonates with ductus-dependent congenital heart disorders. The treatment allows for increased oxygenation and perfusion of vital organs until definitive surgical therapy can be accomplished. However, fever can complicate PGE1 infusion, and adjunct treatments could be required. Intravenous acetaminophen has been demonstrated to be an effective antipyretic, lowering fever without compromising ductal function. This is important because hemodynamic stability is of prime importance in this vulnerable population, and careful monitoring is essential so that untoward effects are not produced during PGE1 therapy, to support the patients optimally until they are stable enough for surgery (Kaya et al., 2024). Besides symptomatic presentation for critical heart disease, healthcare providers must be cognizant of the neurodevelopmental issues in the affected children. Effective management of this population involves more than simple immediate pharmacological interventions, emphasizing close continued monitoring and neurodevelopmental risk factor assessment. Emerging evidence has introduced multiple determinants with effects on the neurodevelopment of this population, including genetic vulnerabilities and environmental determinants. A care integrated model involves prevention and compensation for developmental delays with recommendations on interventions that will enhance cognitive and motor development as the child grows. This emphasizes the pivotal contribution of multidisciplinary teams, who collaborate to personalize management plans that simultaneously meet the cardiac and neurodevelopmental needs of critical congenital heart disease patients, thus optimizing their overall quality of life (Sood et al., 2024). Furthermore, it is impossible to overstate the role that tailored medication plays in treating serious heart disease. Age, weight, and common comorbid diseases are patient-specific factors that are becoming more and more important to optimize as medical therapy and treatment regimens continue to change. These individualized strategies could involve the clever use of drug dosage modification to minimize adverse effects and optimize effectiveness. In neonates and infants with profound heart disease, accurate fluid status, electrolyte, and renal management becomes all-important, particularly in the perioperative period. With the application of clinically established practice guidelines and developing evidence-based practice, clinicians can optimize treatment protocols according to the unique physiological demands of pediatric patients, ultimately optimizing clinical outcomes while reducing post-operative complications. Such an integrated approach is reflective of the interconnectedness and pertinence of a generalized approach of medical management among the pediatric patient population affected with critical heart disease (Sood et al., 2024) (Figure 15.14).

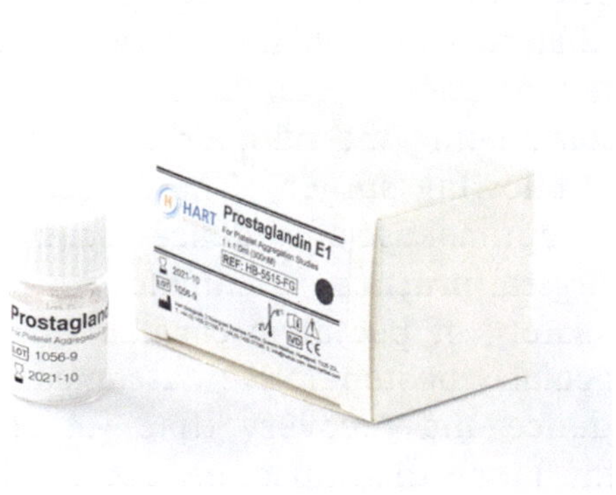

Figure 15.14. Prostaglandin E1.

Source: https://www.hartbio.co.uk/media/products/images/Hart_Bio-0153.jpg.738x499_q85_crop_upscale.webp.

15.4.2. Surgical Interventions

Surgery can play a very key role in the control of severe heart disease in infants and children, primarily concerning congenital heart defects that disrupt normal circulation. Surgery is usually indicated in cases such as aortic coarctation or ventricular septal defects, where the heart chambers beat in discord. Evolution of surgical techniques and the use of cardiopulmonary bypass (CPB) have significantly improved outcomes for these vulnerable patients. Nevertheless, CPB use is not risk-free; it can cause a systemic inflammatory response, which in turn may lead to low cardiac output syndrome (LCOS) and complicate recovery with significant morbidity. Hence, awareness of the balance between intervention gain and inherent complication is still relevant in pediatric cardiac surgery. Recent research emphasizes the need to maximize surgical conditions to achieve the best postoperative recovery in infants and children. For instance, trials of nitric oxide infusion during CPB concentrate on attenuating inflammation and improving myocardial protection. The NITRIC trial, as described in recent clinical reports, demonstrates a stepwise strategy for determining whether the intervention is effective. In this randomized controlled trial, less than two-year-old infants will receive nitric oxide inhalation or standard care, the primary outcome being the number of ventilator-free days following surgery. The research focuses on the optimal use of evidence-based principles in surgical practice, to enhance the efficiency and safety of pediatric cardiac surgery, and particularly postoperative outcomes like LCOS incidence and recovery time (et al., 2019). Furthermore, the impact of successful surgery extends beyond short-term outcomes; it also encompasses long-term quality of life and health for children with critical heart disease. Early intervention is crucial, as evidence shows that early surgical repair can lead to improved developmental milestones and fewer comorbid conditions as the children grow. In considering the totality of surgical procedures, the healthcare costs and resource utilization also need to be considered. Secondary outcomes of the trial, including the length of intensive care stay and hospital readmission, also play a significant role in assessing the overall impact of surgical management. As research advances, attention shifts to enhancing children with heart disease's overall health and survival, forming a comprehensive picture of their course of therapy (Acosta et al., 2020).

15.4.3. Long-Term Care and Follow-Up

Long-term care and follow-up after surgical correction of critical heart disease in infants and children are vital to optimal health outcomes. Patients can endure a variety of complications as a result of the nature of congenital heart disease, including tolerance of challenges in cardiac function, respiratory status, and total growth and development. Routine monitoring enables caregivers to detect any early warning of complications, such as low cardiac output syndrome or pulmonary hypertension. By promoting routine follow-up visits, healthcare teams can implement timely interventions appropriate to each child's unique needs, thus ensuring better postoperative recovery and quality of life. Therefore, implementing a holistic, interprofessional plan of care is required to navigate imminent risk and enhance the long-term prognosis for these vulnerable patients. In long-term care, specific measures must be designed to satisfy the diversified medical, developmental, and psychosocial needs of children with severe heart disease. Follow-through modalities should include regular echocardiograms, cardiac evaluations, and developmental assessments to monitor advancements in more than one area. Pediatric cardiologists, cardiothoracic surgeons, and allied health personnel must collaborate to create a comprehensive follow-up system that enables early detection and control of complications. Parent education and counseling services are also essential since the caregivers most frequently administer complex home care regimens. This integrated model establishes a setting that is favorable to the involvement of families so that they become motivated to participate in their child's treatment and contribute positively to immediate as well as long-term health outcomes. Furthermore, the introduction of novel therapies, such as home oxygen therapy, is the cornerstone of the chronic care of these patients. For example, children with respiratory disease requiring supplemental oxygen are likely to benefit from targeted home oxygen therapy protocols. As noted in recent publications, an effective management plan should have clear guidelines for clinicians and providers of care to optimize delivery of therapy and safety of patients (Balfour-Lynn et al., 2005). Integrating these therapies into the model of long-term care serves not only the direct medical needs of children with heart disease but also supports their overall developmental trajectory. In this way, health care professionals can optimize the long-term resiliency and health status of these children and facilitate successful transition into adulthood (Figure 15.15).

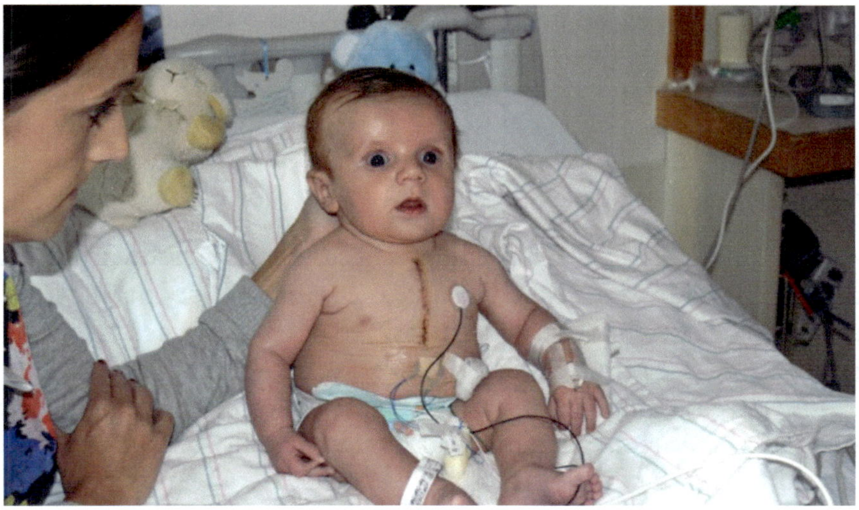

Figure 15.15. Long-term care and follow-up after surgical.

Source: https://mitc.b-cdn.net/wp-content/uploads/2021/11/pcs-banner.jpg.

SUMMARY

Overall, the treatment of critical heart disease in infants and children must be a holistic approach that includes clinical, public health, and socioeconomic perspectives. The discrepancies in results among children with congenital heart disease indicate an urgent need for focused interventions on at-risk groups. Research suggests the significant role of socioeconomic determinants in the poorer prognosis observed among certain racial and ethnic groups, notably Hispanic infants with conditions such as hypoplastic left heart syndrome and dextro-Transposition of the great arteries (Peyvandi et al., 2018). Such identification enables clinicians and policymakers to utilize resources better and develop effective systems of support to enhance the general quality and accessibility of care to affected families. In addition, critical heart disease practice in children must be evidence-based in transfusions.

The expert consensus guidelines highlight the necessity of personalized hemoglobin levels depending on the specific individual child's medical condition. For instance, hemoglobin levels should be at optimal ranges for children with uncorrected heart disease to prevent complications without resorting to unnecessary transfusions (Cholette et al., 2018). Adherence to these standards promotes more effective treatment planning and ultimately improves patient outcomes, illustrating the utility of individualized care in pediatric cardiology. Finally, ongoing research is needed to illuminate further our understanding of critical heart disease in infants and children. Ongoing study of the interplays between socioeconomic status, race, and health outcomes will clarify the systematic impediments influencing care delivery. Besides, as has been proposed by experts, additional studies need to be conducted to identify effective replacements for standard management methods, i.e., blood transfusions, which can be hazardous for critically ill children (Cholette et al., 2018). By investing in research and enabling a collaborative process across health professionals, we can enhance the quality of care provided to children with serious heart disease and ultimately remove disparities that persist across this vulnerable population.

In respect to infant and child critical heart disease, CHD is high on the list as a cause of death in infants. Not only are structural heart defects serious, but complications can also occur during operations. The majority of infants need their problems to be corrected through surgery, which uses CPB techniques. Unfortunately, CPB alone can induce a systemic inflammatory response, causing LCOS, a condition associated with heightened postoperative morbidity and mortality. The NITRIC trial, which was carried out to assess the efficacy of nitric oxide (NO) administration with CPB, gives evidence of a reduction in such inflammatory responses and shorter recovery times by a gain in ventilator-free days (VFD) (et al., 2019). Another critical component of managing infant heart disease is cerebral and somatic oxygen monitoring, particularly following surgery. A promising pilot study highlighted the application of near-infrared spectroscopy to monitor cerebral oxygenation in postoperative high-risk cardiac surgical infants. Despite the controversial evidence for its relationship to mixed venous oxygen saturation, the research suggests cerebral near-infrared spectroscopy can provide valuable information regarding patient status following surgery. Notably, a significant negative correlation between cerebral oxygenation levels and serum lactate, a marker that can indicate complications (Hovarth et al., 2011), was observed. Such findings show the potential of non-invasive monitoring technologies to enhance patient care and guide clinical decision-making in the pediatric cardiac ICU. Last but not least, the evolving landscape of interventions and monitoring strategies in infant critical heart disease reflects the ongoing necessity for research and innovation. The application of therapies such as NO delivery during CPB has the potential to prevent some of the inherent risks of surgeries aimed to repair CHD. In turn, this can be translated into improved outcomes such as fewer mechanical ventilation days (et al., 2019). At the same time, advances in monitoring technology like near-infrared spectroscopy could provide critical real-time data, facilitating postoperative care more appropriately and ultimately improving survival rates and quality of life in this high-risk population (Hovarth et al., 2011). Collectively, these highlights underscore the synergistic interplay between operative techniques, postoperative management, and monitoring technology against the challenges of critical heart disease in infants and children.

A CLOSER LOOK

INNOVATIONS IN SURGICAL TECHNIQUES

Pediatric cardiac surgery has undergone a dramatic transformation in the past few decades, with progressive changes in cardiac surgery. Advances such as minimally invasive surgery and catheter-based interventions have given doctors a tool for treating severe heart disease in infants and children with less morbidity and time to recovery. For instance, techniques like catheter-based balloon valvuloplasty are now common practice, allowing for the opening of stenotic valves without the necessity of a full thoracotomy. It not only minimizes trauma but also allows easier postoperative recovery and less hospitalization, leading to overall better results in pediatric patients. Fetal cardiac interventions are yet another breakthrough in the therapeutic approach to congenital heart disease. The potential to perform procedures in utero is dedicated to the therapy of life-threatening conditions before birth, thus significantly improving prognosis and outcome. The innovation requires intense coordination among multidisciplinary teams, including obstetricians, pediatric cardiologists, and surgeons. This coordination is essential in creating the modalities of safer fetal access and effectively selecting candidates for these new procedures. As noted, early detection and timely intervention are critical for ensuring effective outcomes in such high-risk conditions, underscoring the necessity of integrated care models in further refining pediatric cardiac surgery (Abele et al., 2018). With advancing surgery techniques, the emergence of robotic-assisted technologies has also facilitated fresh avenues for addressing intricate congenital heart disease. Robotic technology allows surgeons to perform , complicated procedures with more accuracy and less invasiveness. Such systems can facilitate advanced repairs, such as aortic or complex valve reconstructions, with minimal patient trauma and maximum recovery. Moreover, the integration of up-to-date imaging modalities and intraoperative surgical simulations during preoperative planning has enhanced the possibility of tailored interventions based on the individual anatomical challenges of infants and children. Both of these advancements demonstrate the significant development being achieved in pediatric heart surgery that will improve outcome and quality of life for affected children (N/A, 1973) (Figure 15.16).

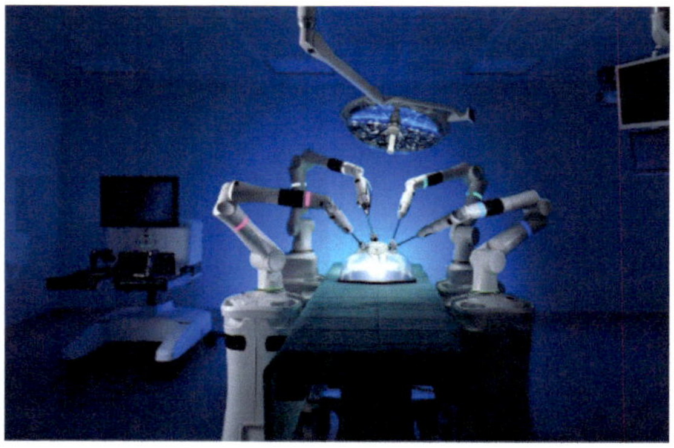

Figure 15.16. Innovations in pediatric cardiac surgery.

Source: https://emag.medicalexpo.com/wp-content/uploads/sites/9/cmr-surgical-versius-clinical-setup-4-arms-00004-1250x808.jpg.

References

1. Meyer-Wittkopf, M., Kaulitz, R., Abele, H., Schauf, B., Hofbeck, M., & Wallwiener, D. (2005). Interventional fetal balloon valvuloplasty for congenital heart disease—current shortcomings and possible perspectives. *Gynecological Surgery, 2*(2), 113–118. https://doi.org/10.1007/s10397-005-0090-zAcosta, S., Azuma, N., Bastos, G. F., Björck, et al. (2020). Editor's choice: European Society for Vascular Surgery (ESVS) 2020 clinical practice guidelines on the management of acute limb ischemia. *Eur. J. Vasc. Endovasc. Surg.*

2. Aiyagari, R., Bhat, P., Donohue, J., Fifer, et al. (2018). A randomized trial of early palliative care for maternal stress in infants prenatally diagnosed with single-ventricle heart disease. *Cardiol. Young.* https://core.ac.uk/download/212864275.pdf (accessed on 29th May 2025).

3. Akah, R. T., Enoh, J. E., & Nkeh-Chungag, B. (2025). The impact of early detection and intervention on congenital heart defects in infants and children: A systematic review. *Recent Advances in Natural Sciences.* https://www.semanticscholar.org/paper/cc71d6435bab22df1811475c35a0f545a5372ac4 (accessed on 29th May 2025).

4. Al Ghadeer, H. A., Alherz, A. H., Albattat, F. S., Alkhamis, M. A., Alamer, M. H., Almulaifi, L. F., Al Ali, A. I., et al. (2024). Pattern and frequency of congenital heart defects among infants of diabetic mothers. *Cureus, 16.* https://www.semanticscholar.org/paper/1437bc00605874617d6ffa4b2e391a77f12d5ba2 (accessed on 29th May 2025).

5. Antzelevitch, C., Yan, G. X., Ackerman, M. J., Borggrefe, M., Corrado, D., Guo, J., Gussak, I., et al. (2016). J-wave syndromes expert consensus conference report: Emerging concepts and gaps in knowledge. *Journal of Arrhythmia, 32*, 315–339. https://doi.org/10.1016/j.joa.2016.07.002.

6. Baer, R. J., Chambers, C. D., Jelliffe-Pawlowski, L. L., Moon-Grady, et al. (2018). Socioeconomic mediators of racial and ethnic disparities in congenital heart disease outcomes: A population-based study in California. *J. Am. Heart Assoc.* https://core.ac.uk/download/323073424.pdf (accessed on 29th May 2025).

7. Balfour-Lynn, I. M., Primhak, R. A., & Shaw, B. N. J. (2005). *Home Oxygen for Children: Who, How and When?* https://core.ac.uk/download/58952.pdf (accessed on 29th May 2025).

8. Bancalari, E., Clyman, R. I., Collaco, J. M., Davis, et al. (2018). *Bronchopulmonary Dysplasia: Executive Summary of a Workshop.* https://core.ac.uk/download/227054384.pdf (accessed on 29th May 2025).

9. BEEP Study Team, Boyle, R. J., Bradshaw, L. E., Brown, S. J., et al. (2020). Daily emollient during infancy for prevention of eczema: The BEEP randomized controlled trial. *Lancet.* https://core.ac.uk/download/287649733.pdf (accessed on 29th May 2025).

10. Beilin, L. J., Chivers, P., Hands, B., Huang, et al. (2014). *Early Infant Feeding and Adiposity Risk: From Infancy to Adulthood.* https://core.ac.uk/download/84111146.pdf (accessed on 29th May 2025).

11. Cholette, J. M., Willems, A., Valentine, S. L., Bateman, S. T., & Schwartz, S. M. (2018). Recommendations on RBC transfusion in infants and children with acquired and congenital heart disease from the Pediatric Critical Care Transfusion and Anemia Expertise Initiative. *Pediatric Critical Care Medicine, 19*, S137–S148. https://doi.org/10.1097/pcc.0000000000001603 (accessed on 29th May 2025).

12. Choudhury, T., Greskovich, S. C., Girard, H., Rao, A. S., Budhathoki, Y., Cameron, E., Conroy, S., et al. (2024). Impact of genetic factors on antioxidant rescue of maternal diabetes–associated congenital heart disease. *JCI Insight, 9*. https://www.semanticscholar.org/paper/8060e58612c8855a32c15984d22cc519a3d33f8e (accessed on 29th May 2025).

13. Dewi, P. D. R., Gunawijaya, E., & Ni, Y. P. V. K. (2022). Early versus late diagnosis of critical congenital heart disease at Sanglah Hospital Denpasar, Bali. *GSC Advanced Research and Reviews*. https://www.semanticscholar.org/paper/16cc0bc06b0120cf7254c66b290badad1096d470 (accessed on 29th May 2025).

14. Forestieri, N. E., Olshan, A. F., Oster, M. E., Ailes, E. C., Fundora, M. P., Fisher, S., Shumate, C. J., et al. (2024). Survival of children with critical congenital heart defects in the National Birth Defects Prevention Study. *Birth Defects Research, 116*(9), e2394. https://www.semanticscholar.org/paper/68cefcbabc6b7e96b15fda198b218eb1aca2f023 (accessed on 29th May 2025).

15. Formosa, M. C. (2008). *Asthma in Childhood*. https://core.ac.uk/download/46602177.pdf (accessed on 29th May 2025).

16. Fraser, C., Jarvis, H., Jha, A., Openshaw, et al. (2016). *Respiratory Syncytial Virus*. https://core.ac.uk/download/77013434.pdf (accessed on 29th May 2025).

17. Gadekar, A., Japzape, T., Lakhkar, B., Suwarnakar, et al. (2013). Accuracy of pulse oximetry screening for detecting critical congenital heart disease in the newborns in rural hospital of Central India. *Images Pediatr. Cardiol.* https://core.ac.uk/download/46603003.pdf (accessed on 29th May 2025).

18. Hovarth, L., Tume, N., MacLeod, M., Meastiz, P., Arnold, P., & Plowman. (2011). Near-infrared spectroscopy after high-risk congenital heart surgery in the pediatric intensive care unit. *Cardiol. Young*. https://core.ac.uk/download/42136645.pdf (accessed on 29th May 2025).

19. Islam, S. M. R., Kwak, D., Kabir, M. H., Hossain, M., & Kwak, K. S. (2015). The internet of things for health care: A comprehensive survey. *IEEE Access, 3*, 678–708. https://doi.org/10.1109/access.2015.2437951 (accessed on 29th May 2025).

20. Kapke, D. R. (2015). *Childhood Type II Diabetes: The Risks and Complications*. https://core.ac.uk/download/58826199.pdf (accessed on 29th May 2025).

21. Kaya, B., Akduman, H., Dilli, D., Kaya, Ö., Çitli, R., & Zenciroğlu, A. (2024). The utilization of acetaminophen for managing PGE1-induced fever in neonates with critical congenital heart disease. *Children, 11*. https://www.semanticscholar.org/paper/9723d7c2f56614e155e638d633f18ecee08504ea (accessed on 29th May 2025).

22. King, J., Lehrnbecher, T., Pana, Z. D., Steinbach, et al. (2017). *Recognition and Clinical Presentation of Invasive Fungal Disease in Neonates and Children*. https://core.ac.uk/download/131024549.pdf (accessed on 29th May 2025).

23. Martinez-Sarria, A., Martín-Martín, J., Van, B. L., & Olano-Lizarraga, M. (2023). The experience of living with congenital heart disease from the perspective of the affected child or adolescent and its family: A systematic qualitative review. *European Journal of Cardiovascular Nursing*. https://www.semanticscholar.org/paper/d3174546588822826ae9e9e9dc0425c3e81460d1 (accessed on 29th May 2025).

24. Morrow, A. L., Goldman, A., Shur, B. D., Lebrilla, C. B., Hadsell, D., Rijnkels, M., Dabelea, D., Raiten, D. J., et al. (2012). *Lactation and Neonatal Nutrition: Defining and Refining the Critical*

Questions. https://core.ac.uk/download/323068342.pdf (accessed on 29th May 2025).

25. N/A. (1973). Focal Spot, Spring 1973. https://core.ac.uk/download/129069200.pdf (accessed on 29th May 2025).
26. N/A. (2000). Focal Spot, Spring 2000. https://core.ac.uk/download/129069317.pdf (accessed on 29th May 2025).
27. N/A. (2009). *Shaping a Healthier Generation: Successful State Strategies to Prevent Childhood Obesity.* https://core.ac.uk/download/71354832.pdf (accessed on 29th May 2025).
28. N/A. (2010). *The Foundations of Lifelong Health are Built in Early Childhood.* https://core.ac.uk/download/71351353.pdf (accessed on 29th May 2025).
29. N/A. (2014). Outlook Magazine, Spring 2014. https://core.ac.uk/download/212869004.pdf (accessed on 29th May 2025).
30. Peyvandi, S., Baer, R. J., Moon-Grady, A. J., Oltman, S. P., Chambers, C., Norton, M. E., Rajagopal, S., et al. (2018). Socioeconomic mediators of racial and ethnic disparities in congenital heart disease outcomes: A population-based study in California. *Journal of the American Heart Association, 7.* https://doi.org/10.1161/jaha.118.010342 (accessed on 29th May 2025).
31. Priori, S. G., Blomström-Lundqvist, C., Mazzanti, A., Blom, N., Borggrefe, M., Camm, A. J., Elliott, P., et al. (2015). 2015 ESC Guidelines for the management of patients with ventricular arrhythmias and the prevention of sudden cardiac death. *European Heart Journal, 36,* 2793–2867. https://doi.org/10.1093/eurheartj/ehv316 (accessed on 29th May 2025).
32. Schibler, A., Franklin, D., Oakley, E., Babl, F. E., Whitty, J. A., Furyk, J., Neutze, J., et al. (2015). Early high flow nasal cannula therapy in bronchiolitis, a prospective randomized control trial (protocol): A Pediatric Acute Respiratory Intervention Study (PARIS). *BMC Pediatr.* https://core.ac.uk/download/41993892.pdf (accessed on 29th May 2025).
33. Siegel, R., & Watanabe, M. (2021). Introduction to the special focus on the development of the autonomic nervous system. *Birth Defects Research, 113.* https://www.semanticscholar.org/paper/51fdc8569e122dd0e7fc13d47e3574a4af6a2225 (accessed on 29th May 2025).
34. Sood, E., Newburger, J. W., Anixt, J., Cassidy, A. R., Jackson, J. L., Jonas, R. A., Lisanti, A., et al. (2024). Neurodevelopmental outcomes for individuals with congenital heart disease: Updates in neuroprotection, risk-stratification, evaluation, and management: A scientific statement from the American Heart Association. *Circulation, 149,* e997–e1022. https://www.semanticscholar.org/paper/85067912037fc3135f74178eee8b27ec9b95fd6a (accessed on 29th May 2025).
35. Vadivelu, S. (2021). From the editor's desk. *TNOA Journal of Ophthalmic Science and Research, 59,* 1. https://www.semanticscholar.org/paper/f71ad2cb26607d0a09257bf48fba1191fe01e8cd (accessed on 29th May 2025).
36. Vagha, K., Taksande, A., Kenjale, S., Vagha, J., & Varma, A. (2023). Neurodevelopmental assessment in children with congenital heart disease by applying the Denver Developmental Screening Test 2: A prospective cross-sectional study. *Cureus, 15.* https://www.semanticscholar.org/paper/36d38dea28b4eda4cc47bebfaaad8f946d5e199d (accessed on 29th May 2025).
37. Winston, C. N., Bowe, M. E., Lee, S., Ranieri, N. R., Ades, A., Gebb, J., Rychik, J., et al. (2024). *Noninvasive Optical Monitoring of Cerebral Hemodynamics Immediately After Birth in Neonates with Congenital Heart Disease.* https://www.semanticscholar.org/paper/394cc3a4a062bcc787596c91a6011d0c12aab0d6 (accessed on 29th May 2025).

INDEX

S

T

V

W

Y